WENNER-GREN CENTER
INTERNATIONAL SYMPOSIUM SERIES

VOLUME 37

FUNCTIONAL BASIS OF OCULAR MOTILITY DISORDERS

Already published in this series:

OLFACTION AND TASTE *Edited by* Y. Zotterman, 1963.

LIGHTING PROBLEMS IN HIGHWAY TRAFFIC *Edited by* E. Ingelstam. 1963.

THE STRUCTURE AND METABOLISM OF THE PANCREATIC ISLETS *Edited by* S. E. Brolin, B. Hellman and H. Knutson, 1964.

TOBACCO ALKALOIDS AND RELATED COMPOUNDS *Edited by* U.S. von Euler, 1965.

MECHANISMS OF RELEASE OF BIOGENIC AMINES *Edited by* U.S. von Euler, S. Rosell and B. Uvnäs, 1966.

COMPARATIVE LEUKAEMIA RESEARCH *Edited by* G. Winqvist, 1966.

THE FUNCTIONAL ORGANIZATION OF THE COMPOUND EYE *Edited by* C. G. Bernhard, 1966.

OLFACTION AND TASTE II *Edited by* T. Hayashi, 1967.

MAGNETIC RESONANCE IN BIOLOGICAL SYSTEMS *Edited by* A. Ehrenberg, B. G. Malmström and T. Vanngard, 1967.

STRUCTURE AND FUNCTION OF INHIBITORY NEURONAL MECHANISMS *Edited by* C. von Euler, S. Skoglund and U. Söderberg, 1967.

GROUND WATER PROBLEMS *Edited by* E. Eriksson, Y. Gustafsson and K. Nilsson, 1968.

PHYSIOLOGY AND PATHOPHYSIOLOGY OF PLASMA PROTEIN METABOLISM *Edited by* G. Birke, R. Norberg and L.-O. Plantin, 1969.

THE POSSIBILITIES OF CHARTING MODERN LIFE *Edited by* S. Erixon *and Assisted by* G. Ardwidsson and H. Hvarfner, 1970.

EVALUATION OF NOVEL PROTEIN PRODUCTS *Edited by* A. E. Bender, R. Kihlberg, B. Lofqvist and L. Munck, 1970.

VESTIBULAR FUNCTION ON EARTH AND IN SPACE *Edited by* J. Stahle, 1970.

THE STRUCTURE AND METABOLISM OF THE PANCREATIC ISLETS *Edited by* S. Falkner, B. Hellman and I. B. Taljedal, 1970.

HUMAN ANTI-HUMAN GAMMAGLOBULINS *Edited by* R. Grubb and G. Samuelsson, 1971.

STRUCTURE AND FUNCTION OF OXIDATION - REDUCTION ENZYMES *Edited by* A. Åkeson and A. Ehrenberg, 1972.

CERVICAL PAIN *Edited by* N. Emmelin and Y. Zotteman, 1972.

ORAL PHYSIOLOGY *Edited by* N. Emmelin and Y. Zotterman, 1972

CIRCUMPOLAR PROBLEMS: HABITAT, ECONOMY AND SOCIAL RELATIONS IN THE ARCTIC *Edited by* G. Berg *et al.*, 1973.

DYNAMICS OF DEGENERATION AND GROWTH IN NEURONES *Edited by* K. Fuxe, L. Olson and Y. Zotterman, 1974.

THE FUNCTIONAL ANATOMY OF THE SPERMATOZOON *Edited by* B. A. Afzelius, 1974.

BASIC MECHANISMS OF OCULAR MOTILITY AND THEIR CLINICAL IMPLICATIONS *Edited by* G. Lennerstand, Paul Bach-y-Rita, C. C. Collins, A. Jampolsky and A. B. Scott, 1975.

ANTIPSYCHOTIC DRUGS: PHARMACODYNAMICS AND PHARMACOKINETICS *Edited by* G. Sedvall, B. Uvnäs and Y. Zotterman, 1976.

GASTROINTESTINAL EMERGENCIES *Edited by* F. R. Barany and A. Torsoli, 1976.

SENSORY FUNCTIONS OF THE SKIN IN PRIMATES *Edited by* Y. Zotterman, 1976.

PHYSICAL WORK AND EFFORT *Edited by* Gunnar Borg, 1976.

NEUROGENIC CONTROL OF THE BRAIN CIRCULATION *Edited by* C. Owman and L. Edvinsson, 1977.

DOPAMINERGIC ERGOT DERIVATIVES AND MOTOR FUNCTION *Edited by* Kjell Fuxe and Donald B. Calne, 1979.

CENTRAL NERVOUS CONTROL MECHANISMS IN BREATHING *Edited by* C. von Euler and H. Lagercrantz, 1979.

STEROID HORMONE REGULATION OF THE BRAIN *Edited by* K. Fuxe, J.-A. Gustafson and L. Wetterberg, 1981

DYSLEXIA: NEURONAL, COGNITIVE AND LINGUISTIC ASPECTS *Edited by* Y. Zotterman, 1981

SPEECH MOTOR CONTROL *Edited by* S. Grillner, B. Lindblom, J. Lubker and A. Persson, 1982

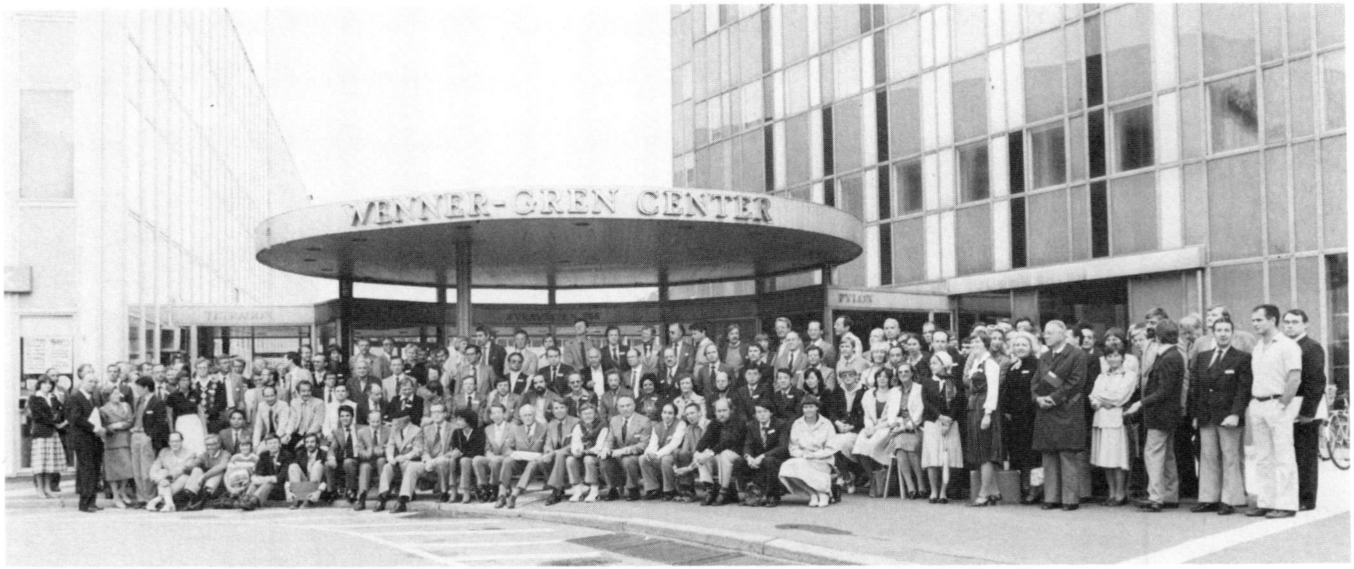

Participants in the International Symposium on "Functional Basis of Ocular MOtility Disorders",
Stockholm, August 31 - September 3, 1981

FUNCTIONAL BASIS OF OCULAR MOTILITY DISORDERS

Proceedings of a Wenner-Gren Center and Smith-Kettlewell Eye Research Foundation International Symposium held in Wenner-Gren Center, Stockholm, 31 August — 3 September 1981

Edited by

Gunnar Lennerstrand

Department of Ophthalmology, Linköping University, Sweden

David S. Zee

Department of Neurology, The Johns Hopkins Hospital, Baltimore, Maryland, USA

Edward L. Keller

Smith-Kettlewell Institute of Visual Sciences, San Francisco, California, USA

PERGAMON PRESS

OXFORD · NEW YORK · TORONTO · SYDNEY · PARIS · FRANKFURT

U.K.	Pergamon Press Ltd., Headington Hill Hall, Oxford OX3 0BW, England
U.S.A.	Pergamon Press Inc., Maxwell House, Fairview Park, Elmsford, New York 10523, U.S.A.
CANADA	Pergamon Press Canada Ltd., Suite 104, 150 Consumers Rd., Willowdale, Ontario M2J 1P9, Canada
AUSTRALIA	Pergamon Press (Aust.) Pty. Ltd., P.O. Box 544, Potts Point, N.S.W. 2011, Australia
FRANCE	Pergamon Press SARL, 24 rue des Ecoles, 75240 Paris, Cedex 05, France
FEDERAL REPUBLIC OF GERMANY	Pergamon Press GmbH, 6242 Kronberg-Taunus, Hammerweg 6, Federal Republic of Germany

First edition 1982

Library of Congress Cataloging in Publication Data

Main entry under title:
Functional basis of ocular motility disorders.
(Wenner-Gren Center international symposium
series; v. 37)
Bibliography: p.
Includes index.
1. Eye—Movement disorders—Congresses.
I. Lennerstrand, Gunnar. II. Zee, David S.
III. Keller, Edward L. IV. Wenner-Grenska samfundet. V. Smith-Kettlewell Eye Research
Foundation. VI. Series. [DNLM: 1. Opthalmology
—Congresses. 2. Eye movements—Congresses.
3. Oculomotor muscles—Physiopathology—
Congresses. W3 WE429 v. 37 1981/WW 410 F979
RE731.F86 1982 617.7'62 82-7548

British Library Cataloguing in Publication Data

Functional basis of ocular motility disorders.—
(Wenner-Gren center international symposium;
v. 37)
1. Eye-diseases and aspects—Congresses
I. Lennerstrand, Gunnar II. Zel, David S.
III. Keller, Edward IV. Series
617.7 RE46

ISBN 0-08-029772-2

In order to make this volume available as economically and as rapidly as possible the authors' typescripts have been reproduced in their original forms. This method unfortunately has its typographical limitations but it is hoped that they in no way distract the reader.

Printed in Great Britain by A. Wheaton & Co. Ltd., Exeter

PREFACE

International symposia concerned with oculomotor and vision research have occurred more frequently in the past few years, but few have deliberately tried to bring the fruits of basic laboratory research directly to the neuro-ophthalmology clinic. The 1974 symposium in Stockholm, sponsored by the Wenner-Gren Center Foundation and the Smith-Kettlewell Eye Research Foundation, was organized with this goal in mind and was highly successful in initiating this difficult process. In 1974 the topics for discussion were selected by laboratory scientists and clinicians were asked to comment upon the basic science presentations.

The present conference grew out of the suggestion originating at the former symposium that the next meeting be planned from a clinical point of view. Therefore, the present conference was organized around specific clinical topics dealing with human oculomotor disorders. An internationally recognized clinician was invited to organize each session around his clinical specialty and to add highly qualified basic and clinical scientists for their particular expertise with the subject. Additional discussants supplemented and broadened each session. Finally, round-table discussions followed the formal presentations of each topic to maximize the opportunity for interchange between clinicians and basic scientists. As a final highlight to the conference David A. Robinson, a scientist who has long exemplified the collaborative spirit between the basic and clinical sides of the oculomotor community, delivered the fourth William A. Kettlewell Lecture.

The presentations made at the conference reflected several trends that have developed in oculomotor research since the last conference. First the clinical community is increasingly using mathematical or computer models to better summarize patient data and also understand the physiological mechanisms underlying disease. Within the group of laboratory workers, a resurgence of carefully controlled lesion studies, particularly in monkeys trained to fixate and follow targets, has led to the development of a number of primate models for human eye movement disorders. Finally, both communities of workers showed a burgeoning interest in the plastic adaptive capabilities of the central nervous system. This theme was highlighted in Professor Granit´s opening presentation and was repeated over and over again throughout most sessions of the symposia. If one topic suggests itself as the subject of a future conference on the oculomotor system, it would probably be the concept of adaptation to disease -- how can these processes be understood at the fundamental level and how can they be channeled for better clinical treatment.

The symposium organizers are deeply indebted to Professor Yngve Zotterman for providing the support and unparalleled facilities of the Wenner-Gren Center in Stockholm. We also acknowledge the generous financial support of the Smith-kettlewell Eye Research Foundation of San francisco, the Swedish Medical Research Council, the Swedish Government and the Swedish Ophthalmological Society.

Gunnar Lennerstrand

David S. Zee

Edward Keller

CONTENTS

Section II Coordinator: R.D. Reinecke

EYE MOVEMENT CONTROL IN STRABISMUS AND AMBLYOPIA

Section III Coordinator: G. Kommerell

CONGENITAL NYSTAGMUS

Section VII Coordinator: J. Dichgans

DISORDERS OF OPTOKINETIC AND VESTIBULAR NYSTAGMUS

Section VIII Coordinator: M.A. Gresty

DISORDERS OF EYE-HEAD COORDINATION

LIST OF CONTRIBUTORS AND INVITED PARTICIPANTS

Richard Abadi
Visual Sciences Laboratory
Department of Ophthalmic Optics
UMIST
P O Box 88
MANCHESTER M60 1QD
England

Larry Abel
Department of Neurology
Case Western Reserve University
University Hospitals
CLEVELAND
Ohio 44106 USA

Robert Baker
Department of Physiology
New York University Medical Center
NEW YORK N Y 10016
USA

Robert Baloh
Department of Neurology
University of California
LOS ANGELES
California 90024 USA

Neal Barmack
Biological Sciences Group
University of Connecticut
STORRS
Connecticut 06268 USA

Graham Barnes
RAF Institute of Aviation Medicine
FARNBOROUGH
Hants GU14 6SZ
England

Pierre Vital Berard
197 Corniche Kennedy
Villa Atalante
F-13007 MARSEILLE
France

Harley Bicas
Department of Ophthalmology
Faculty of Medicine
University of Sao Paolo
14.100 RIBEIRAO PRETO
Est. Sao Paolo
Brazil

Ruggero Bortolami
Department of Veterinary Anatomy
University of Bologna
Via Belmeloro, 12
I-40126 BOLOGNA
Italy

Thomas Brandt
Department of Neurology
Krupp Hospital
Alfried-Krupp-Strasse 21
D-4300 ESSEN 1
West Germany

U.W. Buettner
Department of Neurology
Eberhard-Karls-University
Liebermeisterstrasse 18-20
D-7400 TUBINGEN
West Germany

Ulrich Büttner
Department of Neurology
University Hospital
Moorenstrasse 5
D-4000 DUSSELDORF
West Germany

Emilio Campos
Department of Ophthalmology
University of Modena
Via del Pozzo 71
I-4100 MODENA
Italy

Dante Chiarandini
Department of Ophthalmology
New York University Medical Center
NEW YORK N Y 10016
USA

Ken Ciuffreda
SUNY/College of Optometry
100 East 24th Street
NEW YORK N Y 10010
USA

Alexander Cogan
Smith-Kettlewell Institute of Visual Sciences
2232 Webster Street
SAN FRANCISCO
California 94115 USA

Bernard Cohen
Department of Neurology
Mount Sinai School of Medicine
1 Gustave L. Levy Place
NEW YORK N Y 10029
USA

Han Collewijn
Department of Physiology
Erasmus University
P O Box 1738
3000 DR ROTTERDAM
Holland

Carter Collins
Smith-Kettlewell Institute of Visual Sciences
2232 Webster Street
SAN FRANCISCO
California 94115 USA

Robert Daroff
Department of Neurology
Case Western Reserve University
University Hospitals
CLEVELAND
Ohio 44106 USA

Jacob Davidowitz
Department of Ophthalmology
New YOrk University Medical Center
550 First AVenue
NEW YORK N Y 10016
USA

W. de Decker
Department of Ophthalmology
University Hospital
Hegewischstrasse 2
D-2300 KIEL
West Germany

Louis Dell´Osso
Department of Neurology
Case Western Reserve University
University Hospitals
CLEVELAND
Ohio 44106 USA

Johannes Dichgans
Department of Neurology
Eberhard-Karls-University
Liebermeisterstrasse 18-20
D-7400 TUBINGEN
West Germany

Johathan James Ell
MRC Hearing and Balance Unit
National Hospital
Queen Square
LONDON WC 1
England

Curt von Euler
Department of Neurophysiology
Karolinska Institutet
S-104 01 STOCKHOLM
Sweden

Craig Evinger
Department of Physiology
New York University Medical Center
550 First Avenue
NEW YORK N Y 10016
USA

Steven Feldon
Estelle Doheny Eye Foundation Building
1355 San Pablo Street
LOS ANGELES
Calfiornia 90033 USA

Lars Frisén
Department of Ophthalmology
Sahlgrenska Hospital
S-413 45 GÖTEBORG
Sweden

Michael Goldberg
Laboratory of Sensorimotor Research
Building 36, Room 1 D-18
NIH
BETHESDA
Maryland 20205 USA

Ragnar Granit
Eriksbergsgatan 14
S-114 30 STOCKHOLM
Sweden

Michael Gresty
MRC Hearing and Balance Unit
National Hospital
Queen Square
LONDON WC 1
England

Daniel Guitton
Montreal Neurological Institute
3801 University Street
MONTREAL P Q
Canada H3A 2B4

Lucy Shafik Hanna
18, Champolion Stteet
CAIRO
Egypt

Volker Henn
Neurological Clinic
University Hospital
CH-8091 ZURICH
Switzerland

Nils Gunnar Henriksson
Department of Otolaryngology
University Hospital
S-221 85 LUND
Sweden

David Henson
Department of Optometry
UWIST
19 Park Place
CARDIFF CF1 3DQ
Wales U.K.

Klaus Hepp
Department of Theoretical Physics
ETH
CH-8093 ZURICH
Switzerland

K.-P. Hoffmann
Department of Neurobiology
University of Ulm
D-7900 ULM
West Germany

John Hotson
Department of Neurology
Santa Clara Valley Medical Center
751 South Bascom Avenue
SAN JOSE
California 95128 USA

William Hoyt
Department of Ophthalmology
University of California
SAN FRANCISCO
California 94143 USA

Gunnar Hörnsten
Department of Ophthalmology
Södersjukhuset
S-100 64 STOCKHOLM
Sweden

Masayasu Inagaki
Department of Ophthalmology
Nihon University
School of Medicine
30 Ooyaguchikamimachi
Itabashi-ku
TOKYO
Japan

Hiroshi Ishikawa
Department of Ophthalmology
Nihon University
School of Medicine
30 Ooyaguchikamimachi
Itabashi-ku
TOKYO
Japan

Arthur Jampolsky
Smith-Kettlewell Institute of Visual Sciences
2232 Webster Street
SAN FRANCISCO
California 94115 USA

Edward Keller
Smith-Kettlewell Institute of Visual Sciences
2232 Webster Street
SAN FRANCISCO
California 94115 USA

Christopher Kennard
20 Fortis Green
LONDON N2 9EL
England

Michael King
Department of Ophthalmology
Wilmer Institute
Johns Hopkins Hopsital
601 N. Broadway
BALTIMORE
Maryland 21205 USA

Eberhard Koenig
Department of Neurology
University Hospital
Liebermeisterstrasse 18-20
D-7400 TUBINGEN
West Germany

Guntram Kommerell
Department of Ophthalmology
University Hospital
Killianstrasse 5
D-7800 FREIBURG
West Germany

Birgitta Larsby
Department of Otolaryngology
University Hospital
S-581 85 LINKÖPING
Sweden

John Leigh
Department of Neurology
Johns Hopkins Hospital
601 N. Broadway
BALTIMORE
Maryland 21205 USA

Gunnar Lennerstrand
Department of Ophthalmology
University Hospital
S-581 85 LINKÖPING

Mark Lomas
Visual Sciences Laboratory
Department of Ophtalmic Optics
UMIST
P O Box 88
MANCHESTER M60 1QD
England

James Lynch
Department of Anatomy
University of Mississippi
JACKSON
Mississippi 39216 USA

Ermanno Manni
Department of Physiology
Universita´Catolica
Via Della Pineta Sacchetti 644
ROME
Italy

Keith McNeer
West End Eye Center, Inc.
Suite 110, Grace Medical Village
5700 West Grace Street
RICHMOND
Virginia 23226 USA

E. Mehdorn
Department of Ophthalmology
University Hospital
Killianstrasse 21
D-7800 FREIBURG
West Germany

Otmar Meienberg
Asylstrasse 44
CH-3063 ITTIGEN
Switzerland

Frederick Miles
Laboratory of Sensorimotor Research
Building 36, Room 1D-18
NIH
BETHESDA
Maryland 20205 USA

Sven Erik Nilsson
Department of Ophthalmology
University Hospital
S-581 85 LINKÖPING
Sweden

Lance Optican
National Eye Institute
laboratory of Sensory Motor Research
Building 36, Room 1D18
BETHESDA
Maryland 20205 USA

Wolfgang Precht
Institute of Brain Research
University of Zürich
August-Forelstrasse 1
CH-8029 ZURICH
Switzerland

Robert Reinecke
Department of Ophthalmology
Albany Medical College
ALBANY N Y 12208 USA

David Robinson
Department of Ophthalmology
Wilmer Institute
Johns Hopkins Hospital
601 N. Broadway
BALTIMORE
Maryland 21205 USA

Lucyna Schalén
P.H. Lings väg 15
S-223 65 LUND
Sweden

Dieter Schmidt
Department of Ophthalmology
Univeristy Hospital
Killianstrasse 5
D-7800 FREIBURG
West Germany

Clifton Schor
School of Optometry
University of California
BERKELEY
California 94720 USA

Alan Scott
Smith-Kettlewell Institute of
Visual Sciences
2232 Webster Street
SAN FRANCISCO
Calfironia 94115 USA

Sachiko Sekimoto
Department of Ophthalmology
Nihon University
School fo Medicine
30 Ooyaguchikamimachi
Itabashi-ku
TOKYO
Japan

John Semmlow
Department of Surgery and
Electrical Engineering
Rutgers Medical School
PISCATAWAY
New Jersey 08854 USA

James Sharpe
Yotonto Western Hospital
University of Toronto
399 Bathurst Street
TORONTO
Ontario M5T 2S8
Canada

Lawrence Stark
Department of Physdiological
Optics and Optometry
481 Minor Hall
University of California
BERKELEY
California 94720 USA

Ian Strachan
Department of Ophthalmology
Royal Hallanshire Hospital
SHEFFIELD
England

Tone Suzuki
Department of Ophthalmology
Nihon University
School of Medicine
30 Ooyaguchikamimachi
Itabashi-ku
TOKYO
Japan

Björn Tengroth
Department of Ophthalmology
Karolinska Hospital
S-104 01 STOCKHOLM
Sweden

J. van Hof-van Duin
Department of Physiology I
Erasmus University
P O Box 1738
ROTTERDAM
Holland

Carsten Wennmo
Department of Otolaryngology
University Hospital
S-221 85 LUND
Sweden

Gerald Westheimer
Department of Physiology-Anatomy
University of California
BERKELEY
California 94720 USA

Robert Yee
Jules Stein Eye Institute
UCLA Center for Health Sciences
800 Westwood Plaza
LOS ANGELES
California 90024 USA

Wolfgang Zangemeister
Geffckenstrasse 29
D-2000 HAMBURG 20
West Germany

David Zee
Department of Neurology
The Johns Hopkins Hospital
601 North Broadway
BALTIMORE
Maryland 21205 USA

Yngve Zotterman
Wenner-Gren Center
Sveavägen 166
S-113 46 STOCKHOLM
Sweden

Lars Ödkvist
Department of Otolaryngology
University Hospital
S-581 85 LINKÖPING
Sweden

INTRODUCTION

R. GRANIT

Nobel Institute for Neurophysiology,
Karolinska Institutet, Stockholm, Sweden

We meet at a time when eye muscle motricity for some years has engaged a number of skilful experimenters. Recently an extensive review of vestibular, reticular, and cerebellar control of eye movements occupied 360 pages of a volume from a Symposium at the Scuola Normale in Pisa (Granit and Pompeiano, 1979) and in the same year appeared that excellent book on "Mammalian Vestibular Physiology" written by Wilson and Melvill Jones. Ito´s valuable presentation of "Recent Advances in Cerebellar Physiology" was published in 1978. At this meeting we have an opportunity of consulting an expert on motor control such as D.A. Robinson.

Faced with this avalanche of knowledge an outsider like myself can only offer some reflections on a general feature of motor control that has come to the fore also in many recent experiments on eye movements. I have, of course, been excited by the progress in understanding the role of afferent impulses from the eye muscles as they interact with those from neck and eye afferents in the colliculus and the visual cortex. Nevertheless, at the moment, my present interests stand closer to the new work on the old problem of purposive -- that is goal-determined -- adaptive plasticity. Oculomotricity shares this property with other motor and sensory systems.

I assume the classical findings by Stratton (1897) on the effects of wearing inversion spectacles to be known, likewise those of Kohler (1951) on similar lines. I shall therefore introduce my theme by three recent experiments underlining the parallel with comparable work on the eye movements.

Nashner (1976) placed a man on a platform that suddenly was shuffled backwards inducing in the subject a tendency to fall forwards. This movement stretched the calf extensors that responded purposively with a counteracting stretch reflex. Next the platform was rotated around a horizontal axis crossing his feet, front part turning upwards. This also stretched the same extensors but now the turn of the platform induced a fall backwards apparently checked by vestibular control. The inopportune stretch reflex at first recurred but disappeared after a few successive trials with the platform. It was obviously non-purposive in the new situation.

Evarts and Granit (1976) studied a stretch reflex in the biceps as elicited by mechanical supination of the hand. The subject held a motor driven handle in a firm grip during enforced pronation or supination. To this mechanically elicited stimulus he was instructed to react by himself turning the handle in the direction of pronation or supination. He thus had a pre-determined choice to combine either instruction with either mechanically elicited turn of the handle. Pronation causes biceps inhibition, supination, as stated, excitation, i.e. a stretch reflex. Us interests the fact that when the instruction was to pronate, thus opposing a mechanically elicited supination, the stretch reflex lingered on diminishing in size for a few successive trials but in the end was suppressed as non-purposive in view of the intended voluntary inhibition.

My third example for comparison with oculomotor plasticity is based on the recording of evoked potentials. Fiorentini, Ghez and Maffei (1972) used prisms tilting the target 30 - 40° from the perceived vertical. Adaptive effects were noted already during the first hours of wearing them; virtually complete adjustment to the new vertical was found on the second day. This plastic change was reflected in a decrease of the mean difference between the amplitudes of evoked potentials for the vertical and oblique pattern. Thus, at some site between the retina and the primary visual area in the cortex the purposive plastic adjustment must have taken place.

Parallel experiences from the field of eye motor control have been conveniently summarized int he book by Wilson and Melvill Jones (1979). The relevant material is found in Chaper 8 under the title "Adaptive plasticity in the vestibulo-visual interactive system". I shall briefly review experiments by Melvill Jones and Miles, having had the privilege of seeing their technical arrangements.

From the detailed report of the work carried out in the laboratory of Melvill Jones it emerges that in both human subjects and cats, which are exposed to optical reversal of vision during rotation, short-term and long-term adaptive effects on the vestibulo-ocular reflex (VOR) occur. In the short-term experiments the subjects were rotationally oscillated at 1/6 Hz and 60°/sec angular velocity amplitude, while they were trying to fixate a mirror-reversed image of the surround moving with the turn table. Thus the vestibular drive opposed that requred for visual fixation. One single day of a 16 min exposure to active vision reversal during head rotation produced about 20% attenuation of gain in the VOR. Gain is defined as the rate of peak eye velocity to peak head velocity.

For the long-term effects Melvill Jones used reversing prisms mounted in head-held goggles and worn continously for up to nearly a month (in the case illustrated in the book) while the subject was normally engaged in locomotion. Daily seances of 10 - 20 cycles of rotational oscillation were conducted before, after and during the period of experimentation. In both man and cat an 80% attenuation of gain was induced over the first few days and the change of phase in the sinusoidal compensatory eye movements ultimately came close to reflex reversal. On return to normal vision normal phase was restored in a couple of hours.

Miles and Fuller (1974) using trained monkeys for subjects had recourse to magnifying and diminishing binoculars. With 2.0 x lenses worn for 3 - 4 days gain rose to around 1.8, with 0.5 x lenses it was reduced to 0.65 in otherwise similar tests. This experiment has obvious clinical implications.

However, my interest in experiments of the general type sampled here -- and easily multiplied -- is at the moment merely centred on the very general question of purposiveness in plastic adaptations and its role as criterion for error detection and error correction. In none of the cases selected for introducing the problem was the correction meaningless. The goal was always to produce a purposive response to the demand set by the unexpected behaviour on the part of the environment. Thus the stretch reflex in the first two cases was suppressed because it was useless in the new situation. For vision with its numerous control functions the vertical just has to be vertical. Hence the false information about verticality was corrected. The vestibulo-ocular reflex serves to stabilize the visual image in head movement. Melvill Jones´s experiment made it useless and hence suppressed. In the arrangement of

Miles gain of the VOR adapted to the new requirements.

The common denominator in the reviewed cases is the demonstration on the part of the nervous system to cope with a basic demand for meaningful action. This involves correction of an error. But to insert an error detector in all these examples means that such a signal in each case must be designed according to a hierarchic concept of a goal. Errors have no life of their own. They are defined relative to some desirable achievement. It may well be that a specific centre registers failure or dissatisfaction independently of the where, how, and when of its cause. This we do not know. But it seems to me that the only real explanation of adaptive plasticity lies in its purposive character. Starting from this insight the neurophysiologist has to discover the means employed by the nervous system to realize its aim.

From the neurophysiological point of view error detection seems less of a problem than error correction. This process takes place under the permanent guidance of a goal that has been actualized by being infringed upon by an abnormal mode of stimulation. Elsewhere (Granit, 1977) I have discussed plastic adaptability. My general standpoint is that violation of the criterion of purposiveness in acts of the kind I have surveyed is a sufficient cause for the nervous system to mobilize plastic adaptability in order to contend with the unexpected environmental challenges. For physiologists, used to think in purely mechanistic terms, it may seem a heretic notion that something as abstract as violation of a goal or, in short, antipurposiveness could serve as an internal nervous command to apply a correction. However, a comparison with voluntary motor activity will make it easier to understand my thesis.

We are bound to accept that cur will -- an equally abstract quantity -- in settling for a purpose is capable of transferring its intention to the executive, that is, our motor apparatus. Indeed, the will is a most powerful dictator of motricity. If it demands writing a message it naturally uses hands and fingers, but it can, if forced to do so, produce the wanted message by using a pen fixed to a longish shaft firmly tied to the underarm or even by clamping a pen between the toes. Innumerable motor acts have been developed under voluntary control for satisfying transferred purposes, whatever they may have been. Most of these acts have become automatized. This does not signify that they have lost their purposiveness. It is retained, and when challenged, is capable of asserting its hegemony, as in the experiments reviewed. In fact, what or was the voluntary component in a motor act is its purpose.

Terms such as purpose or goal clearly refer to anticipations related to the environment. But there must also be a corresponding perpetual transfer of the purpose to serve as a criterion during the elaboration of a motor act. I mean that an inside equivalent goal-sensitivity is part of the neural mechanisms. We are programmed for adapting plastically according to a principle of purposiveness and for reacting automatically to its violation. It is an exciting task for neurophysiology to unravel the processes which the nervous system resorts to for making this possible. I would not be surprised if it presupposed understanding of how a voluntary goal is transferred into the language of the motor marionette.

THE WILLIAM A.
KETTLEWELL LECTURE

THE WILLIAM A. KETTLEWELL LECTURE
INTRODUCTION OF DAVID A. ROBINSON

E. L. KELLER

Smith-Kettlewell Institute of Visual Sciences,
San Francisco, California, USA

It gives me very great pleasure to be able to introduce today's speaker for the fourth William A. Kettlewell lecture: Professor David A. Robinson from the Wilmer Eye Institute of the Johns Hopkins Medical School.

David Robinson, or the oculomotor pope as he is commonly known among his many colleagues and associates, is one of the most outstanding examples of individuals who have fostered a collaborative spirit between basic research and clinical application inthe visual sciences - exactly the spirit we have been trying to further with the present meeting. Over the years his work has been firmly rooted in and has had wide application to both communities.

David's far ranging and penetrating influence on the field of oculomotor research might be best put in perspective by a short review of his major research accomplishments over the past 20 years. His publications and lectures have always been paragons of clarity; so technically compact that every sentence carries significant meaning, and at the same time full of wit and picturesque speech. Who has not heard and then began to use such terms as the oculomotor integrator, the repairshop of the brain, the bang-bang pulse-step generator - all these and many others forming the common currency of oculomotor research vocabulary which originated in David's work.

His first memorable contribution in this field was the publication in 1963 of a new and quantitative method for the registration of eye movements. This method has now been widely adapted for use in oculomotor laboratories throughout the world. Today it is considered the premier method of measuring eye movements for animal experiments. Although originally designed for clinical applications, its use in this area has not been as widely distributed, but nevertheless, it has been used when the need for quantitative clinical measurements have required it.

His 1964 papers on the human saccadic and smooth pursuit systems rapidly became classics, widely read and quoted. They are terse, pithy, full of quantitative data and they also introduced us to a new application of the methods of systems engineering to describe the operation of the oculomotor system. While others had pioneered this approach, David's special touch was to require that the model grow out of the data, to summarize, to consolidate, to simplify and to provide insight for future experiments. His models could be readily understood with only a minimum of esoteric mathematical language and we see from this point forward the use even in clinical communications of engineering or computer based models to explain and unify an otherwise bewildering array of data.

In a 1970 paper he pioneered the use of the single-neuron recording technique in the oculomotor system to provide a description of the organization of motoneurons. While other laboratories published similar results at the same time, it was David's contribution to summarize the data in the form of a mathematical expression which pointed out the basic simplicity of organization in the oculomotor neurons pools and formed the base of all future studies into the more central organization.

In 1975, at the previous Stockholm meeting, he again applied his analytic skills to clarifying the confusing accumulation of data that was beginning to emerge from the single-unit recording laboratories - the pausers, the bursters, the burst-tonic units - were all synthesized into a conceptual model of how the saccadic pulse-step generator works at the neural level. This model helps to clarify a cardinal problem - that of the transformation of spatial coding on the sensory side of the visual system to temporal coding on the oculomotor side.

In several papers in the late seventies this model or other models were applied to the deeper understanding of several clinical neuropathological conditions by David and his co-workers. These papers all have obvious diagnostic value. His interest in peripheral mechanisms continued with the development of a static model of eye positions, muscle lengths and orbital forces. This type of work is still in its infancy but holds the promise of significant improvement in the quantitative assessment of strabismus surgery.

More recently he has turned his attention to the problem of plasticity in the organization of the oculomotor system both in the vestibulo-ocular reflex and the saccadic system. Again this field has tremendous appeal both to basic and clinical scientists for its eventual explanation of the enormous regenerative and self-corrective powers of the nervous system.

Thus it can be easily stated that nobody in the oculomotor field has had a wider field of influence than Dr. Robinson. Everyone of us has found some nugget of wisdom applicable to our own field of research in his papers. We are all much the richer for his generalizing and synthesizing approach to this research field. Therfore, it is highly appropriate that he address us today on the topic "A Model of Cancellation of the Vestibulo-ocular Reflex".

A MODEL OF CANCELLATION OF THE VESTIBULO-OCULAR REFLEX

D. A. ROBINSON

The Wilmer Institute, The Johns Hopkins University School of Medicine, Baltimore, Maryland, USA

ABSTRACT

When a moving target is pursued by a head movement, the eyes remain stationary in the head and the vestibulo-ocular reflex (vor) is cancelled. Evidence is reviewed suggesting that cancellation is not done by the pursuit system alone. A model is proposed in which a signal proportional to the velocity of a planned head movement is switched in to cancel the vor. The model appears to reconcile existing data and suggests new experiments and clinical investigations.

KEYWORDS

Smooth pursuit movements; vestibulo-ocular reflex; cancellation of vestibulo-ocular reflex; head tracking; suppression of vestibulo-ocular reflex.

INTRODUCTION

Usually objects moving in the visual environment are tracked with head movements during which the eyes are relatively stationary in the head. In order to do this, the vestibulo-ocular reflex (vor), which would ordinarily move the eyes to compensate for the head movement, must be kept from acting. This behavior is often called suppression of the vor but recordings from second-order vestibular neurons that project to ocular motoneurons show that the vor is not switched off as this term implies but must be cancelled by another equal but opposite signal at the motoneuron. It is commonly assumed that the cancelling signal comes from the pursuit system but evidence is given below that this might not be the case. If so, it is important to recognize the fact since it would influence our interpretation of neural data and provide a clinical test that could have value in localizing a lesion.

DIFFERENCES BETWEEN PURSUIT AND CANCELLATION

Some of the evidence that cancellation is not effected by pursuit has been reviewed elsewhere (Tomlinson and Robinson, 1981) and will only be summarized here:

1. Human subjects cannot, in general, make smooth pursuit movements while attempting to track an imagined target in the dark. They can, however, partially cancel their vor in the dark by imagining a target moving with them. They cancel similarly when given a sound source moving with them in the dark (Schmid, Zambarbieri, and Magenes, 1981) although such a moving sound source does not produce smooth pursuit when the head is still. Presumably, a sound source simply helps one to imagine a target and the two phenomena are the same.

2. Cats have a maximum pursuit velocity of 8 - 20 deg/sec but can cancel at head velocities of 60 deg/sec. Some monkeys cannot pursue vertically faster than 30 deg/sec but can cancel vertically at 60 deg/sec.

3. Cells in the vestibular nucleus behave in a manner during cancellation that cannot be predicted from their behavior during pursuit and the normal vor. If the system were reasonably linear, the behavior during cancellation should be the sum of that during pursuit with the head still and that with the target stationary and the head moving. Such superposition is not found on a variety of cell types in the vestibular nucleus indicating that the circuit mediating cancellation is different in part from the circuit mediating pursuit and the vor.

More recently, additional evidence has been obtained:

4. The torsional vor can be cancelled. You can conduct the following experiment yourself: seat a subject in a rotating chair with head tilted back and eyes fixating a spot directly overhead on the ceiling. Look for torsion eye movements by watching an episcleral vein near the limbus as you slowly walk the chair around in a circle at about 60 deg/sec (6 sec per revolution). You will see a series of slow and quick phases in the first few seconds as the eye rotates about the line of sight - the torsional vor. Now ask the subject to hold a fixation object (a ruler, a piece of printed paper) overhead, so it will rotate as well, and to look at it rather than the ceiling. Rotation now produces no eye movements - the torsional vor is cancelled. Jampel (1981) has recorded such cancellation at head velocities up to 70 deg/sec. Obviously a torsional pursuit system does not exist. The concept is meaningless. Torsional cancellation cannot, therefore, be done by pursuit.

5. In unpublished observations from our laboratory R.J. Leigh, S.A. Newman, D.S. Zee, and N.R. Miller demonstrated a switching phenomenon in cancellation. They examined a patient with total paralysis of one eye but good vision in both. They measured the movements of the normal eye while it was covered, thus opening the loop of the pursuit system. A target attached to a rotating chair was aligned with the visual axis of the immobile eye. The patient had a normal vor in the mobile eye, tested in the dark. When the patient was told to look at the target rotating with him, the mobile, covered eye executed normal movements of the vor but when he was urged to track the target as well as possible, the mobile eye stopped moving. In both cases the visual and vestibular stimuli were identical - the image of the target remained stationary on the retina so that the pursuit system received no visual stimulus - the difference was in mental set. The patient appeared to decide to make an effort that altered the circuitry involved in such a way that the vor was cancelled. This certainly suggests some sort of switching mechanism.

6. Dell'Osso and co-workers (1981) described three patients with dissimilar deficits of pursuit and cancellation. I have heard similar, anecdotal reports from others who examine patients but a quantitative demonstration is still not available.

SIMILARITIES OF PURSUIT AND CANCELLATION

There are two pieces of evidence that seem to imply that cancellation is effected by pursuit:

7. Lesions that cause deficits of pursuit almost always cause deficits in cancellation and vice versa (Halmagyi and Gresty, 1979). Thus, patients as in item 6 above are rather rare. Flocculectomy in the monkey, for example, produces the same quantitative decreases in cancellation and pursuit movements (Zee and co-workers, 1981).

8. Both cancellation and pursuit deteriorate in the same way at high frequencies (0.5 - 2 Hz) during sinusoidal tracking. According to Lisberger and co-workers (1981) both activities are limited by the saturation of an internal eye acceleration signal.

These two considerations indicate that pursuit and cancellation must share common neural circuitry.

A MODEL OF CANCELLATION AND PURSUIT

The model is based on the idea that if a person plans to make a head movement in pursuit of a visual target, it makes a great deal of sense to send a copy of this planned movement as part of the oculomotor command so as to cancel the command that will come from the vor. The vor is working against the goal of eye-head tracking and if not cancelled would make the smooth pursuit system work that much harder to overcome the vor. Thus, if one is tracking with the head a target moving at 150 deg/sec, it is not necessary to assume that the pursuit system is capable of generating velocities of 150 deg/sec (which it normally cannot do) to block the vor. Consequently, any such model can easily generate eye velocities in space that are higher than in the head.

This concept is illustrated in Fig. 1. The summing junction at the right shows that gaze velocity $\dot{G}$ (eye velocity in space) is the sum of head velocity $\dot{H}$ and eye velocity in the head $\dot{E}$. For the frequencies and velocities of interest, the translation of the neural eye velocity command $\dot{E}'$ to actual eye velocity $\dot{E}$ may be considered perfect. $\dot{H}$ is transduced by the semicircular canals (SCC) to an internal copy $\dot{H}'$ that is sent to the eye with a sign reversal to execute the vor. Any signal that causes the eye to do other than $-\dot{H}'$ must be a gaze velocity command $\dot{G}'$ since $\dot{E}'$ is the difference between it and $\dot{H}'$. The summing junction on the left expresses that the velocity of image slip on the retina $\dot{e}$ is the difference between target velocity $\dot{T}$ (in space) and $\dot{G}$. It is generally believed that this activates the pursuit system to create an eye velocity command $\dot{E}'$ (identical to $\dot{G}'$ if the head is stationary). A system that makes planned head movements (head plan) generates an internal signal $\dot{H}_p'$ that is converted somehow (head mech's) into the actual planned head movement $\dot{H}_p$. Total head velocity $\dot{H}$ is the sum of a planned component $\dot{H}_p$ and an unexpected component $\dot{H}_x$ due to external forces.

So far nothing has been said that is not generally agreed upon in oculomotor physiology. The new hypothesis now made is to use $\dot{H}_p'$ as part of the oculomotor command $\dot{G}'$ by adding it to the output of the pursuit system $\dot{E}'$ (cancel path).

One can see at once that a velocity limit just after the smooth pursuit system would limit maximum pursuit velocity in the head but not the cancellation velocity command $\dot{G}'$. During eye-head tracking the smooth pursuit system need only add on any difference, $\dot{E}'$, between head velocity $\dot{H}_p'$ and desired gaze velocity, $\dot{G}'$. One might object by saying that, as has already been pointed out by Young (1977), the pursuit system uses many sources of information, besides vision, to formulate its commands and the use of a planned head movement signal is just another example. This is a valid viewpoint but the essential feature of Fig. 1 is the switch S_1. During many planned head movements one wants the vor to act normally to stabilize gaze in space. Switch S_1 must be open. At other times planned head movements are used to track targets; switch S_1 must be closed. That is the essential feature of the model - a switch which makes the system that cancels different from that which pursues.

Figure 1 illustrates an important point: one does not want to cancel the vor for all possible head movements, only a planned head movement. In fact, the vor works quite well during cancellation if the head is unexpectedly perturbed. An imposed head velocity $\dot{H}_x$ creates a compensatory eye movement $\dot{E}$ via the vor so that actual gaze velocity $\dot{G}$ continues to follow commanded gaze velocity $\dot{G}'$ regardless of the perturbation. This was illustrated well by Lanman, Bizzi, and Allum (1978) by suddenly braking the head during eye-head tracking. The step change in $\dot{H}$ was immediately converted to a step change in $\dot{E}$ by the vor with the result that gaze continued to follow the target. Thus, the system responsible for cancellation cancels planned or predictable head movements, not unpredicted head movements.

To investigate this hypothesis further and test it quantitatively, one must put specific transfer functions into the boxes in Fig. 1. This is done in Fig. 2. The first problem encountered is how to model the smooth pursuit system. Models without internal feedback tend to be unstable because of the 130 msec delay in the system or, if stable, have such a low open-loop gain that their tracking is unrealistically poor. Young proposed, and reviewed the evidence for (1977), an internal

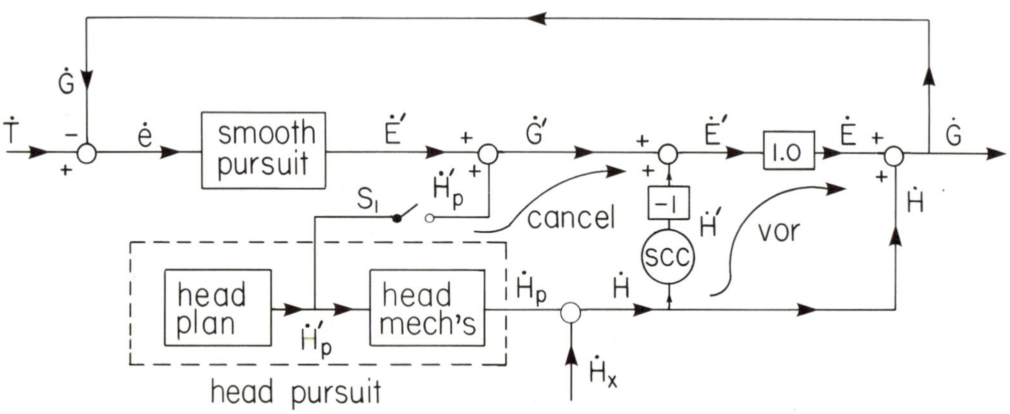

Fig. 1. The basic hypothesis of how pursuit and cancellation interact. $\dot{G}$, gaze velocity; $\dot{H}$, head velocity; $\dot{E}$, eye velocity in the head; $\dot{E}'$, eye-in-head velocity command; $\dot{H}'$, internal copy of $\dot{H}$; SCC, semicircular canals; $\dot{G}'$, internal gaze-velocity command; $\dot{H}_p$, a planned head velocity; $\dot{H}_p'$, the internal command for $\dot{H}_p$; $\dot{H}_x$, head velocity due to external force; $\dot{e}$, velocity of retinal image slip; $\dot{T}$, target velocity in space; S_1, switch to effect cancellation.

positive feedback loop that cancelled the outer negative feedback loop ($\dot{G}$) and made the system stable regardless of delays. The scheme in Fig. 2 employs a modification of Young's idea. One cannot enclose all the delays under a positive feedback loop: a delay of about 50 msec occurs in the retina before the $\dot{e}$ signal enters the brain and there are motor delays between $\dot{G}'$ and $\dot{G}$ of about 30 msec (10 of which is in the muscles) that probably lie peripheral to the point where a copy of $\dot{G}'$ is fed back. Thus, only 50 msec can be included under a positive feedback loop and it can be shown that this is not adequate to make the system stable. But note that when the pursuit system puts out a command $\dot{E}'$, its repercussions on $\dot{e}_d$ are not felt until 80 msec later around the outer loop. If one also delays the inner feedback loop by 80 msec then the two signals arrive at the same time and cancel out. The outer feedback loop is now effectively eliminated and the pursuit system is stable. Put another way, the efference copy signal $\dot{E}_d'$ and the reafference signal $\dot{e}_d$ should be compared at comparable points in time to correctly estimate target velocity with respect to the head, $\dot{T}_h'$. The apparent open loop gain (negative loop only open) of the pursuit system (ignoring nonlinearities) is $1/(1-k)$, the closed loop gain is $1/(2-k)$. If k is 0.9, the gains are 10 and 0.91 respectively. A lag of 40 msec (T_p) is present to account for the observed smooth transition from one velocity to another. Pursuit velocity saturation (PVS) in normal humans is, typically, higher than 60 deg/sec (Schalén, 1980) and we estimate it to be just above 100 deg/sec (unpublished observations). Lisberger and co-workers (1981) point out that high-frequency pursuit is mainly degraded by an acceleration saturation (AS). This occurs on the $\dot{e}$ signal because such a signal is a command for the eye to change its velocity and thus represents an eye-acceleration command. (Note that the positive feedback loop in the pursuit system acts like an integrator; since its output is an eye velocity command $\dot{E}'$, its input may be interpreted as an eye acceleration command.)

When animals became foveate and frontal-eyed it was necessary to get rid of the vor during planned head movements such as those involved in the chase of prey. Before one can plan a head movement to track a target one must first calculate target velocity in space. This is most simply done by adding $\dot{e}_d$ and a copy of $\dot{G}'$ to form $\dot{T}_d'$. Again, one should delay $\dot{G}'$ by 80 msec so that the reafference ($\dot{e}_d$) and motor copy ($\dot{G}_d'$) of a change in $\dot{G}'$ are compared at corresponding times to avoid, among other things, instability. One can now plan to make a head movement of velocity $\dot{H}_p'$ that equals, or is some fraction f, of $\dot{T}_d'$. The decision to track with the head keeps switch S_3 down to pass on the planned head velocity signal. Switch S_1 is closed representing the decision to cancel.

To produce a normal latency for head movements, 50 msec is assigned to planning and 30 msec to the motor periphery. Head inertia is represented by a lag (head mech's) with a time constant T_h that is about 80 msec. The signal actually used for cancelling $\dot{H}_p''$ must first be adjusted by passing it through an internal copy of head mechanics "head mech's" so that it resembles $\dot{H}_p$ rather than $\dot{H}_p'$. Evidence from eye/head ramp tracking at high velocities (e.g. 100 deg/sec) reveals that cancellation does not occur in the first 200 - 300 msec after the start of tracking which may be considered as an unpredictable portion of the tracking when the start of the target motion is not known. Only after a constant target velocity has been observed for some time can it be extrapolated in time and this suggests that the cancellation signal $\dot{H}_p''$ should be delayed by a lag with a time constant T_x of about 0.15 sec.

Through head mechanics, $\dot{H}_p'$ produces the actual head velocity $\dot{H}$ which is transduced by the SCC to $\dot{H}'$. By adding $\dot{H}_p''$ to create $\dot{G}'$ and then subtracting $\dot{H}'$, the vor is cancelled. If $\dot{H}$ is other than $\dot{T}$ (f greater or less than 1.0), $\dot{e}$ will stimulate the smooth pursuit system to move the eye in the head ($\dot{E}'$) so that total tracking ($\dot{G}'$) is correct. Thus, in the steady state, the smooth pursuit system only corrects the error between target and head; it is not required to overcome the vor as well.

So far we have considered the natural situation of tracking a target with eye and head together. Unfortunately, cancellation is usually examined in a highly unnatural situation in which a subject or animal is rotated sinusoidally en bloc while fixating a target fastened to the chair. We talk as though the same mechanisms were involved but clearly this is not so. The model described so far will not cancel a passive head movement. Nevertheless, the vor is cancelled during sinusoidal en bloc rotation and the question arises of how the brain can generate the signal $\dot{H}_p''$ in such cases. It has already been pointed out that the vor is not cancelled for unpredictable head movements so that the essential point would seem to be that for passive, sinusoidal rotations the head velocity is predictable. Thus, we must conclude that predictability is the key for generating $\dot{H}_p''$ just as in the case of planned, active head movements.

Prediction is well known in the smooth pursuit system; in the frequency range 0.5 - 2.0 Hz it raises the gain and decreases the phase lag well below the value that is caused by the 130 msec delay when an unpredictable target is tracked.

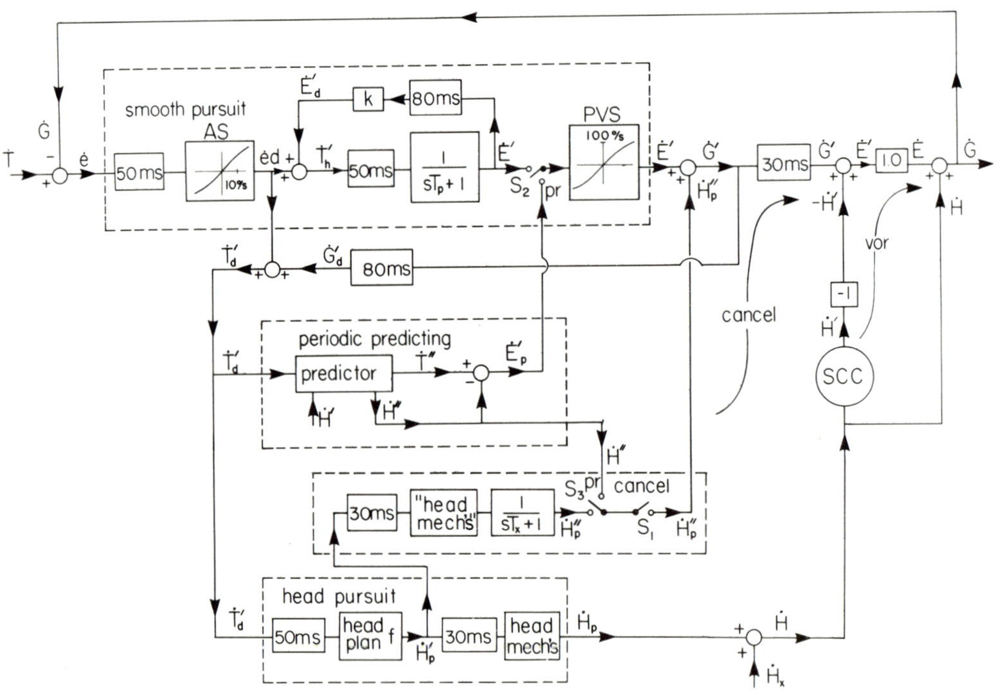

Fig. 2. A model of gaze tracking. Delays are indicated in boxes by the number of ms; AS, an acceleration saturation; $\dot{e}_d$, delayed retinal slip; $\dot{E}_d'$, delayed pursuit command; $\dot{T}_h'$, estimate of target velocity with respect to head; PVS, pursuit velocity saturation; $\dot{T}_d'$, delayed estimate of target velocity in space; $\dot{T}''$ and $\dot{H}''$, predicted estimates of $\dot{T}$ and $\dot{H}$; $\dot{E}_p'$, predictive command for pursuit; S_1, S_2, S_3, switches that reflect an intent to cancel (S_1) or follow predictable, periodic target motions (S_2, S_3 in position pr). Other symbols are as in Fig. 1.

There exist no good models of prediction but it is generally assumed that a prediction mechanism uses the history of a stimulus to predict its future behavior. An obvious example of the use of such an internal clock is group singing and dancing. The predictor generates a signal advanced in time and motor mechanisms are driven by it rather than those provided by vision so that the normal delay of 130 msec is by-passed and the eye no longer lags the target. Lisberger and co-workers (1981) have shown that prediction also occurs during cancellation; the phase lag at, say, 1.0 Hz is substantially less than what would occur otherwise with a 130 msec delay. Thus, we may conclude that the predictor provides a signal for both pursuit and cancellation and this explains why, as cited in item 8 above, pursuit and cancellation deteriorate in the same way in this frequency range since, in either case, such behavior simply reveals the high-frequency properties of the predictor and its inputs.

The predictor in Fig. 2 receives the delayed signal $\dot{T}_d'$, advances it in time by 80 msec (if it is periodic) and produces predicted (anticipated) target motion $\dot{T}''$. Normally, there are two cases: the head is stationary in which case $\dot{T}''$ becomes the command $\dot{E}_p'$ for predictive smooth pursuit, or the subject is rotated <u>en bloc</u> in which case $\dot{T}''$ is identical to predicted head velocity $\dot{H}''$. In case $\dot{H}_x$ and $\dot{T}$ are periodic but not equal, Fig. 2 shows the predictor generating $\dot{T}''$ and $\dot{H}''$ independently (which is why it also receives the canal signal $\dot{H}'$). This would necessitate subtracting $\dot{H}''$ from $\dot{T}''$ to form the predictive command $\dot{E}_p'$ for the pursuit system. Switches S_2 and S_3 are in the predict (pr) setting and S_1 is closed by the intent to cancel. $\dot{H}''$ is now added in to the gaze velocity command $\dot{G}'$ and that will cancel the vor.

The model was simulated on a digital computer to ensure self-consistency and stability. For this purpose the gain of the SCC was 1.0 (correct for frequencies above about 0.1 Hz). The transfer function of head mech's was $1/(sT_h + 1)$. The gain f of head plan was either 0.0 or 1.0 depending on the conditions simulated; the predictor phase-advanced sinusoids by 80 msec; T_p was 40 msec; T_h was 80 msec; T_x was 150 msec; k was 0.9; PVS had a gain of 1.0 at the origin and saturated at $\pm$ 100 deg/sec; AS had a gain of 1.0 at the origin and began to saturate at a value of $\dot{e}$ of 10 deg/sec. This corresponds to an acceleration command of 100 deg/sec^2 considering the gain of 10 created by the positive feedback loop $\dot{E}_d'$. This value is taken from the data of Lisberger and co-workers (1981) for unpredictable target motion.

MODEL BEHAVIOR

The model was used to investigate the problems mentioned at the start by number:

1. In the dark, $\dot{e}_d'$ is missing and in cats and monkey the vor is unimpeded; its gain is about 0.9. In man, for sinusoidal stimuli ($\dot{H}_x$), the vor gain is, oddly, about 0.65 in the dark with mental arithmetic, but rises to 1.0 or falls to 0.35 with the attempt to look at a stationary or moving, imagined target or sound source. It is tempting to speculate that in man, the switch S_1 is not necessarily open or closed but can transmit with gains intermediate between 0.0 and 1.0. Thus, the seemingly irrelevant gain of 0.65 during mental arithmetic may be due to a default, fractional transmission through S_1 in this state that is peculiar to man; a transmission that can be altered by mental effort to 0.0 (so the vor gain is 1.0) when imagining a stationary target, or to 0.65 (so the vor gain is 0.35) when imagining a target moving with the head.

2. The nonlinearity PVS in Fig. 2 allows the pursuit system to saturate at a velocity lower than that of cancellation as observed in cat and monkey (for the vertical system). In humans the limit of pursuit is around 100 deg/sec but the

limit of gaze velocity with head tracking, either horizontally or vertically, remains to be measured. It would not be too surprising if no difference were found since such a fast pursuit system is adequate for most naturally moving targets; the difference becomes more apparent in animals (or perhaps patients) where pursuit itself is rather poor.

3. The failure of the behavior of cells in the vestibular nucleus to obey superposition (cancellation is not the sum of pursuit and the vor) demands the existence of a switch so that the circuit extant during cancellation is not that which mediates pursuit and the vor. The switch S_1 provides this requirement (switches S_2 and S_3 merely choose the sources of command). We cannot say how this switch determines individual cell behavior because we do not know how the signals in Fig. 2 are organized at a cellular level. There is one obvious exception cited by Tomlinson and Robinson (1981): a cell which modulated with E and $\dot{E}$ during pursuit modulated not at all for cancellation during en bloc sinusoidal oscillation. This behavior would be consistent with any cell in the smooth pursuit compartment in Fig. 2. For other cells such as oculomotor-vestibular cells (ibid), details remain unknown but switch S_1 provides an ingredient without which their behavior cannot be explained.

4. Since a torsional pursuit system does not exist, much of the diagram in Fig. 2 does not pertain. Presumably this unusual system can open S_1 (normal torsional vor) or close it (cancellation) during predictable head rotations depending on intention.

5. The behavior of the patient with one immobile eye may be explained by the cancel switch S_1. With vision in the immobile eye during sinusoidal en bloc rotation with $\dot{T}$ equal to $\dot{H}$, $\dot{e}_d$ equals zero. Without strong encouragement to pursue the target, S_1 is left open and a normal vor is seen in the mobile eye under cover. With strong encouragement, the subject, who has an adequate $\dot{H}''$ signal, elects to track, closes S_1, and cancels his vor. This is strong evidence that the position of S_1 represents an internal decision; a decision that can be made more certainly with vision than without it.

6. Lesions involving switch S_1 or $\dot{H}_p''$ will permit pursuit without cancellation. Lesions involving $\dot{E}'$ or $\dot{T}_h'$ will permit cancellation without pursuit. Thus, it is possible to have a lesion that affects one but not the other activity. It might seem odd that a lesion could interfere with cancellation but not pursuit (Dell'Osso and co-workers, 1981) since pursuit ($\dot{E}'$), if available, should be able to counteract $\dot{H}'$ even if $\dot{H}_p''$ is not available to help. But if one tests cancellation above 60 deg/sec (one rotation in six sec) it may appear that cancellation (above 60 deg/sec) is deficient, while pursuit (below 60 deg/sec) is intact. Thus, careful quantitation is needed. The problem remains unexplored, quantitatively, in the clinic.

7. It is very common that lesions that degrade pursuit also degrade cancellation. One should recognize, however, that both activities share elements not shown in Fig. 2. To pursue anything with eye or head, a target must be identified and its retinal slip $\dot{e}$, and no other, must be admitted to the mechanisms in Fig. 2. Should anything go wrong with such an ability both pursuit and cancellation would suffer equally. Thus, it is not surprising that both activities are equally affected by many lesions such as those of the cerebral cortex (Troost and co-workers, 1972). Lesions of the flocculus, which also affect pursuit and cancellation equally (Zee and co-workers, 1981), may involve the premotor addition of the signals $\dot{E}'$, $\dot{H}_p''$ to form $\dot{G}'$ in Fig. 2.

8. The similarity of the high-frequency, sinusoidal behavior of cancellation and pursuit is readily explained by the fact both are determined by the properties

of the predictor and its inputs. The predictor must use the signal $\dot{e}_d$ to detect errors between $\dot{G}$ and $\dot{T}$ whether the head is moving or not. If $\dot{e}$ is underestimated by the acceleration saturation AS, $\dot{T}_d'$ will also be underestimated and tracking will become poor whether it is done by pursuit or cancellation.

9. In addition to the points mentioned earlier, the model also provides an explanation for a phenomenon observed by Lanman, Bizzi, and Allum (1978). They found that for several days to months after bilateral vestibulectomy, monkeys tracked targets with a free head with gaze velocities that were larger than target velocities. The model suggests that if the monkeys attempted to cancel their vor, but there was no vor to cancel, the unopposed cancel signal would drive the eyes at too high a velocity. Specifically in Fig. 2, $\dot{G}$ is the sum of $\dot{H}$, $-\dot{H}'$ and $\dot{H}_p''$. Normally the first two terms cancel out but if $-\dot{H}'$ is missing, $\dot{G}$ will be the sum of $\dot{H}$ and $\dot{H}_p''$ which will be approximately twice target velocity thus accounting for the observed gaze overshoots. Presumably the monkeys eventually learned not to try to cancel.

The model in Fig. 2 raises more questions than it answers and is intended mainly to provoke thought and examination, especially in the clinic. If the basic idea is correct then it is important to try to associate various lesions with quantitated differences and similarities of pursuit and cancellation to see if a clinical test can be devised that would have value in localizing lesions. Possible differences in cancellation between planned and predictable head movements (head free or forced) should also be examined. A problem of nomenclature arises: should one speak of a cancellation system to call attention to its separate neural pathways? I believe so. The entire system in Fig. 2 could be called a gaze pursuit system or eye-head pursuit system. If head movements are not employed, a subsystem conventionally called the smooth pursuit system does the work. When head movements are employed, the smooth pursuit and head pursuit systems both act. Because the vor is also inadvertently activated, the cancellation subsystem is switched in to increase the range and accuracy of gaze pursuit. While cancellation is only a part of a larger oculomotor subsystem, its contribution to gaze pursuit is important and it would seem helpful to recognize it with a separate nomenclature.

ACKNOWLEDGEMENT

I thank J.L. Gordon and H.P. Goldstein for programming and assistance in testing the model. This research was supported by grants EY00598 and EY01765 of the National Eye Institute, The National Institutes of Health of the US Public Health Service.

STRABISMUS AND RELATED DISORDERS

SECTION I

Coordinator: A. B. Scott

EYE MUSCLE STRUCTURE AND FUNCTION

MORPHOLOGICAL VARIATION ALONG MULTIPLY INNERVATED FIBERS OF RAT EXTRAOCULAR MUSCLES

J. DAVIDOWITZ, D. J. CHIARANDINI, G. PHILIPS and G. M. BREININ

Department of Ophthalmology, New York University Medical Center, New York, N.Y. 10016, USA

ABSTRACT

The orbital surface layer of rat inferior rectus muscle was analyzed in serial sections. Fibers of very small diameter (5-7 µm) were found to be multiply innervated fibers (MIFs). They had a prominent endplate-like neuromuscular junction toward the middle of their length and small, superficial junctions elsewhere. The diameter of such MIFs typically increased toward both ends. Sequential sampling by electronmicroscopy of 20 such MIFs reveals consistent patterns of morphological variation. Toward the middle of their length, a well developed sarcoplasmic reticulum (SR) delineates small, distinct myofibrils. Away from that fiber region, the SR gradually decreases and the myofibrils gradually increase in size. Toward both ends, the SR is very poorly developed and the myofibrils are large and/or indistinctly delineated. Mitochondrial content is moderate toward the middle of the fiber and decreases toward both ends. These findings would suggest caution in the assigning of fixed structural profiles to the fiber types of EOM.

KEYWORDS

Extraocular muscle; multiply innervated fibers; rat; sarcoplasmic reticulum; mitochondria; fiber diameter; morphological variation.

INTRODUCTION

As was noted in a recent review of the literature on extraocular muscles (EOM) (Chiarandini and Davidowitz, 1979), the morphology of multiply innervated fibers (MIFs) in these muscles is not as yet clearly established. There is general agreement as to the morphology of one type of MIF that is readily identified in the global region of EOM; these fibers have a poorly developed sarcoplasmic reticulum (SR), large or indistinctly delineated myofibrils, and a low mitochondrial content. There is considerable disagreement among authors, however, with regard to MIFs which occur in the orbital surface layer (OSL) of EOM. Descriptions of the SR range from sparse to moderately developed, and the myofibrils are variously described as being small, medium, large, and indistinct. Descriptions of mitochondrial content range from small to large, and fiber diameters ascribed to these MIFs range from very small to medium size.

When we first began to look at the OSL in rabbit superior rectus we encountered much more variability of fiber structure than could be accounted for by a reasonable number of fiber types. In the attempt to make sense of such excessive variability, we analyzed that muscle layer in serial sections, whereby individual muscle fibers could be reconstructed and sequentially sampled along their length. By means of such serial analysis, it was found that the major population of MIFs in our sample of the OSL displays systematic variation of its morphology along the fiber length, in terms of SR development, myofibrillar size and delineation, mitochondrial content, fiber diameter, and characteristics of the neuromuscular junctions (Davidowitz, Philips and Breinin, 1977, 1980).

We are presently studying the orbital surface layer of rat inferior rectus by means of serial analysis, and have found that rat EOM also contains orbital MIFs that display marked systematic variation of their morphology along the fiber length. These findings were recently reported in abstract form (Davidowitz and co-workers, 1981) and will be described in further detail in this presentation.

METHODS

A white Wistar rat (175 g) was perfused through the heart with 2% glutaraldehyde - 2% paraformaldehyde in phosphate buffer. The inferior rectus was removed intact, fixed in 4% glutaraldehyde, postfixed in 1% osmium tetroxide, dehydrated in graded ethanols, and embedded whole in Epon 812. The muscle was serially thick sectioned at 15 μm in the transverse plane of the muscle fibers. Periodic 15 μm sections were recut for 1 μm and ultrathin sections. The OSL was photographed at 45 μm intervals thereby permitting individual muscle fibers to be followed and reconstructed. The multiple innervation of MIFs was detected by light and electronmicroscopy.

Our objective was to determine whether rat EOM contains orbital MIFs of varying morphology, such as we had seen in rabbit EOM. Among the characteristic features of those MIFs in rabbit EOM are their very small diameter (about 5 μm) toward the middle of the muscle's length, and the presence of prominent neuromuscular junctions within the orbital endplate band. Many fibers with these characteristics were found in the OSL of this rat muscle; these fibers were followed distally and proximally, and were verified to be multiply innervated. The ultrastructure of the 20 longest of these orbital MIFs was sequentially sampled at 62 locations along the OSL. These fibers terminate within the distal 600 μm of the OSL. The overall length of the OSL is about 6.5 mm and all but the proximal 700 μm has been serially analyzed thus far.

RESULTS

Fiber Diameter

The OSL displays a distinct endplate band which is mostly concentrated within the proximal second quarter of the OSL's length. In this region, the majority of orbital fibers are of about 15-20 μm in diameter; these largest diameter fibers had been identified as SIFs by Mayr (1971). Dispersed within this layer are fibers of very small diameter (5-7 μm) which account for about 20% of the OSL fibers (Figs. 1-3). These tiny orbital fibers had been identified as MIFs by Mayr (1971), and this was confirmed by us. The diameter of these MIFs increases to 9-15 μm within the distal 1.0-1.5 mm of their length, in most cases; however, a third of these fibers maintain an essentially constant diameter of about 6-8 μm. Proximally, most of these MIFs increase to a diameter of 8-10 μm, within about 1 mm of the OSL's origin.

Neuromuscular Junctions

Within the endplate band, prominent neuromuscular junctions were frequently seen on the orbital MIFs of very small diameter. In many cases these neuromuscular junctions display: (a) terminal axons lying within scalloped depressions of the sarcolemma, (b) postjunctional foldings which may become moderately developed, (c) subsarcolemmal clusterings of mitochondria, (d) junctional sarcoplasm containing numerous ribosomes, and (e) a soleplate nucleus. However, there is much variability with respect to the presence of these components in the junctions, both among fibers and in sequential samplings of the same junctions (Figs. 4-6). Distal and proximal of the endplate band region, these orbital MIFs have neuromuscular junctions which are characteristically smaller and more superficial.

Variation of the Ultrastructure

The most striking result of this study was the finding that along their length the orbital MIFs consistently display marked variations in the development of the SR and in the size and delineation of the myofibrils. In the proximal second quarter of these fibers, i.e. in the region of the OSL's endplate band, the SR is well developed in the I-band where it delineates small distinct myofibrils which are typically 0.15-0.2 μm in width (Fig. 9). This region of small fibrils is typically about 1.5-2.5 mm long. The A-band is virtually devoid of SR along the fiber length (Fig. 10).

Proximal and distal of the region of small myofibrils, there is a gradual transition to a moderate SR development and an associated increase in myofibrillar size. In the distal direction, the increased myofibrillar size typically stabilizes at about 0.3-0.4 mm width, for a distance of about 1.0-2.0 mm (Figs. 8, 11, 12). Yet further proximally and distally, the SR gradually becomes very poorly developed, and the myofibrils become large and/or indistinctly delineated, i.e. afibrillar (Figs. 7, 13, 14). Distally, this afibrillar segment typically extends for about 0.5-1.0 mm, depending on how far the fiber extends before its termination.

Mitochondrial content is highest in the fiber segment of small myofibrils, and subsarcolemmal clusterings of mitochondria are also often seen in association with the prominent neuromuscular junctions which occur in this region. The proximal and distal afibrillar fiber segments have the lowest mitochondrial content, such reduction occurring most notably in the A-band.

Glycogen content is highest in the fiber segment of small myofibrils. Reduction of glycogen content does not occur to the same degree in the proximal and distal directions. The proximal afibrillar segment retains substantial amounts of glycogen which often appear among the filaments of the I-band. Glycogen content is very sparse, however, in the distal afibrillar segment.

There is no apparent relationship between the variations of ultrastructure and the variations in fiber diameter. Both proximally and distally, comparable transformation to afibrillar morphology occur in all these MIFs, irrespective of whether, or to what degree, they increase in diameter.

DISCUSSION

In a previous study of fiber types in rat extraocular muscle, Mayr (1971) noted that MIFs in the orbital layer tend to be extremely small in diameter and he described such orbital MIFs as having a sparse SR which poorly separates medium myofibrils. While that morphological description would be appropriate for some portions of the MIFs that were serially analyzed in this study, that description would not be consistent with our observation of a well developed SR and quite small myofibrillar width which characterizes our MIF sample in their proximal second quarter.

Teräväinen (1968) studied the neuromuscular junctions in rat EOM and noted that both larger and smaller types of junctions may occur on the same MIF. Our data are in agreement with that finding. Teräväinen (1968) raised the possibility that the largest type of junction on MIFs may be endplates, as such. Our observations regarding prominent junctions on MIFs would be consistent with that possibility.

The morphological variations seen along orbital MIFs in this study are similar in many respects to the variations previously seen along orbital MIFs of very small diameter in rabbit EOM (Davidowitz, Philips, and Breinin; 1977, 1980), though there are differences as well. Those differences include the following. (a) In association with a prominent neuromuscular junction, the rabbit MIFs display a relatively higher localized increase of mitochondrial content within the A-band and I-band, independently of subsarcolemmal mitochondrial clusterings. (b) In the fiber segment of very small fibrils, the rat MIFs typically display a more fully developed SR in the I-band than rabbit MIFs. (c) Distal of the fiber segment of very small myofibrils, the rat MIFs typically exhibit a protracted fiber segment of medium width myofibrils. A comparable fiber segment was not seen in the rabbit MIFs. (d) In rabbit MIFs the changes in organelle content do not occur at the same fiber locations in the distal region of transition to afibrillar morphology, i.e. the reduction in mitochondrial content is completed about 3 mm proximal of where the decrease in SR development is completed. Such displacement of organelle modification is not clearly evident in the much shorter rat MIFs. (e) The rabbit MIFs show a consistent marked diameter increase, from about 5 μm to about 15 μm, toward both their proximal and distal ends: in the rat MIFs, the diameter increase occurs less consistently and to a smaller degree. (f) In rabbit MIFs, the distal fiber portion contains many membrane-glycogen complexes: such complexes were not seen in the rat MIFs.

Most of the literature on EOM fiber types has been based on the tacit assumption that the structure of a given fiber is essentially constant along its length. The above noted findings indicate that such an assumption is not tenable for at least one population of orbital MIFs in rat and rabbit EOM. Depending on where those fibers are sampled they might appear to be of quite different fiber types. It is conceivable that such sampling problems might in part be related to some of the disagreements among various descriptions of orbital MIFs.

Morphological variability along the fiber length is not confined to MIFs. Recent quantitative analysis of orbital SIFs in rabbit indicates that there is a decrease of mitochondrial content and an increase of myofibrillar size about 2-3 mm away from the endplate (J. Davidowitz, unpublished results) as has been suggested earlier (Davidowitz, Philips and Breinin, 1977). Preliminary findings suggest that analogous changes also occur in orbital SIFs of rat EOM, as well. The above findings of morphological variation along orbital MIFs and SIFs suggest that caution is called for in the sampling of EOM and in the assigning of fixed structural profiles to the fiber types of EOM.

It has been suggested that the orbital layer contains MIFs which are twitch fibers capable of conducting an action potential (Bach-y-Rita and Ito, 1966b;Lennerstrand, 1974). In the orbital MIFs described in this study, as well as in the orbital MIFs previously described in rabbit, the SR development and myofibrillar organization does indeed appear to be twitch-like within the portion of the fiber associated with the orbital endplate band. The presence of prominent endplate-like neuromuscular junctions on these MIFs, within the endplate band, would also be compatible

FIGURE LEGENDS

Figs. 1 and 2. Two 1 μm sections through the same group of OSL fibers separated by 2.9 mm. Fig. 1 is within the orbital endplate band. Most of the fibers are of about 15 μm diameter, and many fibers of about 5 μm diameter are seen as well. Four of these tiny fibers (1-4) are among those which were sequentially sampled in this study. Fig. 2: In the OSL's distal fourth, where cells 1-3 increase in diameter by a factor of two or more. Cell 4, however, retains an essentially constant diameter. Scale marker is 10 μm.

Fig. 3. Survey EM at endplate band. The very small diameter fibers (5, 6) are among the MIFs analyzed in this study. Note that the myofibrillar size in these MIFs is similar to that in the largest diameter fibers. Neuromuscular junction on cell 5 is shown in Fig. 4 (X 2,400).

Figs. 4-6. Prominent neuromuscular junctions on orbital MIFs of very small diameter, within the orbital endplate band. Fig. 4: This junction shows significant amounts of postjunctional folding, though the junction is flatly apposed to the fiber surface(X 12,000). Fig. 5: Six branches of the terminal axon in contact with the muscle fiber. Three terminals lie within scalloped depressions of the sarcolemma, but postjunctional folding is negligible. There is an elaboration of junctional sarcoplasm containing numerous ribosomes, and some mitochondrial clustering (X 7,200). Fig. 6: This junction shows much mitochondrial clustering, and considerable amounts of junctional sarcoplasm containing numerous ribosomes (X 12,000).

Figs. 7-14. Sequential samples through one of the orbital MIFs of very small diameter. The prominent neuromuscular junction of this MIF is shown in Fig. 6. The fiber structure associated with that prominent junction is seen in Figs. 9 and 10. Figs. 11, 12, 13 and 14 are respectively 1440, 2085, 2655 and 2835 μm distal of Figs. 9 and 10. Figs. 8 and 7, respectively, are 885 and 1485 μm proximal of Figs. 9 and 10. The magnification in all these figures is 12,000. Fig. 7: In the proximal fourth, the SR is very poorly developed and the myofibrils are large or indistinct, i.e. afibrillar. Mitochondrial profiles are small and sparse, particularly in the A-band. Glycogen content is moderate. Fig. 8: Distal of the afibrillar segment, the SR development increases and delineates myofibrils of medium width. Fig. 9: Plane of section within the I-band, at the prominent neuromuscular munction. For a distance of about 1.8 mm, centered about the prominent neuromuscular junction, this MIF displays small myofibrils (0.15-0.2 μm wide). These myofibrils are distinctly delineated by a well developed SR. The content of mitochondria and glycogen is highest here. Fig. 10: Plane of section within the A-band, at the prominent neuromuscular junction. In the A-band, SR profiles are extremely sparse, so that no myofibrillar organization is evident. This virtual absence of SR in the A-band occurs along the entire length of these MIFs. Figs. 11 and 12: Within the third quarter, SR development decreases and myofibrillar size gradually increases to a medium width of about 0.3-0.4 μm. This myofibrillar size continues in an essentially constant manner for about 1.0 mm in this fiber. These two figures, spaced 645 μm apart, bracket the middle of this region. Figs. 13 and 14: Distal of the region of medium fibrils the SR development gradually decreases to a very low level and the myofibrils become large or indistinct. This afibrillar morphology continues in an essentially constant manner for about 0.8 mm in this fiber. The mitochondrial content is reduced here, and glycogen is very sparse. These two figures, spaced 180 μm apart, are near the middle of this segment.

with the notion that these MIFs are capable of conducting an action potential. As to the functional significance, if any, of the afibrillar portions of these MIFs, that remains a puzzle.

ACKNOWLEDGMENTS

This study has been supported by USPHS grants EY-00309 and EY-01297 and,partially, by funds from the Eye Surgical Fund, Inc. and Research to Prevent Blindness, Inc.

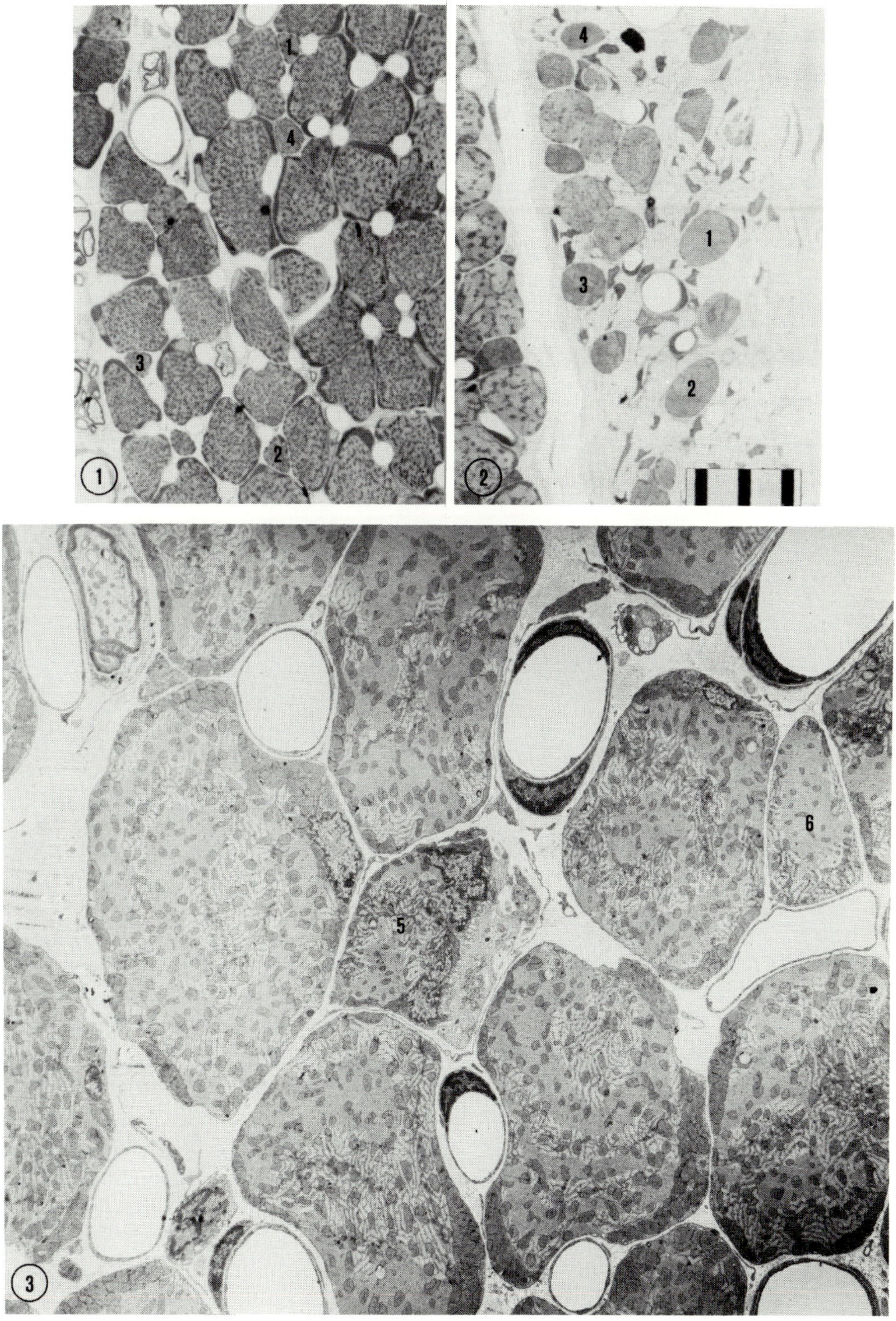
1
4
3
2
1
4
1
3
2
2
5
6
3

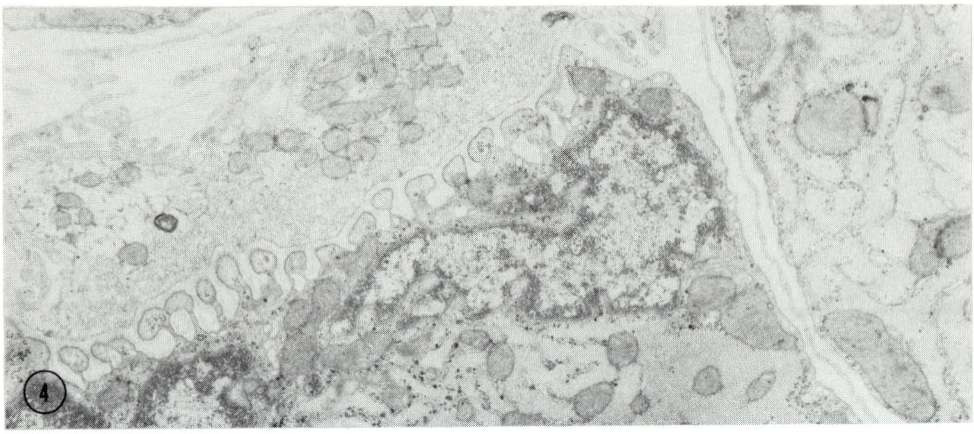

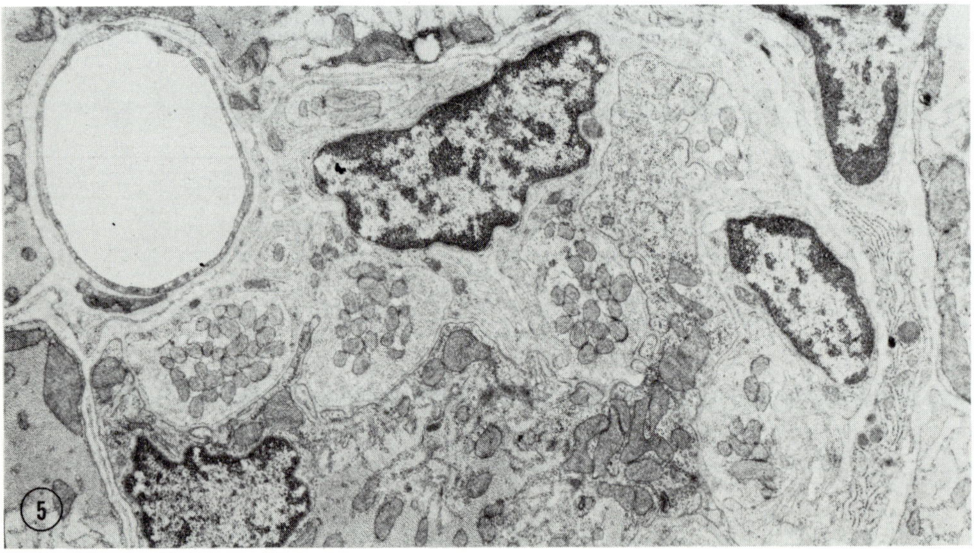

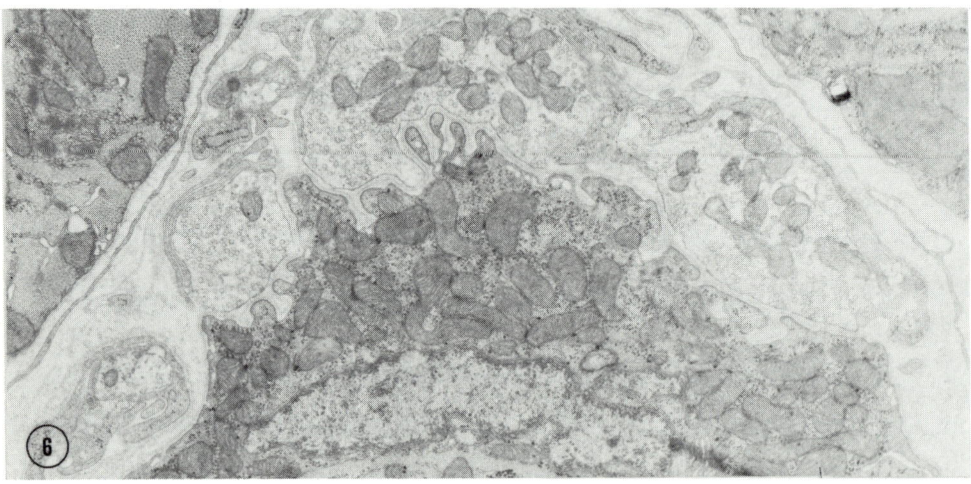

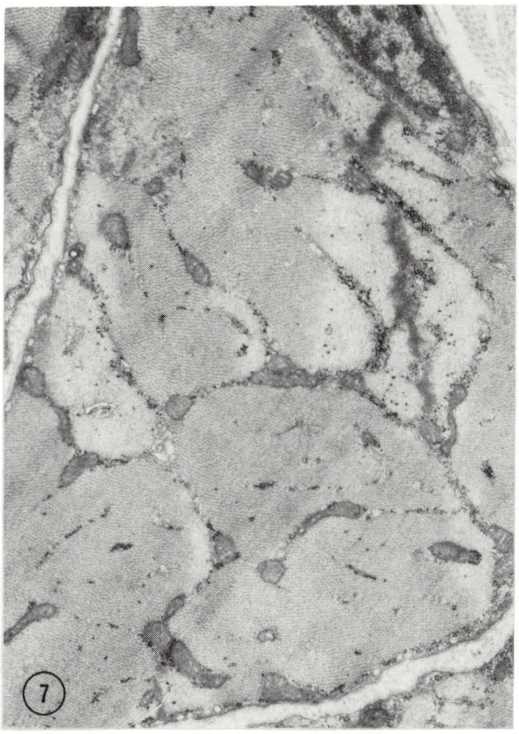
7

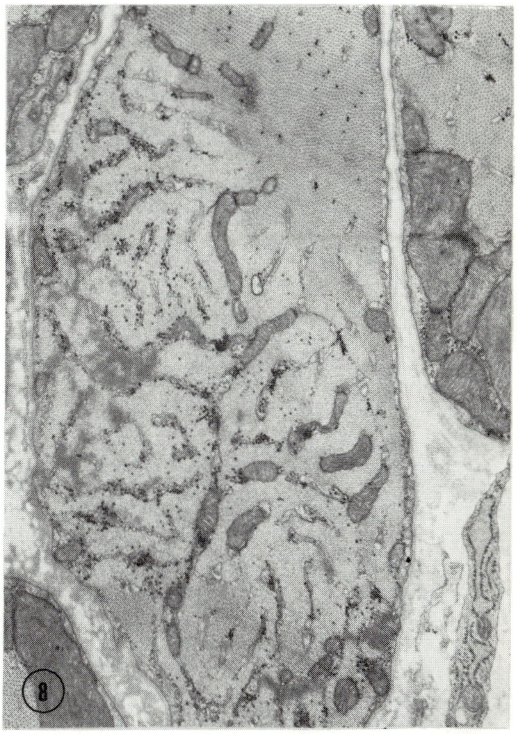
8

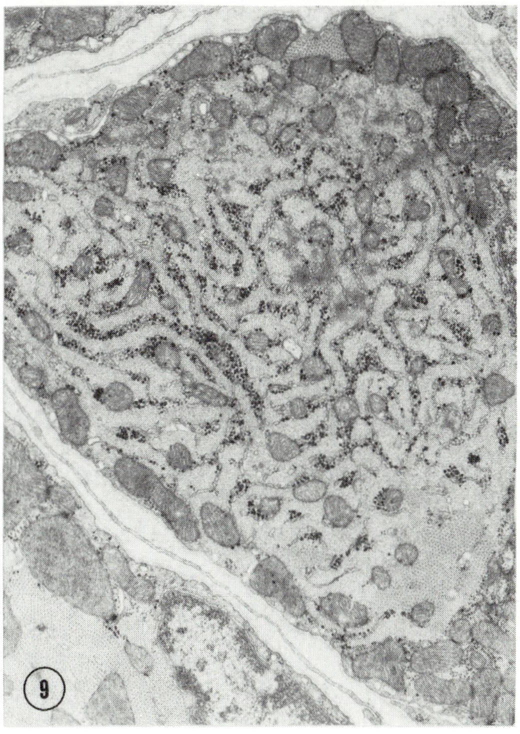
9

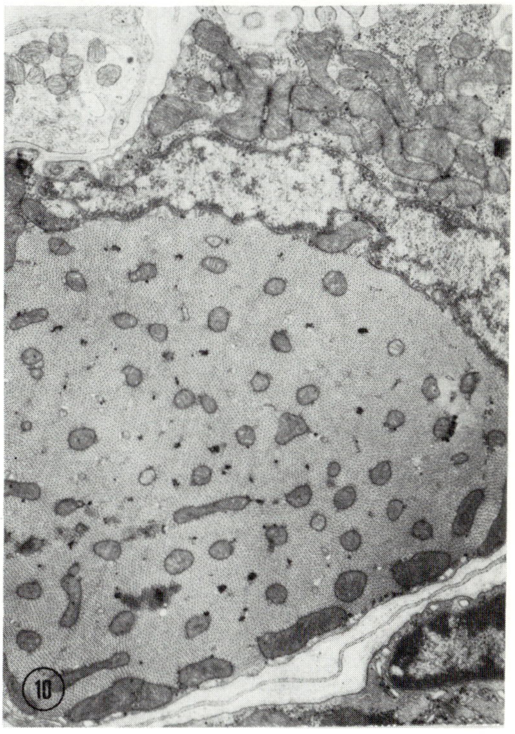
10

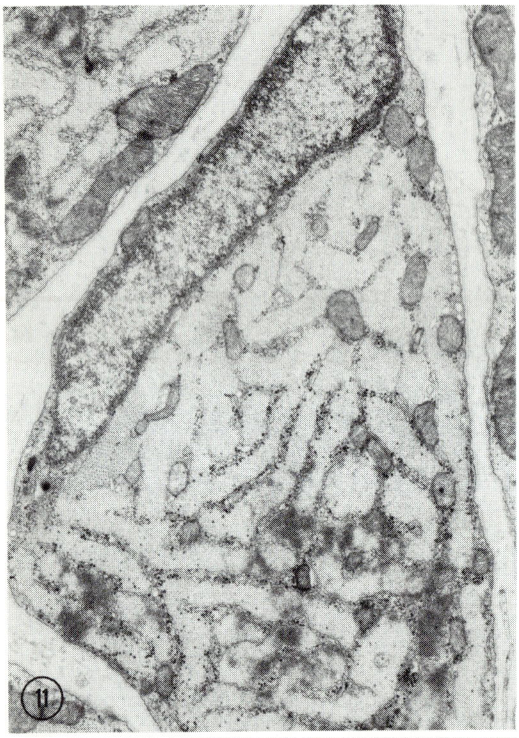
11

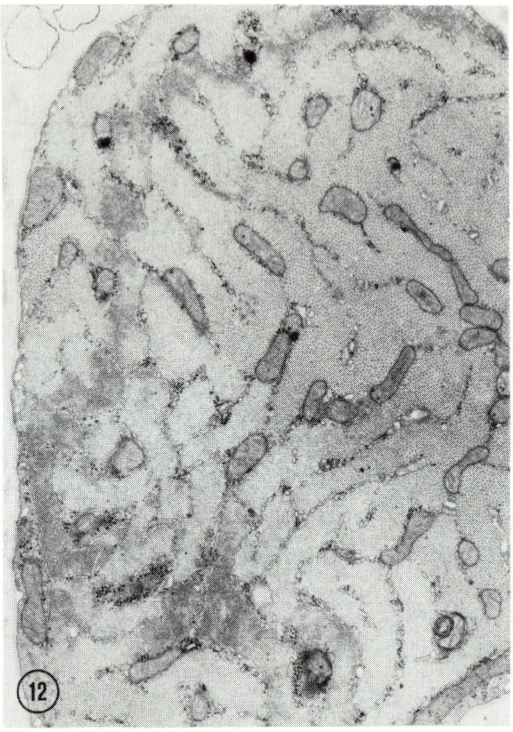
12

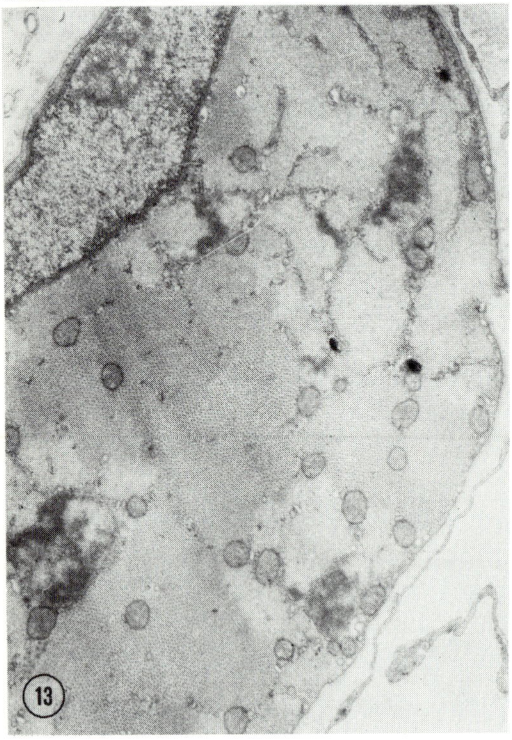
13

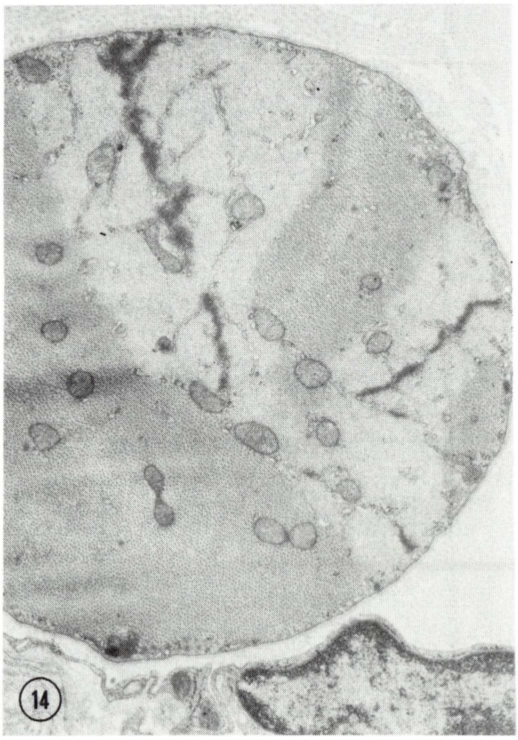
14

THE HISTOPATHOLOGY OF HUMAN STRABISMIC EXTRAOCULAR MUSCLE

K. W. MCNEER* and R. F. SPENCER**

*Departmer.t of Ophthalmology, Medical College of Virginia, Richmond, Virginia, USA
**Department of Anatomy, Medical College of Virginia, Richmond, Virginia, USA

ABSTRACT

There have been many investigations, both basic and clinical relating to histology and histopathology of extraocular muscle. Most of the investigations have been carried out in sub-human species so that anatomical definition, particularly fiber classification, has been based primarily on non-human sources and relied on the criteria established from human and non-human skeletal muscles sources. The definition of normal human extraocular muscle anatomy has suffered accordingly although the extrapolation of non-human to human data has merit. It is therefore difficult to examine specimens of human extraocular muscle and define minimal clinical conditions such as strabismus. Accordingly, human extraocular muscle specimens from both normal and strabismic patients have been examined with a view towards defining normal and abnormal microscopic anatomy. The fundamental alteration in strabismic patients appears to occur in the global layer, slow fiber system and it consists of dense, central mitochondrial accumulation in these fibers.

KEYWORDS

Histology; histopathology; strabismus; human extraocular muscle; central mitochondrial accumulation (coring).

INTRODUCTION

The fundamental histopathologic alteration in human strabismic muscle has not yet been defined. Moreover, anatomic definition of fiber types has never been clear in the human extraocular muscle (EOM). The need to clarify these issues stems from the absence of an adequate frame of reference to separate normal human EOM from strabismic human EOM histopathologically. There have been many investigations into mammalian and other extraocular muscle, though most have been done in sub-human species (Bach-y-rita and colleagues, 1971, 1975; Lennerstrand, 1975) and major contributors have relied on extrapolating lower animal data to human EOM muscle for interpretation.

Electrophysiologists (Breinin, 1971) have demonstrated twitch (presumably fast fiber) and slow fiber response using intracellular electrodes in individual cat lateral recti fibers, activated by electrical stimulation from the abducens nucleus.

Collins (1975) has recorded similar fast and slow fiber response from human EOM using an ingenious electrode inserted into the muscle, but, of course, not employing abducens nucleus stimulation. Yet in only rare instances has the specific fiber being monitored electrophysiologically been removed and examined histologically, (Ozawa, 1969; Bach-y-rita, 1975) and then only in sub-human species.

Data from lower animals indicates two or more fiber types electrophysiologically and at least five anatomically. Moreover, the picture is clouded by an unmanageable variety of published histological muscle fiber classifications, leaving the reader confused upon comparing one paper to another. There is not general agreement among investigators regarding criteria for classifying EOM muscle fibers. Some have chosen fiber size coupled with elaborate anatomical (architectural) descriptions, usually based on randomly sampled portions of an EOM, whereas others have relied on granularity, striations, etc. The architectural and electrophysiologic reference points that serve so well to classify skeletal and other muscle types, are not applicable to EOM (Martinez, Hay, McNeer, 1976). In summary, a review of the literature published on human EOM reveals that:

(1) Histological classification systems of EOM fiber types are inadequate.
(2) There are different EOM fiber types identifiable histologically.
(3) Histologically identifiable fiber types are not fully correlated to electrophysiologically identifiable fiber types.
(4) The bulk of investigative work has been done in sub-human species.

Fiber Classification

The clinical observation of rapid saccadic eye movement and tonic vergence eye movement is quite enough evidence to suspect at least two muscle fiber types, though proving their existence presents problems. Examining human EOM sections permits the viewer to confirm the existence of large pale fibers (fast) and smaller red fibers (slow), plus intermediate zones. Pale fibers seen on histologic section are lighter because they contain less mitochondria. The slow, dark fibers contain more mitochondria and thus stain more intensely. Contraction velocity is inversely related to mitochondrial quantity. Enzyme studies of human EOM confirm slow, fast and also intermediate fiber types. The separation between small and large fiber so characteristic of lower animal EOM persists in the human, i.e., the small orbital fibers surround the larger global fibers proximally, become an incomplete or crescentic envelope at mid-muscle, and disappear at the tendon. There is also an intermediate or mixed zone giving origin to a poorly defined boundary dividing the large and small fibers.

Bormioli and co-workers (1979, 1980) offered conclusive proof that slow fibers (slow myosin) exist in human EOM. The authors' specific antisera immunofluorescence study on human EOM demonstrated the presence of "slow myosin" primarily in the orbital, but also in the global layer. It interested these writers that EOM were the only mammalian muscles containing slow tonic fibers with physiologic properties similar to amphibian slow fibers.

Many problems yet unsolved make it difficult to establish criteria for extrapolating animal EOM histology data to human EOM histology, but the idea is not without merit. Much support and correlation for classifying human EOM fibers derives from lower animal experiments. Basically, there are fast and slow fibers in all mammalian EOM and fiber identification in human EOM holds up upon comparing one slide to the next, but due to the many indirect comparisons between animal, human, skeletal, and eye muscle, the current classification is cumbersome and difficult to commit to memory.

Criteria for muscle classification include features of the following microscopic appearances (Spencer, 1981):

(1) The sarcoplasmic reticulum
(2) T tubules
(3) Size, distribution, and number of mitochondria

It would therefore seem desirable to develop a classification of human EOM using at least one, perhaps all, of these features. Moreover, while histochemistry yields much information about metabolic features of individual fibers, it cannot consistently provide rigorous criteria for fiber classification, particularly on the basis of fiber contractile properties; specifically, whether there are propogated action potentials or not. The distinctive architecture of the sarcoplasmic reticulum and the T-tubules has much value in distinguishing fiber types and has been used reliably for skeletal muscle and sub-human EOM fiber typing. It should be emphasized that in this study, the bulk of the human EOM data was derived from specimens that precluded a thorough evaluation of either and they were accordingly given less emphasis.

Other than electromyography and the work of Collins and Scott on force-length tension characteristics, there currently remains little published electrophysiological data on human EOM. It is easy to perceive the difficulty in reproducing many of the animal experiments with human EOM. Furthermore, the exact proven correlation between the fiber firing on the oscilloscope and that seen under the microscope, even in animal experiments, is missing. Uniform agreement on fiber classification suffers accordingly. It is therefore necessary to work within the confines of available information to characterize human EOM histopathology and thus currently forego a rigorous correlation to electrophysiological data. One salient electrophysiological contribution that deserves attention, however, is the division of labor concept in human EOM derived by Scott and Collins (1973) based on global and orbital EMG recordings. Their findings supported: "the notion that various histological muscle fiber types are functionally differentiated on the basis of the amount of work they do, rather than on the basis of the type of eye movement to which they contribute".

In effect, they suggested that various types of eye movements are not served by separate populations of muscle fibers, rather, there are outer (peripheral) fibers which are recruited early, turned off in extreme gaze, or large saccades, and maintain a steady, low level force for the primary position of gaze. There are deeper (global) fibers, recruited late, of high output, short duration firing during saccadic movement. In short: "The recorded individual motor units changed activity with the need for more or less action of that muscle, no matter what the type of movement.

Thus, significant electrophysiological data indicate a continuous spectrum of fiber activity, suited to demand, rather than a crisp separation into fast and slow fiber, though there appears to be a global-orbital gradient. Histological classifications should be accountable to this point.

Durston likely had the best idea regarding human histological fiber classification when he suggested that the architectural feature or granularity be the basis of distinguishing different fibers. The granular, coarse, and fine fibers owe their characteristic microscopic morphology to mitochondrial distribution. The distinction that makes Durston's classification so appealing is that his system is based on increasing mitochondrial accumulation. On cross section, the fine fiber, having very little mitochondria, shows a virtually uniform pattern of low contrast. The granular fiber appears to have discreet, almost dendritic arrangements of mitochondria resembling bone corpuscle pigmentation in the retina. The coarse fiber has dense accumulations of mitochondria clumped together. Moreover, the coarse fiber has a ring of mitochondrial accumulation about the periphery of the fiber. There appears to be functional organization in that the granular fibers occupy the global and the coarse fibers occupy the orbital layer. The fine fibers are distributed throughout the muscle. There are, of course, intermediate types. The distinction between coarse and granular fibers can be appreciated from the longitudinal section of the muscle. (Plate I). There can be found in coarse fibers mitochondrial accumulations peripherally oriented in a granular pattern. One need only look at the longitudinal section to confirm that the granular pattern is not the dominant feature, rather, there are large longitudinal accumulations of dense pigment coursing in a tube-like fashion, representing aggregates of dense mitochondria, although they might not extend the entire length of the fiber. (Plate I, A.B.)

There is some confusion created in the effort to accept Durston's system: the relationship of muscle fiber morphology to innervation pattern was apparently misinterpreted. Bormioli and colleagues suggested, following their human EOM experiments using slow myosin specific antisera, that Durston, and later Ringel, may have erred in identifying the coarse fiber as multiply innervated! They found the fine fiber to contain slow myosin and the coarse fiber to be multiply innervated. In addition, the fine fiber histochemistry matched that of multiply innervated fibers. Though a minor point, Durston's classification does not take into account the differences in granular fibers. There are light and dark matrix granular fibers, though the reason for this is yet unclear. There are also differences in the size and number of mitochondria, suggesting the intermediate type. (Plate II).

Perhaps the most significant question at this point is as follows: Why are the coarse and granular fibers so organized, complete with intermediate zone, as seen in the complete cross section of human EOM, when they both appear to be singly innervated by histological criteria? One can safely assume that adherents of the classical concept of slow-orbital, fast-global theories will quickly debate the question to conclusion, but such organization does favor the division of labor notion of Scott and Collins. Furthermore, the difference between coarse and granular fibers is sometimes morphologically obscure, suggesting a continuous broad spectrum of fast twitch fibers that, as a function of variations in sarcoplasmic reticulum plus size and number of mitochondria, may differ in the speed of action potential propogation and fatigue.

The organization of the central and peripheral fibers of the extraocular muscle has no corollary in the central nervous system organizational pattern. Moreover, the multiply innervated fine fibers are distributed throughout human EOM muscle and there is no apparent central counterpart to such peripheral organization. There is, however, suggestive organization in the monkey brain stem third nerve dorso medial nuclei. Those small motor neurons innervate the orbital fibers which act as slow fibers (Buttner-Ennever, Akert, 1981; Spencer, Porter, 1981).

Accumulated publications now point to the consistency of mitochondrial alteration, seen at the microscopic level, as the dominant feature of strabismic EOM. Such changes occur also in skeletal muscle pathogenesis. Sections from normal human EOM are not otherwise distinguished from strabismic human EOM under the microscope. There is increasing mitochondrial concentration in the center of the fiber, possibly to produce a more efficient way to utilize energy stores for aerobic metabolism. Perhaps the changes represent a stress response leading to increased utilization of aerobic pathways. Evidence from other histological studies show this type of mitochondrial alteration to be characteristic of muscles undergoing hypertrophy. The clinician's evaluation of EOM overaction is thus histopathologically confirmed as actual hypertrophy. There is also atrophy occurring simultaneously in affected muscles suggesting an active mechanism of breakdown and repair, though it is not yet possible to identify the hypertrophy or atrophy as primary or secondary and thus imply an etiology of strabismus.

Moreover, the affected fiber is the granular fiber which is the singly innervated, aerobic, fast twitch fiber, though it is likely premature to assume that strabismus is a problem confined to the fast twitch fiber system.

Histological Investigation

Since the mitochondrial changes were found originally in clinically overacting muscles (inferior obliques), it follows that the opposing or clinically underacting muscle should be examined to determine if there are corresponding structural alterations.

Pursuant to this thought, a series of biopsies were obtained by the author during routine strabismus surgery. Specimens were obtained using a 2mm Elliott trephine to produce a full thickness (i.e., extending from orbital to global layer) section of the muscle (Plate III). The trephine was applied to the center of the orbital surface several millimeters from the posterior limit of the tendon, and pressed through against a silicone plate. It should be emphasized that the specimens represented the distal segment of human EOM, primarily because of accessibility during routine strabismus operations. Examining distal human EOM specimens precludes a thorough look at nerve endings and the classical orbital-global fiber separation seen at mid-muscle. The excision of the small specimen had no visible effect on EOM function.

The specimens were immediately immersed in phosphate-buffered glutaraldehyde and later processed in the routine fashion (Spencer, McNeer, 1978). Para-phenylenediamine dye was used to stain the specimens because of its superior architectural definition of muscle fibers when examined by phase contrast microscopy.

Eighteen patients yielded a total of thirty-five specimens. There were ten matched specimens of medial and lateral recti of esotropic patients and one set from exotropic patients. Included also were seven clinically overacting medial recti from esotropia and one underacting medial rectus from exotropia. There were eight clinically overacting lateral recti specimens from exotropia and one lateral rectus specimen from double elevator palsy. Two superior rectus specimens from V-pattern esotropia. Finally, the medial and lateral rectus from a sixth nerve palsy were also examined.

The samples afforded the opportunity to examine both the overacting medial rectus and the underacting lateral rectus from the same globe in five esotropic patients. In one exotropic patient the specimens included the underacting medial rectus and the overacting lateral rectus from the same globe.

The global and orbital layer of each specimen was carefully examined for structural alteration under the light microscope. As previously discovered upon examining complete cross sections of clinically overacting inferior obliques, (Spencer, McNeer, 1978) the dominant feature was central mitochondrial accumulation in the granular fiber. (Plate IV). More importantly, the frequency of this finding was much increased in the overacting specimen when compared to the underacting specimen. The mitochondrial alteration was not appreciably different in the overacting medial rectus opposing a paretic lateral rectus (Sixth nerve palsy) when compared to the clinically overacting medial rectus of strabismus (esotropia). Thus, the medial rectus opposing a paralyzed lateral rectus did not differ histologically from a strabismic, clinically overacting medial rectus opposing its ipsilateral antagonist underacting lateral rectus. The medial rectus specimen was obtained six months after the paralysis, though possibly a longer duration would have produced more extensive changes. As expected, the lateral rectus (considered normal as it was not involved) from the double elevator palsy showed no changes.

Central mitochondrial aggregation was of such reliability that the examiner was able to distinguish the overacting specimen from the underacting specimen prior to being informed. The structural alterations were located primarily in the global layer and intermediate zone.

The clinicians' impression of EOM overaction can now be said to have histological support, although the clinically identified underacting muscle cannot yet be distinguished histologically from normal. It should be emphasized that normal human histology investigations have really just begun and more subtle distinctions may arise following future investigations. For the present, however, the characteristic histopathological change of strabismic human EOM is an increased incidence of central mitochondrial accumulation in the global, granular fibers of the overacting muscle. The histology presents other intriguing changes. There is evidence of atrophy and regeneration. Vacuolization and loss of tissue substance are evidence of atrophic change whereas activated satellite cells suggest a regenerative process. Perhaps breakdown and regeneration are a normal cycle of normal muscle and the process becomes accelerated with hypertrophy or increased demand. (Plates V, VI).

Finally, much remains to be done to complete the investigation of human EOM histology and EOM histopathology. The issues brought forth earlier will remain, in part, unanswered here, but there are several points that may be properly addressed again: (1) Normal human EOM histology remains incompletely defined, and human EOM differs appreciably from other mammalian EOM such that comparisons with subhuman species are difficult to make. Fiber classification in all EOM suffers from lack of agreement among investigators and lack of coordination with the electrophysiologists. (2) There are histopathologic changes separating strabismic human EOM from normal human EOM. Both normal and histopathological features of human EOM, furthermore, are quite different from human skeletal muscle, such that criteria used for skeletal muscle characterization cannot be applied to EOM.

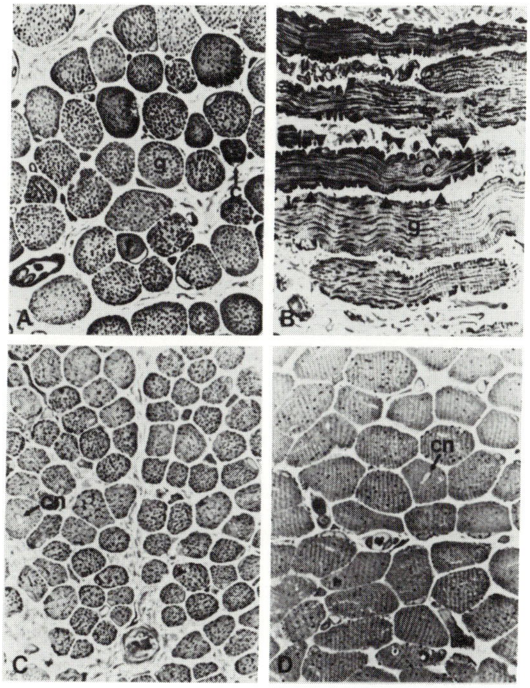

PLATE I

Human extraocular and skeletal muscle stained with paraphenylenediamine and photographed by phase contrast microscopy. A. Cross section of EOM showing coarse, granular, and fine fiber types. (g) granular. (c) coarse. (f) fine. B. EOM longitudinal section. (c) coarse. (g) granular. Arrows above and below coarse fiber delineate subsarcolemmal mitochondrial accumulations. C. EOM cross section. Note central nucleus (cn). D. Skeletal muscle cross section (Biceps). Note striations and absence of mitochondrial pattern seen in EOM plus uniform fiber size. Central nucleus (cn) is considered pathological feature of skeletal muscle, generally associated with muscular dystrophies.

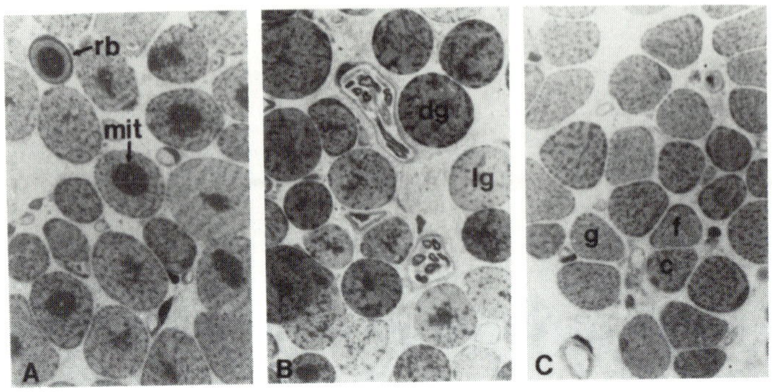

PLATE II

Human extraocular muscle stained with toluidine blue and photographed by brightfield microscopy.

A. Granular cells from global layer showing central mitochondrial accumulation (mit) and ringbinden (rb). The former is evidence of muscle hypertrophy and the latter results from myofibrillar break and contraction leaving an empty annulus within the fiber. It is thought to occur from stress.

B. Granular fibers from the global layer consisting of dark matrix (dg) and light matrix (lg) cells. Basically the same morphological cell type, most classifications have not taken this variance into consideration. Matrix density differences attributable to differences in packing density of myofibrils.

C. The three basic fiber types are illustrated: granular (g), coarse (c), and fine (f). The distinction is based on mitochondrial content and distribution. Coarse fibers have a dense peripheral ring plus large darkly stained clumps of mitochondria. The granular fiber has a peppering of discreet, darkly stained mitochondrial accumulations. The fine fiber is small in diameter and exhibits very little mitochondrial content.

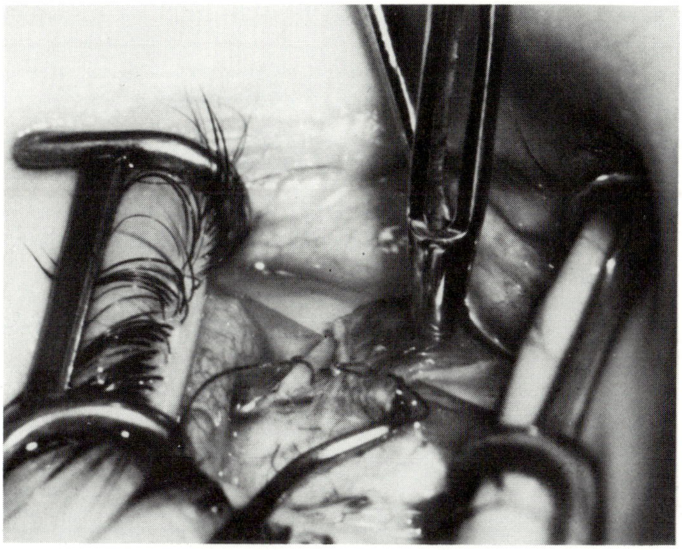

PLATE III

Specimen collection method for tissue used to evaluate mitochondrial alteration in clinically overacting and underacting human EOM. The trephine (t) is passed through the isolated muscle (mr: medial rectus) against a silicone block (s). A full thickness (global-orbital) button (arrow), 2mm in diameter, is obtained

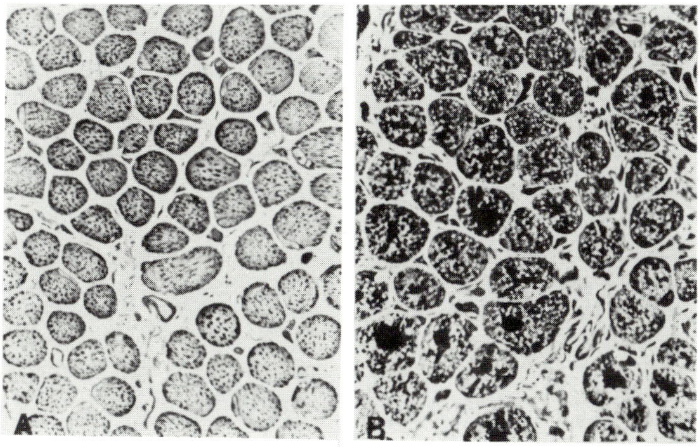

PLATE IV

Human EOM sections of lateral rectus (A) and medial rectus (B) from an esotropic patient. The lateral rectus section shows a group of predominantly granular fibers that are normal in appearance for human EOM. The medial rectus or clinically overacting muscle reveals a large number of fibers with central mitochondrial accumulation and vacuolization indicative of hypertrophy.

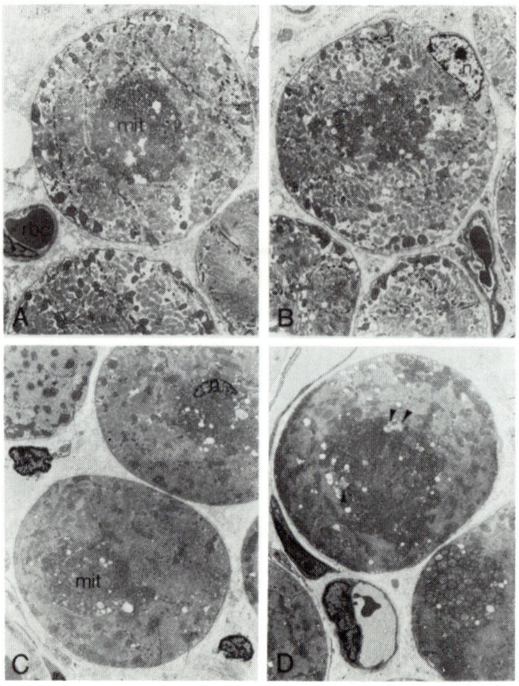

PLATE V

Granular fibers from the global layer of clinically overacting human inferior oblique muscle with central mitochondrial aggregation (mit).

A. Light matrix granular fiber with prominent central core of mitochondria. Red blood cells (rbc) within capillary suggests normal vascular function.

B. Light matrix granular fiber with normal, subsarcolemmal myonucleus.

C. Dark matrix granular fiber with central mitochondrial accumulation and vacuolization. There is also a centrally located myonucleus (n) indicating a pathologic alteration of structure.

D. Dark matrix granular fiber with central mitochondrial accumulation. There is also early loss of mitochondrial structure with disruption of the cristae (arrows). The lost mitochondrial architecture accounts, at least in part, to the formation of vacuoles.

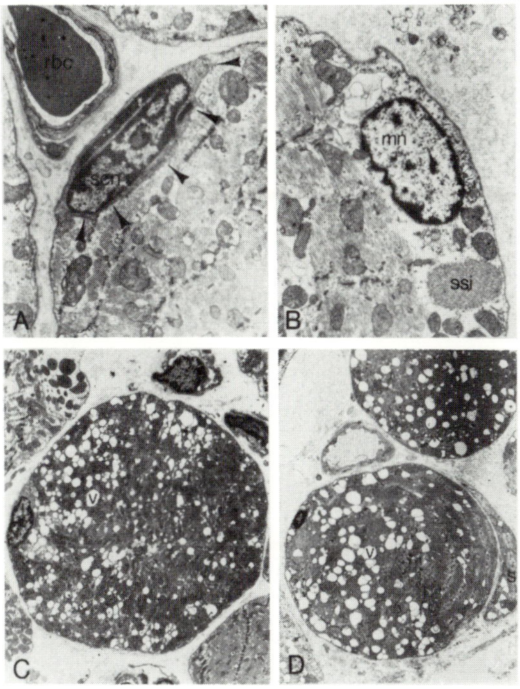

PLATE VI

Human inferior oblique muscle (secondary overaction).

A. Satellite cell within basal lamina of muscle fiber but separated from the fiber by sarcoplasm and plasma membrane (arrows). There is a large, darkly stained nucleus (scn) exhibiting prominent submembranous clusters of chromatin. Satellite cells are embryologically formed as part of the muscle cell wall and are thought to be activated by injury, stress, etc., for the purpose of forming new muscle fiber substance within the basal lamina. rbc: Red blood cell.

B. Muscle cell containing normal myonucleus (mn). It occupies a subsarcolemmal location internal to the basal lamina, surrounded by sarcoplasm but not separated from the fiber. There is a subsarcolemmal inclusion (SSI). Also peripherally oriented SSI have been considered as evidence of latent virus infestation, but they are routinely found in normal and strabismic human EOM.

C. Strabismic muscle cell with extensive vacuolization suggesting atrophy.

D. Split strabismic muscle fiber with absence of complete septum between the main bulk containing vacuoles (v) and the crescentic centrifugally oriented split fiber (sf). Muscle fiber splitting occurs with conditions resulting in hypertrophy or necrosis and regeneration.

POSTNATAL DEVELOPMENT OF EYE MUSCLE FUNCTION

An experimental study in cats with normal and impaired binocular vision

G. LENNERSTRAND

Department of Ophthalmology, Linköping University, Sweden

ABSTRACT

The postnatal development of cat inferior oblique muscle was studied with physiological and histochemical techniques. Muscle fatigue resistance reached adult levels at about 6 weeks of age, while speed of contraction continued to increase up to adulthood. With stainings for ATP-ase and succinicdehydrogenase five muscle fiber types could be identified. All fiber types were seen already in newborn kittens and no age related changes were observed in their relative proportions. Variations with age in contractile properties and in size of the fibers indicate that slow fiber systems of eye muscles mature earlier than fast fiber systems. This might be related to the need for slow eye motor activity in the development of binocular functions and visual resolution.

Cats with defects of binocular vision, due to monocular occlusion with lid suture from age 2 - 3 weeks in domestic cats or to a genetical defect in Siamese (albino) cats, showed slower contractions and lower fatigue resistance of their eye muscles than normal domestic cats. No variations in fiber types or in the relative proportions between types were observed. However, fibers of all types were smaller and the capillary density per fiber was lower in cats with binocular defects than in normal cats.

In guinea pig with poor binocularity also in the normal state, no difference in contractile properties were recorded between normally pigmented and albino animals. This finding lends support to the idea that variations in functional properties between normal cats and lid sutured or Siamese cats depended on the state of binocular vision, and might represent adaptations to the reduced demand for fusional movements in cats with binocular deficiencies.

KEYWORDS

Extraocular muscle; domestic cat; Siamese (albino) cat; postnatal development; contractile properties; histochemical properties; capillary density; lid closure; binocular defects.

INTRODUCTION

The general purposes of these studies, undertaken with physiological and histochemical techniques, have been to

1. describe the normal postnatal development of eye muscles and compare it to that of ordinary skeletal muscle.

2. investigate eye muscles in defects of binocular vision, to see if modified demands on the oculomotor system during development might lead to functional changes in eye muscle structure and function.

Clinically such information would be of importance in evaluating ocular motility problems in children and the patterns of eye muscle adaptation in squint and related disorders.

For a description of the methods used in the experiments and a more detailed presentation of the material reviewed in this paper, the reader is referred to the papers by Lennerstrand and Hanson (1978 a, b; 1979); Lennerstrand (1979, 1980) and Hanson, Lennerstrand and Nichols (1980).

DEVELOPMENT OF CAT SKELETAL MUSCLE

In the cat all hindlimb muscles contract slowly at birth. A differentiation into fast and slow muscles takes place during the first postnatal weeks. Fast muscles steadily increase their speed of contraction until 6 weeks of age when the adult level is reached, while slow muscles retain a low speed of contraction throughout development (Buller, Eccles and Eccles, 1960; Hammarberg and Kellerth 1975 a, b).

The ability to resist fatigue is equally high in all hindlimb muscles at birth. It remains at the same level in slow muscles but declines with age in the fast muscles until the adult pattern emerges at 6 weeks of age (Hammarberg and Kellerth, 1975 a, b).

A histochemical differentiation of fiber types occurs in parallel with changes in speed and endurance of muscle contraction (Nyström,1968a; Hammarberg, 1974). Post-tetanic potentiation of the twitch response is seen in all hindlimb muscles of new-born kittens (Nyström, 1968 b), but in the adult cat it is found only in fast muscles (Buller and Lewis, 1965).

CHARACTERISTICS OF ADULT CAT EYE MUSCLE

Five types of fibers have been identified ultra-structurally in cat eye muscles (Alvarado and van Horn, 1975; see also Table I). Fast and slow twitch fibers with single (focal) innervation of the same kind as in ordinary skeletal muscle are found in eye muscles. In addition there exists two types of slow multiply innervated fibers, resembling the multiply innervated fibers in avian and amphibian muscle, respectively (Chiarandini and Davidowitz, 1979).

It has been possible to differentiate physiologically three types of motor units, one with single innervation and presumably two with multiple innervation (Lennerstrand, 1974; Chiarandini and Davidowitz, 1979). The singly innervated units are fast contracting. Some are easily fatiguing, others show moderate fatiguability (Lennerstrand, 1974). The multiply innervated units are slower in contraction and very fatigue resistant (Lennerstrand, 1974).

Fibers have been morphologically identified in units with single (Lennerstrand and Nichols, 1977) and with multiple innervation (Bach-y-Rita and co-workers, 1977; Lennerstrand and Nichols, 1977). No extensive studies have been made on the postnatal development of eye muscles. It should be noted that such studies on muscles in birds and amphibia with multiply innervated fibers are also lacking.

DEVELOPMENT OF EYE MUSCLE

Normal cat

Physiological properties. Isometric contractions were recorded in the inferior oblique muscle of kittens at different ages and in adult cats. Twitch contractions became faster with age up to the adult stage (Lennerstrand and Hanson, 1978 a). This is in variance with both slow and fast hindlimb muscles, where adult levels are reached before 6 weeks of age, as seen in Fig. 1 A.

Fatigue resistance to a moderate rate of stimulation (100 Hz), applied continously for 30 sec, was lowest at 0 - 2 weeks of age. An increase up to about the adult level had occurred at 6 weeks of age (Fig. 1 B). At higher rates of stimulation (200 Hz) fatigue was most pronounced in kittens below 20 weeks of age. The recovery from a fatiguing stimulation was equally rapid at all ages (Lennerstrand and Hanson, 1978 b).

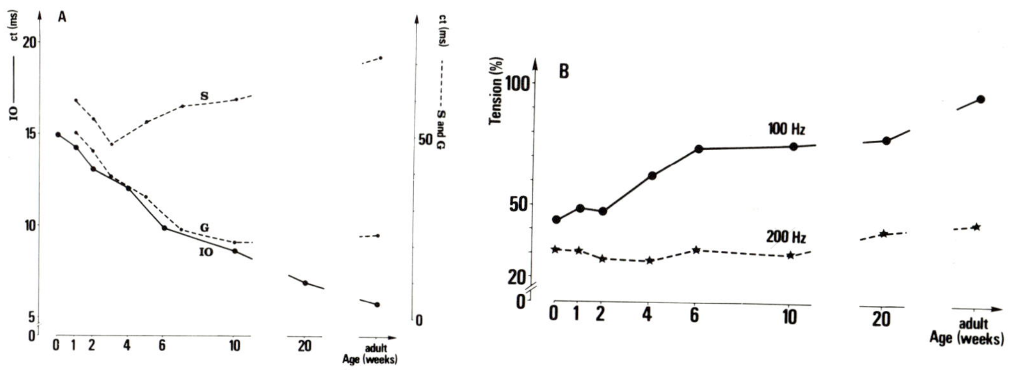

Fig 1 A. Postnatal development of twitch contraction time (ct) in cat inferior oblique (IO), soleus (S) and gastrocnemius (G) muscles. S and G data are from the paper by Hammarberg and Kellerth (1975 a) (courtesy of Prof. J.O. Kellerth). Note different ordinate scales for OI, and for S and G. (Reprinted with permission from Acta Physiol. Scand.)

Fig 1 B. Postnatal development of fatigue resistance in cat inferior oblique. Fatigue resistance expressed as the amount of tetanic tension remaining after 30 sec continous stimulation, in percent of the tension at stimulus initiation. The upper curve obtained with 100 Hz stimulation and the lower with 200 Hz stimulation. (Reprinted with permission from Acta Physiol. Scand.)

These findings and additional ones on posttetanic potentiation (Lennerstrand and Hanson, 1978 b) suggest that the slow fiber systems in eye muscles have reached maturity about 6 weeks of age but that the fast systems continue to develop until the adult stage. It is assumed that fatigue resistance is subserved mainly by the slow fiber systems in kitten eye muscles, as it is in hindlimb muscles (Hammarberg and Kellerth, 1975 b).

Histochemical properties. Histochemical identification of the fiber types with staining procedures for ATP-ase and succinicdehydrogenase (SDH) was first applied in the adult cat. A correlation between previous ultrastructural differentiation (Alvarado and van Horn, 1975) and the present histochemical findings is suggested in Table I.

TABLE I

Suggested correlation between ultrastructural and histochemical types of muscle fibers in adult cat exctraocular muscles.

Electron microscopical data from Alvarado and van Horn (1975) and Alvarado (Personal communication).

EM type	1	2	3	4	5
layer	global	global	global + orbital	global	global + orbital
mean diam. (μm)	30	22	12	23	12
membranous SR + TT	extensive	extensive	moderate	poor	poor
mitochondria	few/small	moderate	many/large	few	many
innervation	single	single	single	multiple	multiple
% of global fibers	38	20	26	15	*
% of orbital fibers	-	-	60-70	*	30-40

Histochemical data from Hanson, Lennerstrand and Nichols (1980)

Histochem. type	II	II	II	I	IIC
layer	global	global	global + orbital	global	global + orbital
ATPase-9.4	++	++	++	0	++
ATPase-fix	++	+,++	+,++	0	++
ATPase-4.35	0	0	0,+	++	++
SDH	0	+	++	0,+	++
% of global fibers	36	24	17	14	9
% of orbital fibers	-	-	54	**	46

*) Alvarado (personal communication) reports occurrance of type 4 fibers in orbital layer and type 5 fibers in global layer but not the relative proportions of each type.

**)3% of orbital fibers were light in all stains and had membrane rifts.

With ATP-ase stainings at pH 4.35 and 9.4 the eye muscle fibers could be separated into three types (c.f. Brooke and Kaiser, 1970); type I stained darkly at pH 4.35 but not at pH 9.4 and was found predominantly in the inner (global) layer; type II stained darkly at pH 9.4 but not at pH 4.35 and was seen in both the global and the outer (orbital) layer; and type IIC stained darkly at pH 9.4 as well as 4.35 and was found mainly in the orbital layer. Studies of cat (Burke and co-workers, (1973) and rat (Kugelberg, 1976) hindlimb muscle fibers have shown type I fibers to be slow, type II fibers to be fast and type IIC fibers to be of intermediate speed of contraction. Both type I and IIC fibers are fatigue resistant (Kugelberg, 1976). A subdivision of the type II fibers could be made with SDH staining (Hanson, Lennerstrand and Nichols, 1980), indicating different levels of fatigue resistance in type II fibers. The relative proportions of fiber types differentiated with histochemical or electronmicroscopical techniques correlated quite well (see Table I). The histochemical properties of type I fibers correspond with those reported for multiply innervated slow fibers in amphibia (Smith and Ovalle, 1973) and histochemistry of type IIC fibers with that of slow fibers in birds (Asmussen and co-workers, 1971).

The fiber types in ATPase staining could be differentiated already in eye muscles of the new-born kitten.The relative proportions of the fiber types did not change with age. Growth in size was more or less linearly related to age for all fiber types up to 20 weeks, but between that age and the adult stage the increase in size was much more prominent for type II than for type I, as exemplified in Fig. 2 for fibers in the global area. This gives further support to the notion that slow eye muscle components mature earlier than fast fiber components (Hanson, Lennerstrand and Nichols, 1980).

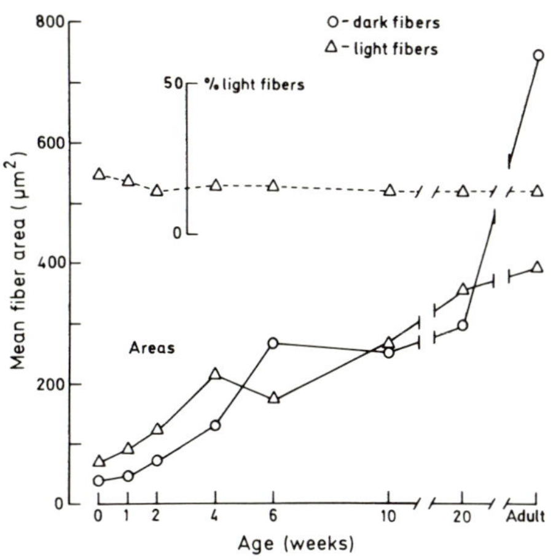

Fig. 2

Postnatal increase in transsectional area of global fibers stained for ATP-ase at pH 9.4 after formaline fixation. Dark fibers are type II and IIC, light fibers are type I fibers. Inset shows the proportions of light fibers at different ages. Dark fibers are significantly larger than light fibers in the adult animal but not at other ages. (Reprinted with permission from Acta Physiol. Scand.)

Functionally this would imply that the eye muscle system for fixation and binocular fusion, presumably subserved by slow and fatigue resistant type I and IIC fibers, would be well developed during the sensitive period for cat visual development between 3 and 10 weeks of age (Hubel and Wiesel, 1970; Blakemore and van Sluyters, 1974).

If eye muscle properties could be altered by manipulation of visual functions, this would be further support for the idea of separate development of the slow and the fast fiber system. It could also give an insight into the adaptational processes in a complex muscle system to changes in functional demands.

Cats with defects of binocular vision

There is an extensive body of experimental data to show that vision and binocular functions are impaired in cats with squint and unilateral amblyopia, and that an amelioration of these defects cannot be expected if treatment is postponed beyond the sensitive period (Hubel and Wiesel, 1965; 1970; Blakemore and van Sluyters, 1974; Yinon, 1976). It is also well known that animals with albinism lack the neural substrate for normal binocular vision due to neuroanatomical defects of their visual pathways (Guillery and co-workers, 1974; Hubel and Wiesel, 1971). The animals with binocular deficits would have normal eye movements except for fusional vergences, which would not be in much demand. Animals with binocular deficits therefore offer an opportunity to study the effects of a restricted and well defined abnormality in oculomotion on the development of eye muscle function.

Physiological properties. Kittens were raised with unilateral lid suture from age 2 - 3 weeks. Their muscle functions were tested at age 20 weeks and at adulthood, and compared with functions in normal cats of the same ages. Adult Siamese (albino) cats were also examined. Speed of contraction was found to be the same in 20 week old lid sutured and normal cats. However, at the adult stage contractions were slower in lid sutured and Siamese cats than in normal cats (Table II). In Siamese cats fusion frequency was also significantly lower than in normal cats. Fatigue resistance was lower in cats with defects of binocular vision than in normal cats of the corresponding age (Table II). These functional changes were more pronounced in Siamese than in lid sutured cats (Lennerstrand and Hanson, 1979).

TABLE II

Speed of contraction, determined as contraction time (ct), half-relaxation time (hrt) and fusion frequency, and endurance, determined as the tension remaining after 30 sec continous stimulation, in normal (N), lid sutured (L) and Siamese (S) cats. p-values from t-tests between N and L groups, and S groups, respectively. (From Lennerstrand and Hanson, 1979; Lennerstrand, 1979).

	20 weeks			Adult				
	N (n=4)	L (n=4)	p	N (n=8)	L (n=10)	p	S (n=6)	p
Twitch								
ct (ms)	7.0 ± 0.3	7.2 ± 0.9	-	5.7 ± 0.6	6.8 ± 1.0	**	7.4 ± 1.4	**
hrt (ms)	11.4 ± 2.3	9.2 ± 1.7	-	7.0 ± 1.0	9.6 ± 2.6	**	11.6 ± 3.2	***
Fusion frequency (Hz)				331 ± 24			292 ± 25	**
Endurance (%)								
50 Hz	138 ± 26	86 ± 20	*	150 ± 35	112 ± 22	**	63 ± 13	***
100 Hz	79 ± 7	57 ± 15	*	95 ± 15	80 ± 8	*	32 ± 8	***

-: $p>0.05$
*: $0.05>p>0.02$
**: $0.02>p>0.01$
***: $p>0.01$

Histochemical properties. The binocular deficiences did not influence the proportions of type I, II and IIC fibers in the global layer, or of type II and IIC fibers in the orbital layer, but they were the same in all groups of cats of the same age (20 weeks or adult). On the other hand the fibers were significantly smaller in the Siamese cats than in normal cats as seen in Fig. 3 **A.** It was further noted that the density of capillaries per muscle fiber was significantly lower in cats with binocular deficiences than in normal cats of corresponding age (Fig.3 B). A correlation is postulated between lowered fatigue resistance and the reduced capillary density, and possibly between speed of contraction and fiber size (Lennerstrand, 1980).

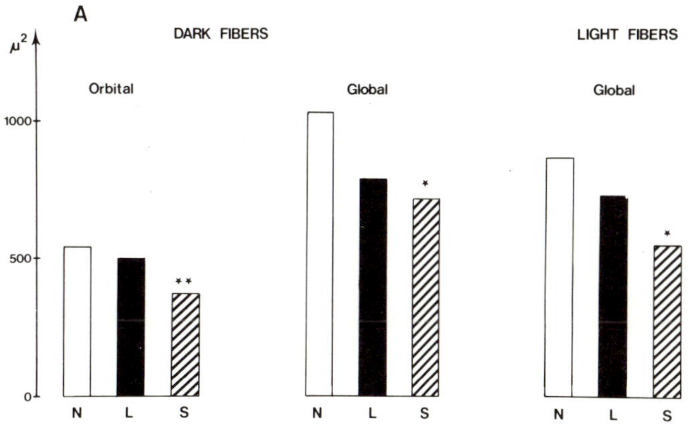

Fig. 3 A

Mean transsectional areas of inferior oblique muscle fibers in adult normal (N), lid sutured (L) and Siamese (S) cats. Dark fibers are types II and IIC, light fibers type I fibers. The fibers in Siamese cats are significantly smaller than in normal cats, in both the global and orbital layers.

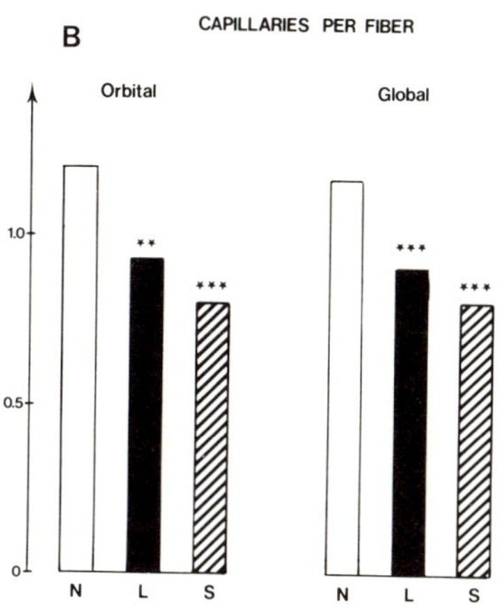

Fig. 3 B

Number of capillaries per fiber in the same groups of cats as in A, in orbital and global layers. Significantly lower capillary densities in lid sutured (L) and Siamese (S), than in normal cats.

Significance levels: * $(0.05>p>0.02)$, ** $(0.02>p>0.01)$, *** $(p>0.01)$.

Functional implications. The reduced demands for fusion movements seemed to lead to a functional adaptation in the eye muscles, reflected mainly in a lowered fatigue resistance. This would point to a functional change in slow fiber properties. However, morphological changes in slow fibers could not be discovered and it is more likely that the adaptation has taken the form of a reduction in blood flow and capillary density. The slower contractions may also indicate subnormal fast fiber development. The functional adaptations had not affected any particular type(s) of fibers but concerned all fibers, in accordance with the idea that specific eye movements not are subserved by particular eye fiber systems but that all fibers contribute to all types of movements (Robinson, 1970; Lennerstrand, 1975). The changes observed in eye muscles resemble those found in other muscles after denervation or immobilization (Lömo, Westergaard and Dahl, 1974; Brown et al,1976). In other muscles these structural changes are reversable with proper training. In eye muscles adaptational effects would therefore probably not compose an obstacle to ortoptic treatment of motor fusion in strabismus, once the sensory substrate for binocular vision had been reestablished.

Animals with poor binocular vision in the normal state

The guinea pig and the rat have laterally placed eyes and insignificant binocular overlap of the visual fields, which implies poor binocular vision even in the normal animals. Speed of contraction of rat and guinea pig eye muscles is approximately the same as in the cat, but the fatigue resistance of the muscles in significantly lower than in normal cats and resemble the values in Siamese cats (Table III). Contractile properties were found to be the same in pigmented and albino guinea pigs (Table III), supporting the idea that dissimilarities between normal and Siamese cats depended on differences in binocular functions and not were genetically determined. Eye muscles of the albino rat did not contain any type I fibers (Hanson and Lennerstrand, 1977). More detailed studies of fiber sizes and capillary density in rats and guinea pigs have not yet been undertaken.

TABLE III

Contractile properties of inferior oblique muscles in pigmented (P) and albino (A) guinea pig, and in albino rat (R).

	P (n=6)	A (n=6)	R (n=8)*
Twitch ct (ms)	6.3±0.7	6.3±0.4	7.8
Fusion frequency (Hz)	325±28	335±27	313
Endurance (%)			
100 Hz	63±24	66±12	-
200 Hz	21±5	18±3	10

*) From Hanson and Lennerstrand (1977)

PROBLEMS FOR FUTURE RESEARCH

The studies just reviewed were performed on the whole muscle and not on individual motor units in eye muscle of kittens at different stages of development. Single units studies would be able to clarify the development of contractile properties in different type of motor units, as shown in hindlimb muscles. It would also be possible to find out if polyneuronal innervation (by different nerve fibers to the same muscle fiber) occurred in eye muscles of young animals, as it does in hindlimb muscles. Polyneuronal innervation disappears at 2 weeks of age in hindlimb muscles (Betz and coworkers, 1979). No such innervation is seen in adult cat eye muscle (Bach-y-Rita and Lennerstrand, 1975). Studies on development of slow motor units in amphibia and birds could further elucidate the age variations in eye muscle properties. It would also be of interest to study the motor unit properties in cats with binocular deficiences.

Investigations of human eye muscle development are still lacking. Such studies would have to be done with non-invasive electrophysiological techniques and would have to include recordings of eye movements and fixational behaviour in children of different ages. Indirect tests on eye muscle function can be made with histochemical methods with the purpose of identifying fiber types and fiber distribution in normal individuals and patients with squint and amblyopia. Ultrastructural changes have been noted in strabismic muscles, as reported by McNeer (this volume), but it is not known at what stage during development they appear.

ACKNOWLEDGEMENTS

These studies were supported by grants from the Swedish Medical Research Council (Nos 3875, 4719 and 3875), Karolinska Institutets fonder, and the Research Committee of Östergötlands läns landsting.

EXTRAOCULAR MUSCLE STIFFNESS IN NORMAL RABBITS, CATS AND VISUALLY DEPRIVED CATS

N. H. BARMACK

Physiology Section, Biological Sciences Group, University of Connecticut, Storrs, CT 06268, USA

ABSTRACT

The rotational stiffness (g/deg) of the eyes of anesthetized and unanesthetized cats and rabbits were made in the horizontal and vertical planes. Values of stiffness for temporal rotations of the globe were: cats, .72 g/deg; rabbits, .11 g/deg. In addition the rotational stiffness was measured for the eyes of six cats which were deprived of binocular vision for 12-14 months by monocular lid closure 10-14 days after birth. The stiffness of the deprived and non-deprived eyes did not differ significantly from normal controls. The stiffness of the eye may be related to binocular vision. However, unlike the powerful influence of visual deprivation on binocular vision, the visual deprivation (monocular lid suturing) employed in the present experiment did <u>not</u> modify the rotational stiffness of the eye of cats.

KEYWORDS

Extraocular muscles stiffness; binocular vision; visual deprivation; monocular lid closure; cats; rabbits.

INTRODUCTION

In human subjects and monkeys electromyographic and electrophysiological data demonstrate a relatively high rate of spontaneous discharge of muscle fibers or motoneurons when the eye is in "primary position" (Bjork and Kugelberg, 1954; Perryman and Breinin, 1971; Fuchs and Luschei, 1970; Scott and Collins, 1973). This spontaneous discharge is present, but has a lower frequency in the rabbit (Barmack, 1977). One consequence of this high spontaneous discharge rate in human subjects and monkeys is the relatively high stiffness with which the globe is controlled. The stiffness of the eye can be measured easily by placing a suction contact lens on the topically anesthetized eye and determining the amount of force which must be applied tangentially to the suction lens to rotate the eye through a known angle (say 5 degrees). Using such a method we have determined that the stiffness of the eyes of normal human subjects, measured in the horizontal plane, is about 1.09 g/deg(Barmack, 1976). The stiffness of the eyes of rabbits is ten times lower than that of human subjects, about .11 g/deg. Rabbits have a poorly developed fovea and only limited binocular vision. Consequently, their eye position control is not as accurate as that of other species which possess foveal vision and which have stiffer oculomotor control system.

It is possible that the development of normal binocular vision is dependent on a concomitant development extraocular muscle stiffness. Indeed the physiology of binocularly driven visual cortical cells in the rabbit differs markedly from that of either the cat or the monkey; lacking columnar organization, having large receptive field disparities, and remaining relatively insensitive to the usually catastrophic effects of monocular visual deprivation (Van Sluyters and Stewart, 1974a; Van Sluyters and Stewart, 1974b). There is no behavioral evidence for true stereopsis in the rabbit, nor has there been a convincing demonstration of visually evoked disjunctive eye movements.

If the lack of a true fovea and the apparent absence of binocular vision reduces the necessity for fine position control in the rabbit, what would be the effects of deprivation of binocular visual experience in an animal which ordinarily has excellent binocular vision? Is it possible that a decrease in extraocular muscle stiffness in an oculomotor system which is ordinarily controlled with a high stiffness may underly certain oculomotor abnormalities? Could low extraocular muscle stiffness be the cause of certain kinds of strabismus in human patients? Consistent with this hypothesis is the observation of decreased numbers of mitochondria in the extraocular muscles of humans afflicted with strabismus (Aichmar and Mayr, 1973). These results imply that there is a lower steady state level of activity in strabismic muscles, and hence a lower active stiffness. Perhaps a binocular neural signal normally enhances the stiffness of extraocular muscles by providing a tonic pre-motoneuronal excitatory input to all oculomotor nuclei. It is possible that deprivation of binocular experience during development may reduce the active stiffness of the extraocular muscles, thereby causing misalignments which ordinarily would not be evident. The consequent misalignment of the eyes would further reduce the stiffness controlled by the hypothesized binocular signal. The consequent reduction in stiffness might render the position control system more vulnerable to anomalous variation in load imposed by other elements of the globe. This possible loss of stiffness might account for the observation that both convergent and divergent strabismus have been detected in cats which had one eyelid sutured during the first 6-12 months of life (Sherman, 1972).

The present experiment was undertaken to test whether binocular visual stimulation is necessary for normal development of extraocular muscle stiffness. The stiffness of the eyes of normal rabbits and cats has been measured and compared. In addition the stiffness of the eyes of cats which have been deprived of normal binocular experience during the first year of life has been measured and compared with measurements obtained from normal cats.

Cats were used as subjects in this experiment because of the extensive physiological and behavioral data which demonstrates the presence of binocular vision in normal animals and the marked influence of monocular lid closure during the first weeks of life on the attenuation of binocular vision (Packwood and Gordon, 1975; Mitchell, Cynader and Movshon, 1977; Weisel and Hubel, 1963a, 1963b, 1965a, 1965b). The measurements contained herein demonstrate that the cat has a globe stiffness of about .70 g/deg, but that this stiffness does not appear to be reduced by monocular lid closure made during the first two post-natal weeks of life and lasting for 12-14 months.

METHODS

Three litters of 3 kittens each were used in this experiment. At 7-12 days after birth the kittens were anesthetized with ketamine hydrochloride (35 mg/kg). One eyelid was sutured closed after removing the outer lid margin. One kitten from each litter was not operated upon. After 12-14 months, each previously operated cat was re-anesthetized and the sutured lid was opened. One month later each cat was re-anesthetized and three stainless steel bolts were fastened to the calvarium with dental cement and anchored to four smaller screws. The bolts mated with a bar which was used subsequently to provide immobilization of the head. At least two days following this procedure, the stiffness of the eye was measured as follows:

Measurement of Eye Stiffness

A 5-0 suture was sewn to the medial and inferior aspects of the corneal-scleral junction of the eye which was topically anesthetized with proparacaine hydrochloride. The suture was attached to a micrometer-stain gauge which gave measurements of force and an optically encoded position signal. The micrometer was then aligned so that one of the two sutures pulled tangentially on the globe in either the superior or temporal directions. Upon completion of the measurements of stiffness in unanesthetized animals, the cats were anesthetized with 35 mg/kg sodium pentobarbital given intraperitoneally and the measurements of eye stiffness were repeated.

RESULTS

Comparison of the Stiffness of the Eyes of Rabbits and Cats

The stiffness of the eyes of 12 rabbits and 9 cats was compared for both temporal and superior rotations of the globe. (Figs. 1 and 2).

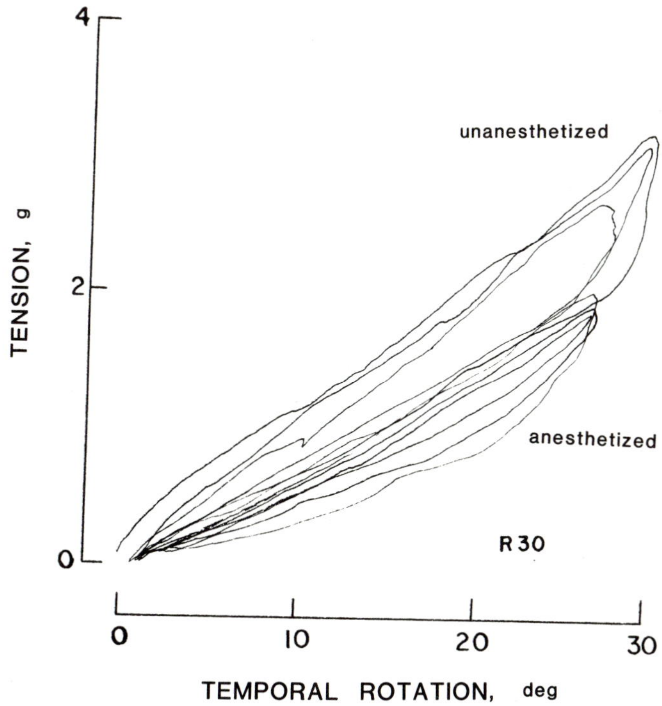

Fig. 1. Measurement of horizontal stiffness of the eye of a rabbit which was unanesthetized and subsequently anesthetized with sodium pentobarbital.

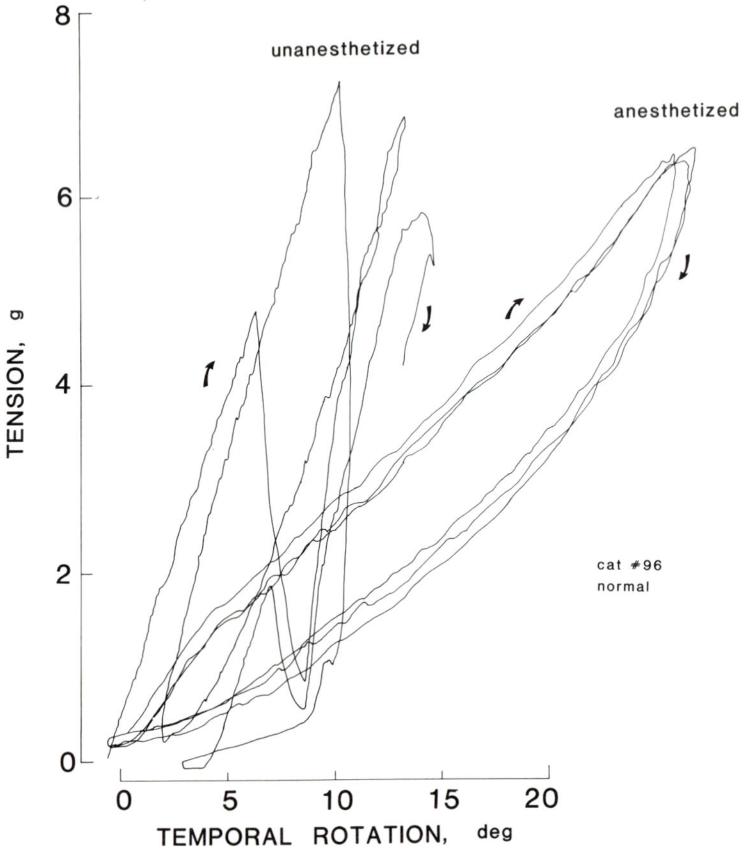

Fig. 2. Measurement of horizontal stiffness of the eye of a cat which was unanesthetized and subsequently anesthetized with sodium pentobarbital.

The stiffness of the eyes of both species was measured while the animals were unanesthetized and subsequently when the animals were anesthetized with sodium pentobarbital. The average stiffness for the eyes of unanesthetized rabbits for temporal rotations of the globe was .11 g/deg (Table 1). The average stiffness for the eyes of both operated and unoperated cats for temporal rotations of the globe was .71 g/deg (Table 1). The previously measured stiffness of the eye of human subjects was 1.09 g/deg. The stiffness of the eyes of both species for superior rotations of the globe were: .10 g/deg for rabbits and .71 g/deg for cats. The stiffness of both species was reduced by the effects of sodium pentobarbital anesthesia, although the reduction in stiffness caused by the anesthesia in cats was much greater (Table 1).

TABLE 1 Rotational Stiffness of Human Subjects, Rabbits and Cats

		Horizontal Stiffness (g/deg)	Vertical Stiffness (g/deg)
Anesthetized			
Cats,	N = 9	.31 ± .08	.33 ± .09
Rabbits,	N = 12	.09 ± .04	.06 ± .03
Unanesthetized			
Cats,	N = 8	.71 ± .08	.72 ± .06
Rabbits,	N = 12	.11 ± .04	.10 ± .03
Humans,	N = 6	1.09 ± .24	

TABLE 2 Rotational Stiffness of Cats with Monocular Lid Sutures and Normal Cats

	Horizontal Stiffness (g/deg)		Vertical Stiffness (g/deg)	
Anesthetized				
Deprived eye	N = 6,	.29 ± .05	N = 6,	.31 ± .09
Non-deprived eye	N = 6,	.33 ± .08	N = 6,	.38 ± .09
Normal eyes	N = 3,	.27 ± .03	N = 3,	.29 ± .08
Unanesthetized				
Deprived eye	N = 6,	.72 ± .09	N = 6,	.71 ± .06
Non-deprived eye	N = 6,	.68 ± .04	N = 6,	.72 ± .02
Normal	N = 2,	.74 ± .09	N = 2,	.73 ± .05

Influence of Monocular Eyelid Closure on the Rotational Stiffness of the Eyes of Cats

The rotational stiffness of the eyes was measured in six cats which had been operated upon before they were two weeks of age. These cats had one eyelid sewn shut for 12-14 months. The rotational stiffness of both the previously closed eye and the unclosed eye were measured one month after the eyelid was opened. This post-operative eyelid opening recovery period was chosen so as to minimize the possible confounding effects of wound healing on the measurement of rotational stiffness. During this one month recovery period no attempt was made to deprive the cats of vision.

The horizontal and vertical rotational stiffness was not modified in cats which had one eye completely sutured shut for a period of at least one year. There was no significant difference between the "sutured eye" and the "non-sutured eye." Nor was there any difference between the stiffness of either eyes of the operated cats from their unoperated control litter mates. The results imply that extraocular muscle stiffness is not modified by the absence of a normal binocular input.

DISCUSSION

The measurement of rotational stiffness of the eyes of both rabbits and cats demonstrated that the eye of the cat is controlled with a stiffness which is greater than the rotational stiffness of the eye of the rabbit by a factor of 7. This might be expected for an animal with frontally placed eyes possessing good binocular vision. However, unlike the marked susceptbility of the central visual system to various paradigms of visual deprivation, the rotational stiffness of the extraocular motor control system of the cat seems immune to the influence of monocular lid closure. This was true for rotational stiffness tested in both the superior and temporal directions. One might have supposed that the medial rectus muscle, because of its role in vergence movements, would be most susceptible to the effects of visual deprivation. However, this is the muscle that is tested most directly during measurements of stiffness for temporal rotation of the globe.

It is possible that visual deprivation caused by monocular eyelid closure may influence other parameters of oculomotor control such as maintenance or modification of an "operating point" on a stiffness curve. This possibility was not examined in the present report. Nor would these data exclude the possibility that a reduced extraocular muscle stiffness may be one of the causes of strabismus.

ACKNOWLEDGEMENT

The author wishes to acknowledge the support of the Oregon Lions Sight and Hearing Foundation for their support of this research which was also supported by the National Eye Institute, EY-00848.

PROPRIOCEPTION IN EYE MUSCLES

E. MANNI* and R. BORTOLAMI**

**Institute of Human Physiology, Università Cattolica S. Cuore, Rome, Italy*
***Institute of Veterinary Anatomy, University of Bologna, Italy*

ABSTRACT

The present report deals with the anatomical and functional organization of the peripheral and central pathways of the eye muscle proprioception. Histological and electrophysiological investigations have shown that the first-order neurons of the extraocular muscle proprioception have their perikarya in the medial dorso-lateral portion of the semilunar ganglion. While the peripheral process innervates the eye muscle proprioceptors, the central one enters the brain stem through the sensory trigeminal root and terminates ipsilaterally in the oral portion of the spinal trigeminal nucleus and in the main sensory trigeminal nucleus. The second-order neurons of the extraocular muscle proprioception are localized in such nuclei and project on the cerebellum and on mesodiencephalic areas. Axons reach the ipsilateral ventrobasal nuclear complex of the thalamus through the ipsilateral medial lemniscus and dorsal trigemino-thalamic tract, abandoning collaterals in the tectum and in the tegmentum of the mesencephalon.
The physiological role of the eye muscle proprioception is discussed.

KEYWORDS

Extraocular muscle proprioceptors; eye muscle spindles; semilunar ganglion; main sensory trigeminal nucleus; spinal trigeminal nucleus; cerebellum; neck muscles; stretch reflex.

INTRODUCTION

The extraocular muscles (EOM) of man and of some animals contain sensory nerve endings which must be considered as proprioceptors. Muscle spindles in particular have been found in the EOM of man, goat, sheep, pig, wild boar and some species of monkeys. No muscle spindles have been demonstrated in the eye muscles of cat, dog, rabbit and guinea pig: however, they contain other receptors which play the role of proprioceptors. Golgi tendon organs too have been shown in different animals.

ENTRY OF OCULAR PROPRIOCEPTIVE IMPULSES INTO THE BRAIN STEM AND LOCATION OF THE CELL BODIES OF THE EOM PROPRIOCEPTIVE FIBRES

Different views have been put forward concerning the entry of EOM proprioceptive information into the brain stem. Several researchers have emphasized the role of the third, fourth and sixth cranial nerves in conducting such impulses. A possible role of the trigeminal nerve was postulated in 1929 by Stibbe who observed ocular afferent fibres in the fifth nerve: since that time connections between the EOM nerves and the trigeminal nerve have been described by others. Also the location of the perikarya of the EOM proprioceptive fibres is debated. According to some researchers they are contained in the trigeminal mesencephalic nucleus (Kosaka, 1912; Freeman, 1925; Cooper, Daniel and Whitteridge, 1953; Batini, 1979 a). However, it is now established that the trigeminal mesencephalic nucleus consists of the somata of the first-order neurons of the masticatory proprioception.
Another view claims that the afferent fibres from the EOM have their bodies in the small ganglia scattered along the trunk of the EOM nerves (Nicholson, 1924; Tozer, 1912) or in the nuclei of the third, fourth and sixth cranial nerve mixed with the motoneurons which provide the EOM (Corbin and Oliver, 1942; Bach-y-Rita and Murata, 1964).

Eye muscle proprioception and the semilunar ganglion. In investigations carried out since more than 15 years we have reached the conclusion that the first-order neurons of the EOM proprioception have their somata in the semilunar ganglion and enter the brain stem through the trigeminal nerve in the Ungulata. Such an assumption has been confirmed by other investigators (Lennerstrand and Bach-y-Rita, 1974; Browne, 1975). Cell responsive to stretching single EOM have been found in the medial dorso-lateral portion of the semilunar ganglion of sheep, pig and calf: they are unaffected either by other trigeminal stimulations or by Nembutal anaesthesia. Their responses to stretch are inhibited during contraction of the muscle, thus they can be considered as muscle spindle afferents (Manni, Bortolami and Desole, 1966, 1968).
Section of a trigeminal ophthalmic branch abolished the responses recorded from the semilunar ganglion to individual EOM stretching and provoked degeneration of the sensitive innervation of the EOM spindles, while this did not occur after section of oculomotor, trochlear and abducens nerves at the basis of the skull, proximally to the cavernous sinus. Cutting the trigeminal root between the semilunar ganglion and the pons did not suppress the unitary responses of the semilunar ganglion to stretching single EOM and did not provoke degeneration of the ipsilateral ophthalmic branch and of the sensitive innervation of the EOM spindles (Manni, Bortolami and Deriu, 1970 a). Contemporary chronic severance of the trigeminal root and of the trochlear nerve (Manni, Bortolami and Deriu, 1970 b) or of the abducens nerve (Manni, Palmieri and Marini, 1971 a) did not eliminate the gasserian responses to the stretch of respectively the superior oblique or of the lateral rectus muscles. Such findings clearly prove that the somata of the first-order neurons of the EOM proprioceptors are really placed in the semilunar ganglion and not in the trigeminal mesencephalic nucleus at least in the Ungulata.
Further demonstration of such an assumption was given by destroying the semilunar ganglion cellular pool which provides the EOM spindles by means of discrete electrolysis. Those experiments (Manni, Palmieri and Marini, 1972 a) were followed by ipsilateral degenerations of: i) EOM spindles; ii) axons in the ophthalmic branch, in the medial portion of the trigeminal root and in the pons reaching the main sensory nucleus and the oral portion of the spinal trigeminal nucleus.
In this way one can reach the conclusion that the semilunar ganglion contains nerve cells whose peripheral processes attain the eye muscle spindles through branches of the ophthalmic nerve; in the Ungulata the sensory processes penetrate the eye muscle from one side, while the motor component reaches it from the opposite side (Winckler, 1956). The central processes enter the brain stem travelling along the medial part of the portio major of the trigeminal root and terminate in the oral portion of the spinal trigeminal nucleus and in the main sensory nucleus.
Histological and electrophysiological investigations have demonstrated a somatoto-

pic arrangement of the EOM proprioception in the medial dorso-lateral portion of the semilunar ganglion of the lamb. In fact both the horseradish peroxidase method and the unitary recording technique have shown that the cells innervating the superior rectus and the superior oblique muscles are localized in the dorsal portion of the proprioceptive semilunar pool, while its ventral layer contains the perikarya which provide sensitive innervation of the inferior rectus and of the inferior oblique muscles. The proprioceptive representation of the medial rectus and of the lateral rectus are placed respectively in the medial and in the lateral areas of the same cellular pool wedging between the dorsal and the ventral layers (Manni and Pettorossi, 1976; Bortolami and co-workers, 1979) (Fig. 1).

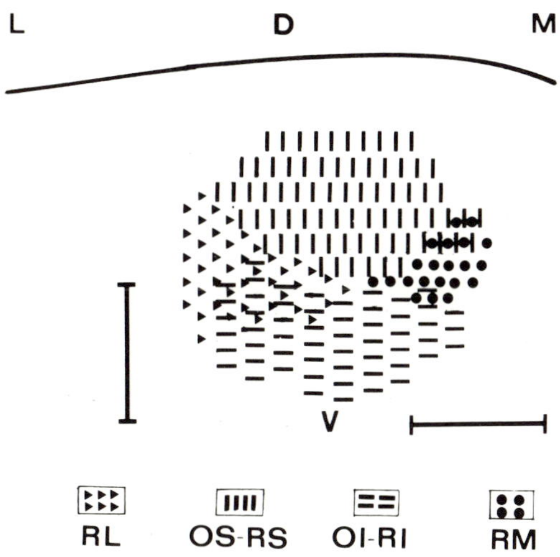

Fig. 1. Schematic diagram of transverse section of lamb semilunar ganglion showing the somatotopic organization of the eye muscle afferents within the proprioceptive cellular pool. L, lateral; D, dorsal; M, medial; V, ventral; RL lateral rectus; OS, superior oblique; RS, superior rectus; OI, inferior oblique; RI, inferior rectus; RM, medial rectus. Calibration: 1 mm (from Manni and Pettorossi, Arch.Ital.Biol., (1976), 114:178-187).

On the contrary other investigators (Batini and Buisseret, 1974), following the old hypothesis of Cooper, Daniel and Whitteridge (1953) and of Fillenz (1956) claim that the first-order neurons of the EOM proprioceptors are located in the mesencephalic trigeminal nucleus. However, horseradish peroxidase injection in the EOM of the cat and rabbit was followed by labelling of a small number of semilunar ganglion cells located in the ophthalmic area of the ganglion itself (Bortolami in preparation,1981). All the authors who suggested that in the cat primary afferent cell bodies of the EOM proprioceptors are contained in the mesencephalic trigeminal nucleus, also report that these cells are very few. On the contrary our data obtained by horseradish peroxidase injection in the eye muscles of the sheep and pig, in which muscle spindles are present show that cell bodies of the eye muscle proprioceptors in the ophthalmic lobe of the semilunar ganglion are very numerous.

Physiological properties of the EOM proprioceptors. They have been investigated by

several researchers in various animals. The conduction velocities of the fibres afferent from EOM spindles ranged between 30 and 110 m/sec in the sheep (Browne,1975). According to Bach-y-Rita and Ito (1976) the conduction velocity of afferents from inferior oblique muscle of the cat ranges between 6.5-52 m/sec with a peak at 10-15 m/sec. Both tonic and phasic responses were recorded to stretching single EOM. In the sheep the presence of two extreme responses to a ramp stretch were identified by Browne (1975) as homologous to the group IA and II of the mammalian neuromuscular spindles, however, intermediate responses were found between these two groups. Some differences in the dynamic properties of the EOM proprioceptors were recognized between cat and sheep. For example a sudden increase in the discharge rate at the beginning of the ramp stretch and a sudden decrease at the completion of the stretch are present in the responses of a certain number of eye receptors of the sheep: however, such a property has not been reported as concerns the eye muscle receptors of the cat (Bach-y-Rita and Ito, 1966a).The properties of the Golgi tendon organs have been investigated in the semilunar ganglion of guinea pig by Lennerstrand and Bach-y-Rita (1974).
EOM spindles of sheep and minipig have a fusimotor innervation, but this is not the case for the EOM of the cat.

EOM proprioception and ganglion cells scattered along the third, fourth and sixth cranial nerves. The hypothesis according to which the ganglion cells scattered along the three EOM nerves could represent the first-order neurons of the EOM proprioception has been controlled (Manni, Desole and Palmieri, 1970). Experiments were performed in the calf, animal in which numerous ganglion cells may be consistently present along the intracranial portion of the oculomotor nerve. Thus such a nerve has been chronically severed on the left side in 9 calves just where it enters the cavernous sinus. Responses to stretch of single eye muscles were picked up from ipsilateral trigeminal ganglion 7-10 days after the operation: they were of the type induced by muscle spindle excitation. On the contrary no responses were registered from the intracranial course of the right oculomotor nerve acutely severed. Histological examination was carried out on the EOM innervated by the left third nerve which had been chronically cut. EOM spindles were normal in 7 out of 9 calves whose central stump of the oculomotor nerve contained only a few ganglion cells. However, a few spindles showed degeneration of sensory fibres in EOM of 2 calves in which the central stump of the third nerve exhibited more than 100 ganglion cells. It is evident that the semilunar ganglion of the calf contains the perikarya of the afferent fibres from the EOM spindles as in lamb and in pig; the ganglion cells scattered along the trunk of the oculomotor nerve may play only a negligible role in innervating the EOM proprioceptors.

CENTRAL COURSE OF EOM PROPRIOCEPTORS

It has been previously pointed out that the central processes of the first-order neurons of the EOM proprioception end in the ipsilateral main sensory trigeminal nucleus and in the oral portion of the ipsilateral spinal trigeminal nucleus of the lamb: the second-order neurons of the EOM proprioception are localized in such nuclei (Manni, Palmieri and Marini, 1971 b). However, some central processes may project also caudally: units influenced by EOM stretch have been recorded in the bulb as well as in the upper cervical cord at the level of the interpolaris and caudalis portion of the spinal trigeminal nucleus (Manni and co-workers, 1975 b). The pontine representation of the EOM proprioception as well is somatotopically arranged in both the oral portion of the spinal trigeminal nucleus and main sensory nucleus (Marini and Bortolami, 1979). The most dorsal layer of the nuclei receives projections of the superior oblique and superior rectus muscles. The medial and lateral recti are represented in the most ventral position, while the projection of inferior rectus and inferior oblique muscles occupies an intermediate layer. Other investigations (Manni, Palmieri and Marini, 1972 b, 1974) analyzed the further course of proprioceptive impulses arising from EOM spindles. Responses to stretching single eye muscles were recorded from the tectum and tegmentum of mesencephalon, along the medial lemniscus and from the ventrobasal complex of the thalamus. Very recent investigations carried out in our laboratories have shown also in the mesencephalon of lamb a somatotopic arrangement of the EOM proprioception (Marini and Bortolami, 1980). In fact (Fig. 2) inferior oblique and inferior rectus muscles are represented dorsally with respect to superior rectus and superior

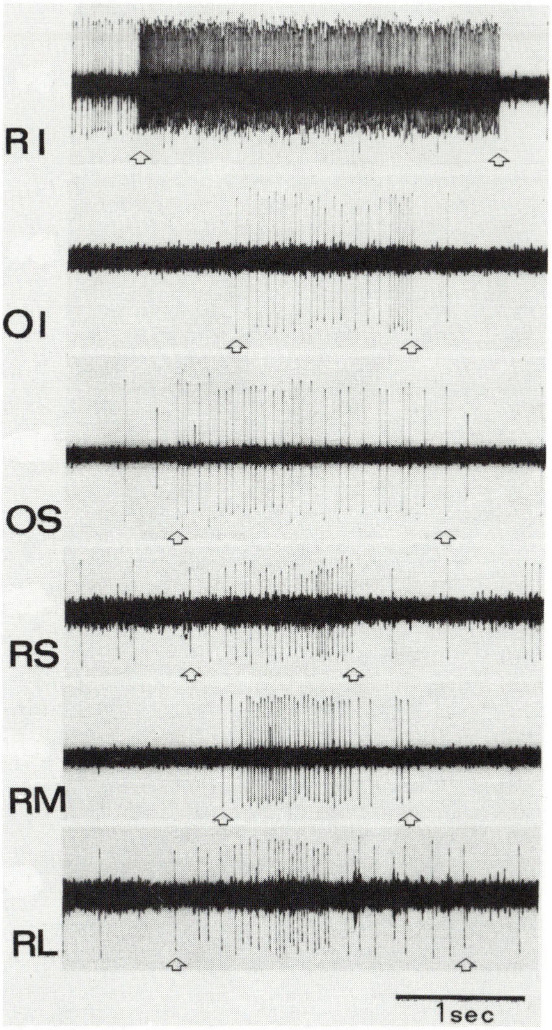

Fig. 2. Records of the unitary discharges in the superior colliculus during stretching (arrows) of single eye muscles. OI, inferior oblique, depth 8100 μm; RI, inferior rectus, depth 8500 μm; RS, superior rectus, depth 9200 μm; OS, superior oblique, depth 9600 μm; RM, medial rectus, depth 10300 μm; RL, lateral rectus, depth 10500 μm. All units were recorded along a single dorso-ventral penetration. Calibration: 1 sec. (From Marini and Bortolami, Exp.Neurol. (1980),69:226-238).

oblique. The medial and the lateral recti project in the most ventral position. Evoked potentials could be recorded from all the above mentioned areas by stimulating the proprioceptive cellular pool of the ipsilateral semilunar ganglion and the ipsilateral proprioceptive representation of the EOM in the oral portion of the spinal trigeminal nucleus and in the main sensory trigeminal nucleus (Manni, Palmieri and Marini, 1974). The latencies were shorter for pontine stimulations (0.30-0.40 msec) and longer (1-1.5 msec) when the semilunar ganglion was stimulated. In the former case no synapse was intercalated along the nervous pathway, while in the latter one, one or more synapses were interposed.

In some lambs discrete chronic lesions were performed in the pontine areas which contain the second-order neurons of the EOM proprioception. Degenerations were identified with Nauta-Gygax method along the ipsilateral medial lemniscus and dorsal trigemino-thalamic tract; they ended in the ventro-basal complex of the ipsilateral thalamus. Thus it seems reasonable to maintain that the second-order neurons of the EOM proprioception terminate in the same thalamic regions in which the afferents from the somatic sensitivity impinge.

Lastly it must be remembered that units influenced by EOM stretch were found at the level of the lateral geniculate body by Donaldson and Dixon (1980) in the cat. Other researchers have been able to identify a cortico-cerebral representation of the EOM proprioception. A projection of the EOM afferents has been shown on the Clare-Bishop area of the cerebral cortex of the cat by Donaldson (1979), however, the responses he recorded exhibited a quick adaptation, while this is not the case for the mesodiencephalic representation in the Ungulata. A representation of the EOM afferents in the visual cortex of the cat has been recently postulated by Buisseret and Maffei (1977), Maffei and Fiorentini (1977) and by Buisseret (1979). Also the cerebellum receives proprioceptive informations (Fuchs and Kornhuber, 1969; Azzena, Desole and Palmieri, 1970; Rahn and Zuber, 1971; Baker, Precht and Llinas, 1972; Batini, 1979 b; Maekawa and Kimura, 1980); this will be discussed later.

PHYSIOLOGICAL ROLE OF EOM PROPRIOCEPTION

Different hypotheses have been advanced by several researchers on the physiological meaning of EOM proprioception.

Sherrington (1918) first suggested that EOM proprioception has a perceptual role. However, Brindley and Merton (1960) demonstrated that only large eye excursions are perceived by human beings. Sherrington's idea of a perceptual role of EOM proprioception was retaken by Skavenski (1972) who elaborated an ingenious technique by means of which he was able to show that subjects could detect the presence of a load and could indicate the direction of pull of their eyes. He provided evidence also that perception of the direction of eye movements is related mainly to the command sent to the EOM and that the proprioceptive information has a scarce influence when the inflow from one eye is in conflict with the command sent to both eyes.

EOM stretch reflex. The existence of EOM stretch reflex is debated. It is generally denied by the great majority of researchers. No muscle contraction following stretch of eye muscles has been consistently demonstrated as is the case for limb muscles. However, it must be pointed out that the presence of a direct trigeminal oculomotor pathway has been postulated (Manni and co-workers, 1981): in fact unilateral section of the trigeminal root without any damage to the cerebral hemispheres in the lamb, pig, calf, rabbit and guinea pig is followed by appearance of degenerated boutons on either the somata or the dendrites of the ipsilateral oculomotor neurons. On the other hand the cut of both oculomotor nerves induces tigrolysis in all the motoneurons of the third nucleus: therefore the presence of internuncial neurons at the level of the oculomotor nucleus is improbable in accordance with Warwick's (1964) observations (Bortolami, in preparation). However, despite of the fact that a true monosynaptic reflex has never been proved, some reflex action of EOM has been reported following EOM stretch. Occasional observations of excitatory or inhibitory responses of EOM have been mentioned by Cooper, Daniel and Whitteridge (1953), Baichenko, Matyushkin and Suvorov (1967) and more recently by Bach-y-Rita (1972). According to Sasaki (1963) stretch of an EOM can hyperpolarize the third nerve motoneurons, however, Baker and Precht (1972) did not confirm such a finding. Goldberg, Hull and Buchwald (1974) showed that interneurons can be orthodromically activated by afferent fibres; however, the intracellular stimulations of these interneurons did not produce any activity in the eye muscles (Goldberg, Lennerstrand and Hull, 1976). Keller and Robinson (1961) did not observe any change on the activity of the abducens nuclei during forced eye movement or during restrained eye. Such a problem has been reinvestigated by Pettorossi and Filippi (1981) in our laboratories (Fig. 3). By selective block of the first-

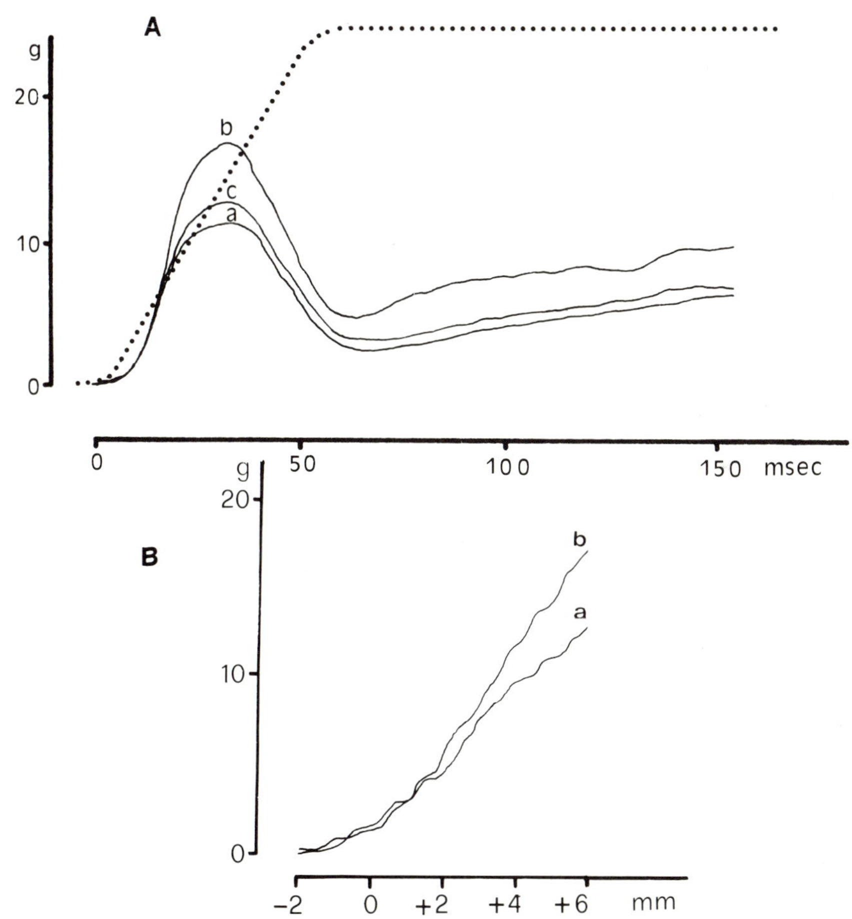

Fig. 3. Tension values of medial rectus muscle during fast (140 mm/sec) A and slow (.8 mm/sec) B ramp stretches. Each trace is the average of 16 single curves. a: before the block; b: 10 min and c: 40 min after the block. In A the dotted line indicates the ramp stretch stimulus. Abscissa: time in msec; ordinate: tension in g. B: abscissa: length in mm; ordinate: tension in g. (From Pettorossi and Filippi, 1981, in press).

order neurons of EOM proprioception in the semilunar ganglion, they observed an increase in the tension of EOM deviated from the primary position more than 18°. Furthermore the spindles of the same EOM could be selectively activated by vibrating the muscle. The electromyogram of the EOM was inhibited. According to Pettorossi and Filippi the EOM spindles seem to influence the eye motility by reducing the resistance of the antagonistic EOM during large and fast eye movement.

Influence of eye muscle stretch on the neck and the limb postural tone. Easton (1971) reported that stretching EOM, in particular the medial rectus, could inhibit the musdes of the neck and the limbs in the cat. According to Easton there is a reflex from eye muscle stretch which could have the physiological meaning of facilitating the labyrinthine reflexes, perhaps timing their oscillations. Manni and co-workers (1975b) confirmed the Easton's findings on the lamb, rabbit and cat. Our observations supported the view that EOM proprioceptors can modulate the extensor muscles of the neck; however, we have seen that impulses from various trigeminal fields could also affect the neck extensor muscles: in fact similar neck responses could be consistently elicited by electrical stimulation of different trigeminal afferents as those running in the maxillary branch, in the supraorbital and infraorbital nerves (Fig. 4). The neck muscles responded also to pinching the

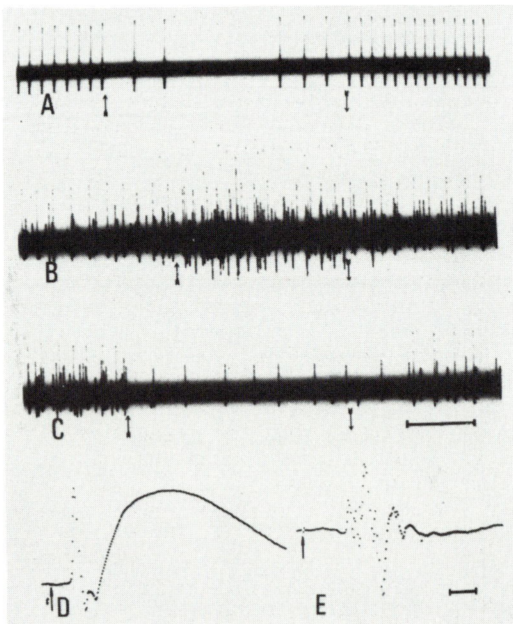

Fig. 4. Three electromyograms recorded from the dorsal muscles of the neck in a lamb. A: inhibition of the electrical activity elicited by stretch (arrows) of the contralateral inferior oblique muscle. B: contralateral activation and C: contralateral inhibition evoked by electrical stimulation of the left supraorbital nerve (0.7 V, 1 ms, 10/s). Calibration: time 0.5 s. D and E: averages of 64 ipsilateral (D) and contralateral (E) responses of neck muscles elicited by electrical stimulation of a medial part of left semilunar ganglion (0.5 V, 1 ms, 1/s). Calibration: time 5 ms. (From Manni and coworkers, Exp.Neurol. (1975), 47, 330-342).

skin of the face and in particular of the eyelid and to digital pressure of the annulus of Zinn at the apex of the orbit. It is evident that the influence of the EOM stretch on the neck extensor muscles is not a specific and peculiar effect of the EOM proprioceptors but it can also be elicited by stimulating other trigeminal afferents. Thus we have suggested another explanation: the neck responses elicited by stimulating the EOM proprioceptors and other trigeminal receptors can be considered as avoiding or defence reflexes of the animal. Such an assumption is supported also by the fact that the reflex responses of the neck extensor muscles were elicited by loading single eye muscles of the lamb with at least 20 g; usually the effect occurred with a load of 30-40 g. However, it must be pointed out that the threshold for activating the eye muscle spindles in the lamb was much lower: 0.5-5 g (Manni, Bortolami and Desole, 1966, 1968). Therefore it is doubtful that the eye muscle spindles play a fundamental role in such a phenomenon; probably it depends upon excitation of the Golgi organs which have a higher threshold than the eye muscle spindles or of the free nervous terminations contained in the extraocular muscles. Such an interpretation is supported also by an analysis of the muscle responses induced by stretching extraocular muscles: they did not cease immediately when the stretch was released as it happens for the responses elicited by muscle spindle excitation, but they persisted for some seconds as an after-discharge (Manni and co-workers, 1975b).

Cerebellum and extraocular muscle afferents. Since the cerebellum is involved in eye movements (Dow and Manni, 1964) several researchers have shown that EOM proprioceptive informations reach its cortex, in particular the lobules V, VI and VII, involving both the mossy and the climbing fibres. Kornhuber (1971) suggested that the cerebellum could exert a control on the eye saccades by transforming space (distance to be moved) into time (neuronal discharge duration) which determines the amplitude of saccades. It has been reported that a certain number of Purkinje cells fire in relationship to eye movements only in the ipsilateral direction. Recent investigations (Batini, 1979) have shown that the latency of the cerebellar EOM projections is compatible with a feed-back loop having a delay short enough to influence the late part of the saccade. The saccadic velocity of stretch seems to be the mechanical parameter for the EOM receptor excitation producing a phasic excitatory or inhibitory response of the Purkinje cells. No velocity sensitivity has been observed; however, the cerebellum could be informed on the plan and direction of eye movement.

The role of the cerebellum in controlling eye movements and in particular saccades has been reinvestigated very recently by Optican and Robinson (1980). Monkeys were trained to fixate small target lights. One horizontal rectus muscle was weakened by tenectomy; saccades made by this weakened eye were hypometric and followed by post-saccadic drift. When the weak eye was viewing, the hypometric saccades became essentially orthometric after 3 days. Total cerebellectomy induced an enduring saccadic hypermetria and post-saccadic drift in the unoperated eye and suppressed all adaptive repair of the saccadic system. Discrete lesions of lobules IV-IX and of the fastigial nuclei created an enduring saccadic hypermetria without post-saccadic drift in the unoperated eye, however, abolished adaptive control of the pulse of innervation. Thus the midline cerebellum is important in repairing saccadic dysmetria but not for repair of post-saccadic drift. Following cerebellar lesions the monkeys were able to make saccades of all amplitudes and direction, however, the pulse and step of innervation were no longer appropriate to target displacement. According to Optican and Robinson (1980) the main cerebellar contribution to saccadic eye movements is the adjustement of the gains of the pulse- and step-generating mechanisms.

EOM proprioception and the superior colliculus. It has been suggested that the representation of EOM proprioception in the superior colliculus could play an important role in the stabilization of perceived objects during eye movements.

Several investigators have analyzed the relationship of the EOM afferents reaching the superior colliculus to visual stimuli (Abrahams, 1979; Batini and Horcholle-Bossavit, 1979; Donaldson and Long, 1980). Units have been identified and localized histologically in the superior colliculus of the cat which responded to moving stimuli presented to the contralateral eye; they were inhibited or excited by electrical stimulation of the nerves to ipsilateral medial rectus and lateral rectus muscles containing afferent proprioceptive fibres. Specifical visual responses were modulated, mostly inhibited by proprioceptive stimulations. On the other hand, proprioceptive responses could be modulated by moving light on some units not responding to specific visual stimuli.

Eye muscle proprioception and visual processes. Quite recently interactions between EOM proprioception and visual processes at the level of area 17 of the cerebral cortex have been claimed in the cat. In the strabismic kittens the proportion of binocularly driven neurons of the striate cortex is drastically reduced even if the animals are deprived of vision from the day when the strabism is induced. A necessary condition for maintaining the normal proportion of binocularly driven neurons of the area 17 is the symmetry of eye motility. Cortical binocular interaction can be impaired by asymmetrical motility of the eye in kittens and in adult cats from artificial strabism even in the absence of vision. Buisseret and Maffei (1977) and Maffei and Fiorentini (1977) reported that binocular interaction in the visual cortex is significantly reduced 15-20 days after interruption of the proprioceptive ocular input in the trigeminal ophthalmic branch.
On the other hand EOM proprioception can affect the visual cortex: electrical stimulation of the proprioceptive afferents at the infraorbital level showed that 25% of cortical units of the area 17 respond to electrical stimulation of the EOM nerves.
In agreement with such a result it must be pointed out that Donaldson and Dixon (1980) were able to identify units of the lateral geniculate body which were influenced by EOM stretch.

CONCLUSIONS

Finally from our present results and from other works in progress in our laboratories it seems possible to conclude that the EOM proprioceptive information of the Ungulata surely projects to the thalamus and probably ends at the level of the cerebral cortex.
While the peripheral and the central course of the EOM proprioception is well defined, it is more difficult to ascertain its true physiological meaning, which is certainly different from the one exerted by limb muscle receptors. In particular there is agreement on the absence of an EOM stretch reflex, although it is likely that the EOM afferents can influence the tension of the EOMs. In addition a direct trigemino-oculomotor connection has been demonstrated not only in the Ungulata, but also in species in which classical muscle spindles in EOMs do not exist. To this direct pathway between the trigeminal ganglion and the oculomotor nucleus can be ascribed the meaning and the value of an effective influence of exteroceptive stimuli on eye motility without any intervention from other nervous centres such as the cerebellum or the mesencephalon.
Convincing evidence has been provided that the cerebellum can utilize the EOM input for controlling the eye saccades. Further investigations are requested for verifying a possible role of the EOM proprioception in the integrative processes at the level of the visual cortex.

ACKNOWLEDGEMENT

Investigations supported by CNR and Ministero Pubblica Istruzione funds. We are indebted to Dr. D. Troiani and Miss A.M. Barazzoni for revision of the English text and to Mrs. B. Zannoni Nicoletti for technical assistance.

DISCUSSION: Session I - Eye Muscle Structure and Function

Monday, August 31, 1981

Participants:

J. Davidowitz
K. McNeer
G. Lennerstrand
N. Barmack
E. Manni

Question:

Do the small muscle fibers found in the orbital layer of the muscle show potentials which are recorded in the usual EMG? What is their place in the rank order of recruitment of extraocular muscle fibers or their special physiologic participation in the various types of eye movements?

Answer:

Davidowitz: Toward the middle of their length, the small diameter multiply-innervated fibers of the orbital surface layer in rat and rabbit appear to be similar to twitch fibers, in terms of the development of the sarcoplasmic reticulum as well as with regard to the prominent neuromuscular junction which they display in this fiber region. We have not as yet examined the histochemical and electrophysiological properties of orbital multiply-innervated fibers in rats. In rabbit, however, Ozawa, Cheng-Minoda, and others in this laboratory did find that some orbital multiply-innervated fibers are capable of conducting an action potential (Ozawa, et al., Documenta Ophthalmologica, 192-201, 1969).

Lennerstrand: In the cat, the mechanical and intracellular electrophysiologic responses of the slow, multi-innervated, nonconducting type of muscle unit is similar to the amphibian. We have not made intracellular recordings of the multi-innervated conducting fibers of the type described today.

McNeer: There is a definite need for relating the multiple approaches to EOM fiber investigation towards the goal of establishing a uniform fiber classification. Currently, the light microscopic classification initiated by Durston appears to be the superior histologic one, though the correlation to electrophysiological studies remains to be done.

Lennerstrand: From the data on cat extraocular muscle fibers it is suggested that the type 1, 2 and 3 identified by ultrastructural features by Alvarado and van Horn are twitch-type fibers which in histochemical terms are type II. Their type ultrastructure 4, a multiply-innervated amphibian-type fiber, is most likely histochemical type I. Their multi-innervated fiber type ultra-structure 5 would probably correspond to histochemical type IIC, similar to avian fibers histochemically.

In human extraocular muscle, where it is much harder to electrophysiologically identify the fibers, the histochemical properties are the most reliable guide and should form the basis of any study which attempts to relate form and function. The panel agrees that interrelationships of histochemical, light microscopic, EM, electrophysiological and mechanical physiologic properties is the next important and necessary step to make existing classifications useful.

Question:

The measured muscle stiffness seems to change with innervation in the cat; however, in human experiments, Collins, et al., showed stiffness to be independent of innervation.

Answer:

Barmack: The measurement of stiffness depends critically on the alignment of the length of the muscle with its normal physiological length. A millimeter error in the measured length of an extraocular muscle near the primary position would change the stiffness of the muscle near the primary position, particularly at low levels of innervation. As a muscle is stretched the stiffness becomes less sensitive to levels of innervation since the major opposing force would be attributable to the passive elastic properties of the stretched (over-stretched) muscle. It is possible that previous experiments on human extraocular muscle may have overestimated the length of extraocular muscles at primary position, and therefore obtained values of stiffness which were abnormally high, particularly around primary position.

Question:

In the human, movement of the eye does not elicit change in the myographic pattern or other measureable function. What are the afferents doing in EOM?

Answer:

Manni: Stretch of muscles generally greatly modulates function, but we agree that this is not true in the extraocular muscles. We have shown that the limb and neck muscle innervational changes due to extraocular muscle stretch originally presented by Easton also result from stimulation of many trigeminal afferents; we believe these to be an avoidance response. It is also worth pointing out that muscle spindles are not present in eye muscles of the cat, and that the stretch threshold for EOM afferents involved in the neck responses is quite high, much more so than for ordinary stretch afferents--these may be free nerve terminations in the muscle.

Granit: The concept of the stretch reflex has changed from that of a single mono- or disynaptic arc to a polysynaptic pathway of long loops with modulation of function several places along the loop. In particular, in the superior colliculus there is interaction of the ocular position, muscle innervation and vision.

Manni: Abrahams, Batini and Horcholle-Bosavit, Donaldson and Long have known that there is convergence of vision and eye muscle proprioception on units in the tegmentum and in the superior colliculus. It may possibly have the function of stabilizing perception during movement; modulation of the vision response from eye muscle stretch and modulation of the stretch response by visual imput have been demonstrated.

Question:

You have shown that there are histological changes in the agonist muscle in strabismus, the medial rectus in esotropia, the lateral in exotropia. What alterations exist in the so-called "contracture" of the antagonist muscle opposite the paretic muscle in acquired paralytic strabismus?

Answer:

McNeer: We have yet to find significant coring or other identifiable changes found by our techniques in these cases.

SECTION II

Coordinator: R. D. Reinecke

EYE MOVEMENT CONTROL IN STRABISMUS AND AMBLYOPIA

ABNORMAL EYE MOVEMENTS IN STRABISMUS AND AMBLYOPIA

L. W. STARK, K. J. CIUFFREDA and R. V. KENYON

Neurology Unit, University of California, Berkeley, USA

ABSTRACT

Precise eye movement recordings in patients with 'strabismus without amblyopia' and with 'amblyopia without strabismus' have revealed quite separate findings as regards their versional eye movements. Amblyopes have increased saccadic latencies, increased fixational drift, abnormal saccadic substitution in small amplitude smooth pursuit tracking---all relatable to sensory deficits. Strabismic patients show saccadic intrusions and latent and manifest nystagmus--- all related to gaze, motor control of the eyes.

Both groups show abnormal vergence eye movements. There is absence of disparity vergence. Instead accommodative vergence dominates together with monocularly driven binocular saccades. Inequality of these saccades is not produced by violations of Hering's Law of equal innervation, but rather by interaction in the extraocular muscles.

KEYWORDS

Strabismus; amblyopia; eye movement recordings; saccadic latencies; fixational drift; abnormal saccadic substitution; saccadic intrusions; latent nystagmus; manifest nystagmus; disparity vergence; accommodative vergence; unequal saccades; Hering's Law; computer simulation.

Strabismus and amblyopia are two common ocular conditions that routinely confront the clinical eye specialist (Buffon, 1746; Burian & von Noorden, 1974). In our research, we sought to determine the eye movement deficits attributed either to amblyopia or to strabismus.

I. VERSIONAL ABNORMALITIES IN AMBLYOPIA

i.- Increased saccadic latency. An important function of the saccadic eye movement system is foveation of peripheral retinal stimuli. Saccadic latency has been extensively studied in normal human subjects, whereas few investigations of saccadic latency have been conducted in subjects having amblyopia and strabismus.

Increased saccadic latencies were observed in amblyopic eyes in six of 11 subjects having amblyopia with or without strabismus (Fig. 1a) (Ciuffreda, Kenyon, & Stark 1978a; 1978b). Significant increases in latency or differences between dominant and nondominant eyes in our two subjects having intermittent strabismus without amblyopia were not observed (Fig. 1b).

We studied targets in the 'near periphery' and found significant effects. Mackensen (1958) used more peripheral stimuli, greater than 15 degrees, and reported no increase (250 vs 225 ms); he theorized that the peripheral retina was little, if at all, affected in amblyopia and turned to eye-hand reaction time measures to study the central retina. He now found dramatic differences in reaction time between the amblyopic and normal eye (325 vs. 225 ms), and this was confirmed by von Noorden (1961) and Goldstein & Greenstein (1971).

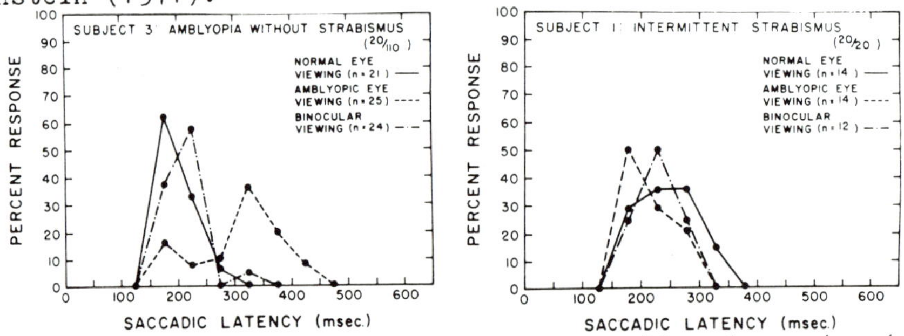

Fig. 1. Increased saccadic latency in amblyopia contrasted with normal saccadic latency in strabismus.

ii.- Increased Fixational Drift. Drift refers to slow movement of the eye during attempted steady fixation. Drift was considered abnormal if the amplitude exceeded 12 min arc and/or the velocity exceeded 20 min arc/sec; these criteria were developed in our oculomotor laboratory following testing of several hundred individuals, including experienced normal subjects, naive normal subjects, and clinic patients. Increased drift was related to the presence of amblyopia, since it was found in amblyopia without strabismus but not in strabismus without amblyopia (Ciuffreda, Kenyon, & Stark 1979e; 1980). Increased drift amplitude and velocity in the amblyopic eye was in strong contrast to monocular steady fixation with the dominant eye or with binocular fixation.

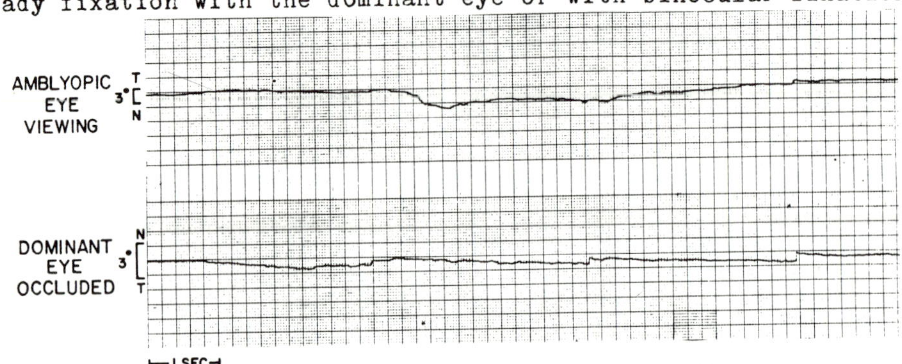

Fig. 2. Increased fixational drift.

Recordings of binocular eye movement during monocular fixation with the amblyopic eye clearly show that the large, slow movement in the amblyopic eye is drift and is not due solely to accommodative vergence, since the movement is largest in the viewing eye (Fig. 2). It is not due solely to smooth pursuit, since the movements are nonconjugate. Finally, it is not due to disparity (fusional) vergence, since the movements are not symmetrical, and they occur with one eye occluded.

The paucity of corrective fixational saccades with amplitudes comparable to the drifts meant that errors created by abnormal drift were generally corrected by drift movements in the opposite direction. This suggests that the microsaccadic system, one of whose normal functions is to correct for drift-induced fixation errors, may be less effective in amblyopic eyes, perhaps related to increased saccadic latencies. Drift may also be due to delayed or reduced velocity error detection in the smooth pursuit velocity-correcting system, or to normal drift characteristics for fixation with a non-foveal region (Zeevi, Peli, and Stark, 1979), as most patients had eccentric fixation. Increased drift might degrade visual acuity not by producing retinal-image motion across the fovea, but by moving the retinal image on to more eccentric positions, while increased drift amplitudes would also contribute to increased variability in any acuity measure.

iii.- Decreased smooth pursuit gain. Pursuit gain for tracking of targets having larger amplitudes (4 and 8 deg) was also of interest. When visual acuity was decreased, low gain pursuit, followed by large saccades correcting for position errors, was observed (von Noorden & Mackensen 1962; Fukai, Tsutsui, & Nakamura 1976; Schor 1975). However, once visual acuity reached 20/25, pursuit gain was generally higher and less variable. Pursuit gain for monocular tracking with the dominant eye generally was within normal limits for our laboratory standards.

iv.- Saccadic Substitution. The results of small-amplitude ramp tracking with the amblyopic eye clearly demonstrated that patients primarily used saccades rather than smooth pursuit movements to follow the target (Fig. 3) (Ciuffreda, Kenyon, & Stark 1979b). Substitution of abnormally large saccades for small-amplitude smooth pursuit movements occurred during small-amplitude, constant-velocity tracking with the amblyopic eye in response to both nasalward and templeward target motions on the retina (Fig. 3).

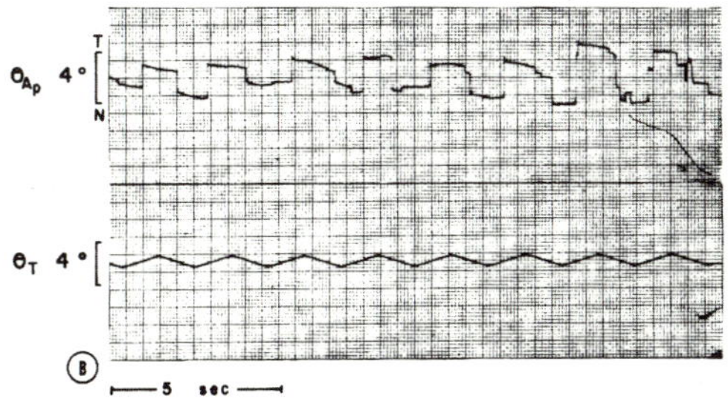

Fig. 3. Abnormal saccadic substitution.

That tracking small-amplitude stimuli binocularly or monocularly with the dominant eye never resulted in abnormal saccadic substitution further points to a sensory rather than motor basis for this pursuit defect.

Although there is no clear mechanism to explain the phenomenon of abnormal saccadic substitution, we may discuss three possibilities. The first is abnormal direction sense in amblyopic eyes. As a result of amblyopia, a depression of the directional-sensitivity gradient over the central retina may occur. This could result in impaired and/or marked variability of direction sense, including errors or biases in estimation of angular distance of targets relative to the preferred fixation locus. In the present situation, overestimation of small-angle target movements on the retina would result in the inappropriately large eye movements exhibited by our patients. It is interesting to speculate that our notion of abnormal direction sense in amblyopic eyes, based upon dynamic test results, may be related to eccentric fixation, which is based upon static test results. Eccentric fixation is found in the majority of amblyopic eyes, and its presence suggests a shift in the zero sensorimotor directional reference point under "steady-state" monocular test conditions. A second mechanism is suppression, commonly found in amblyopic eyes under binocular test conditions. A sensorially depressed central zone would correspond to all or part of the area undergoing suppression in the amblyopic eye during binocular viewing. If this is true, a strategy of placing the target just outside this depressed region might be adopted during monocular tracking with the amblyopic eye. Direction, amplitude, and velocity of target movement could be processed for a longer period of time and could provide a possible explanation for the abnormal tracking response, consistent with other delays in amblyopic eyes. A third explanation might simply be that abnormal saccadic substitution represents a normal phenomenon for small-amplitude pursuit tracking with the peripheral retina. However, the persistence of this abnormal response in one subject whose fixation centralized during orthoptics therapy (see II.4 below) does not lend support to this idea.

v.- Orthoptics. Quantitative eye movement analysis was carried out in an amblyope during an extended period of orthoptics treatment (Ciuffreda, Kenyon, & Stark 1979a). Several aspects of eye movement control improved in the amblyopic eye during treatment: decrease in drift amplitude, decrease in drift velocity, increase in pursuit gain (Fig. 4).

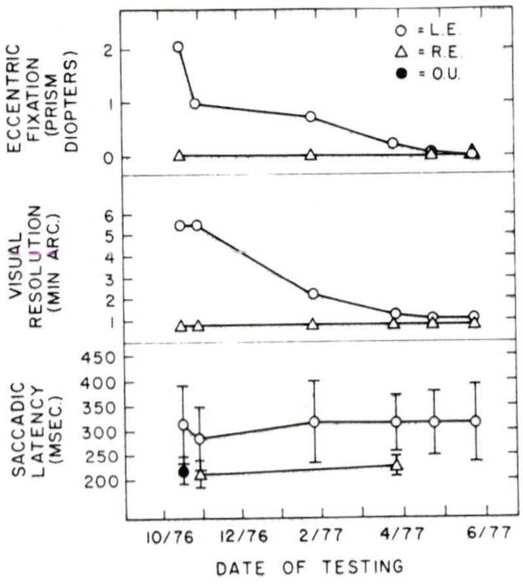

Fig. 4. Orthoptics treatment of amblyope showing amelioration of visual functions without normalization of prolonged saccadic latencies.

These findings demonstrate that as amblyopia decreased and fixation became centralized, certain aspects of eye movement control, primarily under the province of the smooth-pursuit system, could be modified by the orthoptics therapy. Furthermore, the findings suggest that the "critical period" for oculomotor plasticity for these aspects of eye movement our amblyope extended into adulthood.

However, other aspects of eye movement control in the amblyopic eye remained abnormal throughout treatment: increased saccadic latencies, abnormal saccadic substitution, and static overshooting. Perhaps, those neural channels and neural elements for spatial resolution and responsible for eccentric fixation, can be functionally modified in the adult amblyope and require a relatively short course of therapy for recovery (the visual acuity recovery function for our adult amblyope was similar to that measured in a very young amblyope). Perhaps for certain other neural channels and neural elements for saccadic initiation (probably "transient" channels) involved in saccadic initiation, recovery in an adult amblyope is either very slow or no longer possible. The increase in saccadic latencies suggests a processing delay over the central retina in the amblyopic eye involving pathways from the amblyopic eye to centers controlling saccadic initiation, such as the superior colliculus, although involvement of parietal lobe mechanisms underlying directed visual attention remains a distinct possibility.

Although only one patient was studied, we believe that our results and their clinical implications are of interest to those involved in clinical, as well as theoretical aspects of amblyopia.

II. VERSIONAL ABNORMALITIES IN STRABISMUS

i.- Saccadic intrusions. Saccadic intrusions are generally executed in opposite directions separated by 150-500 msec, occasionally less; the second saccade of an intrusion generally brings the eye back towards the baseline, resulting in little net change in eye position (Ciuffreda, Kenyon, & Stark 1979d; 1979e). Average intrusion amplitude was 0.7 degrees with a frequency about 1 per second. In most instances, the baseline position before and immediately after completion of a saccadic intrusion was similar. Subjects were able to follow random target step displacements to the left or right as small as 0.4 degrees in amplitude. In many instances, considerable drift did not precede initiation of the intrusion. When drifts did occur, the accumulated position error was usually corrected by a single saccade. These could be as small as 5 minutes in amplitude, as measured during high-gain recordings. Therefore, it is clear that saccadic intrusions are a pair (sometimes three) of pre-programmed saccades not serving that ocularmotor function of correcting for drift-induced position errors. Since saccadic intrusions were rarely found in amblyopia without strabismus, but typically found in strabismus without amblyopia, the intrusions appear to be related to the presence of strabismus and not amblyopia. Saccadic intrusions are frequently found in patients with neurological disorders, specific dyslexia, and schizophrenia and are also observed less frequently in normal subjects.

ii.- Special maneuvers with saccadic intrusions. Saccadic intrusions were found during monocular fixation with the amblyopic eye in four of five subjects with constant strabismus amblyopia. When a large amount of drift occurred with target fading, saccadic intrusions appear to be unrelated to abnormal eye position or error detection in the amblyopic eye. (The asymmetric dead zone is believed to be due to hemiretinal suppression in the deviated eye.) Saccadic intrusions were not at all the pattern of correction of drift error, but rather this was carried out by one or more unidirectional corrective saccades. Significantly, saccadic intrusions then occurred after reappearance of the target (Fig. 5). Thus there is no evidence to related saccadic intrusions to a 'Lawwill (1968) adaptive phenomenon'---to prevent fading or to 'revive' a faded retinal image.

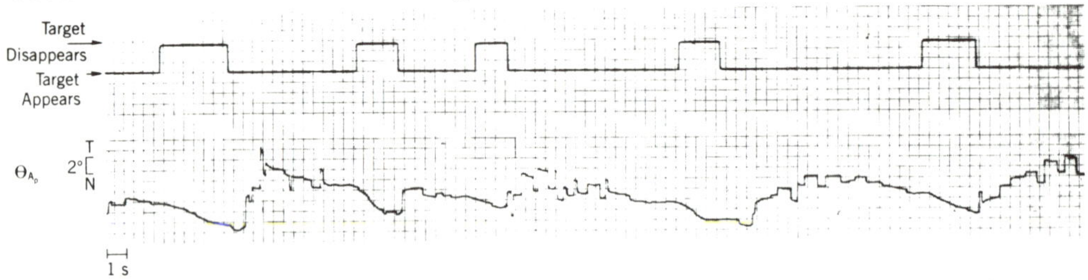

Fig. 5. Saccadic intrusions are not produced when fixation target "fades" or disappears.

Steinman, Cunitz, Timberlake, & Herman (1967) observed that microsaccades could be suppressed when experienced subjects were instructed to 'hold their eye steady' rather than 'fixate' in the presence of a visible target. During the 'hold' command, our patients remarked that they did not pay as much attention to target detail, and perhaps position errors, as they did during the 'fixate' command. However, during both sets of instructions, attention and motivation to perform the prescribed task successfully was high. Some stated that the amblyopic eye seemed more unsteady during the 'hold' command, but that target clarity was similar for both conditions. One patient noted that, at times, she relaxed accommodation and maintained relatively steady, 'saccade-free' fixation by concentrating on the defocused image; at other times, defocusing was not essential to suppress her fixational saccades.

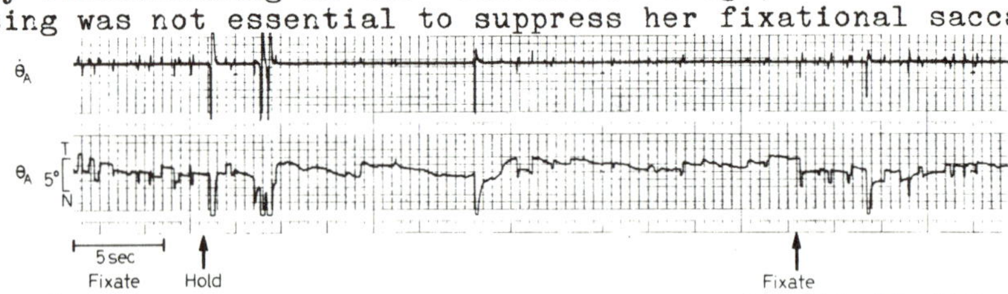

Fig. 6. Saccadic intrusions are suppressed with "hold" command.

The observation most pertinent to our patients was that during the 'hold' command, there was a marked reduction in saccadic intrusion frequency especially easy to see in the velocity traces (Ciuffreda, Kenyon, & Stark 1979c). An earlier report of our work was confirmed by Schor and Hallmark (1978). In contrast, during the 'fixate' command saccadic intrusions occurred at usual rates and amplitudes (Fig. 6). Thus, ocular-motor intentional fixational gaze, rather than a sensory-related phenomenon such as might result from strabismus-induced 'fixation degradation', is implicated in the saccadic intrusion generating mechanism in our strabismus patient. At times saccadic intrusions could be suppressed, but with occurrence of increased drift amplitude and velocity. At other times, and in other patients, suppression of saccadic intrusions was possible without occurrence of markedly increased drift. Again, this implicates an intentional gaze mechanism for saccadic intrusion and relates them to fixational microsaccades that have been suspected to have other than error-correcting functions.

Interestingly, changes in instruction to strabismic or amblyopic subjects from "fixate carefully on the target" to "hold the eye steady" (in the presence of the target) could decrease fixational saccadic frequency by 50% to 90%, similar to that found for normal persons.

iii.- Latent nystagmus. Latent nystagmus is a disorder of the oculomotor system wherein the nystagmus is not present during binocular viewing, but only upon occlusion of an eye; a conjugate jerk nystagmus with the fast (saccadic) phase towards the viewing eye then ensues. The slow phase in the 'gazing' eye is nasal (Fig. 7, left). The term 'gazing' eye is used instead of viewing eye since it is suspected that a motor control deficit and not a sensory abnormality underlies the genesis of latent nystagmus. Evidence for this comes from van Vliet's (1973) experiment with an Ewald pseudoscope; here the latent nystagmus occurred with the slow phase nasally in the eye through which the subject directed his gaze and via which he incorrectly thought he was viewing! The association of latent nystagmus with alternating hyperphoria (Anderson 1954) again suggests a motor gaze deficit and not a sensory one. Burian and von Noorden (1974) prefer the term dissociated vertical deviation to emphasize the noncomitant and nonvergence nature of the deficit wherein "either eye turns up when the fellow eye fixates." Latent nystagmus was found in two out of eighteen patients with strabismus; it was not found in any patients having amblyopia only. Latent nystagmus had a mean frequency of 1.7 Hz, a mean amplitude of 1.0 degree, and a mean slow phase velocity of 2.0 deg./sec.; similar values were found when either the dominant or the non-dominant eye fixated. With our precise recording techniques we could be quite sure that our cases of latent nystagmus did not conceal a manifest nystagmus of very low amplitude (Dell'Osso, Schmidt, and Daroff, 1979).

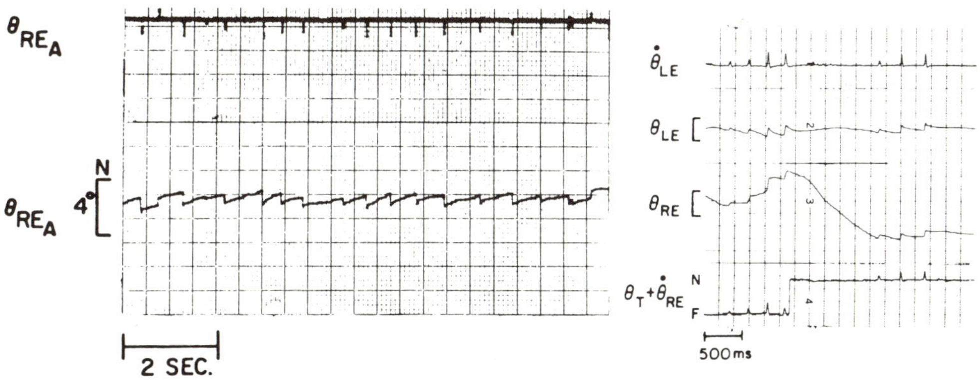

Fig. 7. Latent nystagmus (left) with nasal drift of gazing eye and Manifest nystagmus (right) superimposed on ongoing divergence.

iv.- Manifest nystagmus. Manifest nystagmus is a disorder of the oculomotor system wherein jerk nystagmus is present during monocular and binocular conditions in patients with strabismus. Again, as with latent nystagmus, manifest nystagmus was found in four out of eighteen patients with strabismus, and, in agreement with Gillies (1968), not in patients having only amblyopia (Ciuffreda, Kenyon, & Stark 1979e). Monocular fixation with the amblyopic eye in a patient increased the amplitude of manifest nystagmus to 5 degrees as compared with 1.5 degrees with monocular fixation with the dominant eye or 2.5 degrees with binocular fixation. When one patient changed from fixation in the light to "fixation" in total darkness, mean nystagmus amplitude increased. This suggests that in the light a velocity-correcting system (probably smooth pursuit) requiring visual feedback was operating to counteract the true nystagmus as revealed in the dark; again, evidence pointing to a motor gaze defect rather than to a sensory deficit underlying manifest nystagmus.

When one of our patients with manifest nystagmus made vergence eye movements, the slow phase of the nystagmus summated algebraically with that of a vergence. In the divergence movement (Fig. 7, right) the slow phase of the nystagmus and the accommodative vergence in the viewing eye oppose each other. This interaction counteracts the slow phase of the nystagmus, keeping the viewing eye stationary on the target. With no drift of the eye off the target, the saccadic phase of this nystagmus was absent. This shows that the slow phase in this patient's nystagmus is primary and that the saccade is used to correct for the retinal error produced by the drift.

III. VERGENCE ABNORMALITIES IN STRABISMUS AND AMBLYOPIA

i.- Absence of disparity vergence. Most patients with strabismus and/or amblyopia did not perform normal disparity vergence responses (Kenyon, Ciuffreda, & Stark 1980a; 1981). Although latencies were normal, patients made unequal vergence movements in each eye. Vergence amplitudes were always smaller in the dominant eye than in the fellow eye; the average vergence amplitude of the dominant eye was approximately 18% of that of the fellow eye. The unequal vergences were accompanied by a binocular saccade that served to place the fovea of the dominant eye close to the new target. The combination of this saccade and the small amplitude vergence functioned to place and maintain the dominant eye on the new target (Fig. 8).

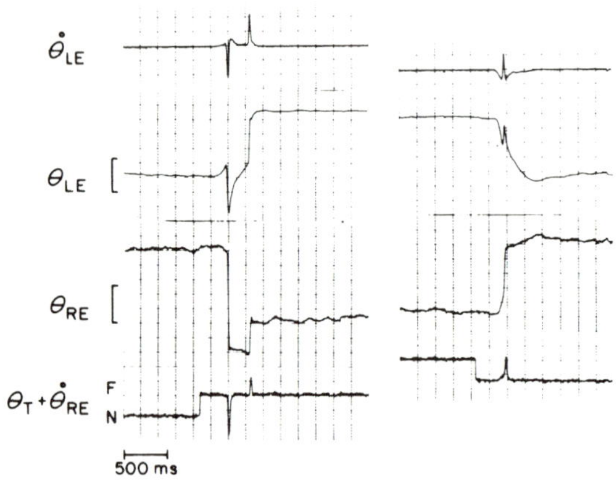

Fig. 8. Abnormal vergence in amblyopia and in strabismus: absence of disparity vergence, with presence of asymmetrical accommodative vergence and monocularly driven saccades; note inequality of saccades due to muscular interaction.

When one eye was occluded, responses of control subjects to the symmetric vergence stimuli resembled responses recorded in our patients under binocular viewing conditions. Each contained unequal vergence with the smaller amplitude occurring in the viewing eye of the control subjects and the dominant eye of the patients. Each used a binocular saccade, triggered by the monocular retinal error in the viewing or dominant eye to bring the fovea of that eye near the new target. In the control subject we know that accommodative vergence produces the unequal vergence amplitudes since occluding one eye 'opens the loop' of the disparity vergence control system. We suspect accommodative vergence is also responsible for the unequal vergence movements in the patients, as will be shown below.

When patients were monocularly occluded, so that only the dominant eye viewed the symmetrically positioned targets, responses agreed both qualitatively and quantitatively with the symmetric vergence responses from these patients under binocular viewing conditions. As with the control subjects, blocking of one eye caused accommodation to drive vergence, producing unequal vergence amplitudes (Kenyon, Ciuffreda, & Stark 1978). The monocular retinal error produced by the target change caused a binocular saccade placing the dominant eye on the new target.

Neither degree of strabismus nor grade of amblyopia in patients with constant strabismus amblyopia had any effect on the responses to the symmetric vergence stimuli. Patients with small-angle strabismus and deep amblyopia produced symmetric vergence responses similar to those of patients who had mild amblyopia and small-angle strabismus. Furthermore, the presence of ARC did not alter the basic response. Within our group of patients three were successfully treated for amblyopia or strabismus. One patient received orthoptics therapy for amblyopia and eccentric fixation in the left eye. After training, his visual acuity increased from 20/110 to 20/20, and his eccentric fixation reduced from 2 prism diopters to zero. His vergence movements, recorded shortly after termination of orthoptics treatment, contained the same characteristic abnormal vergence response recorded in most of our patients. Thus, even after normalization of visual acuity and centralization of fixation, normal disparity vergence responses were never recorded in this former amblyope. Interestingly, some other oculomotor findings such as saccadic latency also remained abnormal in this patient during and subsequent to successfully amblyopia therapy. Patients with a history of strabismus as a child and surgical correction to reduce the strabismus were also included in our sample and again showed the typical abnormal vergence responses. Another patient who now has an exophoria was operated on at age 8 to correct a squint of his left eye. His symmetric vergence responses were similar to those of the other patients in our study having strabismus but who were not surgically corrected. However, still another patient who had an esotropia surgically corrected at age 3 and presently with esophoria, had intermittent episodes of normal convergence interspersed with more frequent abnormal responses. The striking absence of disparity-vergence in our patients may be related to stimulus form. If we had used large field stimuli (Hooten, Myers, Worrall, and Stark, 1979)) or if we had equalized perceptual efficacy of the stimulus to each eye (for example, by using neutral density filters in front of the dominant eye) we might have observed true disparity responses. This possibility is consistent with our notion of suppression as a common factor in strabismics and in amblyopes. Further research with careful eye movement recordings will decide whether the slow, irregular and inconsistent changes clinically observed with patients in amblyopscopes are in fact true disparity-vergence responses.

These results in our patients demonstrate the absence of disparity vergence, and the presence of normal accommodative-vergence, that together with monocularly generated binocular saccades, are able to move the dominant eye onto target.

ii.- Accommodative vergence. Disparity vergence is part of the near triad: accommodation, vergence and pupil (all linked synkinetically by fixed CNS connections). Thus, a disparity stimulus driving vergence also produces a vergence- accommodative response (with a gain of about 0.6 equivalent to a CAC ratio of 0.1 D/prism D); conversely, a blur stimulus driving accommodation also produces an accommodative-vergence response (with a gain of about 0.7, equivalent to an ACA ratio of 4 prism D/D). Maddox (1886) conjectured that ACC-VG was primary and a 'fusion supplement' completed the triadic response; Fincham and Walton (1957) measured the active VG-ACC and speculated that it was primary. Stark, following Donders and Hering (1868), felt that both ACC-VG and VG-ACC were always active and suggested that for a large enough disparity (a few degrees) the stimulus would lie off the fovea and the accommodation system would then be unable to appreciate target blur. This allowed VG-ACC to play a dominant role by providing a mechanism that acts on sensory input and not by changing synkinetic gains. Accommodative vergence was first studied by Mueller (1826) in his famous paradigm experiment; he observed that if one eye were covered, and the viewing eye changed fixation from a far to a near target along its line of sight, the covered eye rotated inward.

During accommodative vergence, binocular vergence movements were first observed and recorded by us in all of the several hundred eye movements analyzed in five subjects. This included viewing with the dominant and non-dominant eye, predictable and nonpredictable stimulus presentations, and for convergence and divergence. These records clearly demonstrate the binocular nature of accommodative vergence (Kenyon, Ciuffreda, & Stark 1978).

Our patient's recordings show the unexpected predominance of accommodative vergence. The absence of disparity vergence leave open the accommodative vergence triadic synkinesis mechanism as a continuing and powerful vergence response controller. The arguments for the presence of accommodative vergence in our patients are that the patients' monocular response is the same as their binocular response, that the patients' monocular response is the same as the normal subjects' monocular response, and that the binocularity of the patients' response is about the same amplitude of the normal subjects' response. The amplitude of vergence in the dominant eye is about 18%, 11%, and 6% of that of the non-dominant eye; in normal controls the amplitude of the viewing eye is about 12% of that of the covered eye.

iii.- Monocular- error- driven binocular saccades. The presence of the monocular driven binocular saccade in our patients is easily understood. Disparity may not be perceived because of the suppression of the non-dominant eye. The retinal eccentricity in the dominant eye is calculated as a horizontal position error that requires a horizontal saccade to correct it. The saccade should, of course, be binocular according to Hering's Law.

iv.- Unequal saccades: not a violation of Hering's Law. The occurrence of monocularly driven saccades upon a background of ongoing accommodative vergence in our patients with striking absence of disparity vergence provided the opportunity for a further exciting observation---the presence of apparently non-Hering's law saccades during vergence (Kenyon, Ciuffreda, & Stark

1976; 1977; 1980c; 1981; Kenyon and Stark 1981; Ono and Nakamizo 1978). These unequal saccades were present in at least 85% of the vergence movements found in all diagnostic groups of patients. In each saccadic pair, the smaller saccade opposes the vergence movement. Saccades that occur before and after the vergence have equal amplitudes, indicating that these unequal saccades are not an artifact of the recording system.

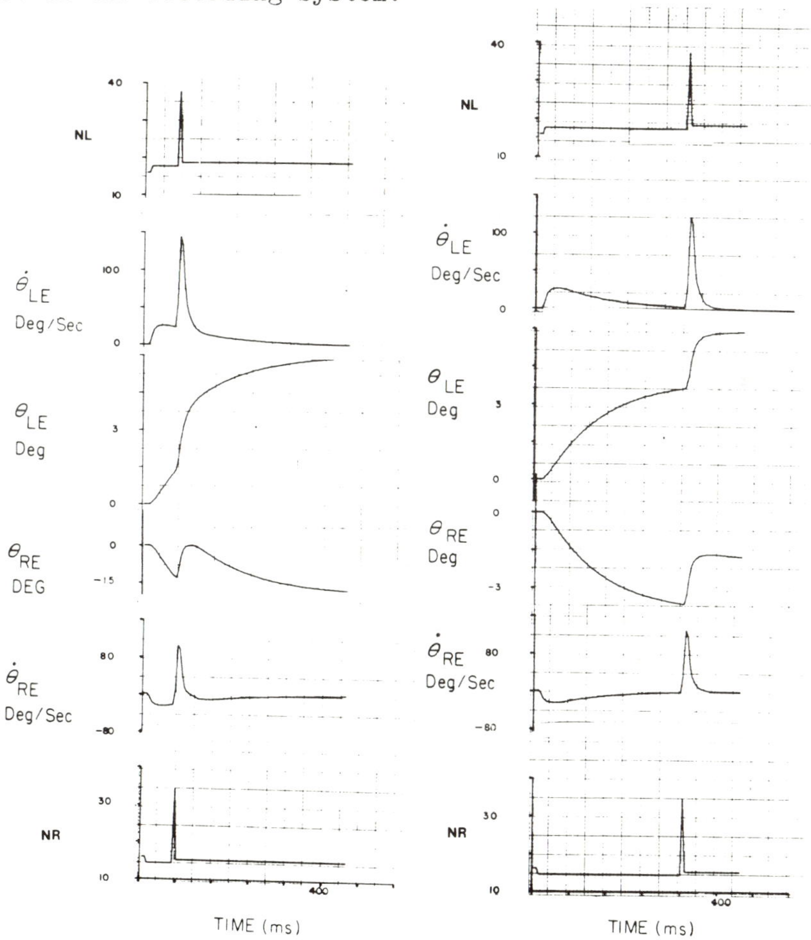

Fig. 9. Simulation producing unequal saccades by muscular interaction. Note linear addition of reciprocally innervated controller signals obeying Hering's law.

The inequalities of these saccades are not restricted to patients, since apparently non-Hering's law saccades are present during vergence movements in normals.

From Hering's Law of equal innervation we would expect binocular saccades to be equal. If the neurophysiological controller signals to the two eyes are different, then this would be a violation of Hering's Law. How can we identify the mechanism of production of the inequality of these saccades? One way is to simulate the interaction with linearly additive saccadic and vergence controller signals, thus obeying Hering's Law, acting on a biomechanical model of eye muscle and globe. Our studies showed (Kenyon and

Stark 1981) the saccades in the simulation to show inequalities similar to those seen in our patient group and in normal subjects with ongoing accommodative vergence or ongoing asymmetrical disparity vergence (Fig. 8). The same qualitative rule applies: saccades directed opposite the vergence are truncated in amplitude and velocity, and the opposite occurs for saccades going in the same direction as the vergence. Since the model obeys Hering's Law of Equal Innervation and uses only linear summation of controller signals, nonlinear summation of saccadic amplitudes with the ongoing vergence seen in these simulations must occur as the result of interactions within the biomechanical mechanisms of the plant model. We conclude that the inequality of saccades is due not to a violation of Hering's law but to a biomechanical interaction in the muscle globe plant.

IV. DISCUSSION

These results provoke many interesting questions. How can our simple separation of amblyopia without strabismus from strabismus without amblyopia be reconciled with more classical classifications? Will our findings be robust to further more extensive surveys with many more patients? What clues to the underlying deficits in neurological control of binocular vision can be extracted from our studies? Is suppression in strabismus and amblyopia the common mechanism blocking disparity vergence? Where are the neuroanatomical loci of the deficits? What are the neuropathophysiological mechanisms?

I would like to thank NASA-Ames Research Center for partial support (NCC 2-86).

VERGENCE EYE MOVEMENTS: BASIC ASPECTS

C. M. SCHOR

*University of California, School of Optometry,
Berkeley, California 94720, USA*

ABSTRACT

Maddox (1893) proposed a hierarchy of mechanisms including tonic, accommodative, fusional and proximal vergence that controlled disjunctive eye movements. Recent studies indicate that one of these mechanisms, fusional vergence, can be divided into 4 subcomponents. Two of these subcomponents, disparity induced and fusional vergence, initiate and complete, respectively, the vergence response to disparate stimuli. A third subcomponent, voluntary vergence, initiates rapid vergence responses to disparate stimuli selected from within complex patterns. A fourth subcomponent, adaptive vergence, maintains the vergence response and reduces stress manifest as fixation disparity, upon the fusional vergence system. There is an additional major component, vergence accommodation, that was unspecified by Maddox. Vergence accommodation and accommodative vergence constitute mutual interactions between the accommodation and convergence motor control systems. These mutual interactions can produce stress upon fusional vergence which can be quantified with steady state equations of accommodative-vergence interactions and displayed with a graphical technique in order to study their influence upon clinical disorders of binocular vision.

KEYWORDS

Disparity vergence, fusional vergence, voluntary vergence, prism adaptation, fixation disparity, Maddox hierarchy, accommodative vergence and vergence accommodation.

INTRODUCTION

In his classical description of disjunctive eye movements, Maddox (1893) proposed that there were four fundamental components of convergence: these being tonic, accommodative, fusional and proximal. He proposed that the combined response of these components resulted in alignment of the visual axes during binocular fixation. The classification was intended to indicate the time sequence of operation for the various components and some of the stimuli for vergence eye movements. It has provided a rationale for the current day clinical analysis of interactions between accommodation and convergence (Sheard, 1930; Fry, 1941; Morgan, 1941; Hofstetter, 1945). However, the classification tends to over simplify the complex organization of mechanisms that control vergence eye movements. For example, recent studies have identified three or perhaps four separate control mechanisms related to fusional vergence. The first of these initiates vergence eye movements in response to retinal image disparities as large as 5° (Westheimer and Mitchell, 1969; Jones and Kerr, 1971) which can be subtended by completely dissimilar forms such as vertical and horizontal lines. When similar and dissimilar disparate patterns are presented in combination, disparity vergence responds independently of target similarity to the smallest disparity in the field (Jones and Kerr, 1971). However, the vergence system is unable to complete its response to dissimilar shapes. Completion and maintenance of a vergence response requires that the uniocular images have similar shape and orientation so that they may be combined into a fused percept (Panum, 1858; Ogle et al., 1967). This end result is suggested by the term fusional vergence.

DISPARITY INDUCED AND FUSIONAL VERGENCE

Disparity induced and fusional vergence have been distinguished from one another by observations of vergence anomalies in stereoblindness. Richards (1970) first reported that some persons with normal stereo acuity exhibited reduced sensitivity to either large crossed or uncrossed disparities presented for very brief durations (80 msec). Jones (1977) observed that many stereoanomalous persons who had reduced sensitivity to one direction of disparity also had a reduced amplitude of vergence eye movements to disparities presented briefly (.2 sec) in the same direction (Jones, 1977). However, when the same persons were given ample time they were able to fully correct their heterophoria with fusional vergence eye movements and thereby obtain binocular alignment. These observations suggest that persons with stereoblindness lack the brisk reflex vergence response to large disparities but are able to complete and maintain vergence responses to small disparities between similar images.

Mechanisms that initiate and complete vergence movements have also been distinguished by a nonlinear effect of stimulus duration upon the direction of the vergence response (Jones, 1977). This nonlinearity is observed in persons whose vergence responses to crossed and uncrossed disparities are unequal in amplitude. When a small disparity is presented to stimulate the weaker mechanism, a brief presentation (.2 sec) causes an incorrect vergence response in the strong direction whereas a long presentation (4.5 s) causes correct responses in the weak direction. These differences in the amplitude and direction of vergence response to transient and continuously presented disparities suggest that there are two distinct processes, one that initiates and another that completes vergence response to disparate stimuli.

VOLUNTARY VERGENCE

A third form of vergence control related to fusional vergence initiates voluntary movements selectively in response to one of several alternative stimuli. These voluntary vergence movements are very fast (Crane, 1978) approaching the upper velocity limit for pursuit eye movements as is evidenced by the speed at which intermittent exotropes can willfully align their eyes. Voluntary vergence movements are essential in seeking out camouflaged surfaces such as those found in random dot stereograms that subtend disparities greater than Panum's fusion limit (Saye, et al. 1975). Vergence movements reduce disparity to within Panum's fusional limit so that the global camouflaged surface can be perceived. Voluntary vergence movements also extend the range of quantitative stereopsis to 24° (Foley and Richards, 1972) which is well beyond the 1° range of quantitative stereopsis found without voluntary vergence movements (Richards, 1977). It is unknown if voluntary vergence is controlled directly by the disparity vergence system or indirectly by voluntary control of accommodation with influences vergence via the accommodative convergence synkinesis (Jampolsky, 1970).

ADAPTIVE VERGENCE

A fourth mechanism related to fusional vergence maintains vergence eye movements by adapting the tonic innervation to convergence in the direction of the fusional vergence response. Adaptation is demonstrated by a change in heterophoria following efforts of fusional con and divergence. Figure 1 illustrates vergence adaptation as a function of the duration that fusional vergence is stimulated. The upper trace shows the relaxation of a 3° convergence response maintained for 5 seconds. When one eye is occluded the eye's position returns within 10-15 seconds to the usual phoria. This rapid decay of convergence is described as an exponential decay with a time constant of 10 seconds (Ludvigh et al., 1964; Krishnan and Stark, 1977). The lower trace illustrates that when convergence is stimulated for a longer duration (30 sec - one minute) the eyes do not relax to the usual phoria posture. The incomplete relaxation of fusional vergence can persist for several hours or for an indefinite period when the disparity vergence loop is opened for example by occluding one eye (Carter, 1965). The adaptation process is very slow, taking 30 seconds to several minutes for horizontal vergence responses (Schor, 1979) and minutes to hours for complete adaptation to vertical vergence responses (Ogle et al., 1967). The time course of adaptation is exponential with most of the effect occurring during the first few minutes that prism is worn (Henson and North, 1980). Reflex fusional vergence has a much shorter response time of 1 second (Rashbass and Westheimer, 1961). Because fusional vergence has nulled or reduced retinal image disparity to less than a minute of arc before vergence adaptation is complete, it is likely that the adaptation does not respond directly to retinal image disparity but rather to the amplitude of the fusional vergence response (Schor, 1979a).

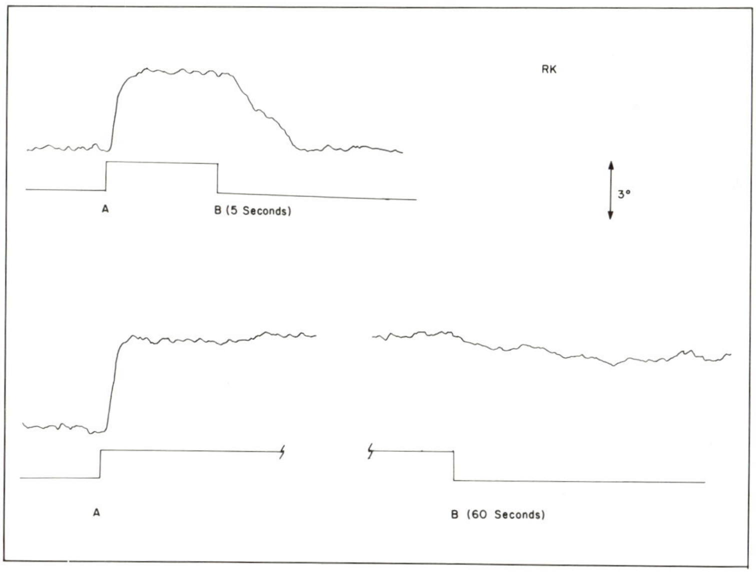

Fig. 1. Disparity-induced vergence, showing time constants for relaxation of fusional vergence after stimulating convergence for 5 sec. (upper trace). A, onset of stimulation; B, occlusion of one eye. Incomplete relaxation of convergence after long-term stimulation of convergence demonstrates vergence adaptation (lower trace).

Adaptation is related specifically to the control mechanism for fusional vergence because accommodative vergence stimulated monocularly does not cause adaptation of the heterophoria. However, binocular stimulation of accommodation does result in vergence adaptation in a direction corresponding to the correction of the heterophoria induced by accommodative convergence interactions. For example, minus lenses that stimulate accommodation and accommodative convergence cause a convergent increase in the phoria. Divergence compensation by the disparity vergence controller results in an adaptation of tonic convergence such that when the minus lenses are removed the phoria has changed in the divergent direction.

Three functional attributes have been suggested for vergence adaptation. Like the emmetropization process that coordinates the optical components of the eye to minimize refractive error, vergence adaptation could underlie similar process of orthophorization that coordinate neuromuscular mechanisms that control binocular alignment (Ogle et al., 1967; Carter, 1965; Crone and Hardowijoto, 1979). This mechanism could account for the high incidence of orthophoria in the normal population (Hirsch et al., 1948; Tait, 1951). If vergence adaptation did underlie the process of orthophorization then most persons demonstrating vergence adaptation should be orthophoric. However, examples have been reported where vergence adaptation occurs in persons with abnormal vertical phorias. In this case, adaptation to prisms adjusts the phoria to the pre-existing abnormal value (Ogle et al., 1967). Adaptation also occurs in people who have heterophorias other than ortho and in at least 75% of these cases the phoria is adjusted to its habitual amplitude while prism is worn (McCormack, 1981). It has been suggested that in these cases, vergence adaptation serves to maintain heterophoria rather than to correct it (Carter, 1957; Crone et al., 1979). A third function suggested for vergence adaptation by Hoffman and Bielschowsky (1900) is to minimize the load or stress upon fusional vergence by substituting the fusional innervational source with a change in tonic innervation to convergence. The source of stress upon fusional vergence is its exponential decay shown earlier (Schor, 1979b, 1980). The decay which is in effect during binocular viewing conditions is compensated for by a small error of convergence referred to as fixation disparity. This small vergence error provides a stimulus to replenish the constantly decaying source of vergence innervation during binocular viewing conditions. Fixation disparity rarely exceeds 6 arc min and is proportional to the amplitude of the fusional vergence response. The decay of convergence can also be eliminated by vergence adaptation that provides a substitute innervational source having little or no short term decay. Thus, when vergence adaptation replaces fusional vergence then the amplitude of fixation disparity, which compensates for the fast temporal decay of fusional vergence, becomes reduced or is eliminated (Schor, 1979b; 1980).

FIXATION DISPARITY

Control mechanisms for fusional vergence and vergence adaptation have been modeled in Fig. 2 as "leaky" neural integrators with short and long decay time constants respectively (Schor, 1979b). Fig. 3 illustrates the proposed trade off of innervation from the fusional vergence integral controller to the tonic integrator controlling adaptation. This model predicts that vergence adaptation should have a negative correlation with fixation disparity. Indeed, such a correlation has been reported (Schor, 1979a); low values of fixation disparity in one direction are usually associated with high vergence adaptation in the same direction of convergence. Occasionally equally low values of fixation disparity occur for both convergent and divergent stimuli even though the associated vergence adaptation is asymmetric. Thus, other motor factors such as the gain of the fast reflex fusion vergence controllers influence the amplitude of fixation disparity. Sensory factors such as central suppression in strabismus may also influence fixation disparity as well as vergence adaptation by limiting the stimulus to vergence eye movements to the peripheral retina (Jampolsky, 1956). The upper limit to fixation disparity is set by Panum's fusional area (Schor and Tyler, 1981). Because these areas increase with retinal eccentricity, central suppression will cause the vergence system to respond to peripheral fusion stimuli and permit greater amounts of fixation disparity without the disturbance of diplopia. Indeed, Ogle et al.(1967) reported that fixation disparity induced by wearing a fixed amount of prism was greater when measured with peripheral than with foveal stimuli for binocular fusion. Presumably central suppression will have a similar effect on the peripheral fusion stimulus.

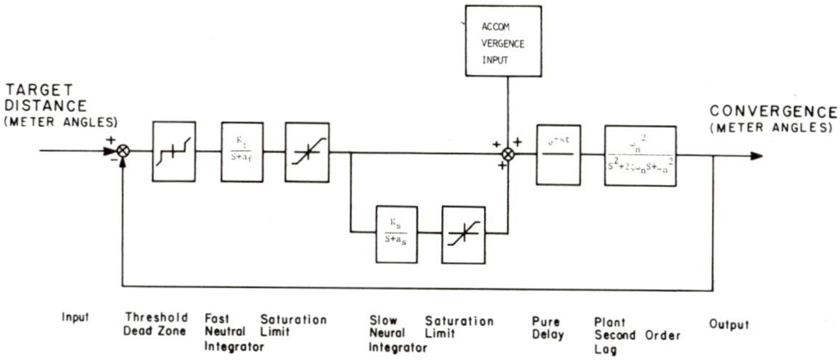

Fig. 2 Block diagram of the dual control mechanism of disparity vergence and its interaction with the accommodative motor system.

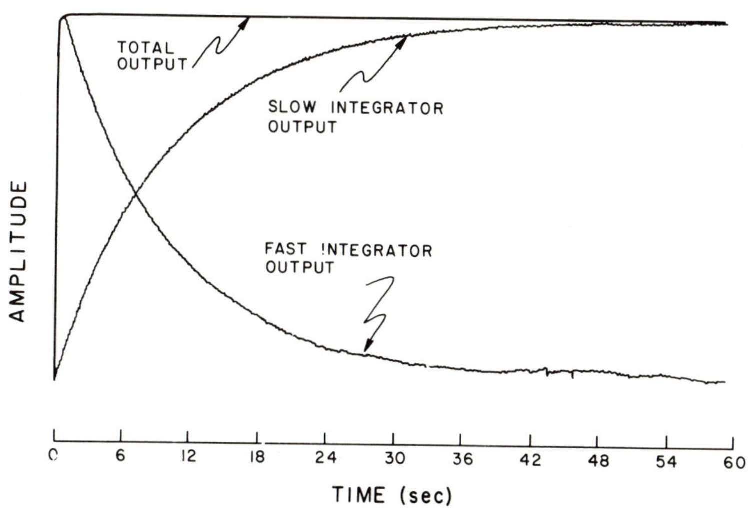

Fig. 3. Total prism adaptation illustrated by an analog computer simulation of the closed loop response of the 2 neural integral controllers of fusional vergence modeled in Fig. 2 and the output of the total vergence system. K_f=2.5; T_f=2.5; K_s=3; T_s=33; K_sT_s=100.

VERGENCE ACCOMMODATION

Another factor that appears to influence the magnitude of fixation disparity is vergence accommodation. Semmlow and Hung (1979) compared forced duction fixation disparity curves measured with a pinhole pupil (accommodation open loop) and with normal pupils (accommodation closed loop). They observed that fixation disparity was reduced by half when the accommodation loop was opened using the pinhole pupil. They conclude that during closed loop conditions forced convergence produced a change in accommodation via convergence accommodation. This change resulted in blur which was corrected by optical reflex accommodation. The correction of blur altered accommodative convergence in a way that increased the stimulus to fusional vergence and the magnitude of the resulting fixation disparity. For example, with forced convergence there is usually an exo fixation disparity. The model shown in Figure 4 illustrates how fixation disparity is increased by convergence accommodation. The convergence effort stimulates accommodation via convergence accommodation and causes an excessive accommodative response. This error, caused by convergence accommodation, is corrected by reducing the output of the controller of optical reflex accommodation. The reduction in accommodative effort also reduces accommodative convergence which in turn increases the phoria in the exo direction. The increase in exophoria increases the amount of exo fixation disparity that resulted from the high prism stimulus to convergence. Opening the accommodative sero loop with the pinhole pupil eliminates the focus errors and their correction caused by convergence accommodation and as a result reduces the amount of fixation disparity caused by prism stimuli for convergence. Thus, interactions between accommodation and convergence are complicated by convergence accommodation during binocular viewing conditions. This additional interaction will cause both lenses and prisms to have a greater effect upon fixation disparity predicted from the AC/A ratio than if the convergence accommodation interaction did not exist.

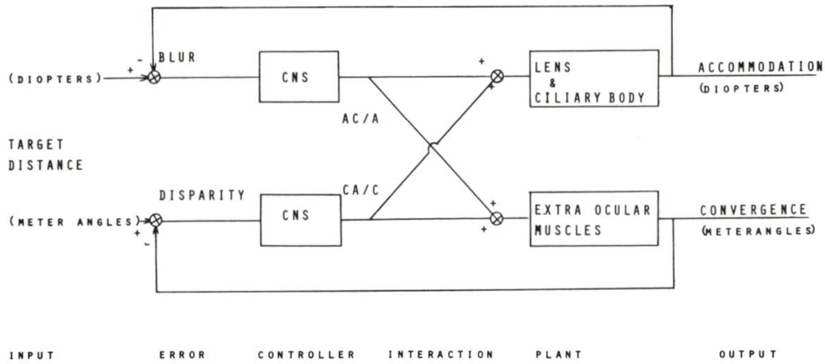

Fig. 4. Systems diagram illustrating the mutual interactions and feed forward cross links between the accommodative and convergence motor control systems.

The total demand upon the accommodative (A_D) and convergence (C_D) controllers under binocular (closed loop) viewing conditions is shown quantitatively by steady state equations 3 and 4 derived below (Schor and Narayan, 1982).

Given: Accommodation Response (AR) = $A_D + C_D \times (CA/C)$ (1)

Convergence Response (CR) = $C_D + A_D \ (AC/A)$ (2)

Where: AR = (1/viewing distance - depth of focus)

CR = (PD cm/viewing distance M) - (Distance Associate Phoria)

AR and CR remain fixed for a given viewing distance since both accommodative and convergence feedback loops are closed.

Then by substitution:

$$A_D = \frac{AR - CR \times (CA/C)}{1 - (AC/A \times CA/A)} \qquad (3)$$

$$C_D = \frac{CR - AR \times (AC/A}{1 - (AC/A \times CA/C)} \qquad (4)$$

The proposed interaction also predicts that the response levels or demands upon accommodation and convergence controllers will always be greater than the stimuli predicted from target distance and the phoria. This is most evident when the CA/C and AC/A ratios are reciprocally related. Under these circumstances the denominators of equations 3 and 4 become zero indicating that the interactions between accommodation and convergence will become unstable since the innervation required for their responses will be infinitely large or reach saturation. The reciprocal relationship between the AC/A and CA/C is approximated whenever either ratio is abnormally high.

The combined effects of convergence accommodation and accommodation convergence can also be illustrated graphically with the accommodation convergence plot shown in Fig. 5 for a person with a high AC/A ratio. The CA/C line is drawn through the associated phoria (X) and the AC/A line is drawn through the reference point representing the fixation distance. The associated phoria, which equals the prism that reduces fixation disparity to zero, is plotted rather than the disassociated phoria because it takes into account the effects of prism adaptation upon the phoria (Schor, 1980). The two lines intersect at a point indicating the amount of fusional vergence and additional accommodation that are necessary to overcome the underlying associated phoria. The horizontal and vertical vectors from the intersection point to the associated phoria indicate the horizontal demand upon convergence and additional adjustments of accommodation respectively (Schor and Narayan, 1982). In this example an associated phoria of 6 eso is corrected by a divergence effort equivalent to 18Δ and an increase in accommodation of 1.5D over the demand of the near viewing distance (2.5D). The closed loop demands upon convergence and accommodation would become extremely large if the AC/A and CA/C lines were parallel to one another. Figure 6 illustrates a similar analysis of a patient having a normal AC/A ratio of 4/1. The lower AC/A ratio results in a smaller demand upon fusional divergence than in the previous example.

CLINICAL IMPLICATIONS

These observations have important implications for accommodative esotropia caused by the combination of a high AC/A ratio and uncorrected hyperopia. The CA/C interaction increases the amount of eso deviation as the eyes attempt to diverge and correct the strabismus. In the case of accommodative esotropia, the high AC/A ratio approaches a reciprocal relationship with the CA/C ratio. Hence, the fusional vergence innervation needed to correct an eye turn caused by a high AC/A ratio may be many times greater than the amount expected for a person with a normal AC/A ratio to correct a vergence error equal to the same angle of deviation. This excessive innervation may account for the need to fully correct the strabismus with lenses and prisms rather than to partially correct the eye turn and leave a small convergence error which would normally be within the physiological

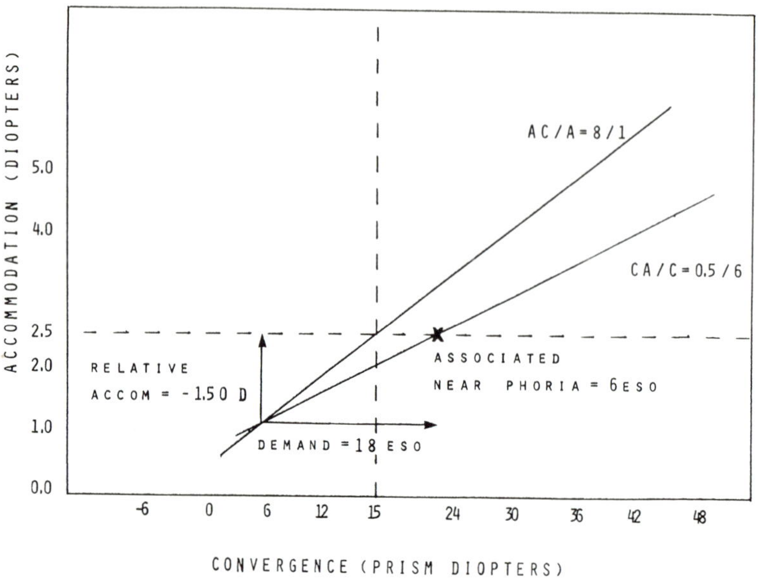

Fig. 5. The CA/C line drawn through the associated phoria (X) and the AC/A line drawn through the convergence accommodation reference representing the near test distance intersect at a point indicating the demand upon accommodation (1.5d) and convergence (18Δ) necessary to correct or overcome an associated phoria of 6 eso for a person with a normal(0.5D/6) CA/C ratio and a high (8/1) AC/A ratio. The demand upon accommodation and convergence controllers will become very large as the slope of the AC/A and CA/C become similar. Note that the reciprocal of the AC/A is plotted.

range of fusional divergence. Convergence accommodation may require a fusional divergence innervation beyond the physiological range of divergence to correct the remaining error. Lack of consideration of convergence accommodation would not discriminate between the two case types shown in Figs. 5 and 6 which have the same errors of convergence but which require markedly different divergence and accommodative efforts for their correction. Thus the mutual interactions between accommodation and convergence result in a greater demand upon fusional convergence than predicted from the traditional Maddox Analysis which disregards both prism adaptation and convergence accommodation.

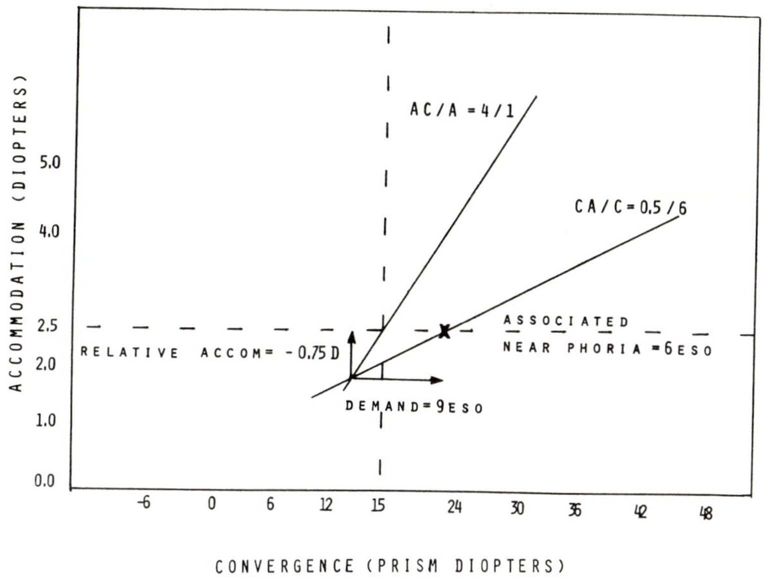

Fig. 6. The CA/C line drawn through the associated phoria (X) and the AC/A line drawn through the convergence accommodation reference representing the near test distance intersect at a point indicating the demand upon accommodation (1.5D) and convergence (9Δ) necessary to correct or overcome an associated phoria of 6 eso for a person with a normal (0.5D/6) CA/C ratio and a normal (4/1) AC/A ratio. The demand upon accommodation and convergence controllers will become very large as the slope of the AC/A and CA/C become similar. Note that the reciprocal of the AC/A is plotted. The lower AC/A ratio in this example results in a smaller demand upon fusional vergence than indicated for the high AC/A ratio in the previous example.

ACKNOWLEDGEMENT

Preparation of this report was supported in part by Grant No. EYO 2573 from the National Eye Institute.

OPTICALLY-INDUCED CHANGES IN THE NEURAL COUPLING BETWEEN VERGENCE EYE MOVEMENTS AND ACCOMMODATION IN HUMAN SUBJECTS

F. A. MILES* and S. J. JUDGE**

*Laboratory of Sensorimotor Research, National Eye Institute, Bethesda and Department of Ophthalmology, The Johns Hopkins University, Baltimore, MD, USA

**University Laboratory of Physiology, Oxford University, Oxford, UK

ABSTRACT

During monocular viewing, when disparity cues are absent, changes in accommodation due to blur cues result in linear changes in vergence: The accommodation-vergence response. Moreover, during binocular pinhole viewing, when blur cues are minimal, changes in vergence due to disparity cues result in linear changes in accommodation: The vergence-accommodation response. We now report that these two open-loop responses undergo adaptive modifications when challenged with optical devices that increase the apparent separation of the two lines of sight. Thus, laterally-displacing periscopic spectacles elicit increases in the magnitude of the accommodation-vergence response and decreases in the magnitude of the vergence-accommodation response, changes which would aid the rapid alignment and focussing of the two eyes.

KEYWORDS

Vergence-accommodation; accommodation-vergence; adaptive regulation; humans.

INTRODUCTION

Transfer of fixation between targets at different viewing distances involves changes in vergence eye movements and accommodation that operate to eliminate disparity and blur, respectively. However, during monocular viewing, when disparity cues are absent, changes in accommodation due to blur cues result in linear changes in vergence: The accommodation-vergence response (Alpern, Kincaid, and Lubeck, 1959; Flom, 1960a; Morgan, 1944). Furthermore, during binocular pinhole viewing, when blur cues are minimal, changes in vergence due to disparity result in linear changes in accommodation: The vergence-accommodation response (Balsam and Fry, 1959; Fincham and Walton, 1957; Kent, 1958; Morgan, 1954). Several studies (e.g., Flom, 1960b; Manas, 1958) have reported changes in the accommodative-convergence to accommodation ratio (AC/A) in response to orthoptics but these changes were very small (<1 prism dioptre/dioptre). Since such changes are within the variability of the normal response (Manas and Shulman, 1954; Westheimer, 1955a, 1955b) there has been some reluctance to accept them as evidence that the neural coupling between vergence and accommodation is subject to modification by learning (Alpern, 1962). The desired coupling between vergence and accommodation

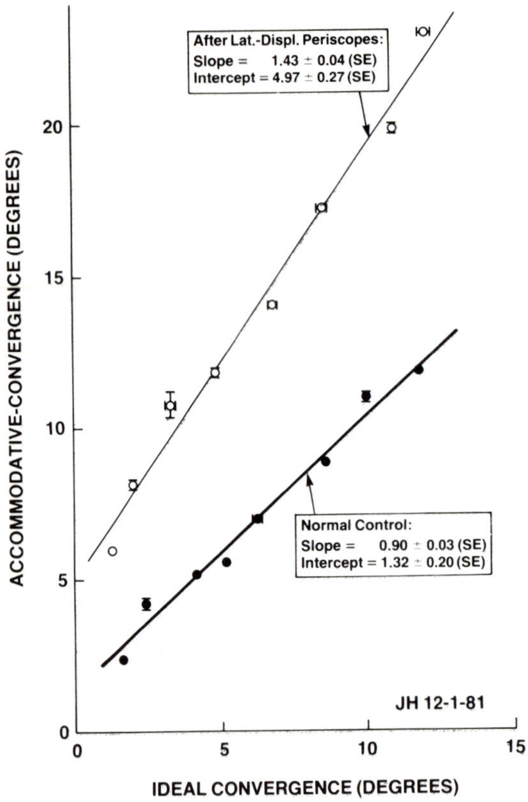

Figure 1. Effect of laterally-displacing periscopic spectacles on the gain of accommodative-convergence. Linear regression lines were fitted by the method of least squares, and the difference in slopes was significant at the .001 level (Student's t). Error bars are SE's. See text for explanation.

under normal binocular viewing conditions is a simple matter of geometry in which the important parameter is the separation of the two eyes: The greater the separation, the greater the required change in vergence per unit change in accommodation. We now provide evidence that the efficacy of this coupling undergoes adaptive modifications when the apparent separation of the two lines of sight is increased with laterally-displacing periscopic spectacles. Some of our preliminary observations on adaptive modification of the stimulus AC/A have been reported elsewhere (Judge and Miles, 1981).

ACCOMMODATION-VERGENCE

For measurement of the accommodation-vergence response, the right eye fixated cross-hairs through a mixing cube and Badal lens, which could provide accommodative stimuli of 0 to 4 dioptres with fixed size and brightness cues. The accommodative state of the right eye was determined with a laser speckle optometer incorporating Badal lens viewing (Charman, 1979; Charman and Whitefoot, 1979; Hennessy and Leibowitz, 1970, 1972; Knoll, 1966). The left eye viewed a screen that was blank except for alignment markings (offset vertically to avoid disparity cues) through a servo-controlled, mirror-galvanometer system that, when aligned by the subject, indicated the horizontal position of that eye.

Figure 1 indicates the vergence responses resulting from accommodative-convergence when a subject fixated targets ranging from 0 to 4 dioptres. The data shown were taken immediately before and after the subject wore laterally-displacing periscopic spectacles, which effectively more than doubled the apparent separation of the lines of sight, for 30 minutes. The measured convergence response (in degrees) is plotted along the ordinate, while the estimated ideal convergence response--that convergence (in degrees) which would be required to maintain correct alignment of the two eyes for each measured state of accommodation--is plotted along the abscissa. The slope of this relationship is a dimensionless parameter that provides a measure of the open-loop gain of the accommodative-convergence response. In the two subjects that were most intensively studied the data were reasonably linear, standard linear regressions yielding correlation coefficients >0.98.[1] The normal variability of the slope from day to day for each individual amounted to <0.15, with standard deviations <0.1. During the spectacle experience, the subject was required to transfer fixation repeatedly between real targets at distances ranging from 0 to 4 dioptres, and make every attempt to achieve single, clear vision. The normal (control) gain for the subject shown in Fig. 1 was 0.90, and this was increased by about 60% (to 1.43) after wearing the spectacles. The second subject showed a similar response to these spectacles, the gain increasing from its normal value of 1.16 to 1.89 (+63%). Since these increases in gain would operate to aid the correct alignment of the two eyes while wearing the spectacles, they can be regarded as adaptive and the accommodation-vergence system can be said to possess adaptive gain control. However, we were unable to decrease the gain of the accommodative-convergence response with medially-displacing periscopic spectacles that reduced the apparent separation of the eyes to zero (cyclopean viewing). Thus, the adaptive mechanism showed considerable asymmetry.

It should be noted that wedge-prism spectacles call for a vertical shift in the whole curve rather than a change in slope. For example, base-out prisms call for an upward shift and this was observed. Similarly, base-in prisms call for a downward shift, and while this too was observed, it was much smaller in extent than that observed with the base-out arrangement. However, some subjects showed a small (up to 20%), transient increase in slope (gain) with the cyclopean and prism spectacles. We attribute this to fatigue of the accommodation response since it was also seen when these same subjects carried out the fixation transfer "exercises" without any spectacles.

VERGENCE-ACCOMMODATION

For measurement of vergence-induced accommodation, each eye fixated cross-hairs in Maxwellian view; blur cues were minimized by using pinhole light sources (less than 0.5 mm diameter) and vergence was varied systematically by rotating the left optical system about the center of rotation of the left eye (c.f. Fincham and Walton, 1957). The accommodation induced by convergence was determined for the right eye with a laser speckle optometer incorporating Badal lens viewing.

Figure 2 indicates the vergence-induced accommodation responses when a subject fused cross-hairs requiring convergence ranging from 0 to 18°. The data shown were taken immediately before and after the subject wore the laterally-displacing, periscopic spectacles for 30 minutes. Vergence-induced accommodation (in dioptres) is plotted along the ordinate, while the estimated ideal accommodative response--that accommodation (in dioptres) which would be required to maintain correct focus of the eyes for each position of convergence--is plotted along the abscissa. The slope of this relationship is a dimensionless parameter that provides a measure of the open-loop gain of the vergence-induced accommodation response. In the two subjects intensively studied the data were reasonably linear for convergence angles >2°, standard linear regressions yielding correlation

1 Since two dependent variables are involved, regression lines were also fitted using the method of Alpern, Kincaid and Lubeck (1959); slopes with this method were within the Standard Error of those obtained with the least squares.

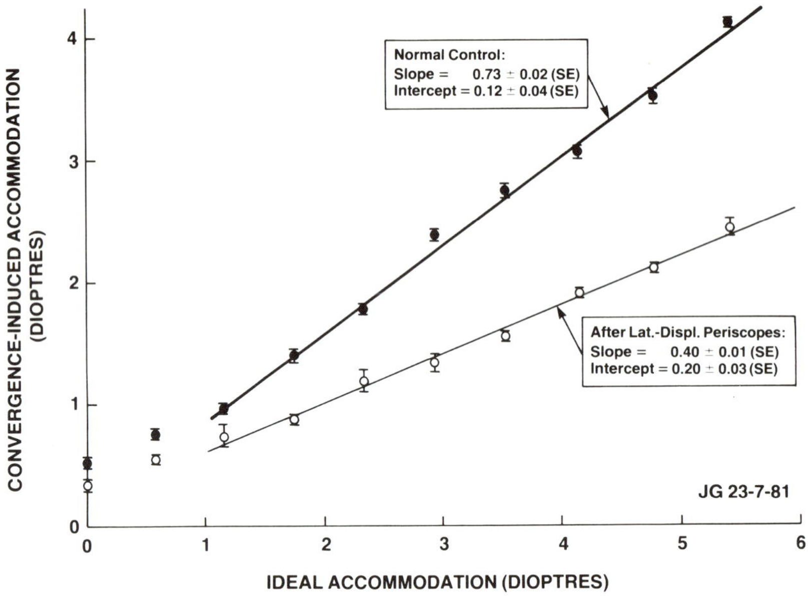

Figure 2. Effect of laterally-displacing periscopic spectacles on the gain of vergence-accommodation. Linear regression lines were fitted by the method of least squares, and the difference in slopes was significant at the .001 level (Student's t). Error bars are SE's. See text for explanation.

coefficients >0.98. The normal variability of the slope from day to day for each individual amounted to <0.15, with standard deviations <0.1. Before the spectacle experience, the gain for the subject shown in Fig. 2 was 0.73 and this was decreased by about 45% (to 0.40) immediately afterwards. In the second subject, the gain decreased from its normal value of 0.86 to 0.41 (-52%). Since these changes would operate to aid the correct focussing of the eyes while wearing the spectacles, they can be regarded as adaptive and the vergence-accommodation system can be said to possess adaptive gain control. Once more, however, the subjects failed to respond adaptively to cyclopean spectacles, while wedge-prism spectacles resulted in vertical shifts of the curves in the appropriate, adaptive direction i.e., downwards with the base-out and upwards with the base-in. Again, the response to the base-in arrangement was less pronounced than to the base-out, which tended to "collapse" into zero. Transient decreases in the slope (gain) sometimes followed sessions with the cyclopean or prism spectacles in some subjects. Since these same subjects showed similar decreases after fixation transfer "exercises" without spectacles, we again invoke fatigue of the accommodation response as the most likely explanation.

ACKNOWLEDGEMENT

It is a pleasure to thank Dr. Lance M. Optican for his invaluable help with the data analyses.

A THEORY FOR CONTROL OF THE OCULOMOTOR NEAR TRIAD

J. L. SEMMLOW

Rutgers Medical School and Electrical Engineering, Rutgers University, Piscataway, New Jersey 08854, USA

KEYWORDS

Vergence eye movements; oculomotor control; binocular vergence; oculomotor balance; near triad.

INTRODUCTION

If any pattern emerges from current oculomotor research, it is that precise motor control is achieved through lavish use of neural control centers. These centers mediate distinct behaviors (saccades, smooth pursuit, vergence), have unique stimuli, and are remarkably independent considering the rich inconnections of neural architecture. Specialization is carried even further in the control of motor responses to near stimuli, where a single oculomotor behavior may be influenced by several different neural centers.

Vergence eye movements assigned to follow changes in target depth are controlled by at least two neural centers: a disparity controller driven by disparate retinal images, and an accommodative controller which senses target blur[1]. Additionally so-called "higher level" controls driven by an awareness, or impression of distance can influence the vergence response. Since in normal binocular vision at least two of these stimuli are always present, near triad motor responses are directed by the coordinated activity of multiple neural control processes.Following a rich history beginning with the theory of Maddox (1886), my lab has been studying the interaction of control processes in the oculomotor near triad.

NEAR TRIAD GENERAL ORGANIZATION

The basic near triad control components and their influences are now well documented. Three distinct oculomotor responses to visual target distance are ocular vergence, changes in lens dioptic power, and changes in pupil diameter. Blur and retinal disparity provide the primary drive and though they are geometrically related, they can be isolated using optical techniques. Under such conditions each stimulus is capable of evoking all three motor responses.

Two of these motor responses directly modify primary stimuli, thus for vergence and lens movement the notion of feedback control applies, wherein lens and vergence movements continue until their respective errors are reduced to some acceptable level. Within this basic framework the "controlled" responses, vergence and lens movement, could be effectively mediated by their separate feedback control systems, each responding to, and compensating for, one stimulus. Nonetheless, it is well known that the two systems interact, perhaps to provide redundancy, or perhaps to achieve some subtle advantage in control. This interaction certainly complicates analysis of the near triad, and may, in fact, extend the influence of abnormal, or failing components. This may explain the fact that near triad malfunctions "form the largest single group of oculomotor disturbances in clinical practice" (Carpenter, 1977).

THEORIES OF NEAR TRIAD CONTROL

A straightforward arrangement of near traid components based on the behavioral features just described is shown in Figure 1. With the addition of quantitative data from experimentation this structure has led to the development of a detailed quantitative theory (Semmlow and Yeager, 1972; Hung and Semmlow, 1980). Earlier theories hinged in the two questions of stimulus dominance and separateness of control processes. In the Maddox theory (1886), later elaborated by Alpern (1962), blur is dominant with disparity providing "fine tuning" (Toates, 1974) for vergence responses. With Fincham and Walton (1957) the reverse is true (disparity dominates and blur supplements accommodation) and only one "near center" is proposed. The "dual interaction" theory (so-called as it explicitly shows both disparity's influence on the lens and accommodation's influence on vergence) represented in Figure 1 is a synthesis of these earlier proposals, and is supported by recent experimental evidence.

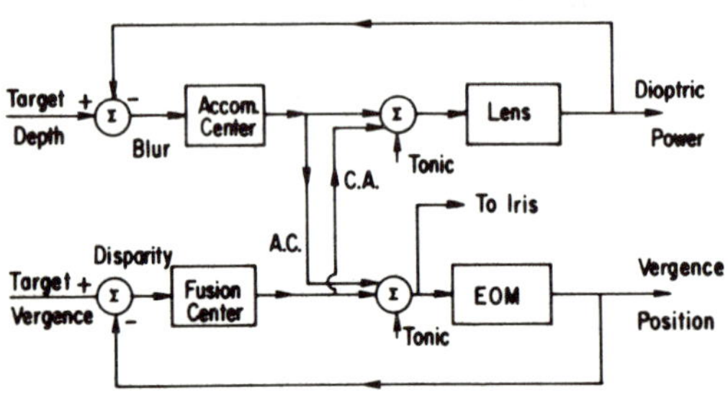

Figure 1. Organization of major near triad components consistent with well established experimental evidence.

The greatest weakness of the Maddox theory is that it does not account for the influences of convergence accommodation, the disparity component which drives the lens. For this reason, the Maddox theory cannot explain the lack of strong correspondence between disassociated (monocular) and associated phoria[2] (Ogle, et al, 1967). Similiarly, it does not predict the presence of a non-zero disparity component during binocular fixation of an orthoporic stimulus (a binocular stimulus where disparity stimulation equals the monocular phoria), (Semmlow and Heerema, 1979). The "dual interaction" theory predicts both these findings and ascribes them to the combined activity of accommodative vergence and convergence accommodation, (Hung and Semmlow, 1980).

The Maddox theory also places more responsibility on blur stimulation than seems justified by experimental evidence. Crone (1973) summarizes arguments favoring the dominance of disparity driven components: CA/C ratios generally exceed AC/A ratios[3], disparity components exhibit less response latency, and the disparity stimulus is more accurate lacking the deadspace and direction ambiquity blur. Additionally, recent experiments comparing disparity vergence dynamics with, and without accompanying blur stimulation show only a small apparent contribution from the blur-driven component (Semmlow and Wetzel, 1979).

The major weakness of Fincham and Walton's proposal also relates to the treatment of the two interactive components. Proposing a single "near center" merely sidesteps the issue of stimulus interaction since this near center must respond in some undefined manner to both blur and disparity stimulation. Further, except for indirect neurophysiological evidence (Jampel, 1959), there is no support for a single functional near center. The existence of separate interactive processes was directly tested in an experiment which isolated blur and disparity components by capitalizing on their differing time characteristics. Results indicate the two interactive components, convergence accommodation and accommodative convergence, could hold different values at the same time, implying separate and distinct neural processes (Semmlow and Hung, 1981). Again, this result supports the dual interactive model, Figure 1.

FUTURE EXPERIMENTATION

Theories and models do service in providing an organizational framework for observations and study. Quantitative models also make specific predictions, some of which can be experimentally verified. Binocular accommodative vergence movements found in experiments by Semmlow and Venkiteswaran (1976) were first noted in early simulation runs of the dual interactive model (Semmlow and Yeager, 1972). More recently, model simulations predicted the influence of open- and closed-loop accommodation on fixation disparity (Semmlow and Hung, 1979). A quantitative model can also evaluate methodology before, and aid data evaluation during, experimentation. Pre-experimental simulations of the dual interactive model confirmed the validity of a new statisical technique for isolating response components (Hung, Ciuffreda and Semmlow, 1981).

Some implications of the dual interactive model have not yet been experimentally tested. Most important is the issue of stimulus dominance. While the dual interactive model provides for response contributions from both stimuli, the functional importance of these contributions depends heavily on the strength of the interactive processes, accommodative vergence and convergence accommodation. Model simulations show that the percent contribution from each stimulus component depends, in large part, on the combination of AC/A_s and CA/C ratios (Hung, Semmlow and Ciuffreda, 1981). Taking the nominal range of these ratios, the model suggests that for most subjects, most of both lens and vergence responses are controlled by disparity-driven components. This prediction of disparity dominance is a consequence of generally higher CA/C ratios and a more tightly controlled (higher loop gain) disparity feedback system.

As mentioned previously, experimental findings to date support this prediction, but the evidence is largely circumstantial. Major new findings will likely depend on innovation. For example, new analytical techniques are being developed which use the unique statistical properties associated with individual components to isolate them from coordinated motor responses (Hung, Ciuffreda and Semmlow, 1981a). Such a technique provides direct information on a component's contribution (which may not be constant throughout the response) to the binocular response.

Experimental verification might also be achieved by comparing lens responses to disparity-only, blur-only, and combined binocular stimulation. Again, new technology is required as these critical experiments are restricted by available instrumentation; eye movement associated with normal disparity or binocular stimulation generates substantial artifact in current dynamic optometers. Advances in optometer design to permit artifact free recording of lens power on a moving eye would be a significant contribution to near triad research.

FOOTNOTES

[1] In keeping with the terminology suggested by Stark, Kenyon and Ciuffreda (1980) we term the motor movement driven by disparite retinal images, disparity vergence, and the movement driven by blur, accommodative vergence.

[2] Associated phoria as defined by Ogle, _et al_ (1967) as the disparity stimulus required to produce zero fixation disparity.

[3] When expressed in analagous units such as meter angles and diopters.

VERGENCE DISORDERS

R. D. REINECKE

Department of Ophthalmology, Albany Medical College, Albany, New York, USA

ABSTRACT

The major clinical categories of strabismus are classed either as vergence-set disorders or vergence-movement disorders. The differences between the two classes become apparent as age of onset, prognosis for straight eyes and stability of the conditions are considered. The new classification may allow research to proceed more logically as to the genesis of strabismus.

KEYWORDS

Vergence disorders; strabismus, clinical types;treatment, strabismus; optokinetic nystagmus

INTRODUCTION

Eye movement disorders may be divided conveniently into: (a) conjugate eye movement disorders such as pareses of lateral conjugate gaze; (b) disconjugate paretic disorders such as III, IV, or VI cranial nerve paralyses and inter-nuclear ophthalmoplegias; and (c) vergence disorders such as non-paralytic strabismus. Only the latter, vergence disorders, is our present topic. Vergence disorders can be subdivided into (1) a vergence-set disorder such as a typical esotropia of 20 prism diopters and skew deviation, and (2) vergence-movement disorders such as paralysis of divergence, paralysis of convergence, accommodative esotropia, intermittent esotropia, intermittent exotropia, and alternating sursumduction. These vergence movement disorders manifest themselves as a lack of synchronization in respect to the vergence demands for a particular distance from the patient. The purpose of this paper is to examine and contrast the salient features of the two vergence disorders.

This study was supported in part by a training grant (EY07037) from the National Eye Institute, National Institutes of Health, and by a research grant from Research to Prevent Blindness, Inc.

BACKGROUND

Vergence-set disorders can be viewed as a well adapted, stable strabismic condition. In contrast, the vergence movement disorder class is reasonably unstable because of dissimilar causes, or identical causes, but occurring at a time when adaptation is less. Since we are to carefully inspect these two groups as to eye movement anomalies which might lead to strabismus, it would be well to inspect briefly the vergence movements of normals. The vergence movements of normals typically function as follows:

a. If asymetric vergence totalling x^o is required to refixate an object binocularly on the horopter, $x^o/2$ will be provided vergence of each eye, and $x^o/2$ will be provided by a simultaneous corrective saccade of each eye.

b. If symetric vergence alone is required, no saccades will occur.

c. The gain of the vergence system can be considered one if it responds at all times with $x^o/2$ in each eye. Thus if a new object is in the midline, but closer to the subject, each eye will converge $x^o/2$ and no saccades will occur. If the new object is on the visual axis of one eye but nearer to the subject, each eye will converge $x^o/2$ and be followed by saccades of $x^o/2$ of each eye which will bring the one eye back on target, and bring the other eye the remaining distance to the target.

d. If marked asymetrics of vergence are required, as is the case when an exotropic eye is brought on target, the gains will differ between the eyes in the following manner: The gain in non-fixing eye will be greater than one, and be less than one in the fixing eye, but the saccadic refixation will always be present with each vergence response when asymetric vergence is required.

e. The vergence response will have a shorter latency than the saccadic response unless a saccadic response is used to switch fixation to the other eye before the reflex begins.

f. The mechanism of dampening of the responses made by the fixing eye is not known.

g. Divergence and convergence behave similarly and follow the above rules.

Since any time one visual axis is off target the above rules apply in returning the eye to the target, a fault in the vergence system or the saccadic system could conceivably result in an inability to align the visual axes binocularly on the target. The saccadic system is resistant to damage and no good examples of isolated saccadic disorders leading to strabismus are available to study the effects of an inadequate system. Conversely, the saccadic responses in strabismic patients is usually normal.(Fricker, 1971) Since the saccadic system drives each eye equally, central problems such as cerebellar disorders cause a lack of precision in aligning both eyes on the target, but the visual axes remain parallel. An example of such a patient is a boy age 8 who has difficulty in suppressing the vestibulo-ocular reflex. Mild ocular dysmetria is present and the patient has to steady his head while reading. Movement of the head causes the VOR to interfere with the fixation pattern of reading and difficulty ensues, but no strabismus occurs.

When convergence or divergence paralysis occurs, the patient typically can fuse at either distance or near and suitable prisms allow the eyes to function at the troublesome distance. No comitant tropia develops for all distances. Indeed, if the patient is given prisms or surgery, even the fusion reserves return to normal. Such a patient has lost the usual AC:A ratio but vergence otherwise is normal.

What if pursuit problems develop? It is of interest that marked monocular asymetric of OKN exist in many strabismic patients.

This clue should be further investigated. The eye movement recordings show binocular following movements of OKN of a strabismic patient, but remarkably asymetric pursuit and substitution of of saccades when the OKN is monocular. (See Fig. 1) Many strabismics do not show this feature.

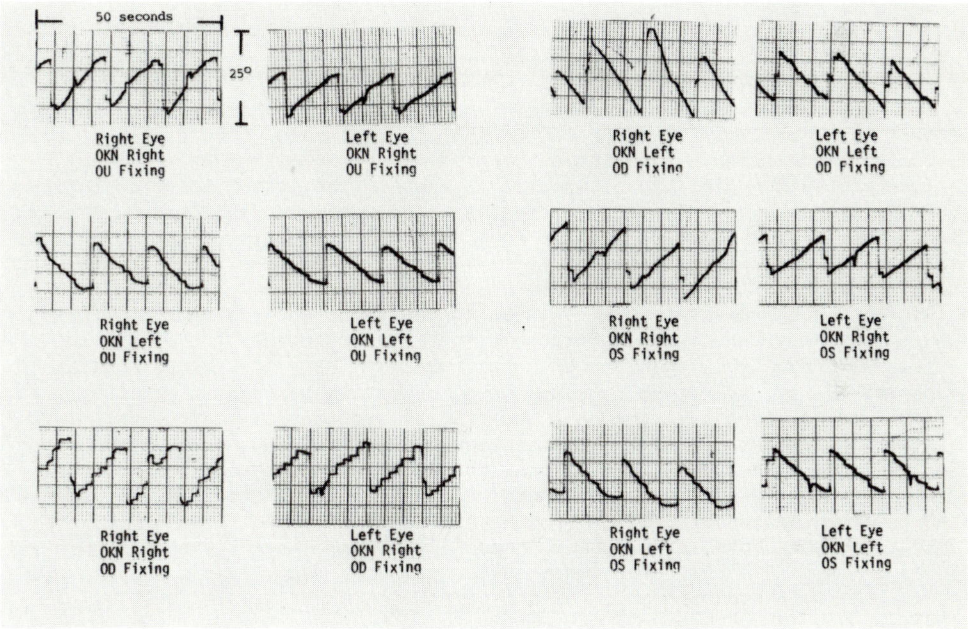

Fig. 1. 32 year old white female with congenital esotropia, several surgical procedures prior to age 8, and 4 prism diopters esotropia. Note the monocular asymetric nasal movements that show substitution of saccades for following movement.

The dichotomy of the vergence-set and vergence movement disorder classes of strabismus will now be characterized.

VERGENCE SET DISORDERS

These disorders are characterized by a constant deviation of the visual axes. The deviation tends to mimic orthophoria, namely, that most attempts to change the deviation result in failure. For example, if prisms are applied to such deviations, the angle of strabismus changes so that the angle with the prisms in place is comparable to the angle prior to the application of the prisms.(Scott, 1977;Bagolini,1976 b) The patient often has abnormal retinal correspondence which implies the patient to be well adapted to the angle of strabismus.

The salient mechanism most likely in use with these patients was hypothesized by me in this conference six years ago and seems to be even more valid now than ever.(Reinecke, 1975) For reasons unknown, the patient adopts a mismatch in the retinal signal versus the afferent muscle signal (or efferent muscule copy). The mechanism is similar to a phoria, excepting for the lack of motor alignment of the visual axes.

VERGENCE-MOVEMENT DISORDERS

The Vergence-movement disorders include those strabismic disorders which are comitant but variable, as opposed to the constant ones just described which are comitant but fixed. Examples of vergence-movement disorders are many, but the intermittent tropias are of special interest. The intermittent deviations sequentially act like normals then tropias. The vergence movements used to change the tropia position are the same as those exhibited by the normal who is stressed by the application of a 4 diopter prism. Such normals and intermittent tropias first use vergence then saccades as many times as necessary to achieve either the position of tropia or the position of fusion. Such patients may have a strong psychological factor in that the perception of nearness may invariably initiate or break fusion. The remarkable stability of fusion of many exotropies at near vs. the almost constant exotropia at distance has not been explained. A superficial explanation of the above is to say the patient has a high accommodation-convergence to accommodation ratio (AC:A). Careful measurements will show the AC:A's of such patients to usually be within normal limits. Prolonged occlusion of one eye of such patients often reveals the latent near deviation to equal the overt distance deviation. If vergence movements are recorded in such patients, they will act as phorias if stressed with a 4 diopter prism base-in, but will respond as a tropia with suppression and exhibit only bilateral saccades if tested with base-out prisms.

It would seem helpful to characterize these two classes of vergence disorders by examining each specific disorder as to its time of onset, usefulness as an adaptive mechanism, stablity and responsiveness to treatment.

SPECIFIC CASE CONSIDERATION OF VERGENCE-SET DISORDERS

Infancy - Skew deviation of neonates

The occasional neonate who has bonafide self-correcting esotropia under 3 months of age is noteworthy. Every strabismologist has seen such children. Creig Hoyt (1980) observed that such children evidence a temporary skew deviation. (In Table 1, this is termed "skew deviation of neonates".) As the eyes straighten, the skew deviation subsides.

Table I

Vergence Set Disorders	Vergence Movement Disorders
Diagnosis:	
a) Skew Deviation of Neonates b) Congenital Esotropia c) Acquired Constant Esotropia d) Constant Exotropia e) Monofixational Phoria-Tropia f) Small Angle Esotropia g) Small Angle Exotropia h) Skew Deviation of Adult	1. Accomodative Esotropia 2. Nystagmus Blockage Syndrome 3. Intermittent Exotropia 4. Intermittent Esotropia 5. Spasm of Convergence 6. Divergence Paralysis 7. Convergence Paralysis 8. Dissociated Vertical Divergence
Angle of Strabismus:	
1)Relatively constant at all distances	1) Variable with a) Distance b) Accommodative demands c) Light balance to each eye d) Attention to detail
Adaptation to Prism:	
1) May be slow, but usually present Exceptions: (h) Skew deviation of adult	1) Frequently do not adapt 5 - 8 2) Frequently do adapt 1 - 4
Diagnosis amenable to Vergence Training:	
Typically no response	Intermittent Exotropia - fair response Intermittent Esotropia - usually poor response
Predictability of Response to Surgery:	
Poor	Reasonably good

Age most common:

Under 3 months	
a) Skew Deviation of neonates	Generally later
Under 6 months	
a) Congenital Esotropia b) Congenital Exotropia	1) Accommodative ET 2) Nystagmus Blockage 8) Alternating Sursumduction
Under age 3	
c) Acquired Constant Esotropia e) Monofixational Phoria-Tropia	
Under age 6	
f) Small Angle Esotropia g) Small Angle Exotropia d) Constant Exotropia	
6 - 10 years	
	3) Intermittent Exotropia 4) Intermittent Esotropia
10 - 20 years	
	5) Spasm of Convergence 7) Convergence Paralysis
50 years	
h) Skew Deviation of Adulthood	6) Divergence Paralysis

Congenital Esotropia

The eyes are uniquely designed to handle physiologic diplopia. (All physiologic diplopia is horizontal.) As the eyes align on an object in the horopter, all objects off the horopter become diplopic. However, the high acuity sensitivity of the macula and fovea attract our attention so much that we easily discount the remaining blurred environment which often is horizontally diplopic. The congenital esotropic child has not learned that it is unusual for the visual scene to change rapidly in the fovea. When the eyes of a congenital esotropic infant with cross fixation are alternately occluded, the infant will continue to stare at whatever the uncovered eye finds on its fovea. Only with movement or other attention directing efforts will the child redirect the eye towards the original object of fixation. With further alternate occlusion, the same sequence occurs. Even the older child and occasionally an adult evidences a to-and-fro movement of the eye which has just been uncovered as the other eye is occluded. The patient seems to be using a rapid scanning to settle the fovea on the original object of fixation.

Normally,eyes function without vertical disparity. Hence, any vertical disparity could pull the second image into consciousness (as is done clinically to produce diplopia in amblyopia follow-up in infants) and permit alternation to occur.(Wright)

A skew (vertical) deviation would permit diplopia and thus allow re-alignment of the eyes. Perhaps that is the role of skew deviation in the neonatal esotrope. As an esotropic child ages, various strategies are utilized to orient the patient in the visual world. A vertical deviation, and resultant diplopia which would only be present when the eyes came into conflict as to which eye's image were real, could be a useful means of visual orientation. Since it is known that the normal person will evidence dissociated vertical divergence if the occlusion is prolonged (Bielschowski 1938), it is hardly surprising that this mechanism might be utilized by the esotropic patient. The gradual onset of DVD seems consistent with this mechanism. As suppression is established with an esotropia, the only means of momentary diplopia is with a vertical dissociation. As this is repeated, the vertical movement becomes larger and larger. While vertical diplopia can be easily elicited in the neonate esotrope, the older patient with DVD requires larger and larger prisms. This drifting up of the eye (dissociated vertical divergence) has been resistant to surgical treatment and only by recessing the superior rectus by what was considered crippling amounts, can the eyes be made to remain level.(Scott and Braverman, 1977) Verhoeff (1941)predicted that unilateral large recessions will cause the opposite eye's DVD to worsen. Hence, the surgery should be bilateral. An occasional esotropic patient will resolve the esotropia by early DVD, but will retain the attending alternating sursumduction with abnormally large amounts of vertical fusional reserves.

From the above, we must ask ourselves, could the induction of a large temporary or intermittent vertical deviation in infancy eliminate the positive adaptive strategy described by Fred Miles in this conference.

The observation that OKN's are asymetric in congenital esotropes is of some interest. Inasmuch as this is the first oculomotor anomaly which seems to be fairly consistently associated with esotropia. The observation that this asymetry disappears with age of the patient is also of some interest. The following case description is of a 36 year old white female who had onset of esotropia earlier than age two and eye muscle surgery at age 7. Examination revealed the patient to have an 18 prism diopter esotropia. A suspicion of poor pursuit movements prompted an EOG which revealed binocularly fair tracking movements, but monocularly slow and a noteworthy OKN response. The OKN binocularly was reasonably symetrical. Monocular readings showed staircase following movements when the target moved temporally in either eye. Saccades were normal. We have seen numerous patients with cerebellar dysfunction who have lost pursuit movements in all directions and substituted saccadic movements. Such patients have no symptoms unless they are carefully queried as to reading road signs while riding in a car. The above-mentioned strabismic esotrope with an asymetric specific tracking disorder is dissimilar to cerebellar patients. It is tempting to speculate that the asymetric tracking disorder with only adducting tracking intact can in someway be related to the esotropia's etiology. Such an etiology might be plausible in those rare esotropias which march steadily to ever increasing esotropia irrespective of treatment excepting crippling surgery.

The further question of why a strabismus of 18-20 prism diopters being the most common amount of esotropia is difficult to rationalize excepting a randomized search for a non-competitive retinal-macular relationship. This has been the traditional explanation of this angle strabismus which is appropriately called the blind-spot syndrome.(Swan, 1947) Certainly the stability of this deviation as opposed to exotropia is well known.

The remarkable occasional success resulting from surgical treatment of an adult esotropic patient is also noteworthy. Consider the 32 year old white male who has had a documented history of lifelong esotropia. Surgery at age 28 resulted not only in straight eyes but also the attainment of stereoscopic vision. Similarly, there are several instances of the development of fusion, good vision in each eye and stereoscopic vision in microstrabismic patients in their twenty's.(Keiner, 1978) These results contrast sharply with our expectation from surgery or orthoptics. Jampolsky (1971) has stated that the "sensory shock" of the new eye position resulting from surgery gives us the needed treatment. Other possibilities exist such as threshhold change of muscle tonus and the subsequently changed afferent signal which, in turn, might then cause the changes in the foveal relationships.

CONCLUSIONS

The various eye movement strategies and mechansims have been examined and only the following show promise at this time:

1. Pursuit mechanisms involved with OKN are notably defective unidirectionally in children with strabismus and occasionally in adults.

2. Vertical misalignment may be a diplopia-producing mechanism in the neonate (skew deviation) and in the strabismic patient. An explanation of the mechanism of dissociated vertical divergence might be uniquely productive in the management of strabismus.

3. The vergence-set disorders are stable and resistant to treatment.

4. The vergence-movement disorders are in a plastic state and are amenable to surgery.

5. Perhaps this new classification of eye alignment problems will be helpful in bringing about more logical treatment modalities.

DISJUNCTIVE MOVEMENTS IN COMITANT STRABISMUS

B. BAGOLINI and E. C. CAMPOS

Clinica Oculistica dell'Università di Modena,
via del Pozzo 71, Modena, Italy

ABSTRACT

The compensation or eating up of prisms in comitant strabismus is discussed. This phenomenon, practically consisting of disjunctive movements, appears to have similar characteristics with normal fusional movements. Its relationship with anomalous retinal correspondence (ARC) is considered in detail. It is suggested that compensation of prisms may be interpreted as motor fusion - although of anomalous type. It is thus defined anomalous fusional movements (AFM). It constitutes a sensori-motor sequela of strabismus. On one side it interacts with ARC in maintaining an anomalous type of binocularity; on the other side it is a major handicap for a restoration of orthotropia both with prisms and surgery.

KEYWORDS

Strabismus; vergence movements; motor fusion; prisms; anomalous retinal correspondence; binocular vision.

INTRODUCTION

The existence of fusional movements in the central field of strabismic patients with anomalous retinal correspondence (ARC) was pointed out by Halldén (1952). More recently, disjunctive eye movements in strabismus have been analyzed in detail in our Laboratory, following an observation by Bagolini (1967). This was done by examining the behavior of strabismic patients whose angle of deviation was corrected with prisms. It is well known since Travers (1936) that strabismic patients tend to compensate for such correction, or eat the prisms up. In other words, the patient tries to go back to his/her original deviation. This phenomenon does not take place immediately after prisms are put in front of the patient's eyes. It may take seconds, minutes or even hours to fully develop.

PERSONAL STUDIES ON DISJUNCTIVE MOVEMENTS

An analysis of vergence movements in esotropic patients was done by Bagolini (1971) and then expanded five years later (Bagolini, 1976b). Eighty five over 100 consecutive patients compensated an exact correction of the angle of deviation, by means of base-out prisms. Forty eight patients compensated - partially or totally - an overcorrection of their angle of deviation ranging from 20 to 30 prism diopters. All cases showed ARC as tested with the striated glasses.

In summary, particularly patients with small-angle strabismus and ARC, tend to compensate for a prismatic correction of their angle of deviation. Disjunctive movements are used by these patients to stabilize the angle of strabismus to which they adapted from the sensory point of view.

A further analysis was done on a group of 30 esotropic patients with ARC, to evaluate the possible presence of disjunctive movements even in diveregence and verticality (Campos and Zanasi, 1978). Twenty two patients compensated - totally or partially - for 10 base-in prism diopters. Therefore, they showed divergence movements. Thirteen over 17 patients compensated prisms based up or down (of 5-7 diopters), showing disjunctive vertical movements.

Finally, in a study of 6 esotropic patients with ARC at the striated glasses it was shown that an increase of the angle of deviation in time is observable even at the synoptophore (major amblyscope), using various types of targets (Campos and Catellani, 1978).

COMMENT

Some general statements are appropriate before an interpretation of the phenomenon can be attempted. Normal binocular vision (NBV) is sustained from the sensory point of view by normal retinal correspondence (NRC); from the sensori-motor point of view by normal fusional movements (NFM). Normal fusional movements are those disjunctive movements elicited by stimulation of disparate retinal elements with sufficinetly equal images.

An anomalous type of binocular cooperation has been described in small-angle strabismus (Bagolini and Capobianco, 1965; Bagolini, 1967; Bagolini, 1976a). This binocularity is made possible from the sensory point of view by an anomalous overlapping of the visual fields of the two eyes, sustained by ARC and is called anomalous binocular vision (ABV). Therefore, similarities exist between ARC and NRC. In fact, the latter supports a normal overlapping of the visual fields of the two eyes, which is however much stronger than the one supported by ARC (Bagolini and Campos, 1977). A comparison between NFM and disjunctive movements in strabismus was made possible by our observations. These movements were thus interpreted as anomalous fusional movements (AFM).

Common Features Between NFM and AFM

-in both cases there is a variation in the muscle tonus due to a shift of retinal images
-they are both sensori-motor entities
-both exist in convergence, divergence and verticality.

Differential Features Between NFM and AFM

-AFM are much weaker and slower than NFM
-AFM are less precise than NFM, i.e., often there is not a full compensation of the prismatic power, as it happens for NFM
-NFM tend to bring equal images over normally corresponding retinal elements; AFM tend to bring roughly equal images over retinal elements corresponding in an anomalous way.

Thus, it makes sense to state that ABV is sustained from the sensory point of view by ARC and from the sensori-motor view point by AFM. However, ARC and AFM are not as strictly interconnected as NRC and NFM are. There are patients with ARC and without AFM. Moreover, AFM are still present in some cases when ARC is interrupted and diplopia or suppression are artificially elicited through sensorial obstacles.

We believe that ARC and AFM are both a sequela and not a cause of strabismus. The input for these two entities follows a common path; nevertheless, each has a separate further processing. This can be inferred by the fact that they develop and may be eliminated rather independently (Bagolini, 1976b).

Aside from the shift of the spatial localization properties of the retinal elements, represented by ARC, there is a shift of the motorial value of such elements, e.g., the two foveas do not bear either the same localization property or a zero motorial value. In strabismus with ARC and AFM such properties are acquired by the fovea of the fixing eye and an eccentric area of the deviated eye, which can be quite extended (Bagolini, 1976a).

The finality of AFM is to maintain the angle of deviation which makes ABV possible. Any attempt to disturb this situation is hampered by AFM. They tend to avoid spontaneous fluctuations of the angle of deviation and are an obstacle to treatment of small-angle strabismus.

AFM may probably explain the pathogenesis of various syndromes, including horror fusionis, diplopia-phobia, the "repulsion des images", the blind-spot syndrome. We refer to previous publications for an exhaustive discussion of this subject (Bagolini, 1976b; Campos and Zanasi, 1978).

STEREOPSIS AND OPTOKINETIC NYSTAGMUS

J. VAN HOF-VAN DUIN and G. MOHN

Department of Physiology I, Erasmus University, Rotterdam, The Netherlands

ABSTRACT

Stereopsis and optokinetic nystagmus (OKN) were assessed in normals and in subjects with impaired stereovision. OKN was elicited by whole field and by small field (20^ox 30°) stimulation.Directional asymmetries were found to be present in stereoblind subjects with convergent strabismic amblyopia, anisometropic hypermetropic amblyopia, and non-amblyopic strabismus divergens. Since monocular OKN was found to be directional asymmetric in all stereoblind subjects, a connection seems to be present between binocularity and symmetry or asymmetry of monocular optokinetic responses.

KEYWORDS

Stereopsis; optokinetic nystagmus; direction asymmetry; binocularity; amblyopia; strabismus divergens; anisometropic hypermetropia.

Studies on visually deprived cats have suggested a relation between the loss of binocular cortical neurons and the presence of asymmetrical optokinetic responses. Monocular OKN has been found to be impaired in these animals when the stimulus is moving in a nasal-to-temporal direction (Van Hof-van Duin,1976, 1978a, 1978b, Hoffmann 1979). Recently, similar impairments in monocular OKN have been found in amblyopic humans when small field stimulation was used (Schor and Levi, 1980).

In the present study optokinetic responses of stereoblind subjects were compared with those of normal humans. Visual acuity was measured in all subjects, and correction, if necessary, was worn by all subjects during testing. None of the subjects showed manifest or latent nystagmus.
Stereovision was tested with several tests: Titmus and Randot tests were used at 40 cm distance; the Random dot E test was used from near to 6 m distance; projected Julesz stereograms were viewed from varying distances; in the 3-rods test binocular and monocular performances were compared; the sensitivity for 'motion in depth' was tested in a set up in which the sideways movement of two projected shadows of a moving pin is perceived as motion in depth when stereopsis is present.
OKN was elicited by whole field and by small field stimulation. With whole field stimulation OKN was studied by recording the electro-oculogram while subjects were seated in the centre of a rotating drum (diameter 120 cm, height 120 cm). The pattern

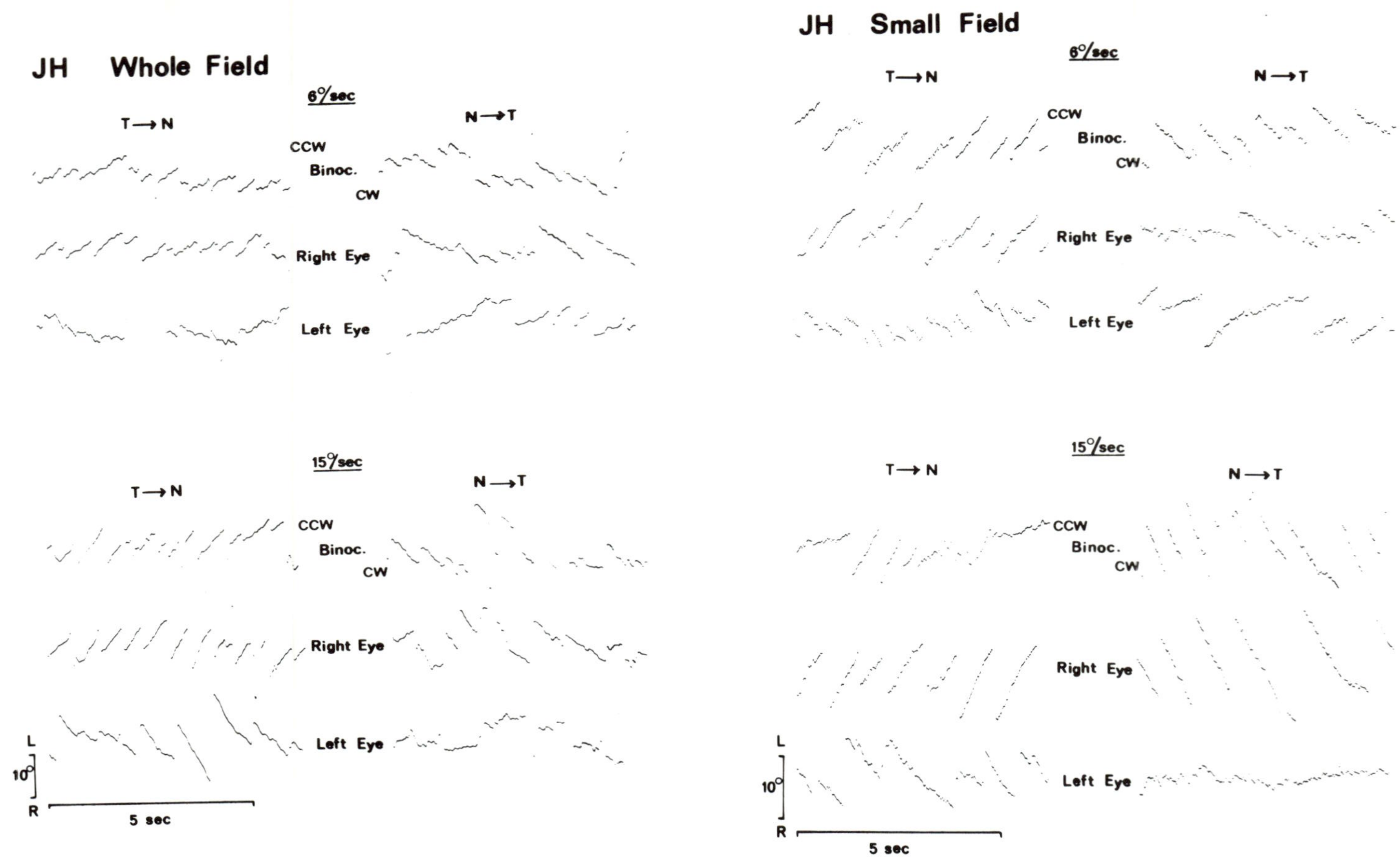

Fig. 1. Comparison of OKN elicited with whole field (left) and with small field (20° x 30°) stimulation (right) in a non-amblyopic stereoblind alternating divergent strabismic subject. Binocular and monocular horizontal OKN in response to patterns drifting at 6o/sec and 15°/sec in temporal-to-nasal (T→ N) and nasal-to-temporal (N→ T) directions.

on the walls of the drum consisted of black and white checks, each measuring 1 cm^2 (spatial frequency 0.5 cy/deg). Small field OKN was stimulated with a 0.5 cy/deg square wave grating drifting horizontally in a $20^o \times 30^o$ rectangular field, viewed at 57 cm distance. Gratings were formed on a CRT using a standard raster technique. Gratings had a mean luminance of 160 cd/m^2, and contrast of 65%. Horizontal velocities used in all experiments were 3, 6, 15 and $30^o/s$. OKN was tested binocularly as well as monocularly, with both clockwise and counterclockwise stimulus movement. Subjects were asked to stare at the center of the moving field and keep the drifting pattern visible. EOG-signals were recorded on magnetic tape and analysed by means of a computer programme which eliminated fast eye movements and produced measures of the slow phase velocity of the OKN, as well as calculated gains.

Results obtained in 4 stereoblind subjects were compared with OKN of normal subjects who reached stereoacuity values of 20" - 50" in the Randot test. Binocular and monocular OKN of normal subjects appeared to be symmetrical in response to temporal and to nasalward target motion, both with whole field and with small field stimulation. As described by Schor and Narayan (1981), increasing field size was found to be related with increasing sensitivity to higher velocities. Whole field stimulation with $3^o/s$ failed to elicit OKN in most normals, $30^o/s$ however, resulted in regular OKN. With small field stimulation, OKN in response to target velocity of $3^o/s$ was regular, but to $30^o/s$ variable.

Compared to normal subjects, monocular OKN of all stereoblind subjects was found to be impaired. Examples of an alternating divergent strabismic subject with normal visual acuity in both eyes (6/6), are shown in Fig. 1. Binocular and monocular OKN to whole field (Fig. 1, left side) and to small field (Fig. 1, right side) stimulation are shown for pattern velocities to $6^o/s$ and $15^o/s$. Compared to normal, responses to $6^o/s$ target motion were found to be reduced, both binocularly and monocularly. With $15^o/s$ whole field stimulation regular OKN was elicited only by the right eye and then only by nasalward target motion (T→N, Fig. 1). All further monocular and binocular responses showed impairments, i.e. reduced slow phase velocity, reduced fast phase frequency and irregularities. With small field stimulation this subject exhibited besides reduced OKN, marked asymmetries in response to temporal target motion for each eye with $6^o/s$, $15^o/s$ (illustrated in Fig. 1) and with $30^o/s$.

Directional asymmetry with reduced slow phase velocity of monocular OKN in response to temporal stimulus motion was also found in 2 stereoblind convergent strabismic amblyopes, confirming Schor and Levi's results (1979, 1980). In both subjects asymmetries were obvious in response to whole field as well as to small field stimulation. Furthermore, OKN was recorded in a stereoblind anisometropic hypermetropic amblyope (correction OD +3.25, -0.5 170°: V 6/50; OS -0.25: V 6/6). Monocular OKN response to small field stimulation with $6^o/s$ target velocity was found to be reduced and irregular in both directions. With a stimulus velocity of $15^o/s$ clear directional asymmetries were evident: for each eye slow phase velocity and fast phase frequency were reduced in response to temporal target motion.

Summarizing, 4 stereoblind subjects (1 non-amblyopic divergent strabismic, 2 amblyopic convergent strabismics and 1 non-strabismic anisometropic amblyope) showed reduced OKN, with asymmetries especially in response to higher velocities.

The results obtained in stereoblind subjects lend support to the idea that in the human, as in the cat, there is a connection between binocularity, measured here as stereopsis, and symmetry or asymmetry of the monocular optokinetic responses. As in the cat (Hoffmann, 1981) binocular cortical neurons appear to be necessary also in humans for the presence of normal monocular OKN in response to stimulus movement in the nasal-to-temporal direction.

DISCUSSION:

In response to the question of the practicality of the clinical measurement of the convergent accommodation to convergence ratio (CA:C), Dr. Schor responded that the utility was as yet unknown, but the measurement of CA:C can be practically done with some ease. Dry (or dynamic) retinoscopy is used to measure the accommodative state of an eye as the convergent demands of the eyes are varied with prisms of varying powers. Hence, a gradient change in accommodation is obtained as a function of the prism stimulus to convergence.

Dr. Schor emphasized the differences in the measurements of the accommodative convergence to accommodation ratio (AC:A) when the gradient method is used in comparison to the calculated AC:A based on the phorias measured at two different distances. The difference between the two ratios is usually attributed to the proximal factor of convergence, but he acknowledged that the CA:C might play a role but to date there is no data to confirm or deny such a relationship. Until that data is forthcoming, it would be better to stay with the conventional explanation of proximal convergence as being the explanation of the discrepancy.

The discussion then turned to the presentation of Dr. Miles and whether the changes which he was able to show in the AC:A had any potential for permancy and thus clinical usefulness. He was skeptical as to its clinical utility, but felt that the changes demonstrated did explain the tendency of the AC:A to increase and to seldom decrease. The adaptation causing the changes in the AC:A ratio could be measured as long as 8 hours following the training session, but these changes were under the condition of keeping the loop open, i.e. keeping one eye patched. If the subject is allowed to become binocular, the adaptive changes are wiped out within minutes. Dr. Miles pointed out that the view that the AC:A is not modifiable is based on just the latter observation, namely that if the person is permitted to become binocular immediately after a training session aimed at modifying the AC:A, the AC:A will be found to be unchanged. In the course of the discussion, Dr. Miles pointed out that past studies are often not clear as to whether a change in the AC:A was being sought or merely a change in the baseline. For example, if prisms are placed in front of a subject, the base is simply shifted in that the convergent demands are changed for all distances. Whereas in his experiments, the eyes are functionally further separated, thus demanding changing AC:A for effective near viewing as compared to no change for effective distance viewing. He went ahead to point out that if a subject had a need for an adaptive change and the change was in the direction of an increase in the AC:A, then the daily requirement would surely cause the change to occur. Thus, training would not be needed. It was emphasized that the past argument that the AC:A cannot be decreased nor the CA:C increased and thus cure an accommodative esotropia should not be used to say that these ratios are unchangeable. In point of fact,the ratios are difficult to change in those directions and the adaptability is largely in the reverse direction. This ability to adapt in one direction is fortunate since the increasing convergent demands occur with the increasing interpupillary distances with growth.

Some concern was expressed in regard to Dr. Stark's paper in respect to the treatment of adult amblyopic patients. Clinicians had seen such patients develop irreversible diplopia. Since a patient who has amblyopia treatable at age twenty years of age will respond to treatment at age sixty or any age should the good eye become impaired, the risk hardly seems justified. Dr. Ciuffreda, co-author of Dr. Stark, assured the audience that special considerations led to the treatment of patients mentioned in the paper and concurred on the inherent danger of diplopia in this group of patients. He emphasized that their interest was in the finding that in the course of the treatment of the amblyopia, some eye movements were noted to change. He went on to note that the degree to which vergence movements responded to disparity stimuli was dependent upon the disparity targets. Thus, differing investigators must carefully note their stimuli and have the stimuli comparable if the results are to be compared. His experimental paradigm is to use small disparities and only the central retinal areas. Both of these factors must be included as to their quantity if we are to compare results.

Dr. Stark continued the discussion and emphasized his findings that under their experimental design they were unable to find disparity vergence with strabismic or amblyopic subjects. The recorded vergence in his charts was thought to be accommodative vergence. Others were surprised at the short latencies of the vergence response which he classified as accommodative. Dr. Stark went on to point out that although accommodative vergence is binocular, it is not symmetric and has only about 12% of the amplitude in the dominant eye as compared to the non-dominant eye. The panel noted that Dr. Stark's experiments used a design of changing both accommodation and convergence demands simultaneously and it was thus difficult to readily distinguish the disparity from the accommodative vergences.

Discord between the clinicians and the non-clinicians became apparent in the definition of vergence. The clinicians have a need for a term which includes the changing alignment of the visual axes in respect to convergence and divergence, no matter what the time course of this change. Dr. Stark emphasized that he wished vergence to be used only in respect to a brief time base. No resolution of this disagreement was reached. Dr. Semmlow also noted the difficulty of distinguishing disparity vergence from accommodative vergence when the experimental design changed demands on both systems simultaneously. He went on to emphasize that although the two can be measured independently, what is needed is a system to change both, as occurs in a natural environment, but with some parameters to enable one to sort the two apart. Simply opening the loop on one or the other system is sufficient. Others present noted that that other paradigms such as placing a prism in front of a patient to evaluate only the disparity vergence had its shortcomings as well. In that artificial system, disparity vergence has an extremely short latency and is always accompanied by saccadic corrective movements, unless equal vergence demands are presented simultaneously to each eye.

As the panel discussed Dr. van Duin's paper, emphasis was made that most of her subjects were patients with normal binocular vision, excepting being stereoblind. The asymmetry of optokinetic response found in these subjects was a reduced gain of the slow phase in the nasal-temporal direction, but not the gross absence of this nasal-temporal OKN as noted in many congenital esotropes. Several of the panel noted the importance of using small field OKN to study the asymmetries of OKN since these asymmetries may be masked by the full field OKN stimuli such as that occurring when the subject is centered in a rotating environment.

When Dr. Stark queried the clinicians about the acceptability of his scheme of classification, the reaction of the clinicians was strong in that they felt that any classification should include sufficient descriptors so that a variety of unrelated conditions will not be lumped together. This is the problem with simply classifying all patients as having strabismus and/or amblyopia. There are a variety of both strabismic and amblyopic conditions which are unique unto themselves. The vital element in classification and the reporting of patients is the inclusion of sufficient data about each subject or patient that other investigators can appropriately interpret the data. This means not only the angle of strabismus, the visual acuity of each eye, but also the sensory adaptation to the misalignment of the eyes and the recorded eye movements to both normal and stressed conditions.

SECTION III

Coordinator: G. Kommerell

CONGENITAL NYSTAGMUS

CONGENITAL NYSTAGMUS CLINICAL ASPECTS

D. SCHMIDT

Univ.-Augenklinik, Freiburg, Federal Republic of Germany

ABSTRACT

In this survey clinical data on frequency, heredity, earliest occurrence, prognosis, and head movements in congenital nystagmus are presented. In differential diagnosis, spasmus nutans, paroxysmal familial nystagmus, seesaw nystagmus, and gliomas of the optic nerve and chiasm are pointed out. According to clinical case histories, latent nystagmus seems to be not congenital.

KEYWORDS

Congenital nystagmus; congenital cataract; albinism; achromatopsia, spasmus nutans; gliomas of the optic nerve and chiasm; latent nystagmus.

INTRODUCTION

All kinds of nystagmus observed within a few days of birth are generally called congenital nystagmus (CN).

Two main groups of CN can be differentiated: an 'idiopathic' nystagmus and a nystagmus occurring with *anomalies* of the eyes and/or the CNS.

An 'idiopathic' nystagmus is a nystagmus without any obvious neurological or ocular defect. It is probable, that many patients are included in this category, simply because of a failure to detect the presence of an underlying neurological defect (including vestibular system dysfunction).

An 'idiopathic' CN may be observed clinically as a horizontal, vertical or rotatory type of nystagmus. The analysis of the nystagmic *waveform* does not allow to differentiate between CN with and without eye anomalies (6, 44).

Before a nystagmus can be categorized as an 'idiopathic' one it has to be examined carefully.

Sometimes, there is a family history of nystagmus, but even then an underlying inherited *'occult' ocular disorder* could be possible. 'Occult' ocular disorders commonly exhibit an *autosomal recessive mode* of inheritance (18) as for example Leber's congenital amaurosis, congenital cone dysfunction, optic atrophy, and macular hypoplasia - except for ocular albinism which is inherited as an x-linked recessive disease.

Sometimes it is necessary to make electrodiagnostic tests, particularly ERG or VER.

As mentioned by Wybar (43) 8 of 45 cases with 'idiopathic' nystagmus were initially regarded as having extremely poor vision, or even as being completely blind. This was refuted, however, by electrodiagnostic tests.

Heredity of 'idiopathic' CN: The *irregular dominant x-linked type* is more common than the *recessive x-linked transmission*. In literature, pedigrees of CN are also mentioned with *regular dominant autosomal* inheritance and with *autosomal recessive* inheritance (12). Some authors (14, 9) especially stress the vertical component of the nystagmus in families with autosomal dominant CN.

Frequency of 'idiopathic' CN: Forssman and Ringnér (1971) calculated the frequency of CN: One case with CN in 1000 males and one case with CN in 2800 females. Hemmes (20) calculated only one case with CN in 5032 males and once case in 10.596 females.

Frequency of CN in ocular anomalies: Cataract: A nystagmus occurs in 50 - 75% of patients with complete cataracts, whereas patients with partial cataract exhibit a 30 - 50% incidence of nystagmus. In patients with unilateral cataract, there is likewise an incidence of 30% (16).

Albinism: A nystagmus is present in most patients. Ohm (1930) reported that the reduction of the central visual acuity cannot be the main cause of nystagmus, as there exist also cases of lack of pigment without nystagmus. There are even pedigrees of albino families in which some members have nystagmus and others have not (40).

Achromatopsia: The collection of all case reports combined with additional patients (16) show an incidence of nystagmus of at least 65% in 321 cases with achromatopsia. (Probably in reality the incidence of nystagmus is much higher than 65%).

EARLIEST OCCURRENCES OF CN

Many authors have found that their patients' nystagmus first occurred shortly after birth. Fisher (11) for example, wrote:

> 'The father who was stated to be affected with the same peculiarity had noticed the abnormal movements of his child's eyes, when he first looked at it, within a few hours of its birth.'

In contrast, Nettleship (31) wrote that in the case of some *albino* patients, the oscillations have 'certainly not been noticed until the child was many weeks or even some months old'. Usually a nystagmus is not present in patients with *cataracts* until several months of age (36). In contrast to O'Neill's observations, Goddé-Jolly and Larmande found two patients with both cataract and nystagmus *at birth*. In a case of a baby with *aniridia* (10), no nystagmus was observable at 8 weeks. A nystagmus of a horizontal, variable jerk-type was, however, evident at the age of 4 months.

It has also been reported that nystagmus primarily occurred in the first months of life in *achromatopsia* (19). Likewise, in most cases nystagmus was first observed after several months or years, however, in a few cases already at birth (16).

PROGNOSIS

A long-term prognosis of 'idiopathic' nystagmus is more favourable than the one of 'occult' ocular disorders (18). In two affected families, a complete disappearance of the 'idiopathic' nystagmus during childhood in two out of four boys was reported (23). Nystagmus can also diminish in certain ocular disorders in the course of years. This also holds for *achromatopsia* (30, 16). François et al (15) reported a tendency of reduction or even of disappearance of the nystagmus with age which could be observed regularly in all their patients. Usually this improvement develops in the second decade of age.

We also observed a disappearance of the nystagmus as the following case history proves. Case I: B., Th., born on Dec. 2, 1969.

> He was first seen in the University Eye Clinic Freiburg in July 1977 with a coarse horizontal pendular nystagmus and a photophobia together with an achromatopsia.
> In December 1978, no nystagmus could be observed any more. In December 1980, an ENG was performed which showed normal smooth pursuit movements of the eyes, normal optokinetic responses, and normal saccadic eye movements. There was no spontaneous nystagmus in primary position. However, during gaze holding to one side (20° or 30° right or left gaze) high frequent (8 Hz) pendular movements of very low amplitude for a very short period (2-3 sec) occurred.

The visual acuity of patients with achromatopsia does not improve considerably after the disappearance of the nystagmus.

There are also indications that nystagmus decreases in *albinos*. Krill (27) noticed this phenomenon, particularly in albinos who develop more pigment with age, noting that the nystagmus may eventually disappear altogether. The visual acuity may also eventually increase slightly. Especially in the case of incomplete Tyrosinase-positive oculo-cutaneous albinism, nystagmus, and photophobia are less marked and decrease with age (42).

It has been observed that patients who have undergone *cataract* surgery (36) show a decrease of nystagmus during several months after proper aphakic correction. The association of nystagmus with congenital cataracts is a poor prognostic sign regarding the visual outcome. A better prognosis can be obtained by preoperative absence of nystagmus (37, 16).

HEAD MOVEMENTS

Forsythe encountered a 10-year-old boy with nystagmus and head movements since birth. He also observed a patient, whose head movements began early in infancy and disappeared at 8 years. Another of his patients was conscious of these movements and could stop them for short periods of time. The head movements disappeared during sleep, but the nystagmus persisted.

Gresty et al (17) noticed that the associated head nodding was quite prominent in childhood but had largely disappeared in adult life. The occasional appearance of head nodding without nystagmus in a particular patient, whose family exhibited hereditary nystagmus was reported by Käser (22).

DIFFERENTIAL DIAGNOSIS

Spasmus nutans (Sp. n.) is mentioned in the differential diagnosis of CN with head movements. Sp.n. consists of the following triad: frequent nystagmus, head movements and head tilt occurring usually between the age of four and 12 months or even up to the age of three years. This disorder seldom lasts less than two months, and it can persist until the age of eight years (32). It is characteristic of sp.n. that all its signs disappear spontaneously.

The diagnosis of sp.n. in comparison to that of CN, is made of
1) the age at which the disease begins. Sp.n. begins later than CN.
2) the form of eye movements. In sp.n. there is a characteristic high frequency

nystagmus (6-8 Hz or faster, 32, 17) which is commonly asymmetric or unilateral (32).

3) the form of head movements. In sp.n. head movements seem to be a *learned behavioural pattern* which nullifies the pathological nystagmus. In contrast to this, head movements in CN were found to be of two types: an adaptive response which improves vision and a bizarre waveform ('tremors') (17).

Paroxysmal familial nystagmus which sometimes can be associated with vertigo, oscillations of the head, limb tremors or even ataxia has to be considered in the differential diagnosis (38, 41).

Gliomas of the optic nerve and chiasm represent another very important differential diagnosis to CN and to sp.n. in early infancy. These tumors can also lead to a pendular nystagmus which may be either unilateral or bilateral, vertical or horizontal, and may occasionally be accompanied by abnormal head movements (4).

In patients with vertical pendular nystagmus associated with rotatory eye movements it is necessary to consider the possibility of a *seesaw* nystagmus which can occur congenitally or can be caused by a tumor of the sella region.

LATENT NYSTAGMUS (LN)

Frequency: Lang (28) observed LN in approximately 0,5% of 37.515 patients. (He found 198 patients with LN). Kornhuber (25) calculated a frequency of 0,6% in the average population. Lang (28) found a strabismus in 99% of the 198 cases with LN.

Contrary to this, he found a strabismus in CN, however, only in 30% of his patients.

According to Verhage (39) page 211 and Ishikawa (21) there are only few persons with LN who have *no strabismus* at all who even have orthophoria.

In 60 patients with LN a predominance of male patients was found (63,4%), thus, showing a relationship of almost 2:1 between males and females (26). This could point to the importance of a hereditary factor in LN or in the usually accompanying strabismus. Until now, it is not clear, whether LN is a hereditary disorder as has been presumed in literature (25). There is no answer to the questions: Is strabismus or is LN hereditary?

From our studies of literature, we found many remarks referring to insults of the CNS or the eyes shown at an early infant age. The best example for an acquired disorder, is the report of Abramson (2) on the presence of LN in only one out of two identical twins. The twin with LN had suffered from a febrile convulsion at the age of 9 months, and Abramson states that LN may be caused by 'postnatal insults' to the CNS.

Other acquired causes of LN found in literature: Appearance of LN after longstanding purulent conjunctivitis with corneal impairment, after birth trauma as well as after chorioretinitis.

Our own observation can confirm the findings in literature for an acquired LN as the following case may show:

CASE II: L.J. born on June 27, 1967:

A hemophthalmus was found in both eyes after birth injury in consequence of face presentation. The hemophthalmus was observed on the 9th day after birth in the examination in the University Eye Clinic Freiburg. At that time, no nystagmus could be observed. The blood in the anterior chamber and vitreous was resorbed very slowly. A pendular horizontal nystagmus appeared after several months. The analysis of the nystagmus showed an additional LN when closing one eye at a time.

The observation that LN occurred with CN in four patients with retrolental fibroplasia is a further sign of an early infantile insult (8). In addition, we recently examined three more patients with retrolental fibroplasia and LN with CN. Here is another example of an acquired LN:

CASE III: H.J. born on September 19, 1967:

We also observed a boy in the University Eye Clinic Freiburg with hydrophthalmus of both eyes who presented an esotropia and a LN at the age of one year.

According to all these findings it is apparent that LN cannot be congenital.

PROGNOSIS OF LN

Ohm (1936) observed an essential decreased intensity of LN in a patient who was reexamined nystagmographically after an interval of six years. Another patient is reported in literature (26) who showed an unequivocal LN when five years old, but he did not show a LN any more when controlled eleven years later. Verhage (39) collected 30 cases from literature and added 31 own cases. He remarked that there was hardly any patient with LN in the age of presbyopia. Anderson (3) also stresses that in some of his patients LN appeared to decrease with age but in contrast no diminuition of alternating hyperphoria was observed.

SURGICAL THERAPY OF ALTERED HEAD POSTURE

Anderson-Kestenbaum's principle of treating abnormal head postures in patients with CN is generally recognized.

Periodic alternating nystagmus is a contraindication to Kestenbaum's operation (24). There were several authors who mentioned an increase in visual acuity postoperatively (7). In addition a broadening of the neutral region and an overall reduction in nystagmus in all gaze angles is reported (7). However, there was no improvement in vision in other patients (24).

The surgical treatment of slight abnormal head tilt and the treatment of changing direction of the head posture requires an immobilization-operation ('Faden'-Operation) (29). Several authors perform combined operations (5, 29).

CONSERVATIVE TREATMENT

This consists mainly of prismotherapy. A treatment of CN with prisms seems to be advisable for many patients, however, it has been mentioned that in a series of 120 cases, there were only three patients with 'idiopathic' nystagmus who appeared to be suitable for it (43). Besides treatment with medicaments, the method with after-images, low vision aids with telescopic spectacles, and contact lenses were used in patients with CN. The new method of auditory feedback technique (1) seems to be successful but it has yet to be applied in more patients. Concerning the control of nystagmus, Ohm (33) described a girl with albinism who was aware of her nystagmus and was able to modify it for very short intervals.

CONGENITAL NYSTAGMUS: BASIC ASPECTS

L. F. DELL'OSSO

Ocular Motor Neurophysiology Laboratory, Veterans Administration Medical Center and Department of Neurology, Case Western Reserve University, Cleveland, Ohio, USA

ABSTRACT

Studies of the underlying mechanisms responsible for oscillations of the ocular motor system have provided insights into the normal functioning of this system and resulted in therapeutic benefits to patients afflicted with one such instability. Congenital nystagmus (CN) is the manifestation of a high-gain instability in the slow eye movement (SEM) subsystem which is initiated by fixation attempt. The CN oscillations cause the eyes to move away from and back to the target with any of several waveforms. It is possible to identify a distinct portion in each of these waveforms which corresponds to target foveation. Waveform analysis enables us to distinguish true CN from another congenital form of nystagmus which is mechanistically and phenomenologically different. Accurate detection of null angles in patients with CN can be used to therapeutically intervene to reduce their nystagmus and thereby increase their visual acuity.

KEYWORDS

Congenital nystagmus, genesis, foveation, waveforms, SEM instability, nulls, and acuity.

INTRODUCTION

The last decade has seen the application of two powerful tools to the study of congenital nystagmus (CN): a) accurate ocular motility recording techniques, and b) control system analysis. Preceding this unique two-pronged attack on a mystifying clinical problem was, with a few isolated exceptions, a collection of anecdotal observations, unsubstantiated myths, and benign clinical neglect. The clinician was not in an enviable position because he lacked the following: the ability to differentiate the various CN waveforms; the equipment to accurately locate null angles or to differentially diagnose CN from another common, but largely unrecognized, congenital form of nystagmus; and knowledge of the relationship between the CN waveform and target foveation. Thus, attempts at therapy were few and success stochastic. The level of understanding at that time is best illustrated by the following:

"Never write on nystagmus; it will lead you nowhere." Wilbrant (1921).

"A lot of intensely intelligent and highly dedicated workers have given their lives to this subject of nystagmus and very little has come out of it." Distinguished American neurologist (1965).

and, with tongue in cheek,

"So much has been written about nystagmus that there are only two unresolved questions about nystagmus: 1) the origin of the slow phase, and 2) the origin of the fast phase." Unknown source.

In this chapter, I will confine myself to two of the forty-one distinct varieties of nystagmus which have recently been identified (Dell'Osso, 1980). My discussion of the basic aspects of CN will be divided into several sections: genesis, foveation, waveforms, mechanism, nulls, and acuity. In addition, latent/manifest latent nystagmus (LN/MLN) will be discussed. MLN is a congenital form of nystagmus, but it is not a form of CN; although both are present at birth, they are two distinctly different types of nystagmus. Without the aid of accurate ocular motility recordings MLN is often difficult to distinguish clinically from CN and therefore, is often misdiagnosed as CN.

GENESIS

As with all forms of true nystagmus, a slow eye movement (SEM) is responsible for the genesis and continuation of the oscillation (Dell'Osso, 1980). The cause of the SEM is one of the parameters which differentiate the various types of nystagmus. It may be a rotating visual field, rotation of the subject, a vestibular imbalance, or a brainstem lesion. In 1973 fixation attempt was identified as the stimulus responsible for generating the initial slow eye movements of CN (Dell'Osso, 1973 a,b). Prior to that time, the literature contained contradictory anecdotal observations which attempted to link the genesis of CN with such things as lid position and/or retinal illumination. Since most patients do not attempt to fixate behind closed lids but could be expected to do so with eyes open in a darkened room (especially if not totally dark) it was not unusual to observe that CN "disappeared behind closed lids but remained with lids open in darkness." By carefully controlling fixation attempt, we showed that neither of these conditions were related to the genesis of CN. As increased fixation attempt results in a nystagmus with increased intensity, so does the presence of various psychophysiological inputs. A chain consisting of increased fixation attempt causing increased nystagmus causing decreased acuity causing further increased fixation attempt results in a vicious positive feedback loop which makes it difficult for the patient with CN to see clearly details which are near the level of his maximal acuity (Dell'Osso, 1973b). The clinical implications of this are that one must minimize fixation effort in whatever therapeutic method is employed so that visual acuity can be maximized.

In the past, it was assumed that one type of CN was caused by an afferent defect in the visual system: this was called, "sensory-defect CN." The inference that a sensory defect could cause CN was made because of the association between CN and one or more afferent defects which were present in many, but not all, patients. This confusion of genetic association with true causality was unfortunate and resulted in further muddying of the waters when attempts were made to relate etiology to assumed waveform; this will be discussed later. It should be clearly stated, however, that an afferent defect and the presumed failure to develop fixation reflexes cannot possibly explain a motor oscillation which is present at birth. The reasoning behind the assertions that non-vectorial defects such as aniridia, blurring due to cataracts, ocular albinism etc., should invariably result in the highly-vectorial horizontal CN, is obscure at best. Since many patients with CN have absolutely no sensory defect, it is obvious that such a defect is not a necessary condition for CN. Also, since many patients who have the above sensory defects do not have CN, these defects are not sufficient conditions for CN. Since they are neither necessary nor sufficient, they are not causal. Further discussion of the genesis of CN appears in the section on mechanisms.

FOVEATION

Early descriptions of CN, based on clinical observations, stated that the oscillation was centered about the target or intended gaze angle. Thus, the image of the target on the retina of a person with CN supposedly slid rapidly back and forth across the fovea, never coming to rest in this most important area. Such a description completely ignored a commonly known piece of clinical evidence; patients with CN could have visual acuities in the 20/20 to 20/40 range. Since it is necessary for a target to be imaged in the foveal area for approximately 100 msec to achieve an acuity of 20/20, this clinical description of the CN oscillation was clearly in error. Using both retinal cinematography (with a laser beam as a target) and accurate eye movement recordings, the exact relationship between foveal motion and target position was discovered (Dell'Osso, 1973a). It was shown that in CN the eyes oscillate away from and back to the target such that one peak of the oscillation (be it either pendular or one of the many jerk waveforms) corresponds to target position. Only in this way can the eyes come to rest when the image of the target is directly on the fovea and good visual acuity be possible.

The preferred side of this fixation bias is idiosyncratic as is the frequency with which this bias reverses (i.e. the eyes oscillate to the other side of the target). The bias is conjugate, as are the fixation bias shifts, so that the image of the target always falls on corresponding parts of both retinae. Furthermore, one can see with accurate eye movement recordings that, in the interest of target foveation, most CN waveforms are flattened at those peaks which correspond to target foveation. Thus, the ocular motor system maximizes the amount of time during which the eyes are motionless and the target is foveated (Dell'Osso, Flynn, and Daroff, 1974; Dell'Osso and Daroff, 1975). Note that maintaining target foveation in the face of an instability capable of driving the eyes off target with SEM velocities of several hundred degrees per second requires extremely powerful fixation reflexes not poor, underveloped reflexes as was postulated by the proponents of the sensory-defect idea. In many CN waveforms, target foveation is obtained by foveating saccades which are part of the waveform (Daroff, Troost and Dell'Osso, 1978). Immediately following such saccades, one finds the flattening of the waveform described above (See Fig. 1).

The discovery of the existence of a fixation bias and of shifts in the side of the fixation bias in patients with CN, has uncovered a method to assess foveal function in these patients (Dell'Osso and Daroff, 1975). If the fovea is functioning normally, then the flattened peaks of a CN waveform which correspond to target foveation (with the fixation bias to one side) are at a corresponding gaze angle when the flattened peaks are on the opposite side of the oscillation (after the fixation bias has shifted to the other side). If, in addition to CN, the patient also has foveal dysplasia, there would be a difference of several degrees between where the target is foveated when the oscillation is biased to one side and the position in space where foveation occurs when the bias shifts to the other side. Thus, by observing the shifts in fixation bias, one can assess foveal function in a patient with CN.

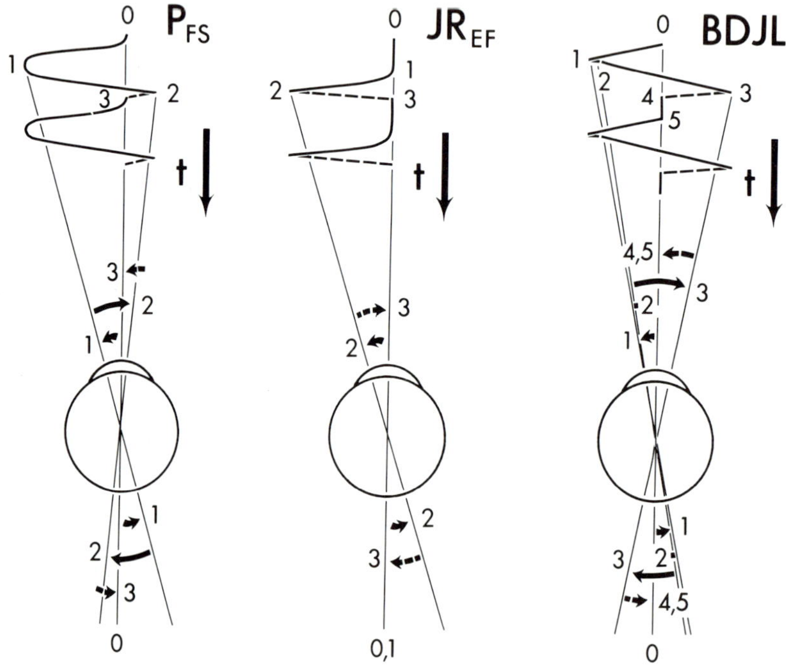

Fig. 1. Illustration of the foveation "strategy" employed during pendular nystagmus with foveating saccades (P_{FS}), jerk right with extended foveation (JR_{EF}), and bidirectional jerk left (BDJL) nystagmus. Target is foveated for extended periods of time resulting in good acuity. Saccades 2-3 (P_{FS}) and 1-2 (BDJL) are braking saccades. Saccades 2-3 (JR_{EF}) and 3-4 (BDJL) are foveating saccades. t, time scale.

WAVEFORMS

Accurate eye movement recordings have been used to identify the twelve distinct waveforms exhibited by patients with CN (Dell'Osso and Daroff, 1975; Dell'Osso, 1976). They fall into three categories: there are 3 pendular waveforms, 8 jerk waveforms, and 1 dual-jerk waveform. Furthermore, the 8 jerk waveforms consist of two groups; 4 are unidirectional and 4 are bidirectional. The classic pure jerk waveform (sawtooth) is extremely rare in CN and more commonly consists of an increasing-velocity SEM off target (slow phase) followed by a foveating saccade (fast phase) which returns the eyes to the target. There are many subtleties about these waveforms which can only be revealed through accurate ocular motility recordings and which are impossible to see clinically. One of the most important of these subtle movements is the small braking saccade. Braking saccades serve to stop (or brake) the classic runaway SEM characteristic of CN. The identification of braking saccades in the study of CN waveforms pointed out a stimulus for saccades which was unknown prior to that point. That is, saccades could serve to stop a runaway SEM in addition to their normal role of repositioning the eyes to bring a target to the fovea (Dell'Osso and Daroff, 1976). In CN waveforms, braking saccades are sometimes also foveating saccades (Fig. 1).

Since the four bidirectional jerk waveforms and pseudo-cycloid (a unidirectional jerk waveform) are clinically indistinguishable from the three pendular waveforms, it became clear that, prior to accurate ocular motility recordings, there was a strong tendency to over-diagnose pendular CN and under-diagnose jerk CN (Dell'Osso and Daroff, 1975). This point becomes extremely important when one considers the attempts which have been made in the past to infer etiology from waveform. The erroneous couplets of sensory-pendular and motor-jerk, which unfortunately still permeate the thinking of many ophthalmologists, became extremely suspect when we realized that these misconceptions were the result of clinical observations alone. They are not supported by accurate eye movement recordings which differentiate the truly pendular waveforms from bidirectional or pseudo-cycloid forms. In fact, no such correspondence exists (i.e. one cannot infer etiology from waveform). We have shown, by the study of a single family with a common genetic heritage, that the manifestation of their CN could take many forms, both pendular and jerk (Dell'Osso, Flynn and Daroff, 1974). Subsequent studies of over two hundred CN patients have confirmed our initial findings.

MANIFEST LATENT NYSTAGMUS

While studying the waveforms of CN, it became clear that there existed another congenital form of nystagmus which was not CN. Many patients referred to our laboratory with the diagnosis of CN had, in fact, a latent nystagmus which was present with both eyes open. Although both eyes were open, the patient was only using one eye to view the world (i.e. he was suppressing the other). Since image suppression is equivalent to occlusion, nystagmus present under these conditions was designated, "manifest latent nystagmus" (MLN) by Kestenbaum (1961). We studied thirty-one patients with MLN (Dell'Osso, Schmidt and Daroff, 1979); some, whose MLN was clearly visible, were misdiagnosed clinically as having CN and others, who appeared to have no nystagmus with both eyes open, were diagnosed clinically as having latent nystagmus. In fact, all had MLN and we have not yet recorded a patient with true LN (i.e. no nystagmus recorded with both eyes open). Since the slow phase of the MLN oscillation is a decreasing-velocity exponential, it is easily differentiated from CN with the aid of accurate eye movement recordings but it is almost impossible to do so by clinical observation alone. MLN is, therefore, nystagmus present with both eyes open, but with only one eye viewing, which has a decreasing-velocity exponential slow phase and a fast phase in the direction of the viewing eye.

The high probability of a misdiagnosis in these cases is important clinically when one is considering therapy (especially surgical therapy). Another way in which accurate eye movement recordings can differentiate between CN and MLN is in the behavior of the oscillation at the various gaze angles. CN usually has a null at some gaze angle and the oscillation increases in intensity to either side of that gaze angle. MLN does not have a null except that, in accordance with Alexander's Law, it may diminish as gaze is directed in the direction of the slow phase. Knowing the distinctions between the slow phase waveforms and the behavior of the nystagmus with different gaze angles, it becomes relatively easy to use accurate ocular motility recordings to diagnose differentially CN, MLN, or various forms of acquired nystagmus (Dell'Osso, Schmidt and Daroff, 1979). Since CN and MLN are distinct types of nystagmus, it should be noted that a patient may have both. We have recorded many patients with both CN and MLN to varying degrees.

Important facts which relate to the mechanism of MLN are as follows: a) the direction of the conjugate slow phase exponential drift is <u>always</u> nasal to the viewing eye and is independent at gaze angle, strabismus angle or tropia type (i.e. ET or XT); b) in some patients MLN can also be recorded in the dark with no retinal input. Thus, any hypotheses aimed at explaining MLN must apply equally to ET's and XT's, must apply with the fixing eye in full adduction as well as abduction and should not rely on a mechanism requiring retinal input. Consistent with these constraints we have put forth the hypothesis that MLN is caused by a confusion between the perceived egocentric direction associated with binocular vision ($\theta_P = \frac{\theta_R + \theta_L}{2}$) and that associated with monocular vision ($\theta_P = \theta_R$ or θ_L). Such a confusion will always result in a conjugate nasal exponential drift toward the improperly perceived version angle (a simple step-response of the ocular motor plant). This nasal drift is independent of gaze angle or tropia and is independent of retinal input. Theories which rely on pursuit asymmetries and/or lateral gaze-holding inabilities fail to explain the directional constancy of MLN under all combinations of the above variables. The MLN of an XT (25% of patients we have seen with MLN are XT's) is exactly the same as that of an ET (i.e. direction, waveform and variation with gaze angle). All evidence points to a single mechanism causing MLN in both ET's and XT's that is distinctly different from the mechanism causing CN.

MECHANISMS

The initial evidence supporting the hypothesis that a high-gain instability of the SEM subsystem caused CN, came from observations made in a variable feedback experiment (Dell'Osso and colleagues, 1972). It was found that a patient with CN was able to pursue more rapidly moving targets than normal subjects could. This prompted the use of variable artificial feedback to change the overall loop gain. A normal subject will brake into a repetitive series of back and forth saccades under these conditions; the patient with CN developed a high-gain pendular oscillation. This response indicated that his SEM subsystem was responding in the abnormal experimental situation. Additional evidence, given the fact that the SEM subsystem and fixation are closely linked (if not unitary), consists of the following: fixation attempt is responsible for generating the nystagmus oscillation; the CN patient is locked in a positive feedback loop in which increasing his effort to see results in an increased nystagmus oscillation; and the waveforms of CN are either pendular (sinusoidal) or consist of increasing-velocity SEM runaways. Taken together, these data suggest to the control system engineer, two distinct types of feedback system instability.

One can describe a feedback control system by its system transfer function, which is the ratio of two polynomials in the variable (s) which describe input and output behavior (gain) over all frequencies. The polynomials can be factored into roots where the roots of the numerator polynomial are called, "zeroes", and the roots of the denominator polynomial, "poles." As the gain of a feedback control system is changed, so are the positions of the poles when plotted on the s-plane (i.e. real $s=\sigma$ on the X-axis and the imaginery $s=j\omega$ on the Y-axis) (Daroff and Dell'Osso, 1979). The mathematical background to understand clearly the positions and migration of these system poles and their relationship to oscillations in a closed-loop system is too extensive to be discussed here. Suffice it to say that when two of these poles are on the imaginery axis ($j\omega$-axis poles) the system oscillates in a sinusoidal manner and, when a pole exists on the positive-real axis (σ-axis poles) an increasing-velocity SEM runaway results. Since these poles migrate with various values of gain, it is not surprising that a system (or a patient) may manifest either one or both types of instability. We have observed many patients with CN who have both pendular and jerk waveforms.

The exact manner in which high gain affects SEM stability is unknown. If the instability merely results from high gain and a negative feedback loop, then the transfer function must be non-minimum phase (i.e. a pole or a zero must exist on the positive σ-axis). It is also possible that the rising gain alters the basic nature of the loop by changing a normal inhibitory junction into an excitatory one and, in so doing, creates a local positive feedback loop which would allow for positive-real pole positions without having been a non-minimum phase system. In a patient, increasing the gain (or fixation attempt) appears to drive the poles up the $j\omega$-axis, since the frequency of the oscillation may increase along with its amplitude. In a similar manner, increasing effort (gain) seems to drive a pole further into the right-half plane (on the σ-axis). The behavior of CN patients with a dual-jerk nystagmus waveform supports the contention that the pendular and jerk waveforms are independent oscillations caused by different types of instability. Usually dual-jerk is a high-frequency, low-amplitude pendular oscillation superimposed on a low-frequency, high-amplitude jerk nystagmus. One or the other component can be independently reduced or eliminated or, one component may spontaneously diminish or increase.

Initially, it was thought that the high gain of the SEM subsystem resulted from a primary defect in the saccadic subsystem (Dell'Osso and colleagues, 1972). This hypothesis arose from observations of saccades which were smaller than those required to refixate new targets. However, subsequent studies, made after identification of the relationship between waveform and target foveation, showed conclusively that the new targets were always accurately foveated by a combination of the ongoing oscillatory waveform and a saccade. Thus, the calculation of required saccadic amplitude was accomplished by the saccadic subsystem using information from the oscillating SEM subsystem, truly an impressive feat requiring precise amplitude and phase information. Whatever the reason for the high gain in the SEM subsystem, it can safely be said that it is not due to a deficient saccadic subsystem. Pendular CN may merely result from increasing the loop gain of an otherwise normal SEM subsystem with its inherent transport lags. Similarly, jerk CN may be the result of too much gain occurring in the normally present positive feedback loop around the neural integrator. Zee, Leigh and Mathieu-Millaire (1980) proposed the existence of such a loop when discussing cerebellar-induced gain changes which caused increasing-velocity runaway slow phases in nystagmus acquired by a patient with cerebellar dysfunction. Since no lesions have ever been associated with CN, it is reasonable to hypothesize that CN results from high gain in an otherwise normal neurological control loop.

The clinical phenomenon of inversion of the optokinetic reflex and the relationship between the head oscillation of patients with CN and their CN waveforms are topics which deserve mention in this section on mechanism. Over the past ten years, I have observed that the null angle of a CN patient (normally stationary unless he has periodic alternating nystagmus) was a function of eye velocity as well as position. That is, during SEM tracking the null would shift in a direction opposite to the pursuit direction (unpublished observations of many CN patients). The amplitude of the shift need not be equal in both directions and could be related to the pursuit velocity. Such a shift can be seen in Fig. 6 of Dell'Osso and colleagues (1972) but it was not discussed and, until recently, has remained only a curiosity tucked away in my bin of interesting findings which should be studied further. Since I and several other colleagues in our laboratory failed to connect this observation with any clinical findings or significant mechanistic hypotheses, it remained a low-priority item. However, Halmagyi, Gresty and Leech (1980) have recently made the critical connection. They discovered this virtually unknown phenomenon and used it to show that the reversed optokinetic nystagmus found in patients with CN was due to the patient's own gaze-modulated nystagmus shifted to the primary position by the optokinetic stimulation. These workers demonstrated the modulation of a CN patient's nystagmus by attempted smooth pursuit. Thus, the null agle in patients with CN is a function of both intended eye position and intended eye velocity. It should be noted here that presentation of an OKN stimulus to a CN patient cannot be equated with an adequate OKN stimulus to his retina. The latter requires stabilizing the image motions due to the CN and then imposing the OKN retinal image drift (a very difficult task). Thus, inferences about the functioning of the basic OKN system of a CN patient made by studying responses to simple OKN stimulus presentations must be highly suspect. The resulting eye movements may be modified CN, CN plus OKN or modified CN plus OKN but they will not be OKN alone. As a final thought on this subject, it would not be surprising to discover (when we are able to properly study it) that the basic OKN reflex of a CN patient has been modified since the retina has constantly been exposed to horizontally moving images which must be perceptually stabilized. Such a finding, which has not yet been satisfactorily shown, would in no way imply cause and effect (i.e. an OKN asymmetry causing CN). CN is present at birth (before foveation reflexes develop) and in the dark (where the possible existence of an OKN asymmetry is irrelevant).

It has long been claimed that the head motion, seen in some patients with CN, was compensatory. For this to be true, the patient's vestibulo-ocular gain would have to be reduced to a value of zero (Daroff, Troost and Dell'Osso, 1978). It has now been shown that the head oscillation is not a compensatory movement (Gresty, Halmagyi and Leech, 1978). Rather, it has a common pathological origin with the CN and does not affect the periods of target foveation found in the CN waveform because of the normal vestibulo-ocular reflex acting to cancel the motion induced by the head oscillation.

Since CN is caused by a high-gain instability in the SEM subsystem, one might expect persons with CN to be able to pursue moving targets at least as well as normals. Indeed, CN patients have no trouble (personal observation) with such sports as handball, racquetball, baseball, etc., all of which make high demands on the pursuit subsystem. However, uncritical observation, by either man or an unsophisticated computer algorithm, of ocular motility records on attempted pursuit by CN patients might lead one to doubt that they can pursue at all. The apparent paradox is easily resolved if one understands the mechanism of CN as it relates to actual target foveation. It is only during the flattened portions of most CN waveforms that the eyes are motionless and on target. During the remaining portions they are either being irresistably drawn off target with ever-increasing velocity or they are being directed back towards the target by a saccade. Thus, the only times one might accurately assess the integrity of smooth pursuit in the CN subject is during these otherwise motionless foveation intervals. If one imagines a simple jerk waveform (constant in amplitude and frequency) added to a perfect ramp tracking eye movement, what results bears no resemblance to the good smooth pursuit of a normal but would reflect the good smooth pursuit of a patient with such an ongoing nystagmus. But we know that with gaze angle changes, as well as attempted pursuit, CN waveforms change in type, amplitude, frequency and direction. Although the resultant eye movement records look nothing like good normal pursuit, they may actually represent good pursuit, given an ever-present CN. Evaluation of smooth pursuit (or the response to an OKN stimulus) must be done with full recognition of the inherrent changes in CN which accompany the responses of a CN patient to either stimulus. It cannot be done by simple computer algorhithms which identify saccades (excluding small braking saccades, which they miss) and construct simple linear links between the end of one saccade and the beginning of the next. Such artificial data are unrelated to the true eye movements of a CN patient and conclusions drawn from analysis of such data are so suspect as to be meaningless.

NULLS

The use of ocular motility recordings has enabled us to accurately define the null angle and/or convergence angle which results in a nulling of a patient's CN (Dell'Osso and colleagues, 1972). This can be directly translated into the size of prism required or, in cases where the null angle is too large, the exact amount of surgery to be performed. Accurate eye movement recordings have been used to identify the shift in null position with occlusion of each eye, commonly called the latent component in CN, and are also useful in documenting the null shift with time in periodic alternating nystagmus (Daroff and Dell'Osso, 1974; Dell'Osso, Flynn and Daroff, 1974). Additionally, ocular motility recordings have documented the stationarity (during fixation) of the null angles in patients with CN both pre-operatively and post-operatively (Dell'Osso and Flynn, 1979). Anecdotal comments concerning a mysterious revival of a new null angle, after surgical intervention had supposedly shifted the original null to the primary position, have been laid to rest. When properly done, surgery permanently shifts the null angle to the primary position; this has been documented by ocular motility recordings made immediately post-operatively and null stationarity has been documented by periodic recordings. If the initial surgery was inadequate, the new null angles will also appear immediately post-operatively; the adoption of a new head position may take several days. These will remain stationary until a second operation is performed. Information about other effects of CN surgery has also been provided by accurate ocular motility recordings. It has been found that, in addition to shifting the null, surgery broadened the null and decreased the intensity of the nystagmus at off-null gaze angles (Dell'Osso and Flynn, 1979). Follow-up on some cases that we have studied pre- and post-operatively has shown the null to remain stationary at the new position for many years (Flynn and Dell'Osso, 1979).

ACUITY

One of the important results of our studies of CN using accurate ocular motility recordings has been the realization that acuity of CN patients could be improved; in many cases they had previously been the objects of benign neglect. The therapeutic benefits resulting from such studies of CN have been significant. They range from very simple things, such as seating a child in the center of a classroom to maximize angle at which he views the board (thus minimizing the horizontal shrinkage caused by his horizontal oscillation) to the more complex realization that post-operative visual acuity can be greater than pre-operative acuity at the null (Dell'Osso and Flynn, 1979). Surgical rotation and prism rotation are not mere substitutions for head turning. Both considerably reduce the "effort-to-see" or "fixation attempt" and permit optimal acuity at-a-glance;

this is the aim of good CN therapy and is also why post-operative, primary position acuity can be better than pre-operative acuity at the null angle. Studies of waveforms (Dell'Osso, Flynn and Daroff, 1974; Dell'Osso and Daroff, 1975) revealed the importance of foveation time and the distortion of the oscillatory waveform which was imposed by the ocular motor system in an effort to increase foveation time. An analysis of foveation time and CN has also been presented by Abadi and Sandikcioglu (1974).

In addition to the use of prisms and the utilization of CN surgery, auditory biofeedback has been proposed as a method to diminish CN intensity and thereby permit greater acuity (Abadi, Carden and Simpson, 1979). This latter method takes advantage of the effects of psychophysiological inputs on the intensity of CN (Dell'Osso, 1973b). While useful in the laboratory, biofeedback has not yet been shown to be beneficial over long periods of time. Although the use of biofeedback is promising, it must be demonstrated that CN patients can voluntarily diminish their oscillation without the aid of biofeedback in real life situations. It should be noted that, if this can be demonstrated, the ability to calm oneself and diminish an existing CN is not dependent on the biofeedback which facilitated the learning process. Thus, other methods (yoga, tanscendental meditation, etc.) could also be used. The success of such "mind-set" altering therapies would probably be highly idiosyncratic.

IS HEAD POSITION IMPORTANT IN CONGENITAL NYSTAGMUS?

M. S. LOMAS, R. V. ABADI and C. M. DICKINSON

Department of Ophthalmic Optics, University of Manchester Institute of Science and Technology, Manchester M60 1QD, UK

ABSTRACT

Congenital nystagmus waveforms recorded for various combinations of head and eye position were compared. Results indicated that head rotation itself did not modify the waveform and that eye position was the important parameter.

KEYWORDS

Congenital nystagmus; idiopathic; albino; eye position; head position.

INTRODUCTION

A variation with gaze direction and the frequent association with head turns must have been two of the earliest observations made on congenital nystagmus (CN). It has been generally assumed that any head rotation merely brings the "null position" or position of least nystagmus into the more useful straight ahead direction. This study sets out to examine if the CN depends only on eye position or if the head rotation itself has some modifying effect. Obviously such findings would be important to consider for present surgical CN procedures.

METHODS

Thirteen subjects with CN were studied, seven oculocutaneous albinos and six idiopathic cases. Their ages ranged from 12 to 48 years. Both albino and idiopathic subjects showed typical CN waveforms and presented a history of nystagmus from early infancy. The experiments consisted of examining the CN waveform obtained with different combinations of horizontal head and eye positions:-

a) Eye rotation only - with the head in the primary position gaze was directed at LED's positioned centrally and at intervals every 10° out to $\pm 30^{\circ}$. These targets subtended 15' arc when viewed from 114 cm.

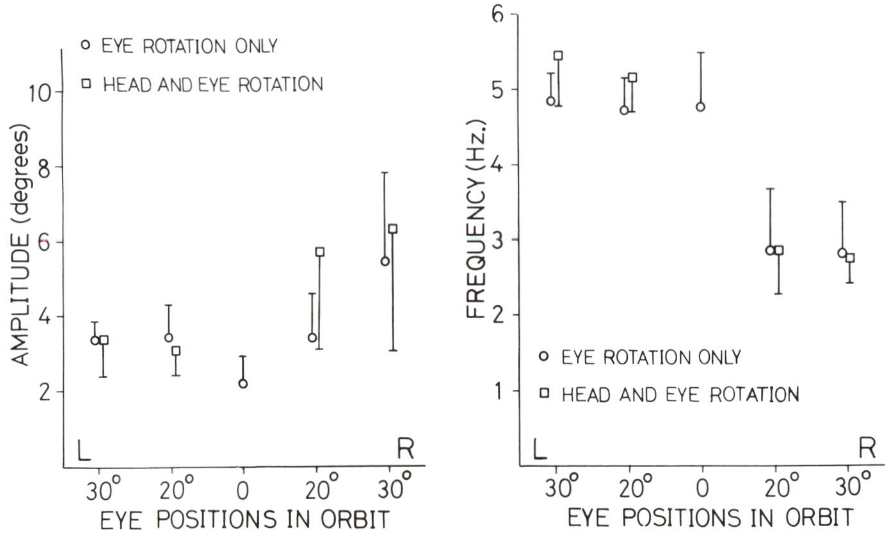

Fig. 1. Manual analysis for one albino subject illustrating nystagmus peak-to-peak amplitude and frequency variation for orbital eye positions reached by eye and combined head/eye rotations. No significant trends are present.

b) Head and eye rotation - with fixation maintained on the central LED, the head was turned ± 10°, 20° and 30°.

c) Head rotation only - with the head turned 30° to right or left while fixating, the LED positioned at the same angle as the head rotation.

Horizontal movements of both eyes were measured using DC electro-oculography and calibrated in the usual manner. Both chart and magnetic tape recordings were made of the responses. A tightly fitting adjustable head band attached to a light aluminium frame permitted horizontal head rotations centred about the approximate head/neck centre of rotation, so that a linear potentiometer attached to the frame and a large calibration protractor enabled head rotation measurement.

Analysis

For each orbital eye position a comparison between the CN recorded as a result of eye rotation alone and combined head/eye rotation was made using three techniques-

a) Qualitative analysis - using Dell'Osso's waveform classification (Dell'Osso and Daroff, 1975).

b) Manual quantitative analysis - mean amplitude and frequency were calculated from chart recorder measurements. Harmonic components present in some waveforms made such analysis difficult.

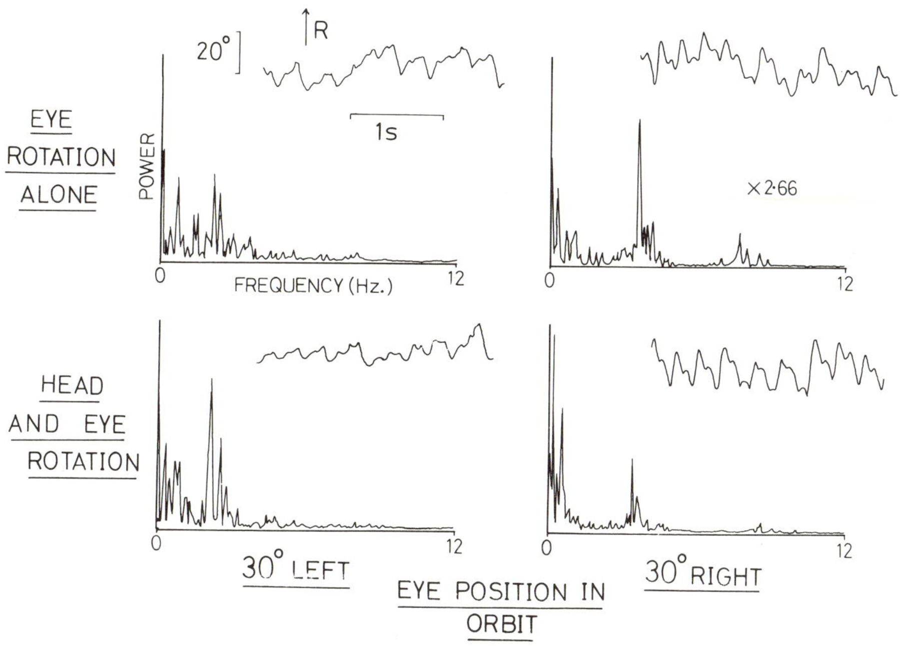

Fig. 2. Fourier analysis and nystagmus waveforms for one idiopathic subject. For each orbital eye position, the power spectra show similar frequency components of comparable amplitudes for both eye and head/eye paradigms. The use of different scaling factors explains the amplitude differences in the 30° right position. Multiplication of the lower trace values by 2.66 equalizes power scales. The nystagmus waveforms are also qualitatively similar; a dual jerk right being obvious for the right orbital position.

c) A discrete fast Fourier transform was performed on the recorded data for the 30° eye and head/eye rotation positions. Using PAFFT overlay to Daquan MS program, the PDP 8 computer produced a bandwidth of 0-15 Hz from continuous 17 second data samples. As the aim was again one of comparison, no attempt at calibration of the power spectrum in absolute terms was undertaken.

DISCUSSION AND RESULTS

Gresty (1977) mentions three consequences that head rotation could have on central nervous system activity -

a) mechanical distortion of the brainstem

b) circulatory disturbances in the vertebral and possibly spinal arteries

c) initiation of proprioceptive signals from the neck's joint and muscle receptors.

If any of the above factors were to have an influence on the CN then it would seem reasonable to expect an increasing or at least consistent effect with increasing neck torsion. Hence any isolated, even if obvious differences between eye and head/eye rotation instances would most likely just be due to unconnected CN variations as alertness and fixation attempt vary. As a second check, any differences found should also be apparent in the head rotation alone paradigm.

For all subjects examined no qualitative or meaningful quantitative differences could be found between the CN for any orbital eye position attained by either eye or head/eye rotations (Figs. 1 and 2). Head rotation alone resulted in waveforms similar to that found with central head and eye positioning. If any contribution from head rotation was present it was too small to be extracted from the random CN fluctuations found in all subjects. Hence for the degree of head torsions used the three factors mentioned above presumably had minimal effects on the neural mechanisms responsible for the CN. The above conclusions held for both idiopathic and albino subjects irrespective of the presence of any habitual head posture. Additionally outside the study group, two cases of manifest latent nystagmus (Dell'Osso, Schmidt and Daroff, 1979) and two post-operative idiopathic subjects also showed that head rotation played no part in deciding their CN characteristics.

ACKNOWLEDGEMENTS

This work was supported by an MRC Project Grant No G979/1025/N and Christine Dickinson received an MRC studentship award No 77/7291. The Wellcome Trust kindly provided assistance with travelling expenses.

INVERTED AND ASYMMETRICAL OPTOKINETIC NYSTAGMUS

R. V. ABADI, C. M. DICKINSON and M. S. LOMAS

Department of Ophthalmic Optics, University of Manchester Institute of Science and Technology, Manchester M60 1QD, UK

ABSTRACT

Large field optokinetic responses of subjects with congenital nystagmus (CN) were examined. If the stimulus moved in the same plane as the CN then under binocular viewing conditions the spontaneous nystagmus was present in a gaze - modulated form for both albino and idiopathic subjects. Monocular responses, however, differed for the two observer groups.

KEYWORDS

Congenital nystagmus; albino; idiopathic; optokinetic nystagmus; inversion; asymmetry.

INTRODUCTION

When normal observers view a drifting pattern, the resultant involuntary conjugate eye movements are most distinctive. Linear slow phases in the same direction as the motion of the stimulus are interrupted by fast opposing saccades giving rise to the classic optokinetic nystagmus (OKN). However, sometimes, the OKN response can show irregularities and in the past clinicians have attempted to correlate these irregularities with particular CNS disorders. For example, it seems generally accepted that a reversed OKN is pathognomonic of congenital nystagmus (Barany 1921, Brunner 1933, Dichgans and Jung 1975). The aim of this paper is therefore two-fold - to examine this diagnostic assertion and to uncover any other possible deviations from the norm.

SUBJECTS AND METHODS

All observers had congenital nystagmus (CN); seven oculocutaneous albinos and five classified as idiopathic. Records of how the spontaneous nystagmus altered with gaze were made using DC electro-oculography (EOG). With the help of velocity traces the nystagmus waveforms were classified in keeping with Dell'Osso and

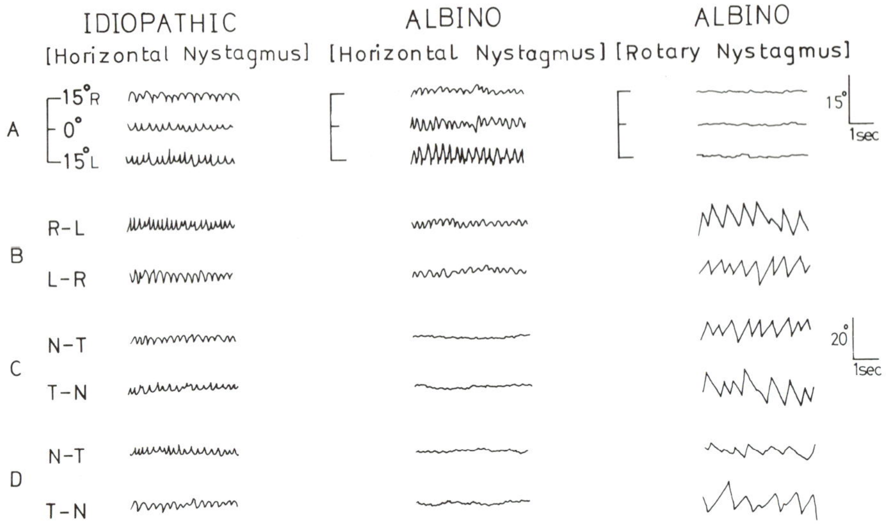

Fig. 1. Optokinetic responses (OKR) for 3 observers with congenital nystagmus (CN). Trace A - spontaneous gaze evoked CN; B - binocular OKR for right to left (R-L) and left to right (L-R) stimulus movement; C and D - monocular OKR for right and left eyes respectively for nasal to temporal (N-T) and temporal to nasal (T-N) stimulus motion. Pattern velocity was 50°/sec.

Daroff (1975).

The optokinetic stimulus consisted of low spatial frequency stripes moving horizontally across a semi-cylindrical field (180° x 42°) at one of four velocities 10, 30, 50 or 80°/sec. Both monocular and binocular viewing conditions were examined. Each subject was instructed to gaze into the centre of the pattern and keep the bars clear. The horizontal eye movements of both eyes were simultaneously recorded by EOG.

RESULTS AND DISCUSSION

The responses of the idiopathic subjects clearly followed recently reported characteristics. That is, if the stimulus field moved right to left, the spontaneous nystagmus habitually found on looking to the left was present even though the eyes were directed towards the primary position; if it moved from left to right the right gaze oscillation became apparent (Fig. 1) (Halmagyi, Gresty and Leech 1980). The higher stimulus velocities were more likely to initiate this response. Though the induced nystagmus often beat in an anomalous direction it was not a true reversed OKN. This was because the slow phase of the nystagmus did not show constant velocity and it did not show the familiar saw-tooth waveform. A better description would be inverted OKN (Yee, Baloh and Honrubia 1980 , Le Liever

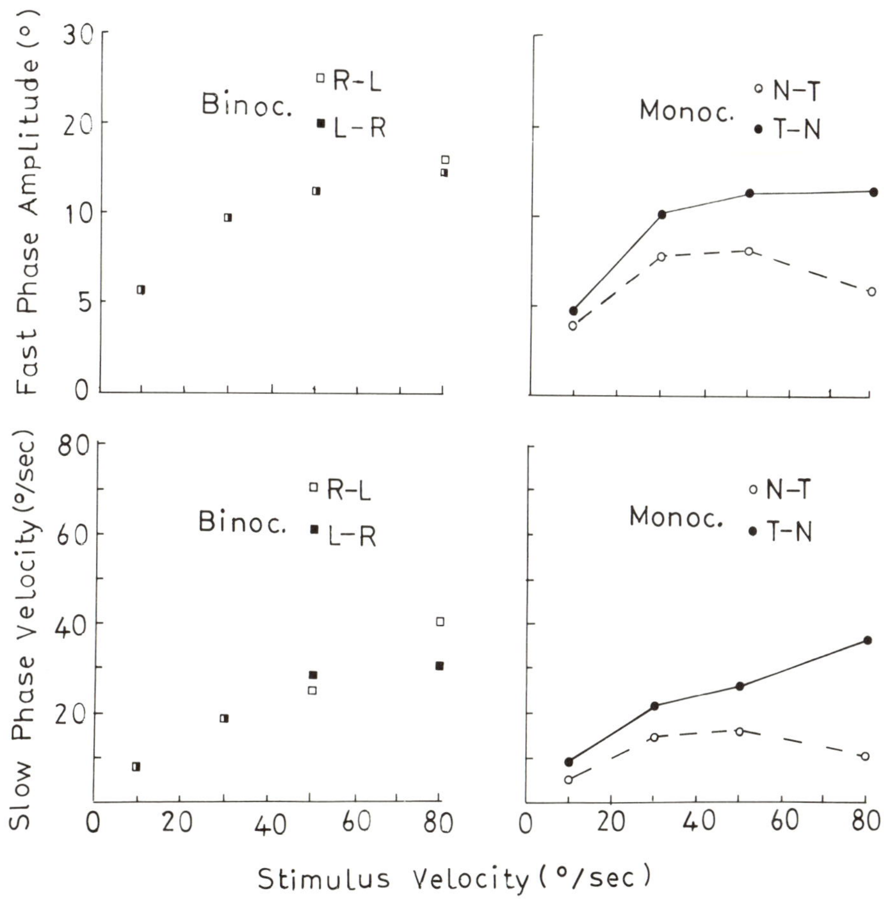

Fig. 2. An albino observer with rotary CN shows monocular asymmetrical responses.

and Barber 1981). The monocular responses showed the same pattern.

All four of the albino observers with horizontal CN showed binocular responses similar to the idiopaths. However the monocular responses, irrespective of the direction of the stimulus, tended to show persistence of the primary position CN in a highly irregular or diminished form (Fig. 1). In both groups it was impossible to report any directional asymmetries for monocular viewing. On the other hand, one albino with a rotary nystagmus showed a normal saw-tooth waveform shape for both binocular and monocular conditions. Moreover monocular stimulation gave rise to asymmetrical OKN responses (Figs. 1 and 2). It therefore seems that an inversion is pathognomonic of CN only when the stimulus moves in the same meridian as the spontaneous CN, thus verifying a suggestion made by Jung and Kornhuber in 1964. To test this further we examined the horizontal OKN of a subject with an idiopathic vertical CN. There was no inversion nor asymmetry of the responses. This would imply that OKN asymmetry is related to foveal function (Baloh, Yee, Honrubia 1980b).

ACKNOWLEDGEMENTS

This work was supported by an MRC Project Grant no G979/1025/N and Christine Dickinson received an MRC Studentship award no 77/7291. The Wellcome Trust kindly provided assistance with travelling expenses.

CONTROL OF NYSTAGMUS USING EYE MOVEMENT AUDITORY BIOFEEDBACK

K. J. CIUFFREDA, S. G. GOLDRICH and C. NEARY

State University of New York/State College of Optometry, 100 East 24th Street, New York, N.Y. 10010, USA

ABSTRACT

Eye movement auditory biofeedback was used in weekly training sessions to control nystagmus in 5 adult patients. Visual, psychological, and cosmetic benefits were accrued by all patients. Persistence of this conditioning effect was demonstrated.

KEYWORDS

Nystagmus, biofeedback, fixation, eye movements, visual acuity

INTRODUCTION

Nystagmus, abnormally-large rhythmic movement of the eyes, is a common clinical ocular condition involving the sensory-motor system. Several methods have been used to aid in the control and treatment of nystagmus (Ciuffreda, Goldrich, and Neary, in press), but none have had wide appeal. The goal of extraocular muscle surgery and composite prism glasses is to "shift" the null zone into primary position. This permits attainment of maximum visual acuity without necessity of a concomitant head turn. While extraocular muscle surgery has produced good functional and cosmetic results, it does require careful patient screening and necessitates use of sophisticated eye movement instrumentation for evaluative purposes. Further, transient or even permanent post-surgical diplopia can occur. Cosmetic acceptability and image degradation limit the amount of prism used in composite prism glasses. After-image training allows the patient to use visual feedback to monitor directly changes in eye position and velocity. It is believed that availability of this information to the oculomotor system allows for rapid learning of error reduction, initially in the null position with gradual expansion into contiguous regions of visual space. However, contrary to initial expectations, it has met with only limited success. Orthoptics has improved vision function in some cases. Instructing patients to "hold the eye steady" rather than to "fixate accurately" while looking at a target has reduced nystagmus in selected patients. Reduction of nystagmus with concomitant slight improvement in contrast sensitivity has been reported recently (Abadi, Carden, and Simpson, 1980) in 3 patients following eye movement auditory biofeedback training at home for 6 months. The present paper reviews and expands upon our recent findings (Ciuffreda, Goldrich, and Neary, 1980, 1981, in press) using eye movement auditory biofeedback in weekly laboratory sessions to train control of eye position and velocity in 5 patients having either congenital jerk or acquired pendular nystagmus.

METHODS

Methodology has been detailed elsewhere (Ciuffreda, Goldrich and Neary, 1981, in press) and will only be briefly described here. Horizontal eye position of one eye, during either monocular or binocular viewing and with refractive correction in place, was monitored by a photoelectric technique (Stark et al, 1977). The audio-feedback unit received electrical input from the eye movement monitor through an adjustable level detector integrated circuit whose output signal controlled a voltage regulated audio oscillator integrated circuit having a frequency range of 500 to 5000 Hz. Output signal was amplified and played back to the patient through a loudspeaker. Characteristics of the tone reflected eye position and steadiness during midline fixation, i.e., the patient "heard" his nystagmus. Therapy was administered in weekly (3 to 13 weeks) one-hour training sessions. Following baseline recording of fixation, the auditory biofeedback was added, and the patient was instructed to "do something" to reduce the jerkiness of the tone. Distance Snellen visual acuity with unlimited viewing time was evaluated at the beginning and end of each session with patients using the newly-learned training strategy, but without auditory biofeedback, to reduce nystagmus and maximize visual acuity.

RESULTS

Our findings are summarized in Table 1, and representative recordings are presented in Figure 1. Average maximum group reduction of nystagmus amplitude, peak slow-phase velocity, and frequency was 82, 86, and 34%, respectively, with addition of eye movement auditory biofeedback. Some reduction of nystagmus was evident at the initial training session. Further, after 2 or 3 sessions, all patients were able to reduce nystagmus for several minutes with audio cues removed. Outside the test/training apparatus, patients were able to control their nystagmus rapidly and at will (our goal was to get the patient to reduce nystagmus on cue within a few seconds). This was based on study of videotape recordings as well as by careful visual observations made by us in the laboratory and by friends of the patients at work and in the home. It should be emphasized here, however, that nystagmus reduction was only accomplished by conscious, concentrated effort by the

TABLE 1 RESULTS OF EYE MOVEMENT AUDITORY BIOFEEDBACK TRAINING

Patient No.	Visual Acuity Initial/Final (20/)	Mean Amplitude (deg) Nystagmus Without/With Biofeedback	Mean Frequency (Hz) Nystagmus Without/With Biofeedback	Mean Peak Slow-Phase Velocity (deg/sec) Nystagmus Without/With Biofeedback
1	$50^{-2}/40^{-1}$	2.2/0.4	2.6/1.8	20.0/2.8
2	$30^{+3}/15^{-1}$	1.2/0.2	2.8/1.4	27.7/1.3
3	$50^{+1}/40^{+1}$	1.0/0.2	3.4/1.5	7.0/1.2
4	100/50	3.8/0.4	2.6/2.4	22.0/2.5
5	$25^{-3}/15^{-1}$	0.8/0.2	3.1/2.4	12.0/2.8
$\overline{X}$ =		1.8/0.3	2.9/1.9	17.7/2.1

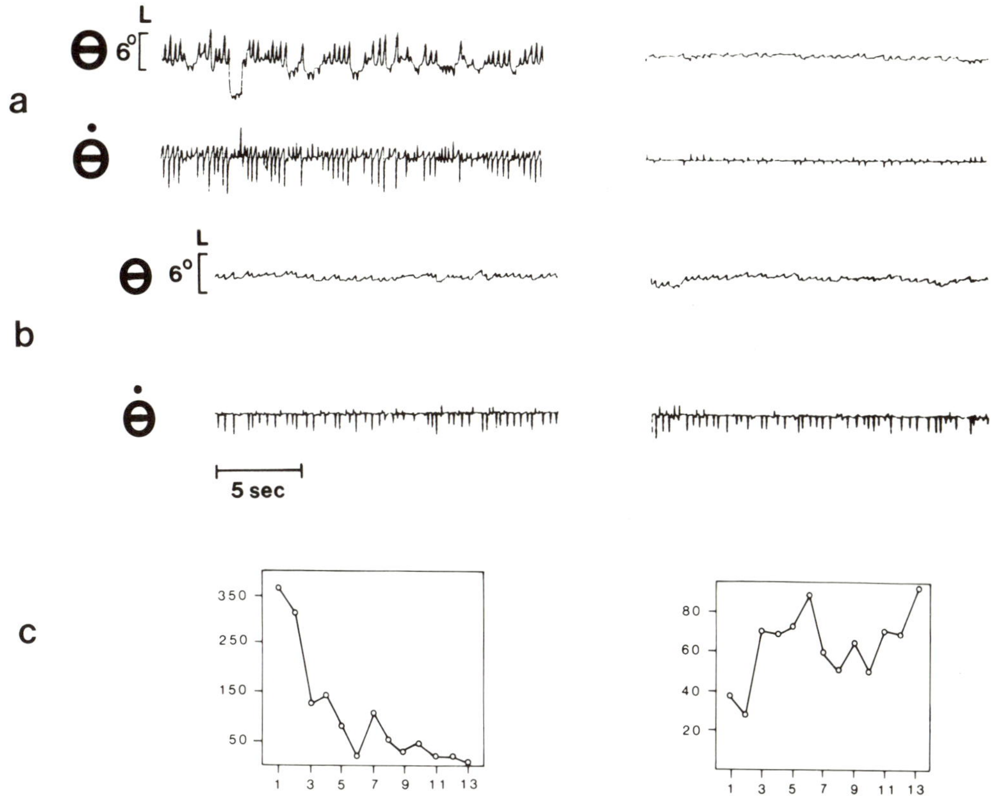

Fig. 1. Results for patient 1. (a) Eye position (Θ) and velocity ($\dot{\Theta}$) as a function of time. Fixation without (left) and with (right) auditory biofeedback. Reduction of nystagmus is evident when audio cues added. (b)Eye position (Θ) and velocity ($\dot{\Theta}$) as a function of time. Fixation with auditory biofeedback provided (left) and subsequently withdrawn (right). Similarity of responses demonstrates ability to maintain reduced nystagmus following feedback withdrawal. (c) Performance with auditory biofeedback as related to weekly session number. Left graph shows time in seconds to reduce nystagmus to specified criterion level, and right graph shows percent time at this reduced nystagmus level, as training progressed.

patient (it is of interest that speech therapists report that most stutterers must continuously maintain conscious effort while using breathing techniques which reduce stuttering). Thus, our training did not alter the baseline nystagmus characteristics per se, but rather involved the influence of conscious higher-level control on the basic neural discharge pattern producing nystagmus. Visual acuity was measured at the end of training with the patient attempting to reduce nystagmus in the absence of the audio information. Gains, found in each patient, ranged from 1 to 4 lines Snellen. Of 2 patients retested several months later, one was able to reduce nystagmus significantly without eye movement auditory biofeedback, while both could markedly reduce nystagmus within a few seconds when audio information was subsequently provided. Visual acuity remained improved in both patients. Thus, the post-training eye movement and visual acuity results suggest persistence of the basic conditioning effect.

DISCUSSION

The results of our investigation were encouraging and clearly demonstrated the effectiveness of eye movement auditory biofeedback in the control of nystagmus. All patients received visual, psychological and cosmetic benefits from the training. Nystagmus could frequently be reduced so that it was barely detectable by our recording system and undetectable to the naked eye, with concomitant improvement of vision. Improvement of visual acuity in some of our patients may have been greater if not for the reduced neural sensitivity of the visual pathways resulting from abnormal experience, i.e., the habitually increased retinal-image motion. In addition, patients were now able to reduce the nystagmus at will for the first time in their lives resulting in obvious psychological and cosmetic benefits. One of us (S.G.G.) is continuing this research, with inclusion of additional training procedures such as the emergent textural contour stimulator (Goldrich, 1981) which provides visual feedback regarding eye position, eye movement, and eye focus during fixation and scanning of targets. Results have been positive and further studies are planned using a broader clinical base.

ACKNOWLEDGEMENTS

This project was supported in part by grants from The Optometric Extension Program Foundation (Project Number 80-81-1), The Optometric Center of New York Research Foundation, and The American Optometric Foundation.

EFFECT OF BACLOFEN ON CONGENITAL NYSTAGMUS

R. D. YEE*, R. W. BALOH** and V. HONRUBIA***

**Jules Stein Eye Institute, Department of Ophthalmology, UCLA School of Medicine, Los Angeles, California, USA*
***Department of Neurology, UCLA School of Medicine, Los Angeles, California, USA*
****Division of Head and Neck Surgery, UCLA School of Medicine, Los Angeles, California, USA*

ABSTRACT

Baclofen produced a subjective improvement in visual function and an objective decrease in nystagmus in four of seven patients with congenital nystagmus. Pursuit, optokinetic responses, vestibulo-ocular responses and visual-vestibular interactions were improved in some patients.

KEYWORDS

Baclofen; congenital nystagmus; optokinetic nystagmus; pursuit; vestibulo-ocular response; visual-vestibular interaction.

INTRODUCTION

Baclofen (beta-parachlorophenyl gamma-aminobutyric acid) is a derivative of GABA (gamma-aminobutyric acid). GABA is an inhibitory neurotransmitter in the mammalian nervous system, but does not penetrate the blood-brain barrier since it is a polar, hydrophilic compound. Baclofen is a less polar, lipophilic compound that does cross the blood-brain barrier. It has been reported to be effective in decreasing spasticity resulting from cerebral palsy, multiple sclerosis and spinal cord injuries (Milla and Jackson, 1977; Brogden and co-workers, 1974; Sachais and co-workers, 1977; Feldman and co-workers, 1978). However, it is not clear whether or not its therapeutic effect results from its GABA-minergic activity (Davidoff and Sears, 1974; Curtis and co-workers, 1974; Fukuda and co-workers, 1977; Potashner, 1979). Halmagyi and co-workers (1980) reported that baclofen was effective in decreasing nystagmus and oscillopsia in three of four patients with periodic alternating nystagmus. In this report the effect of baclofen on nystagmus and other types of eye movements in patients with congenital nystagmus is described.

SUBJECTS AND METHODS

Seven, young adult males with congenital nystagmus were treated with baclofen 20 mg PO tid. Snellen visual acuity and eye movements were measured before treatment was begun and during treatment. Four patients had congenital nystagmus associated with ocular albinism. Eye movements were recorded with DC electro-oculography. The recording system had a bandwidth of 0-35 Hz (-3 dB), and has been described in detail previously (Baloh and co-workers, 1980). Nystagmus was recorded while patients were instructed to fixate an intense, red, 1° laser target on a white screen placed 1 meter in front of them. Nystagmus was recorded in the gaze position of least nystagmus (null position), center gaze and horizontal, eccentric gaze at 5° intervals. Nystagmus intensity was calculated as nystagmus amplitude X frequency (Hz^{o}). Pursuit was induced by the laser target moving sinusoidally (0.2 Hz, 22.6^{o}/sec peak velocity). Optokinetic responses were produced by placing patients within a full-field drum that rotated at constant velocity of 30°/sec and sinusoidally (0.05 Hz, 60°/sec peak velocity). Vestibulo-ocular responses (VOR) were induced by rotating patients in the dark, while they were seated within a motorized, Barany chair moving sinusoidally (0.05 Hz, 60°/sec peak velocity). Visual-vestibular responses (VVOR) were produced by rotating patients sinusoidally within the stationary optokinetic drum (synergistic interaction) and by rotating patients in the dark with fixation of a small, red light-emitting diode attached to the chair (antagonistic interaction).

VISUAL FUNCTION AND NYSTAGMUS

No significant side-effects were reported, except for slight to moderate fatique and drowsiness. All patients described feeling tired for the first few days of treatment. This symptom persisted in one patient (Patient 3). As shown in the Table, four patients reported an improvement in vision, that was described as improved clarity of vision at distance and during reading. A slight increase in visual acuity at distance was found in these patients. Most of these patients reported that less effort was required for clear vision, and that their reading comprehension had improved. A decrease in nystagmus intensity in the null position of gaze was found in these patients.

TABLE VISION AND NYSTAGMUS

Patient	Visual Acuity[1] Pre-Rx	On Rx	Subjective[2] Vision	Nystagmus[2] Intensity
1	20/40-1	20/20-2	+	+
2	20/30-1	20/30+2	+	+
3	20/20-2	20/20-3	o	o
4*	20/50	20/40	+	+
5*	20/60-2	20/50-2	+	+
6*	20/60+3	20/60-1	o	o
7*	20/200	20/100	o	o

1 Binocular, Snellen visual acuity in null position.
2 + indicates improvement in subjective vision or decrease in nystagmus intensity on treatment and o indicates no change.
* congenital nystagmus associated with ocular albinism.

In the patients who had decreased nystagmus intensity, the decrease in amplitude was greater than that in frequency, and the decreased intensity was present in all positions of gaze. Nystagmus in center gaze in Patient 1 is shown in Fig. 1A. The amplitude prior to treatment (top line) was greater than that on treatment (bottom line). Nystagmus in center gaze in Patient 2 is shown in Fig. 1B and C. He could voluntarily produce a right esotropia, decrease the nystagmus and improve his vision. Before treatment his right eye converged 22°. On treatment nystagmus intensity was decreased and only 11° of convergence were needed.

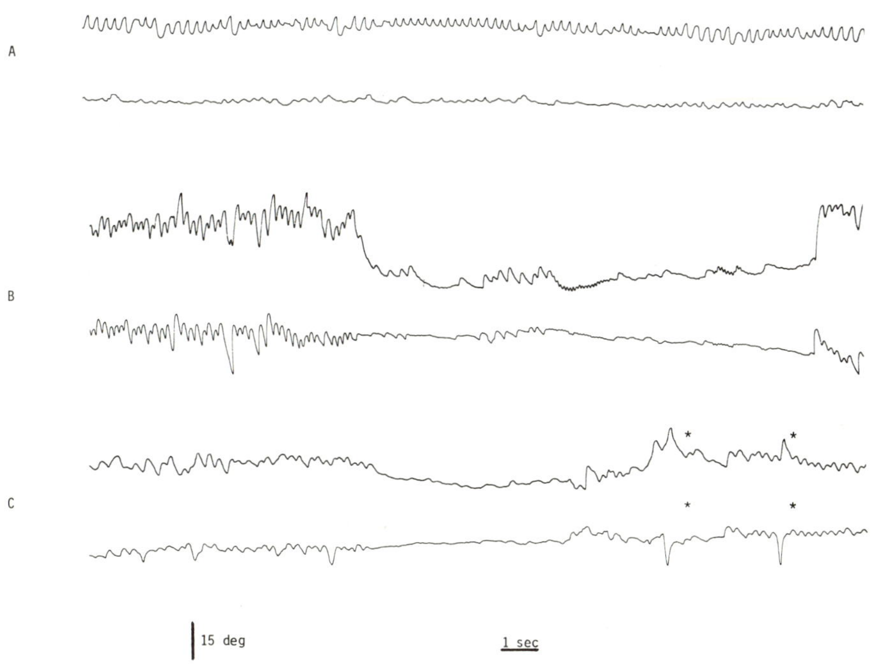

Fig. 1. Nystagmus in center gaze. A- right eye of Patient 1 before (top) and on treatment (bottom). B- right (top) and left (bottom) eyes of Patient 2 before treatment. C- Patient 2 on treatment. * eyelid blink artifacts.

The location of the null position did not significantly change on treatment. However, the interval of gaze in which the nystagmus intensity was the least (null zone) increased. Figure 2 presents the relationship of intensity and gaze position before and on treatment in Patient 1.

OTHER EYE MOVEMENTS

Improvement in other types of eye movements was found in most patients who had a decrease in nystagmus. In most of the eye movement tests the improvement could be attributed to the decrease in nystagmus. Pursuit in Patient 1 is shown in Fig. 3. Pursuit is most improved during target motion to the left, the direction of the patient's null position.

Optokinetic responses in Patient 2 are shown in Fig. 4. During drum rotation to the right at 30°/sec, one of the forms of "inverted" optokinetic responses, that have been described in other patients with congenital nystagmus (Yee, Baloh and Honrubia, 1980), was observed. The smooth movement of the response was toward the left, and had a decreasing velocity trajectory. During drum rotation to the

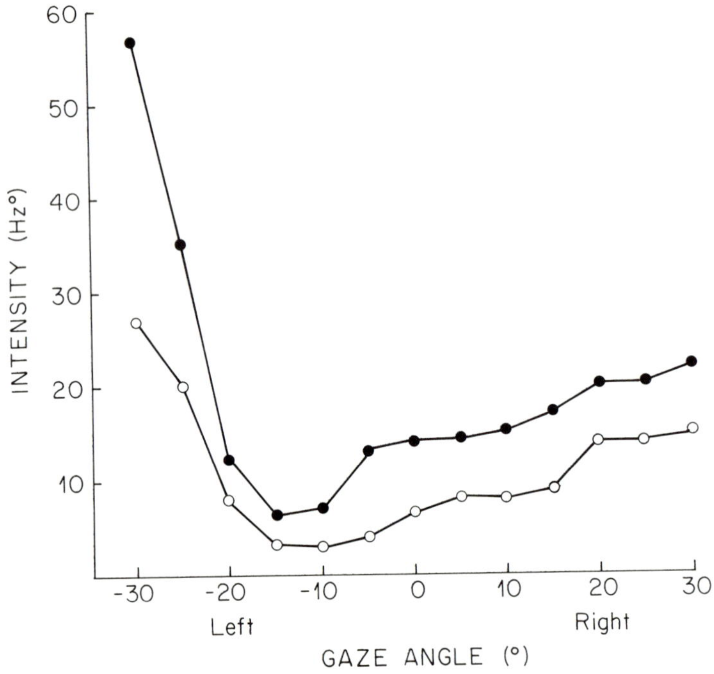

Fig. 2. Nystagmus intensity and gaze position in Patient 1. Closed circles are before treatment and opened circles are on treatment.

left, leftward smooth movements had low velocity and short periods of high velocity smooth movements to the right were present. On treatment the inverted smooth movements were still present during rotation to the right, but were of lower velocity. During rotation to the left, smooth movements were of higher velocity and had ramp-like, constant velocity trajectories. The center gaze positions are marked in the Figure, and indicate that the changes in the optokinetic response are not due to changes in the position of the eyes in the orbit.

VOR to rotation in the dark is basically normal in most patients with congenital nystagmus (Yee and co-workers, 1981). If nystagmus is present with eyes opened in the dark, its smooth movement velocity summates with the velocity of the VOR. The VOR slow component velocity during sinusoidal stimulation in Patient 6 before treatment is shown in Fig. 5. The asymmetry of the response was due to a DC bias to the left of 8°/sec, that correlated with the velocity of a spontaneous nystagmus in the dark. With the DC bias removed, the VOR gain (slow component velocity/chair velocity) was within the low-normal range for our laboratory. Figure 6 shows the VOR slow component velocity on treatment. There was no significant DC bias or spontaneous nystagmus in the dark. Interestingly, nystagmus intensity with fixation in the light was not decreased on treatment in this patient. Improvement in the augmentation and suppression of the VOR during the VVOR tests could also be correlated with a decrease in nystagmus in some patients.

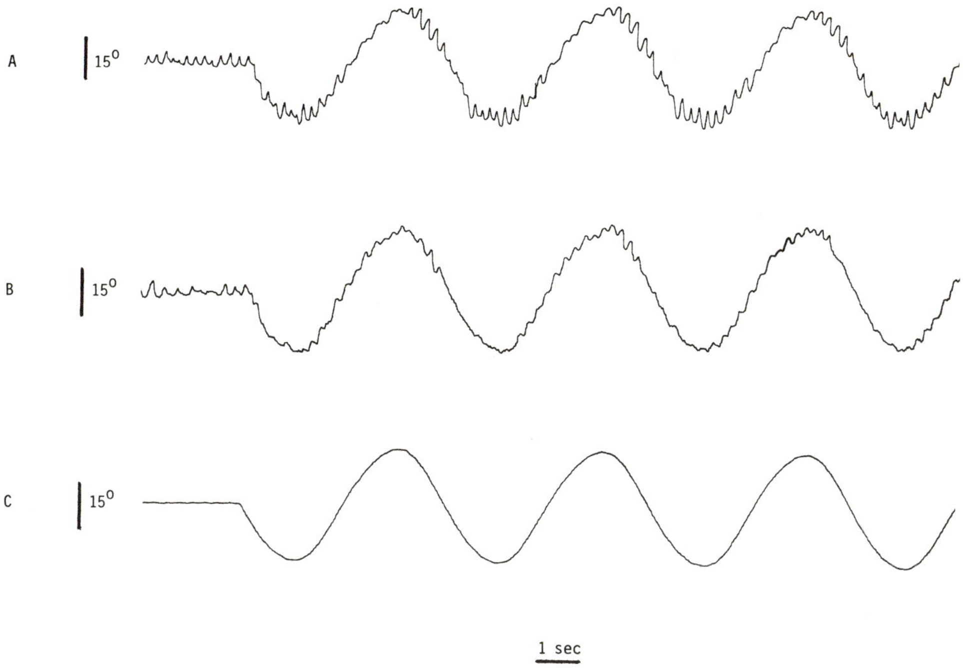

Fig. 3. Pursuit in Patient 1. A- right eye before treatment. B- on treatment. C- target position.

DISCUSSION

Bender and co-workers (1946) demonstrated that small doses of phenobarbital and amobarbital given intravenously can decrease nystagmus and improve visual function in patients with congenital nystagmus. Gay and co-workers (1969) reported that small doses of phenobarbital given orally decreased nystagmus, improved visual acuity and improved vestibulo-ocular responses to caloric irrigation in one patient. However, barbiturates have not been used routinely in the treatment of congenital nystagmus. These drugs have been shown to impair optokinetic responses and produce gaze-paretic nystagmus in normal subjects and in patients with many forms of nystagmus, and probably act as central nervous system depressants. Hypnotic effects and tolerance can limit the effectiveness of chronic therapy.

Baclofen appears to be moderately effective in decreasing nystagmus and improving visual function in some patients with congenital nystagmus. The increase in visual acuity in four patients was slight. However, a marked change in visual acuity might not be expected in our patients. Visual acuity was measured with binocular vision and the preferred null position of gaze. If nystagmus were decreased, but not abolished, the patient could achieve the same stabilization of retinal images on treatment with less eccentric gaze and/or convergence. The subjective improvement in visual function could reflect a decreased effort required to obtain clear vision. The objective findings of decreased nystagmus intensity and improved ocular motor function suggest that the effect of baclofen on nystagmus underlies the improvement in vision.

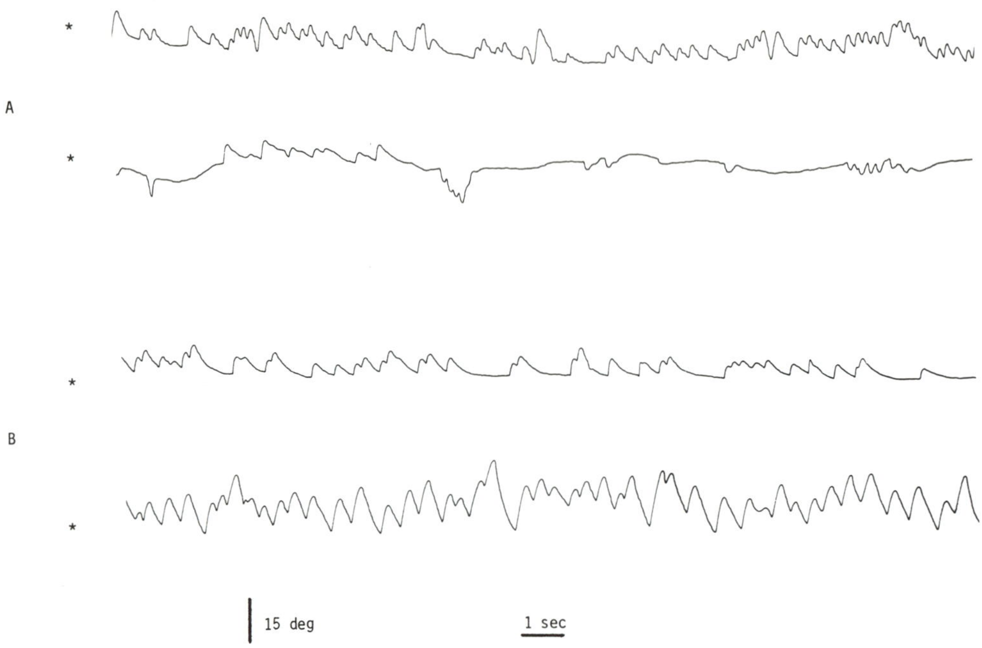

Fig. 4. Optokinetic responses in Patient 2. A- before treatment. Top- drum rotation to right, bottom- drum rotation to left. B- on treatment. * marks center gaze position.

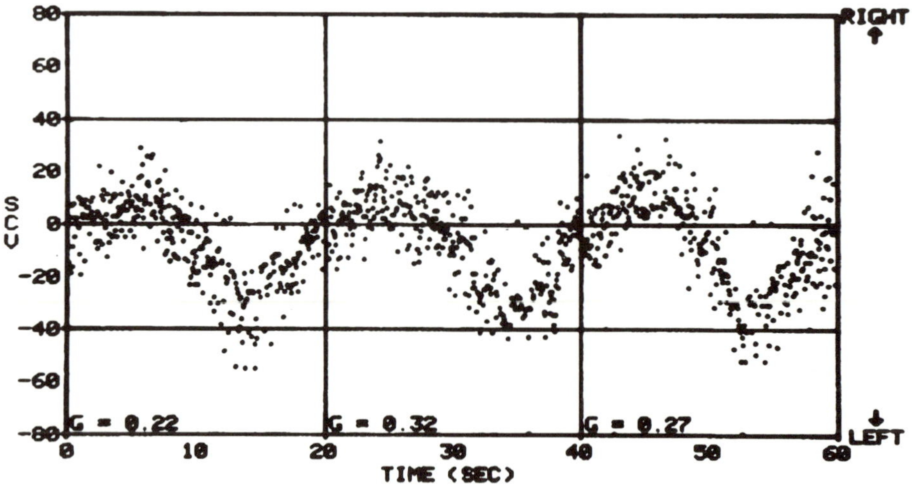

Fig. 5. VOR slow component velocity during sinusoidal rotation before treatment in Patient 6. SCV- slow component velocity (^{o}/sec). G- VOR gain after 8°/sec DC bias was removed.

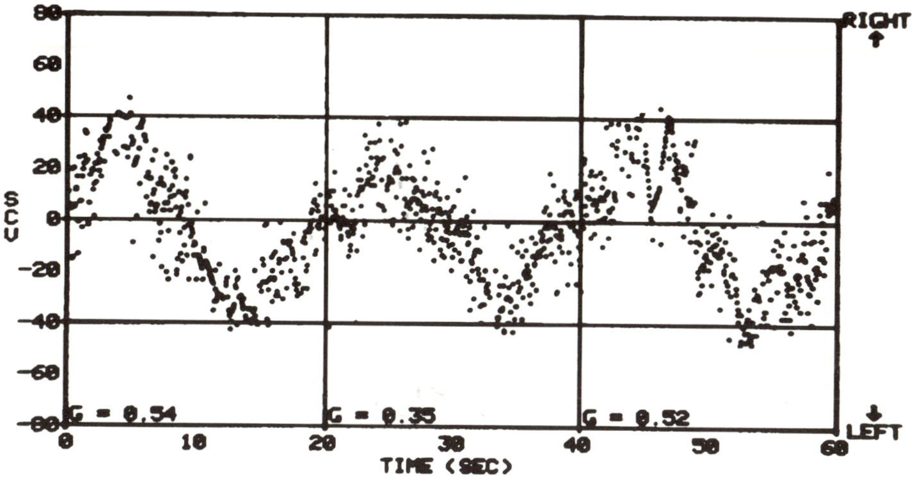

Fig. 6. VOR slow component velocity during sinusoidal rotation on treatment in Patient 6.

The possibility that the changes in vision and eye movements were due to a placebo effect was not investigated. In most patients visual function and eye movements were measured after cessation of treatment, and were found to have returned to their pretreatment levels. In the four patients who had had improvement on treatment, re-institution of treatment again produced improvement. However, a masked study is required to adequately assess the effect of baclofen. Baclofen did not benefit all of the patients, and nystagmus was still present in those that it did help. We do not recommend treatment of children or potentially child-bearing women with baclofen until its side-effects with chronic use are known and its efficacy is established. Hopefully, a more effective drug will be found as an alternative or adjunctive therapy to surgery and prisms.

IS AN OPTOKINETIC DEFECT THE CAUSE OF CONGENITAL AND LATENT NYSTAGMUS?

G. KOMMERELL and E. MEHDORN

University Eye Clinic, Freiburg, Federal Republic of Germany

ABSTRACT

On the basis of the large intraindividual and intrafamilial variability of nystagmic waveforms on the one hand, and the universal absence of adequate optokinetic (OK) responses on the other hand, we suggest the hypothesis that a defect of the OK system may be the basic abnormality of congenital nystagmus (CN). The OK defect represents a lack of the control loop which normally prevents drifting of the eyes. Absence of the OK control loop in the developing brain of infants could allow for a permanent establishment of irregular nystagmus generators which would normally be suppressed by the retinal slip they produce. Correspondingly, a partial defect of the OK system with reduced responses to monocular naso-temporal stimulation could allow for the development of latent nystagmus (LN).

KEYWORDS

Congenital nystagmus; latent nystagmus; optokinetic nystagmus.

CONGENITAL NYSTAGMUS (CN)

Introduction

Reports in the literature have demonstrated that the nystagmic waveforms are very variable among patients with CN (Caussé, 1936; Dell'Osso and Daroff, 1975; Dichgans, 1969; Jung and Kornhuber, 1964; Ohm, 1929; Yee and others, 1076), but common to all patients is a defect of the OK system (Brunner, 1921; Halmagyi and others, 1980; Yamazaki, 1979; Yee and others, 1980). The vestibulo-ocular reflex is basically normal in the majority of cases (Yee and others, 1980). On the basis of electronystagmographical investigations in 86 patients with CN, we confirm the great intraindividual and intrafamilial variability of nystagmic waveforms and corroborate the absence of adequate OK responses. We suggest that the defect of the OK system is the basic abnormality in patients with CN, and that the ocular oscillations develop secondarily in the absence of feedback control.

Methods and Results

During the last twelve years, we have collected dc-electronystagmograms (ENGs) of 86 patients with CN. In most cases, the reason for recording the ENG was to assess whether a surgical correction of abnormal head posture was indicated. This brought about a selection in that only six cases with eye diseases were investigated, and the majority (80) had normal eyes. Records were taken when the patient fixated at various positions along the horizontal meridian, and when horizontal OK stimulation was applied. In most cases, vertical positions of gaze and vertical OK responses were also tested. The OK pattern was produced by casting shadows of seven degree wide stripes on to a half cylinder which covered most of the visual field. Most patients were stimulated binocularly at 60°/s, but occasionally additional parameters were used. The instruction was to look attentively at the stripes in the middle of the screen.

A considerable variation of nystagmic waveforms occurred in several patients during a given fixation task (Fig. 1).

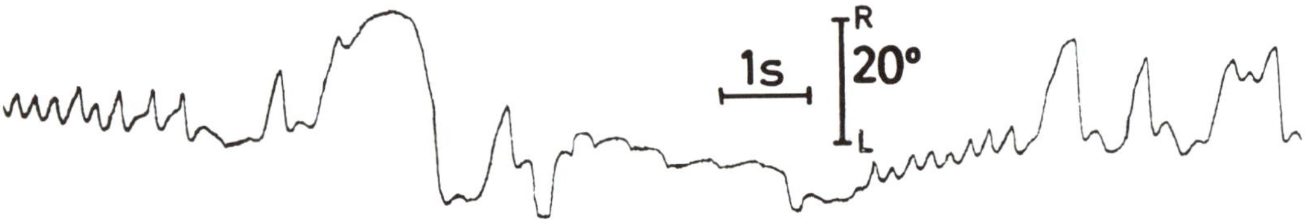

Fig. 1. Variation of waveforms. The patient looked at a target 20° on the left. CN with normal eyes (GS 201157; ENG, 0.5-20 Hz).

This spontaneous variability rendered the assessment of OK responses difficult. To overcome this difficulty, we applied OK step stimuli in our last 15 cases. The patients were asked to observe the middle of the OK pattern, which was at first stationary. Then, the pattern was abruptly set in motion (60°/s), or the motion was abruptly inverted. In none of the numerous trials was an adequate OK response elicited in the horizontal plane (Fig. 2 and 3).

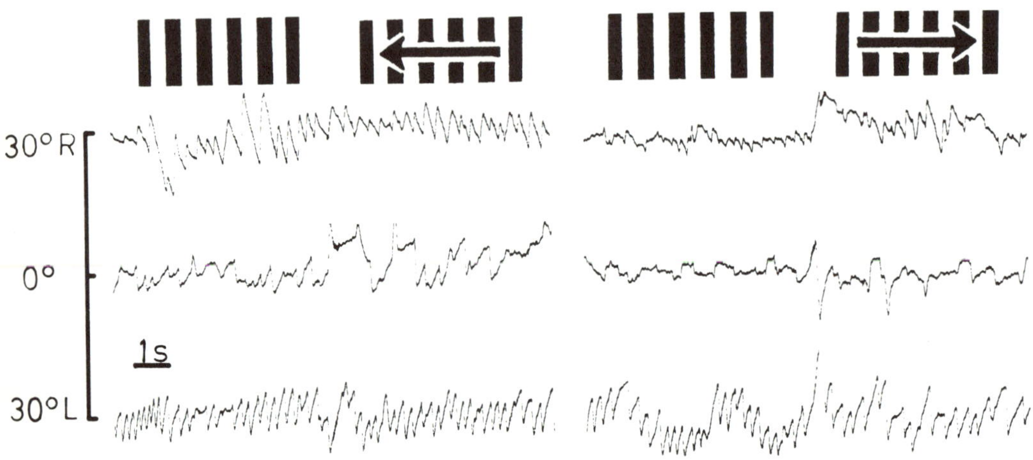

Fig. 2. Absence of responses to OK step stimuli (60°/s) in three directions of gaze. OK stimulation does not shift gaze evoked N patterns to the primary position as in the cases with "reversed" OKN reported by Halmagyi and others (1980). CN with normal eyes (AM 261261). ENG, 0-20 Hz.

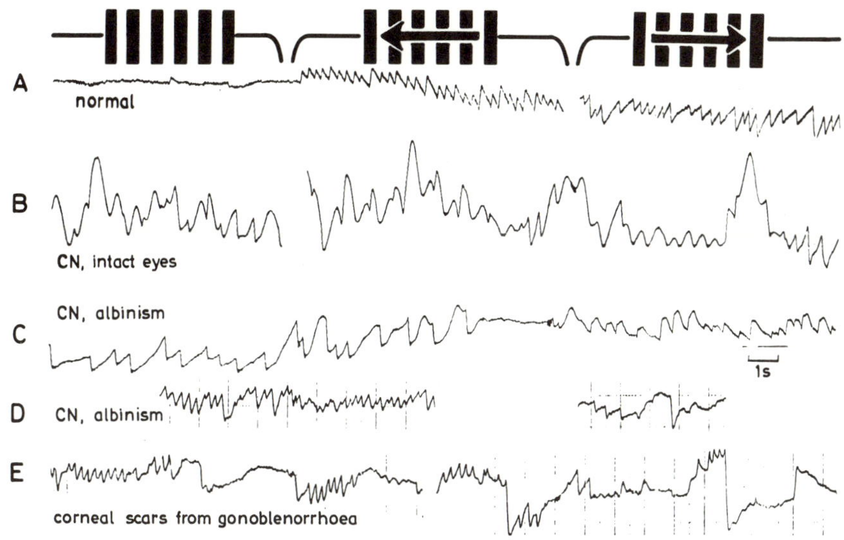

Fig. 3. OK step stimuli applied to four patients with CN (RT 100970, EJ 011265, PJ 190467, GS 200746); ENG, 0-20 Hz.

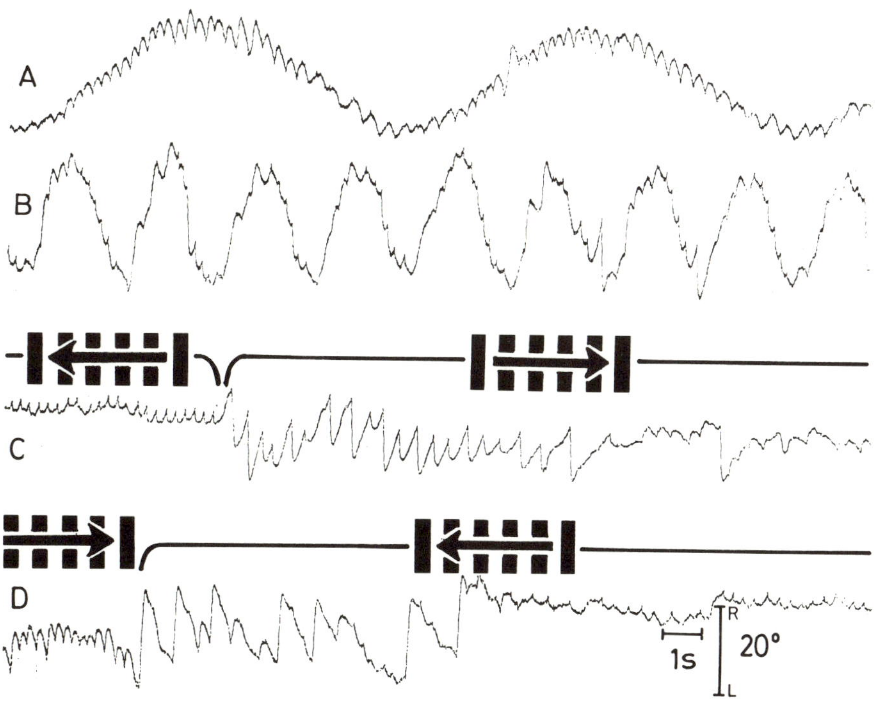

Fig. 4. The strategy of *leftward* pursuit switches from rightward cycloids at low target velocity (A) to leftward cycloids at high target velocity (B). OK step stimuli produce asymmetrical cycloids resembling normal OKN (C and D). However, with continued OK stimulation, the waveform relapses to symmetrical cycloids. CN with normal eyes (HF 130744); ENG, 0-20 Hz.

The response which was closest to a normal OKN is shown in Fig. 4 C and D. The patient was able to modify his cycloid N for about eight seconds when the OK stimulus was abruptly reversed. One branch of the cycloid became elongated and the other shortened. Similar waveforms were elicited when the patient tried to track a sinusoidally moving target (Fig. 4 A and B). At higher velocities to the left, the patient switched from rightward cycloids to leftward cycloids. This shows that the spontaneous N is not simply superimposed on smooth pursuit movements.

Occasionally, the response to OK stimulation looked like a reversed OKN, as in the albino of Fig. 3 C. This might represent an analogy of the reversed OKN in albino rabbits which occurs when the anterior 60 degrees of their visual fields are selectively stimulated (Collewijn and others, 1978). But in human albinos, a reversed OKN is certainly not a constant finding (Dichgans, 1969). The albino brother (Fig. 3 D) of the patient mentioned above showed only a slight reduction of his N when the OK stimulus was moved in the direction of the slow phases.

Discussion

The lack of proper OK responses in patients with CN represents a defect of the feedback system which normally prevents drifting of the eyes. Even in normal adults, linear drifts occur when the visual feedback is removed in darkness (Kamei and Kornhuber, 1974; Mulch and Lewitzki, 1977; Skavenski and Steinman, 1970), and blind patients are unable to maintain steady eye positions (Leigh and Zee, 1980).

In the developing brain of infants, eye drifts initiated by internal "noise" of the ocular motor system cannot be cancelled if there is a lack of the OK control loop. Thus, N generators might establish themselves permanently and might cause the complex waveforms of CN. This hypothesis is also compatible with the intrafamilial variability of nystagmic waveforms which has been observed by several workers (Jung and Kornhuber, 1964; Yee and others, 1976; our own observations in three families), because not the N itself is thought to be transmitted genetically but rather the OK defect.

As we instructed our patients to look attentively at the stripes when they were set in motion, we stimulated presumably the foveal pursuit system together with the global OK system. The unspecific responses indicated that both of these systems were defective. However, in a few of the patients, we investigated the pursuit system separately and in accordance with Halmagyi and others (1980) and with Yamazaki (1979), we consistently found a gross impairment of foveal pursuit. The coarse following responses which could be elicited did not simply constitute a superposition of smooth pursuit and spontaneous N (Fig. 4 A and B). The mechanisms which allow patients which CN to keep their line of sight relatively close to a moving target require further investigation, using a recording system which allows accurate monitoring of the position of the fovea versus the position of the target.

If the OK and pursuit defects indeed represent the disposition, and the nystagmic oscillations the secondary sequelae, one should assume that CN is usually not present at birth but becomes manifest only after some time. Unfortunately, the information about the beginning of "congenital" N is vague both in the literature (Schmidt, this Symposium) and in our own experience. Many parents did not observe their child's N before the age of three months when normal fixation was expected to develop, and this would support our hypothesis. On the other hand, the few cases in which N has been observed at birth do not refute our hypothesis, because the disorder which might usually be confined to a disconnection of the OK and pursuit pathways, could exceptionally also produce the N generator directly.

In the experimental animal, our hypothesis could perhaps be supported if elimination of the OK system shortly after birth produced an instability of gaze to CN. In the cat, an appropriate structure to be destroyed could be the nucleus of the optic tract (NOT). However, species differences may be of importance.

What is the pathogenesis of the N in patients with congenital eye disease? These patients show the same variability of nystagmic waveforms, and the same OK defect, as the cases with CN and normal eyes (Yee and others, 1976, 1980). We suggest that the so-called ocular, or sensory N is due to a mal-development of the OK system secondary to the sensory deprivation. A coincident, or parallel dysplasia of the intracerebral OK connections could perhaps be suspected in metabolic malformations, e.g. in albinism and in congenital cataracts; but N also develops in cases with exogenous blurring of the retinal image. In this respect, Ohm's (1958, p. 28) observation of N in four infants with corneal opacities after neonatal gonorrhoic infection are of particular interest. Ohm found N on the 27., 42., 44., and 99. day of life. We have investigated an adult with corneal opacities from neonatal gonorrhea who had a very irregular N, and no OK responses (Fig. 2 E).

The generators which cause N in patients with normal and with abnormal eyes cannot be controlled by the retinal slip which they produce. However, the N generators can be influenced by non-visual factors such as general excitement, the effort to look, the gaze angle, and the vergence. These influences can be utilized therapeutically.

LATENT NYSTAGMUS (LN)

LN is defined as a jerk N whose rapid phases are directed to the side of the visually dominant eye. With the left eye occluded, both eyes drift to the left, and with the right eye occluded, both eyes drift to the right (Fig. 5). It has long been observed that patients with LN show a nasal-temporal asymmetry of the OKN on monocular stimulation. Pattern movement from nasal to temporal is less effective than pattern movement from temporal to nasal (Doden, 1961; Keiner and Roelofs, 1955; Kornhuber, 1960; Loewer-Sieger, 1962; Nicolai, 1959; Roelofs, 1928). In pronounced cases, OK stimulation from nasal to temporal may even be unable to overcome the temporo-nasal slow phases of LN (Fig. 6). In moderate cases, the velocity of OKN slow phases is markedly reduced with pattern movement from nasal to temporal (Fig. 7). Correspondingly, patients with LN show impaired pursuit from nasal to temporal (Schor, 1981; Fig. 8). The asymmetries definitely exceed the very subtle nasal-temporal asymmetry which was recently detected in normal subjects (van Die and Collewijn, in print).

We suggested the hypothesis that the marked nasal-temporal asymmetry of the OK and pursuit systems might be the cause of LN (Kommerell, 1978). According to this concept, the temporo-nasal vector of the OK and pursuit systems would be tonically preponderant, even in the presence of stationary patterns. This directional preponderance could drive the slow phases of LN as soon as only one eye is admitted to vision. Total occlusion of one eye would be the strongest means to skew the OK and pursuit systems, but as most patients with LN also have strabismus, part of the directional preponderance would become manifest with spontaneous suppression of the squinting eye (Dell'Osso and others, 1979; Kestenbaum, 1961; Roelofs, 1928; Verhage, 1942). With binocular viewing, the well-functioning temporo-nasal components of both eyes could complement each other, and would prevent drifting of the eyes.

There are two analogues of LN in which a directional preponderance of the OK and pursuit systems may also cause spontaneous N. The first is a brainstem lesion which leads to downbeat N (Zee and others, 1974), and the second is a lesion of the cerebral hemispheres which leads to slow phases directed to the contralateral side (Sharpe and others, 1979).

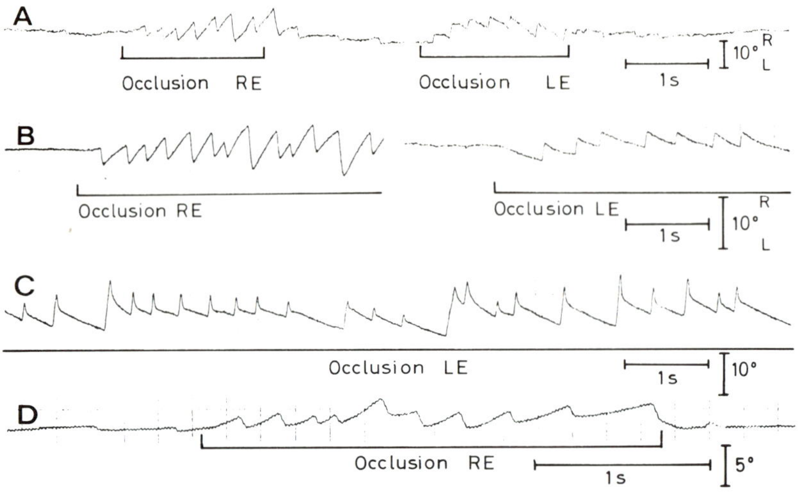

Fig. 5. Latent nystagmus. Various shapes of slow phases: in case A linear, in case B decreasing velocity, in case C linear after dynamic overshoot of the rapid phase, and in case D increasing velocity. Recording technics: binocular EOG (0-20 Hz) in A, infrared reflection system (0-100 Hz) of Bouis and others (1975), applied to the viewing eye, in B, C, and D. (FU 180771, AZ 020874, WM 061150, HF 201170).

Possible Objections

(A) The shape of the slow phases. The slow phases of LN are variable. They may be linear, as would be expected from a pure imbalance of the OK system, but exponentials of decreasing or increasing velocity also occur (Fig. 5). Decreasing velocity exponentials (Dell'Osso and others, 1979) may be produced by a gaze-paretic component which is obvious particularly in strabismic infants with crossed fixation (Kommerell, 1978). A decreasing velocity exponential restricted to the beginning of the slow phase represents dynamic overshoot of the rapid phase (Dell'Osso and others, 1979; Fig. 5 C), and the ensuing linear drift is compatible with the concept of "pursuit N". Increasing velocity exponentials also occur (Fig. 5 D). This deviation from linearity may also be produced by interference with components which are not necessarily related to LN.

(B) LN in darkness. In some patients with LN, the slow phases can be reversed by occlusion of one eye in the dark (Kornhuber, 1960; Jung and Kornhuber, 1964; Schor, 1981; van Vliet, 1973). We confirmed this in three out of four specifically tested patients (Fig. 9 B). This observation is compatible with the wellknown influence of mental imaging on the OK system and could be analogous to the capability of trained subjects to elicit an OKN by visual imagery of a moving stimulus pattern (Zikmund, 1966).

(C) Looking through Ewald's "pseudoscope". Van Vliet (1973) reported that some of his patients, looking through Ewald's pseudoscope, showed LN with rapid phases in the direction of the eye which they thought they were using, although the contours were in fact imaged on the contralateral retina. We are grateful to Dr. van

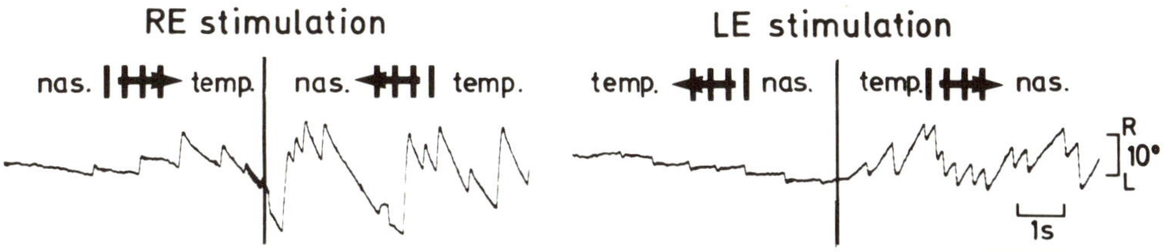

Fig. 6. Pronounced nasal-temporal asymmetry of the OKN on monocular stimulation (60°/s) in a patient with LN. Movement of stripes from nasal to temporal does not even overcome the slow phases of the LN. Binocular EOG (0-20 Hz). (CW 130360).

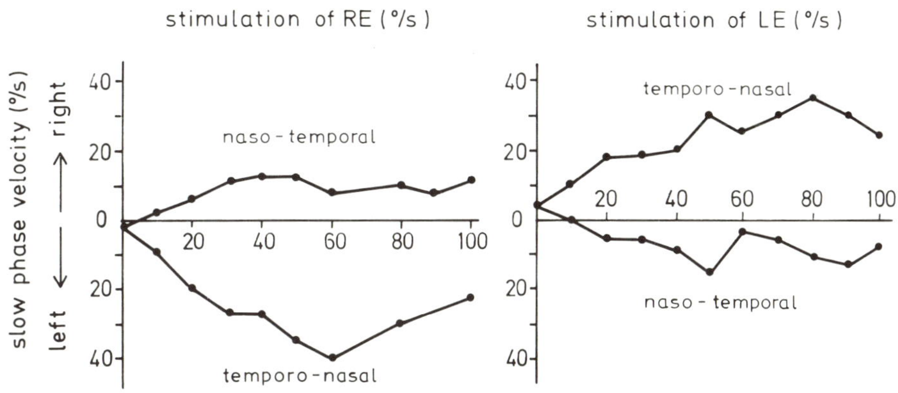

Fig. 7. Moderate nasal-temporal asymmetry of the OKN on monocular stimulation in a patient with LN (UD 110671).

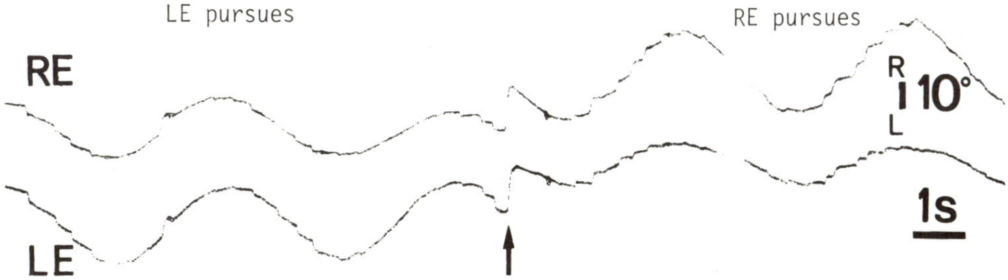

Fig. 8. Impaired smooth pursuit from nasal to temporal of a patient with LN tracking a sinusoidally moving target with one eye occluded. At the arrow, the occlusion is switched from the left to the right eye, and the patient performs a saccade to pick up fixation with his right, esotropic eye. The reduced amplitude of the non-fixing, esotropic eye (first LE, and then RE) is mainly an artefact caused by the non-linearity of the *monocular* EOG (0-20 Hz).(Same patient as in Fig.6 CW 130360).

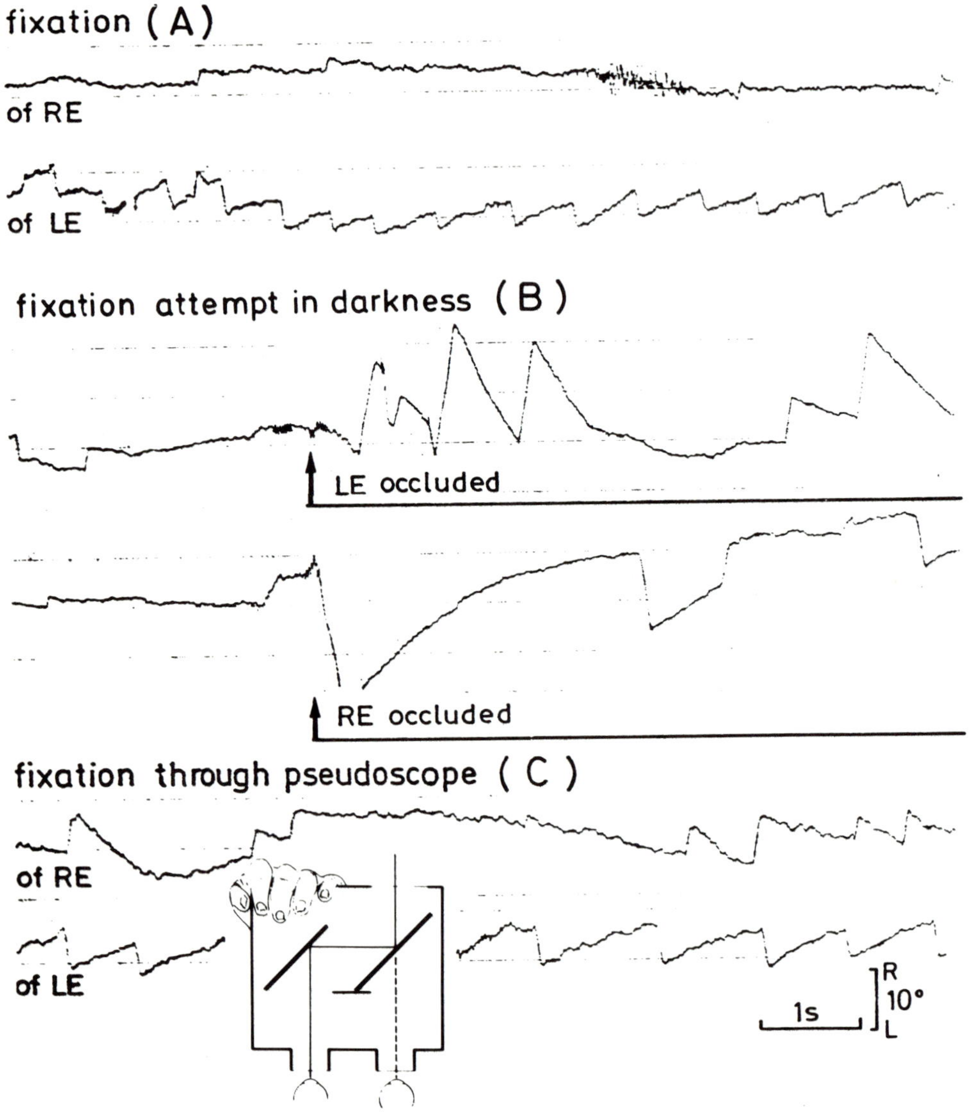

Fig. 9. Latent nystagmus. The directional preponderance becomes manifest not only with monocular fixation of a real target (A), but also with monocular "fixation" of an imaginary target in darkness (B). With monocular fixation of a real target through a "pseudoscope" (inset), the direction of LN corresponds to the eye which is actually exposed, and not to the side of the instrument which is uncovered (C). Binocular EOG (2-20 Hz). (JK 051067).

Vliet for lending us his pseudoscope which we used in eight patients. As van Vliet's instrument provides only a very narrow visual field, we constructed a modification with a wider visual field (inset of Fig. 9 C) which we also used in the eight patients. With neither of these instruments were we able to reproduce van Vliet's results. The direction of the LN was always determined by the actually viewing eye. We cannot fully explain the different results, even after having communicated with Dr. van Vliet about them, but we suspect that some of van Vliet's patients may have had difficulties in adjusting the small visual field of Ewald's pseudoscope to their eyes. Moreover, some of van Vliet's patients may have had CN rather than LN, as van Vliet's Fig. 6 shows pendular and cycloid waveforms instead of sawtooth N.

Association of LN with Strabismus

The occurrence of LN is highly correlated with strabismus (Kornhuber, 1960; Lang, 1978; Verhage, 1942). On the basis of this correlation, the hypothesis has been suggested that the lack of proper binocular vision leaves the OK system on an atavistic level of animals which constitutionally lack binocular vision (van Hof - van Duin, 1978). Such animals, as the rabbit, show nasal-temporal asymmetry of the OKN (Dubois and Collewijn, 1979; Precht, this symposium), as do patients with LN. This hypothesis is supported by the demonstration of nasal-temporal asymmetry of the OKN in normal infants during the first three months of life (Atkinson, 1979; Naegele and Held, 1980), the persistence of nasal-temporal asymmetry of the OKN in cats which were reared in the dark (van Hof-van Duin, 1978a) and of cats which were deprived of binocular vision by occlusion of one eye early in life (van Hof-van Duin, 1976).

LN has not been documented in cats deprived of binocular vision. This fact could be accounted for if one assumes that the nasal-temporal imbalance of the OK system can be compensated by other parts of the ocular motor system in cat, but not in man.

Although early deprivation of binocular vision appears to be an important pathogenetic factor of OK asymmetry and LN in man, a lack of binocular vision is not an absolute determinant of LN, and, conversely, the presence of binocular vision does not absolutely exclude LN. We have seen a patient (SW 250672) with a unilateral hypoplasia of the optic nerve who had congenital squint, and certainly never had binocular vision. Nevertheless, we found only a subtle nasal-temporal asymmetry of the OKN, and LN was absent on ophthalmoscopic examination. On the other hand, we have seen exceptional cases with LN who had binocular vision with only slightly reduced stereopsis (JK 051067). These observations show that factors other than defective binocular vision play a role in the manifestation of LN. These factors can be compensatory, or aggravatory.

Supported by the Deutsche Forschungsgemeinschaft, SFB 70, B4.

DISCUSSION

Optokinetic Responses in Patients with Congenital Nystagmus (CN)

Drs. Abadi, Dell'Osso, Gresty, and Yee agreed that the so-called inversion of the OKN in patients with CN usually represented a nystagmic waveform which also occurred with fixation of a stationary target in the lateral field of gaze. Such transpositions of nystagmic waveforms from the lateral field of gaze to the center tend to occur only at higher stimulus velocities (Dr. Gresty). Dr. Yee feels that there are exceptional cases of true inversion of the OKN.

Dr. Dell'Osso doubts that moving a drum in front of a patient with CN really stimulates his optokinetic (OK) system, because, in normal subjects, the stimulus which keeps an OKN going is a *slow* shift of the retinal image, and in the presence of CN, the shift of the retinal image may be too fast to be adequate. Therefore, according to Dr. Dell'Osso, the absence of specific OK responses does not allow the inference that the patient has a defective OK system.

Abnormal Head Posture in Patients with CN

Dr. Kommerell agreed with Dr. Lomas that the adoption of a specific gaze angle was the mechanism which reduced the intensity of CN, and that the abnormal head posture was only a secondary phenomenon which allowed the patient to use his optimal gaze position. He had obtained a simple proof of this by asking patients with CN to read a small distant letter while their trunks were being gradually turned on a swivel-chair. The patients then tended to keep their head and eyes in the same position of space, and the nystagmus did not increase, although the neck afference was changing.

Treatment of CN with Auditory Feedback

Dr. Abadi reported on very similar results as those obtained by Dr. Ciuffreda, when the patients had been trained in the laboratory. However, when the patients had taken the instrument home for further training, Dr. Abadi's results had not been as good and as permanent as Dr. Ciuffreda's.

Dr. Kommerell found it amazing that the artificial auditory feedback should work as a specific therapy, whereas improvement and deterioration of vision, being at the patient's disposal as a natural and lifelong feedback to conscious experience, was not effective. As a control experiment, to exclude a placebo effect, he suggested the use of an auditory signal taped at a previous session, and played back without any correlation to the patient's actual nystagmus.

Dr. Ciuffreda said that he had not yet tried the control experiment suggested by Dr. Kommerell. Nevertheless, he felt that the improvement with auditory feedback was a specific effect, and he mentioned two reasons in support of his opinion. First, he had been recording eye movements in many nystagmus patients over periods of weeks during which auditory feedback was not given. Nystagmus characteristics remained relatively constant without gross changes, certainly not even beginning to approximate the reduction of nystagmus evident when auditory feedback was added. Second, some patients had been asked to "hold" rather than "fixate" the target (i.e., the Steinman hold/fixate paradigm), and this had resulted in a reduction of nystagmus amplitude and/or frequency no greater than 25%. Thus, he had been considering only reductions of greater than 25% to be a direct effect of auditory feedback.

As to the question why patients with CN did not use their *visual* feedback more effectively, Dr. Ciuffreda believed that these patients had a reduced neural sensitivity as a result of their abnormal visual experience, i.e., the congenital, habitually occurring increased retinal image motion. According to Dr. Ciuffreda, the patients, when trained to use auditory feedback, may learn some "internal higher-level strategy" to reduce the nystagmus. As evidence for this, Dr. Ciuffreda mentioned that the patients following training had reduced their nystagmus in the absence of audio information, and that the "baseline nystagmus", when they had not been trying any of the newly-learned "tricks" had not changed during the course of training.

As further evidence for "higher-level strategies", Dr. Ciuffreda mentioned two patients who had reduced their nystagmus; the first, by imagining he was looking into his null region (10° to the left) as he actually fixated the midline target, and the second, by imagining he was looking merely with his better eye during *binocular* viewing.

SECTION IV

Coordinator: A. Jampolsky

NEW CONCEPTS IN TREATMENT OF STRABISMUS AND RELATED DISORDERS

THE "FADEN" OPERATION

W. DE DECKER

Department of Orthoptics, The University Eye Clinic, Kiel, Federal Republic of Germany

SUMMARY

Fadenoperation is like an artificial palsy with a slight exponentially increasing effect. It cannot replace a well indicated recession, but most cases of congenital strabismus show changing angles and respond to Fd much better than to recessions. Additional recessions are necessary only when the passive abduction under anaesthesia is found to be restricted, and should be added with extreme care: the Fd doubles the effect of recessions. Fd is a good tool in the treatment of acquired palsies (counter-paresis to the yoke muscle) when the surgeon wishes to influence that field of action only. Practical hints are given by referring to the results of about 400 cases of congenital alternating strabismus and 22 cases of nystagmic amblyopia, who failed with occlusion therapy, on whom we have operated using these principles.

KEYWORDS

Fadenoperation, artificial palsy of extrinsic eye muscles, dynamic strabismus, counterparesis.

1. TECHNIQUE

Cüppers (1974) published the original technique, which contains an obligatory dissection of the muscle from its insertion. When we began to use the "Faden" (Fd) we strongly felt that a technique without a disconnection would give us more freedom, as many patients with complicated strabismus need surgery on more than 2 recti. Our own technique (1975) fixes the muscles by the edges only (Fig. 1), preserving blood supply. In addition we found it easier, even in reoperations, as it produces less scaring between the two insertions. We prefer the same procedure also when an additional recession is necessary. Technical details are extremely important for successful cures. Nobody should begin with this operation, unless he is an experienced retinal surgeon. The main points are:

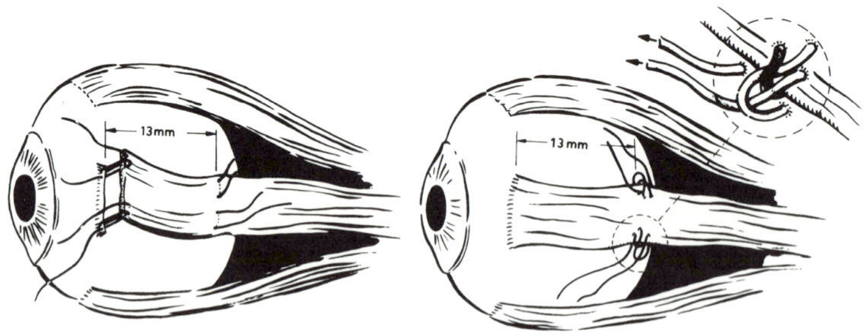

Fig. 1. Left : Fadenop. after Cüppers
right: Author's technique

1.1 An excellent view of the sclera and muscle is essential, and this is aided by the use of hooks of different widths (Fig. 2).

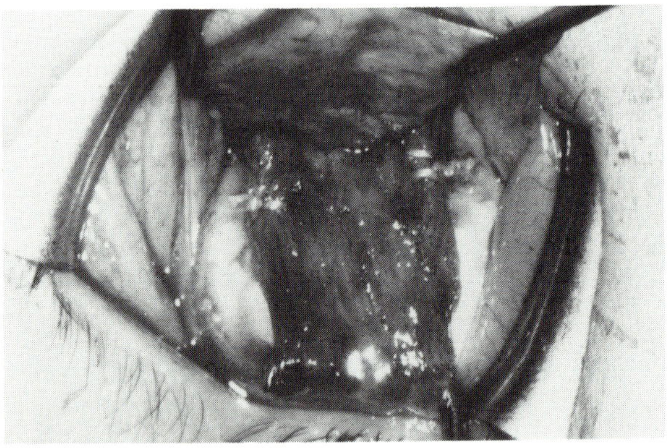

Fig. 2. Correct posterior attachment

1.2 Inexperienced surgeons fail to reach 13 mm, and in addition they produce pulley problems by loose sutures. We therefore perform 3 stitches through the muscle and sclera, which is safer than one. Only 3 perforations have been produced in 1000 operations without serious consequences.

1.3 Care should be taken that one does not produce adhesions to the Tenon tissues, which makes it impossible to close the conjunctiva without producing limitation in the horizontal ocular motility.

1.4 Any associated recession is fastened using an interwoven whipped suture. If this is neglected the muscle withdraws from both new insertions and the reoperator will find a block scar.

1.5 A minor complication, a prolapse of orbital fat, may occur in patients with small globes. We have had to reoperate on the conjunctiva in about 1%. The best way to avoid this is to prepare all the Tenon tissue in one flap, to hold it wet and to restore it carefully, but without sutures.

1.6 Bleeding from an injured vortex vein can produce severe proptosis (Fig. 3).

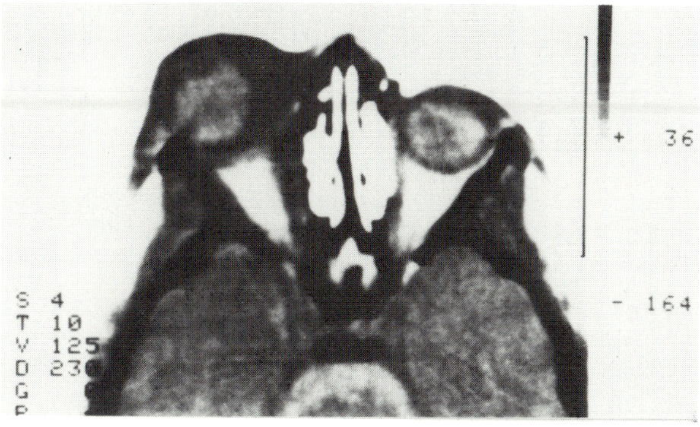

Fig. 3. Proptosis from injury to a vortex vein

1.7 It has been suggested that it might be possible to destroy the anterior portion of the muscle as a substitute for a Fd, but Cüppers (1981) and other surgeons who do the Fd routinely feel very reluctant about adopting such a procedure. This raises the question of how much destruction a regular Fd creates. We have recorded the EMG from a lot of muscles during reoperations. Figure 4 demonstrates that, after cutting or reinforcing, the "bridge" between the 2 insertions is still well innervated, while after several reoperations in severe cases paretic signs can be observed. The records were done by tefloncoated platinium wires, a technique which we learned from A.B. Scott (de Decker 1979). In terms of mechanical symptoms it can be summarized that after cutting a Fd with additional recession one half of the functional reduction remains, while after cutting a simple Fd, 2/3 of the action will recover.

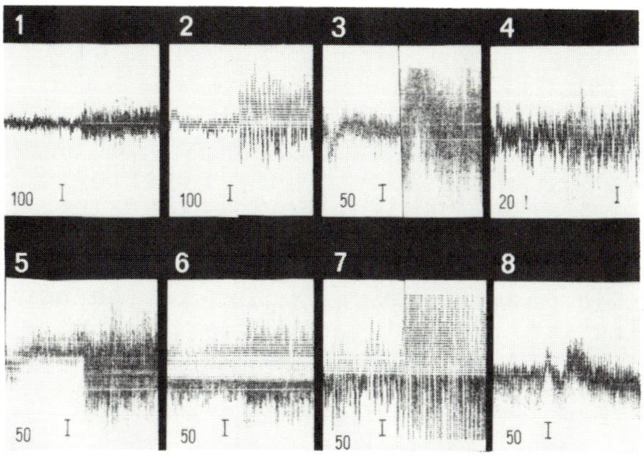

2. INDICATIONS

The Fd produces an artificial palsy, which makes it inadequate for problems which truly need recessions. 5 groups of indications respond very well to Fd, 4 of which affect the congenital strabismus syndrome (Ciancia 1962, Lang 1967). The changing angle in cases of convergent strabismus shows 3 different partial functions which have to be assessed separately (Conrad and Treumer 1981).

2.1 Instability in the course of time.

2.2 Overconvergence. Here it is extremely important to ensure that our patients do not belong to any refractive or accomodative overconvergence types. A special pitfall is the hypoaccommodative group exhibiting small pupils on near fixation, and requiring bifocals!

2.3 Overadduction. This is the smallest group but gives, especially in combination with the other symptoms, the best results. On the other hand we sometimes do not dare to operate on adults with changing angles as we are afraid to reduce the adduction ability too much, which would cause a divergent position in side gaze, with diplopia.
Sometimes dissociated vertical divergence (DVD) is part of the congenital syndrome.

2.4 Unilateral manifested DVD gives an excellent indication for the Fd, which we, in contrary to Sprague, Moore, Eggers and Knapp (1980), perform without any recession. From 30 cases of the year 1979 we could improve 28, while 2 failed. The bilateral types have been reported as generally successful by Knapp and coworkers, but the only two cases we ever did were not successful. We feel that the reason for this may be that every weakening procedure to one superior rectus alone may stimulate the contralateral elevators, following Hering's law.

2.5 Finally, some cases of paretic strabismus require a Fd to weaken the yoke muscle. Here again a careful decision has to be made. If, for example, after tucking the superior oblique, in the primary position a nearly constant vertical angle remains, a recession to the contralateral inferior rectus would be the indication of choice. But when an increasing VD is found only in downgaze a Fd to the same inferior rectus is the better operation. In straight translation from the German we call this a counterparesis. I would like to give one sophisticated example to point out what such a Fd can do. Frequently a misdirected innervation follows a III-N-palsy. Suppose that the upper lid can be raised only in adduction. Then a Fd to the contralateral lateral rectus, with or without recession, not only reduces the horizontal incomitance but forces the patient also to increase the innervation of this lateral rectus. This stimulates the paretic contralateral medial rectus, following Hering's law, and the lid will rise (Fig. 5).

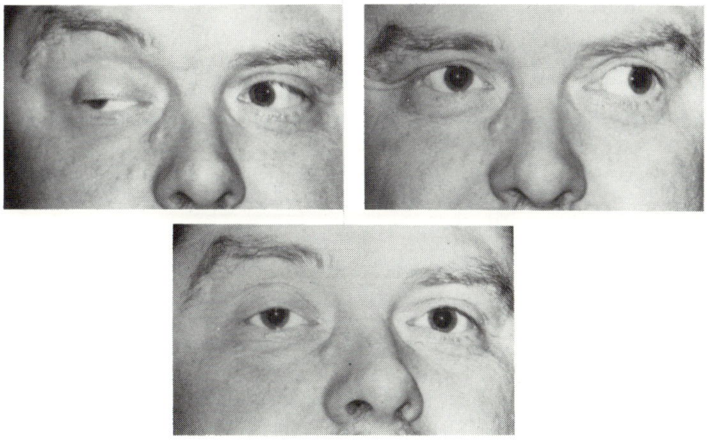

Fig. 5. Upper: Levator function depending on direction of gaze

Lower: Improvement following counter-paresis

I cannot leave this chapter without a few comments on nystagmus (N) problems.

a) In congenital esotropia the normal finding is an abductional N of the latent type. A bilateral Fd to the medial recti therefore must reduce not only the overaction mentioned above but also reduces the slow phases, which make the eyes drift into the field of action. Again, one example may explain our practice. A young man had undergone 3 squint operations during childhood, but still had a poor cosmetic appearance. He adducted the dominant right eye in order to calm the latent N while, due to the previous operations, the left eye was straight but elevated by DVD. We performed a Fd of 14 mm to the right medial rectus, a recession of 10 mm to the left lateral rectus and a Fd of 12 mm to the left superior rectus. The result was not excellent but satisfactory (Fig. 6).

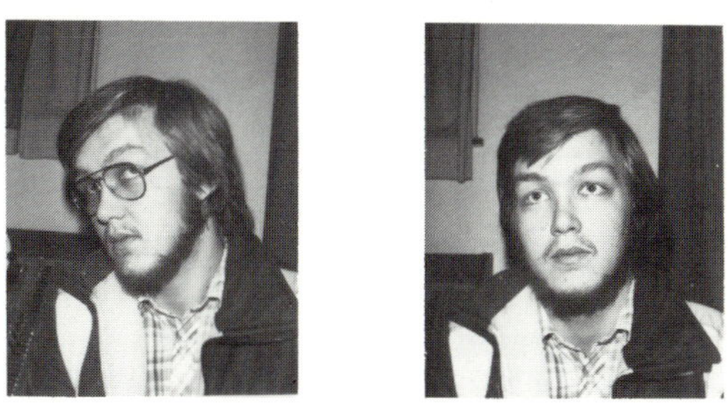

Fig. 6. Head posture before and after correction on 3 muscles

b) Pendular nystagmus normally does not mean a good indication for Fd. The nystagmus is not the cause, but the result of the hidden visual congenital obstacle. There is, however, one exception. Normally patients with congenital nystagmus do not experience oscillopsia, as they have a compensatory sensorial mechanism. However, some shake their heads indicating that this compensation is incomplete. Fixing on a flashing light, they report a "dancing view", like a sailor watching a lighthouse at night. In these circumstances, the light never blinks from the expected direction, as man lacks a sense for the position of his eyes in deep darkness. Patients with pendular nystagmus see interruptedly: during their dark phases the eyes move and here also the flashing light appears from an unexpected direction. This, in my opinion, is the only indication for reducing the pendular nystagmus by Fd on all 4 horizontal rectus muscles. As the amplitude of pendular nystagmus movements is small, the Fd has to be placed very well back on each muscle to have a significant effect - and there is therefore very little danger of overcorrection.

3. CLINICAL PRACTICE AND RESULTS

Alternating congenital strabismus and unilateral squint with severe nystagmus of the latent type which does not respond to occlusion therapy are two important ocular motility problems for which the Fd has much to offer.

3.1 Changing angle

It appears very scientific to measure the angles of squint with the prism cover test, but this gives only the maximum values. Most patients who seem to have constant deviations show short periods of relaxation, which can be detected by either:

1) Careful observation.
2) Asking the parents, which we found very helpful.
3) Knowledge of the smallest angle of anomaly.
4) Considering the other symptoms of congenital strabismus.

We proved this with a simple test some years ago. A group of 27 children with obvious dynamic angles underwent Fd with fair or moderate results, while a control of 20 of the congenital type, whom we never saw relaxing, reached good corrections also. The conclusion we made was that most patients do not need additional recessions, in opposition to the argument of Mühlendyck and Linnen (1975), Quéré et al. (1978), Spielmann and Laulan (1978), Behrens-Baumann and Wölz (1978). The following results with about 400 children are based on operations from 1978. Since that time we have followed constant principles, and can now analyse our results retrospectively. 235 patients have had bimedial Fd only, any oblique problems being operated upon separately (Fig. 7). The diagram shows that a bimedial Fd of 11 mm corrects maximum angles about 10° - 15°. 12 mm are adequate for 15° - 20°, and 13 mm give good result up to 25° max. angle. About 80% look well corrected in these groups. If the angle exceeds 25°, the rate of success decreases to 50%, which indicates, that there an additional recession is necessary. In only 69 patients did we find it essential to add recessions. The results are, in cases with angles up to 25°, about the same but clearly better in extreme maximum angles (Fig. 8).

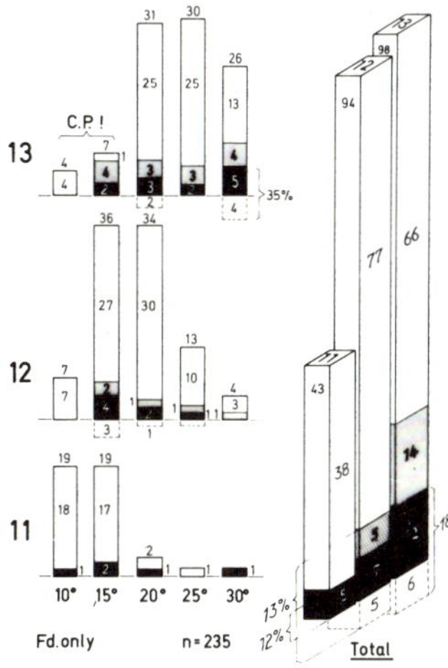

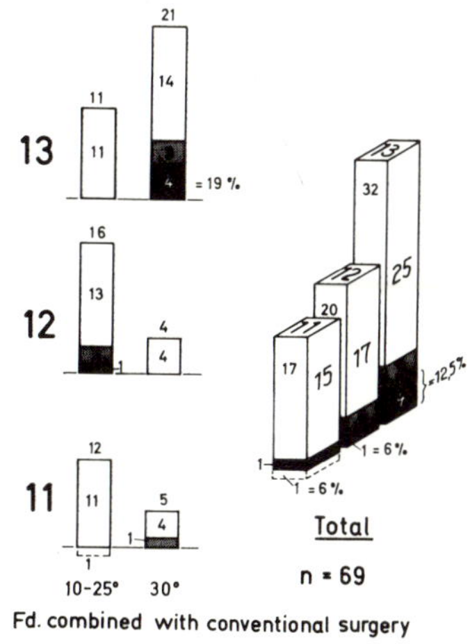

Fig. 7. Results of Fadenoperations only (left)
Fig. 8. Results of Fd combined with conventional surgery (right)

The decision, whether or not to add a recession is often made under anaesthesia, as a limited passive adduction indicates that Fd alone would not be enough. The evidence of parallelism under anaesthesia is not a satisfying proof that Fd alone would be successful. The number of longlasting overcorrections is very small (4,7%) (Fig. 9).

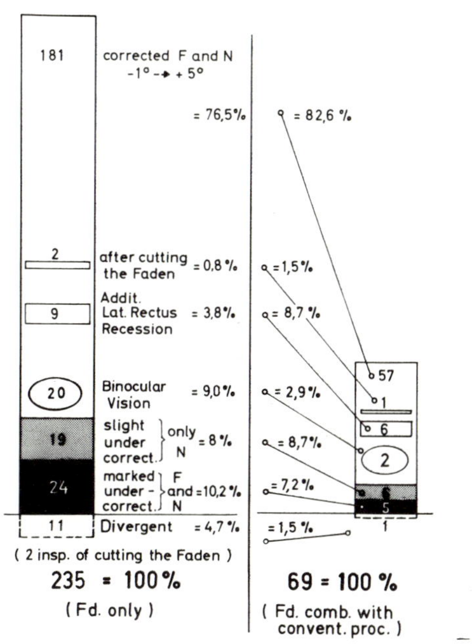

Fig. 9. Results of all operations

Overcorrections following Fd have two different characters: very few cases show a severe adductional palsy, which forces us to cut the Fd within 3 - 4 days. More often the motility is found to be sufficient, and the eye position is the same on near and distance fixation or is even less divergent at near. In this situation we do not sacrifice the Fd but recess one or both lateral recti some months later, after prismatic correction. This leads to very good results and reinforces the influence of the Fd on near fixation, by rotating the point of effective attachment of the muscle more posteriorly. Figure 10 indicates that the best results were obtained when small basic angles were ascertained together with NRC or microanomaly. The ascertainment of one of these factors alone also gives a good likelihood of a fair result and even in the absence of these specific indications the procedure often achieved good results. Figure 10 also shows the number and type of reoperations in detail.

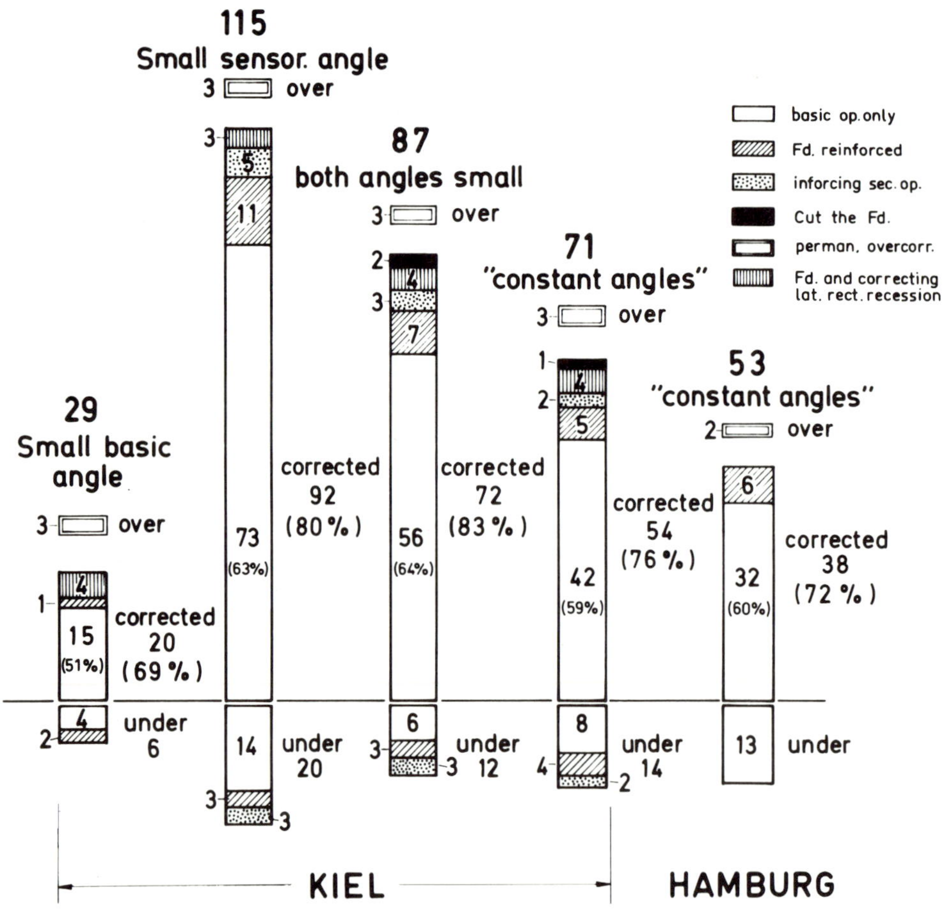

Fig. 10. Results related to preoperative findings, and distribution of second operations

Unilateral Fd are not so successful, even when the squint is unilateral. Within these limitations, the results are better when the angle of squint is small and additional recessions are not required. (Table 1)

TABLE 1 Unilateral Fd

		correct. -1^0 to $+5^0$	not correct.	failures %
Total :	81	59	22	27 %
Fd. only	39	30	9	23 %
Fd. comb. Conv. surg.	42	29	13	31 %
Max. angle	46	39	7	15 %
Angle $20^0 - 30^0$	35	20	15	43 %
Fd. only Max. angle	26	23	3	11,5 %

Results of 81 operations

- unilateral Fd. -

Only small angles give good results

3.2 Unsuccessful occlusion therapy (Nystagmic amblyopia)

We see 4 - 5 infants yearly, among 130 new amblyopes, who fail with occlusion. Overadduction and nystagmus of the latent type cannot be overcome by occlusion, which creates even more adductional impulse. In these patients we performed a unilateral Fd, in extreme cases with additional recession. When even this failed, we reoperated and set the medial rectus back to 13 mm in 2 patients. This means that we reduced the lever arm as in a Fd. 22 of those patients, operated in 1975 - 1978 at an age of about 18 months have been followed up and showed fair results in 1980 (de Decker and Henning 1979). The early Fd is not too dangerous a procedure. We have made some experiments with newborne rabbits and have demonstrated that the segment of the globe under the operated muscle continues to grow normally (de Decker and Henning 1979).

4. MECHANICAL PROBLEMS

Two special questions rise whenever Fd-problems are discussed; motility and effect upon the basic angle.

4.1 The profile of action is that of a slight exponential increasing palsy (Conrad and Treumer 1981, Cüppers 1981) (Fig. 11). This is welcome in the few cases with overadduction, while in the majority with changing angles and some overconvergence only it means a side effect, which is tolerable in most children, but normally not in adults. Bilateral Fd to both medial recti produces a motility which is much smoother, for which reason we prefer bilateral Fd today. On the other hand the character of a palsy again is welcome when the Fd acts as a counterparesis. Cüppers recently (1981) pointed out that the profile of action after Fd to the yoke muscle should ideally follow the curve of the resting function of the paretic agonist. But up to now nobody has shown how this goal could be reached, and our dosage of counterparesis is more or less guesswork.

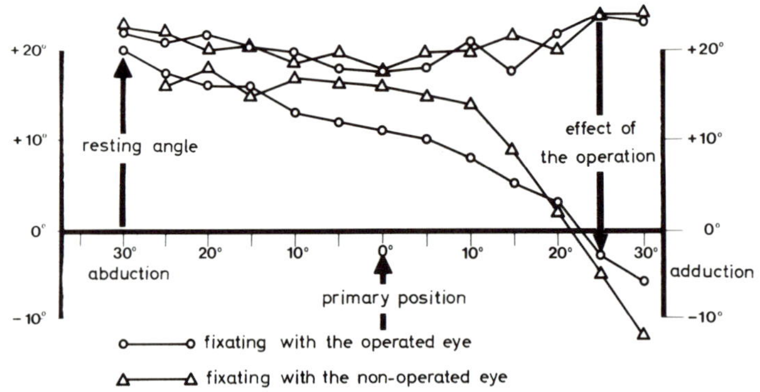

Fig. 11. Profile of action of a Fd on a medial rectus

4.2 Cüppers has stated for years that Fd normally does not touch the primary position. But clinicians (Haase and coworkers 1978) have seen such an effect, and our own experience confirms this observation. If we placed the Fd as far posteriorly as the fovea, the lever arm would be reduced to zero. Without any doubt the antagonist would then turn the eye until the active and passive forces came to a new equilibrium. A similar but slighter effect must be produced by any amount of Fd. My coworker Conrad found not only the expected exponential increase of the effect with increasing angles of side gaze, but also an influence upon the eye position in primary position; and even in 20° of abduction the influence had not decreased to zero. (Fig. 12). What happens when a recession is added to a Fd? Conrad's finding was that the profile of action was less prominent compared to Fd alone, but the eye position had been markedly shifted. (Fig. 13).

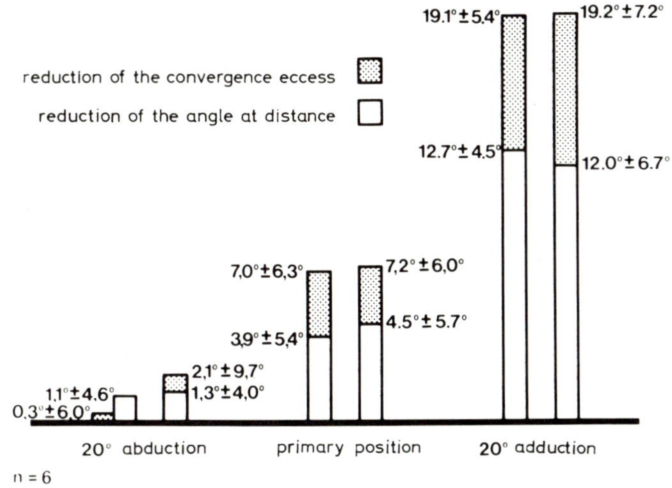

Fig. 12. Unilateral Fd on a medial rectus influences the eye position and motility more in adduction but also slightly in abduction

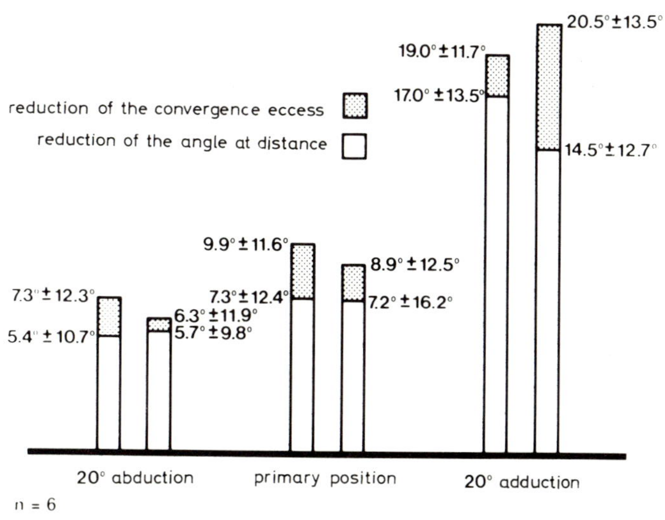

Fig. 13. The combination with a recession decreases the efficiency of the Fd

This brings us to a last question. Why does a Fd increase the mm - degree - ratio of an additional recession so much? The fact is well proven in the literature and in clinical discussion. Suppose we would perform a recession alone, then all the length of the muscle is able to take up the slack in the orbit. Consequently an isolated recession never gives an effect that equals the 5°/mm, which should be expected from the circumferential angle of the globe. The effect is more or less 2°/mm. This effect increases even when a resection of the antagonist is added. A Fd is different from a large recession as it does not relax the muscle, and no slack can be taken up as there is none. Looking upon the "Fd anatomy", (Fig. 1) we see that the posterior fixation even forces the muscle to make a little more way in the orbit. The amount of a recession will influence the position of the eye. We can make the calculation for the combination of both. Suppose that the unfixed parts of the muscle are able to develop a slack and take it up later. One third of the muscle becomes fixed to the globe and cannot take part in the changes in length. One third of the 5°/mm for the circumferential angle therefore should be added to the 2°/mm we normally can reach. With this calculation we would come to $3,7^{o}$/mm. In clinical practice the surgeon should anticipate that the addition of a Fd to a recession will roughly double the effect of the recession upon the basic angle. An example may point this out more clearly: the smallest angle ever seen may be 10°, which should be valid under general anaesthesia also. The largest angle may be 25°. In that case, following these priciples, a bimedial Fd of 13 mm should be aided by a unilateral recession of 2,5 mm to the medial rectus of the non - leading eye ($4 \times 2,5^{o}$/mm = 10

OBJECTIVE CALCULATION OF STRABISMUS SURGERY

C. C. COLLINS and A. JAMPOLSKY

Smith-Kettlewell Institute of Visual Sciences,
San Francisco, California, USA

ABSTRACT

We have developed a simple method for calculation of the amount of strabismus surgery required in selected cases based on objective physical measurements of globe and muscle stiffness. We have utilized instrumented length-force forceps at surgery to determine the tissue stiffness of the intact eye, of the isolated globe (medial and lateral rectus muscles detached), and of the individual medial and lateral rectus muscles. Thus evaluating the patient's own oculomotor model, we have derived simple equations using these readily measured stiffness values to calculate the amount of surgery to be performed on the medial rectus and, separately, the lateral rectus muscle to correct a strabismus deviation. The calculations agree with the amount of surgery actually performed by the surgeon guided independently by clinical intrasurgical assessments on strabismus patients. The method should provide a more precise and rational basis for strabismus surgery as well as unique, fundamental human oculomotor data on functions of the eye muscles and their restraining tissues before, during and after strabismus surgery.

KEYWORDS

Strabismus, muscle physiology, bioengineering, patient models, surgical planning.

ACKNOWLEDGEMENTS

These investigations were supported by NIH Grants EY 03915, EY 01719, EY 01186, 5 S01 RR05566, and The Smith-Kettlewell Eye Research Foundation. The authors thank Mrs. Maureen Clarke for writing the control and data collection programs and helping to record and reduce the data. We also thank Andre Gordon for his help in taking and reducing the data. We thank Gerald Dittbenner for applying strain gauges to the length-force forceps, and Albert Alden for design of the electronics and continued maintenance of the length-force forceps. We thank Steven Chung for A/D converter and computer I/O design, fabrication and maintenance. We thank Dr. Elbert Magoon for clinical observations and consultation, and Dr. Harley Bicas for helpful critical comments on the measurement techniques. Special thanks to Dr. David Robinson for emphasizing the necessity of the more difficult measurements on the awake patient.

INTRODUCTION

Even a moderate improvement in understanding and care of strabismus will have major value in a field where thousands of such operations are done monthly with a reoperation rate of 20-50 percent for the average clinician (1,2). It is our conviction that the application of quantitative principles of engineering physics to ocular motility disorders in strabismus will lead to better understanding of the oculomotor system, resulting in improved diagnosis and management.

We will show that the muscle and globe restraining mechanical components in the orbit can be readily understood, quantitatively measured, and directly applied to the real life clinical situation. Objective physical measurements guided by a rational framework of knowledge of the oculomotor system (a simple model) have already been valuable in diagnosis, and now promise to provide an improved quantitative guide to strabismus surgical planning.

That these measurements can be clinically useful to predict and guide strabismus surgery has been shown by direct comparison of the calculated amounts of strabismus surgery that the model predicts "should be done", with the successful amount actually done by an expert strabismus surgeon using his own independent, clinically derived, assessments and judgments. These agree remarkably well in selected cases.

Specifically, as a result of the development of forceps movement and force measurement techniques and of simple static oculomotor modeling to handle the data, it now appears possible to compute the optimum surgery to be done from objective quantitative measurements made at surgery. This would solve a major clinical diagnostic and management problem, with tremendous health care delivery benefits for human strabismus.

METHODS

At surgery, we have utilized instrumented length-force (length-tension) forceps which have been previously described (3) to determine the tissue stiffness of the actively innervated intact eye before anesthesia and subsequently, under anesthesia, of the isolated globe and of the individual medial and lateral rectus muscles of strabismus surgical patients. We report here the results from our latest five patients ranging from 9 to 33 years in age.

The force the forceps apply to the eye is measured with strain gauges attached to the shanks of the forceps tips. Displacement of the eye by the forceps is measured by micro-sonar. A small microphone with an opening attached near the tip of the forceps receives 40 kilohertz ultrasonic pulses produced by a small electrostatic transducer held fixed with respect to the head. The time of flight of these sound pulses from the ultrasonic source to the microphone (receiver) on the forceps provides a sonar signal proportional to the distance the tip of the forceps moves. Thus, we can directly produce length-force plots.

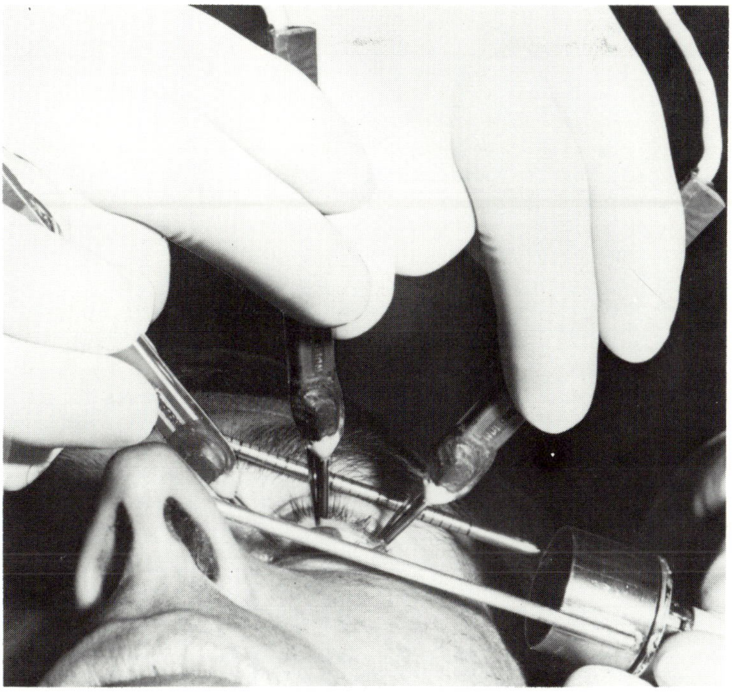

Fig. 1. Successive views showing proper use of the length-force forceps.

Figure 1 illustrates use of the length-force forceps on a patient. The surgeon places the open end of two parallel spacing rods on the bony ridge of the nose and the ultrasonic source transducer (loudspeaker) attached to the other end of the rods is braced against the bone of the cheek which keeps the plane of measurement of the ultrasonic transducer fixed at an optimal angle with respect to the head and eye (a plane tangent to the eye at about 20° temporal gaze position). Distance indication is strictly linear in the nasal quadrant and up to 20° temporal gaze position because the ultrasound beam diffracts around the eye in the nasal quadrant to fill the sound shadow of the eye. The sound path traverses an essentially circular arc following the contour of the eye and the forceps movement beyond tangency of the ultrasonic beam with the globe. From 20° to 50° temporal rotation the straight line ultrasonic path length measures the circular arc of eye and forceps movement to within 5% accuracy.

The surgeon grasps the limbus with the forceps and rotates the eye first nasally and then temporally. The forceps are held radially to the eye, that is such that an extension of their long axis would pass through the center of rotation of the globe at all times during measurements. The sonar microphone tip is located 2 mm above the tip of the forceps grasping the eye. The consequent 14.5 mm radius readings of the sonar system are converted to correspond with the 12.5 mm radius of the eye in a computerized calibration procedure.

The resulting pre-calibrated, on-line, real-time length and force measurements are converted from analogue to digital form, stored in (an Apple II) microcomputer memory, permanently archived on floppy disk and subsequently plotted to yield the length-force diagrams shown in the Results section (Fig. 4). Grams of force are recorded vertically and millimeters displacement (equivalent degrees of eye rotation) horizontally in such records of strabismus patients.

The slope of such a curve represents tissue stiffness in grams per degree (or, if preferred, in grams per millimeter). By observing the indicated geometric constraints in the protocol of tissue stiffness measurement, force and length errors tend to cancel each other and thus overall errors are generally held to less than 5%.

Using these readily measured stiffness values we can evaluate each of the static mechanical parameters of the patient's own oculomotor model, from which we have derived simple equations to calculate the amount of surgery to be performed on the medial rectus and, separately, the lateral rectus muscle to correct a strabismic deviation.

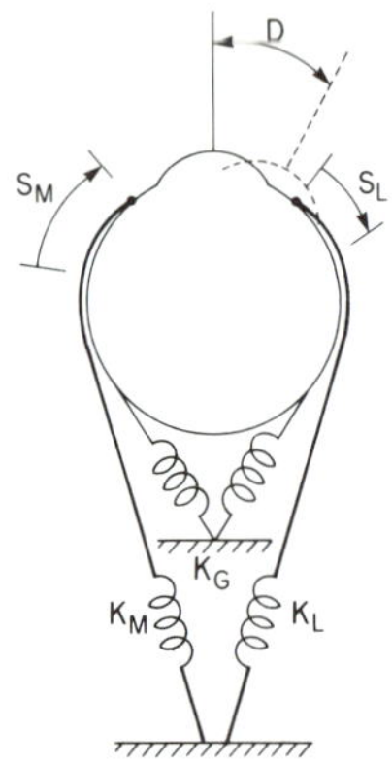

Fig. 2. Anatomical patient model.

Figure 2 is the linear, clinical two-muscle model of the patient's static oculomotor plant which has proved adequate for these calculations. The springs represent the passive stiffness of the globe restraining tissues (K_G), the medial rectus muscle (K_M), the lateral rectus muscle (K_L). The parallel sum total of all these elements represents the stiffness of the intact eye (K) of the awake patient. D is the strabismic deviation and S_M and S_L represent the medial and lateral rectus muscle surgery, respectively.

A linear model is justified since the stiffness and net innervation of actively innervated human muscles for which surgery is calculated, has been shown to be quite linear (4,5,12). The intact eye of awake human subjects also displays a constant stiffness with a linear length-force relationship (10,11) and the passive tissues of the isolated globe, which make up only about 20 to 30% of the stiffness of the intact eye, are found to be approximately linear to within about 10% over most of the field of gaze (4,5), thus contributing only about 2 to 3% nonlinearity to the entire system.

We can derive equations for the amount of muscle surgery in two steps. First we assume symmetrical surgery of S mm on each muscle of similar stiffness and derive the total amount of surgery, 2S, required to surgically put the globe in the primary position. The surgically altered muscle force (in grams), F_M, required to rotate the globe straight, is set equal to the total tissue force, F_G, which deviates the globe from the primary position, i.e.: $F_M = F_G$. The corrective muscle force is equal to the surgical change of length of each muscle, S, times the stiffness of the muscle:

$$F_M = SK_M + SK_L = S(K_M + K_L).$$

The force producing the strabismic deviation equals the deviation, D, (which can be expresed in mm as prism diopters x 0.1) times the stiffness of the intact eye of the awake patient, K.

Thus: $F_G = DK$.

Solving; the symmetrical surgery on each muscle is equal to the deviating force divided by the combined muscle stiffnss:

$$S = DK/(K_M+K_L).$$

However, it has proved impractical to directly measure the stiffness of the detached and innervated individual muscles while the patient is awake, but the combined stiffness of the innvervated muscles can be derived indirectly by subtracting the isolated globe stiffness (measured in the anesthesized patient with muscles detached) from the stiffness of the intact eye measured with the patient awake.

Thus: $K_M+K_L = K-K_G$.

Substituting, the required symmetrical surgery on each muscle is:

$S = DK/(K-K_G)$, which is the equation we utilize.

The second step involves properly apportioning the total surgery into the individual amounts of surgery to be performed on each muscle for the general case of a non-symmetrical strabismus operation (involving unequal muscle stiffnesses). In patients without mechanical restrictions the total surgery, 2S, can be divided between two muscles of unequal stiffness in inverse proportion to the individual stiffness of each muscle (i.e., a stiffer muscle requires less surgery to produce a given strabismus correcting force). Thus, one can derive equations for the optimal amount of strabismus surgery on each muscle. This divides the <u>force</u> equally between the two muscles. In this case:

$$S_M^* = (2S)\ K_L/(K_M+K_L), \text{ and } S_L^* = (2S)\ K_M/(K_M+K_L);$$

where S_M^* and S_L^* are the optimal mm amounts of medial and lateral rectus muscle surgery respectively. $S_M^*+S_L^* = 2S$, the total amount of surgery.

For the purpose of dividing the total amount of surgery between the medial and lateral rectus muscles, one can utilize the ratio of the stiffness of the passive, non-innervated muscles within their normal range of movement. If measured near extreme gaze lengths, the stiffness of human oculorotary muscles has been previously shown to approximate their stiffness when fully innervated by voluntary effort (4,5,6). This is not true of animal experiments utilizing constant frequency, fixed pulse-width electrical stimulation which elicits a completely different type of recruitment pattern (6,7,8). Using a <u>ratio</u> of the passive muscle stiffness measurements rather than their individual absolute values to apportion the total surgery (which has been calculated from innervated stiffnesses) further enhances the accuracy of the method.

When a restriction or muscle contracture prevents the muscle or globe from moving through the entire range of gaze, we must often deviate from this optimal surgical combination to apportion the amount of surgery and muscle force differently between the medial and lateral rectus muscles. One method of choice is to center the useful range of elasticity of the contractured muscle upon the primary position of the globe (the useful range of elasticity can be defined as the length of muscle extension up to its point of restriction, where extension requires 40 grams or more). This choice is made in order to permit the eye to have equal movement to either side of primary position.

Assume that this dictated choice of surgical change of muscle length is S_L for a contractured lateral rectus muscle. The amount of surgery on the other muscle is then found from a more general equation which expresses the new altered MR surgery, S_M, as a function of the deviation, the new S_L and ratios of muscle stiffnesses:

$$S_M = D\ (K/K_M) \ - S_L\ (K_L/K_M).$$

In the converse case: $S_L = D\ (K/K_L) \ - S_M\ (K_M/K_L).$

This relationship is perhaps better visualized graphically as in Fig. 3, where S_M is plotted against S_L and the resulting straight line represent all combinations of recess-resect surgery which would result in the necessary force, F_M, to correct the strabismic deviation. We call this line the constant corrective force line, or surgical locus. (This is the locus of constant corrective force due to the net difference in muscle force or torque which will rotate the globe straight). In Fig. 3, 5 mm of MR recession and 5.6 mm of LR resection would suffice as would also 2 mm recession and 12.4 mm resection, or 3.8 mm MR recession and 8.9 mm LR resection, etc. Note that surgical combinations above the line would overcorrect and combinations below the locus would result in undercorrection of the deviation. The optimal surgery in this case (for patient #2) was calculated as S_M = 3.8 mm MR recession and S_L = 8.9 mm LR resection. The parameter evaluations for these calculations are given in Table 1.

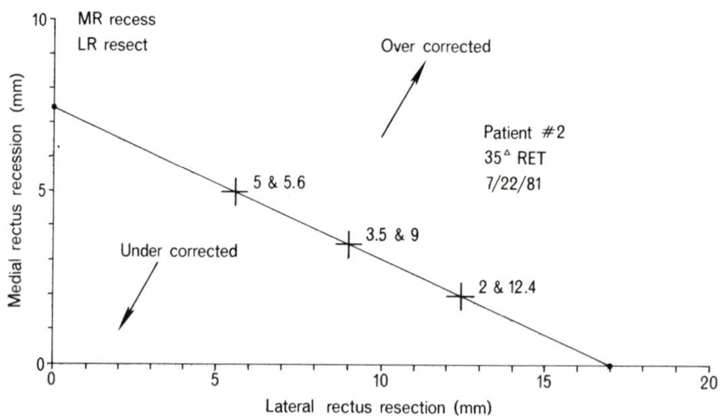

Fig. 3. Calculated surgical locus of all recess-resect combinations which would correct the deviation of patient #2.

RESULTS

We present all graphical information on a single, consistent data set comprising patient #2 (Figs. 3, 4 & 5). Typical results of these investigations are shown in Fig. 4. These examples of the technique illustrate a previously operated patient, with a 35 prism diopter right esotropia. Figure 4 is a complete set of length-force (L-F) curves shown with superimposed scales of eye position and force. The 35 prism diopter esotropic deviation is also shown as a vertical dashed line. It can be seen that the curves are shifted in the direction of and tend to center on the strabismic deviation.

The L-F curves for passive muscles show a marked increase in stiffness (steepness of the curve) beyond extreme gaze length in the normal situation (nasal quadrant in Fig. 4). This expresses the natural "tether" effect of these tissues. In the pathological case of a restriction or contractured muscle, the stiffness increases sharply <u>within</u> the normal range of gaze (temporalward in this patient). The intact eye (the top record of Fig. 4) is restricted in abduction to 12° of temporal rotation (a mechanical limitation of -3 on the Jampolsky scale).

In these L-F measurements one also sees the passive mechanical hysteresis and viscosity of the length-force relationships manifest as open loops (10). The force these tissues exert in opposition to being stretched to a given length is greater than the force they exert, at the same length, as they passively shorten (as a simple spring; and as seen in the "springback" test (9,13)). We have chosen to measure the stiffness of these tissues being extended (as an antagonist load on a contracting agonist muscle).

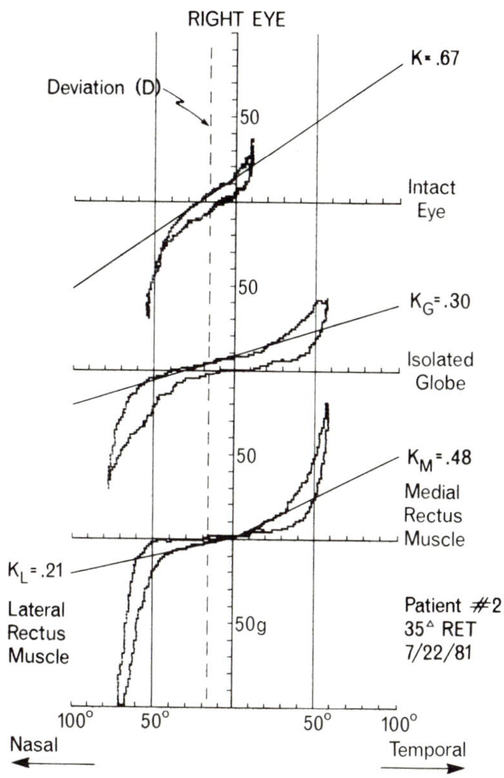

Fig. 4. (Top) Active length-force (L-F) record of the intact right eye of a fully awake 35 prism diopter esotropic patient (#2). The eye appears normal in adduction but is severely restricted in abduction with an abrupt, extremely stiff restriction at 12°. (This later proved to be scar tissue which was removed at surgery).
(Middle) L-F record of the isolated globe which shows a gradual restriction in abduction (40 g at 50°).
(Bottom left) L-F curve for the lateral rectus muscle which appears normal (20 g at 50°).
(Bottom right) L-F of the medial rectus muscle which exhibits a restrictive tether (20 g at 33° nasal extension) limiting the normal range of gaze, and 50 g at 50°.

In Fig. 4 (top), the stiffness, K, for the awake, intact eye is the slope of the top L-F curve, which can be measured as 0.67 grams per degree. (Grams per degree is the more conventionally used metric by oculomotor model physiologists).

The center curve in Fig. 4 is the L-F record for the passive, isolated globe with the medial and lateral rectus muscles detached. Note the much smaller stiffness, K_G = 0.30 grams per degree (but increasing beyond the 12° restriction). Most of the passive stiffness of the intact eye is attributable to the muscles. They generally contribute about two thirds of the total stiffness; the passive globe restraining tissues ordinarily contribute only about one third.

On the bottom left is the L-F record of the passive lateral rectus muscle (K_L = 0.21 grams per degree within its operational zone). Note the stiffness increases only beyond the normal range of gaze. The passive muscle force is only about 20 grams at 50° extreme gaze. This muscle appears normal.

On the bottom right in Fig. 4 the length-force curve of the detached, passive medial rectus muscle is shown (K_M = 0.48 grams per degree from primary to 30° temporal rotation). Note the passive stretching forces become large within the normal range of gaze (50 grams at 50°). 40 grams is the average maximum force a short, maximally contracted active agonist muscle can exert (4,5) to move the eye against the sum of both muscle and globe restraining loads, hence this stiff MR muscle, combined with the globe restraining stiffness, would restrict temporalward eye movement beyond about 30° (where the sum of their forces is about 40 grams).

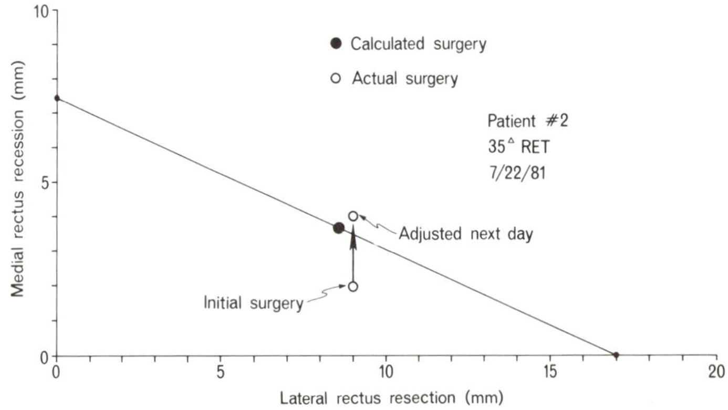

Fig. 5. Comparison of calculated optimum and actual surgery for patient #2.

The calculated optimal surgery for this patient is shown as the solid black disk in Figure 5. The results of the actual surgery performed on this 35 prism diopter esotropic patient are shown as the open circles plotted with respect to the surgical locus introduced in Fig. 3. The initial surgery was 9 mm LR resection and 2 mm MR recession but this surgery resulted in an undercorrection (as calculations indicated). The next day adjustable sutures permitted a better result which approached the correcting force line. The final successful surgery came very close to the calculated theoretical optimum as can be seen.

It should be pointed out that our calculations were made after the surgeon independently performed the surgery which he arrived at using only his usual clinical intrasurgical assessments of each strabismus patient. Thus, our calculations in no way affected what the surgeon actually did in practice.

		PRISMS	GRAMS/DEGREE				CALCULATED			ACTUAL			RESULTS
DATE	PATIENT #	D_X	K	K_G	K_M	K_L	S	S_M	S_L	S	S_M	S_L	1 DAY POSTOP
7/15/81	1	35 RET	.69	.23	.29	–	**13.5**	**7.2**	–	**13.0**	**7.0**	–	2 RET
		LE	–	–	–	–		**6.3**	–	–	**6.0**	–	
7/22/81	2	35 RET REOP	.67	.30	.48	.21	**12.3**	**3.8**	**8.6**	**13.0**	**2.0→4.0**	**9.0**	ORTHO
8/5/81	3	25 LET REOP	.89	.41	.23	–	**9.2**	**4.6**	–	**9.5**	**3.5→6.5**	–	3 RET
		RE	–	–	–	–		**4.6**	–	–	**3.0**	–	
8/12/81	4	40 RET	.95	.44	.30	–	**14.9**	**5.1**	–	**15.0**	**6.0**	–	ORTHO
		LE	1.29	.60	.45	.34		**5.0**	**4.9**	–	**5.0**	**4.0**	
8/15/81	5	30 RXT REOP	.55	.35	.50	.43	**16.6**	**7.7**	**8.9**	**14.5**	**5.5**	**9.0**	10 RXT

Table 1.

Table I shows the diagnosis, parameter evaluations (in grams per degree), surgical calculations in millimeters, actual surgical treatment in millimeters, and clinical post-surgical results for five patients (including three reoperations). The accuracy of these calculations was based on the final surgical outcome measured the next day (including adjustments, if made). There were 4 ESO cases and 1 EXO case. In all but one of the five patients, calculated surgery agreed within 10% of the amount of actual surgery performed independently. In all cases where calculations agreed with actual independent surgery, corrections fell within the criterion for satisfactory surgical results (ortho to 5 prism diopters). The one disparate case was undercorrected and calculation would have suggested that the surgeon do more surgery.

DISCUSSION

We have collected data from over 30 strabismus patients to date. Although much work remains, the significant success shown in the typical results of the five most recent cases reported here make the method appear quite promising.We have demonstrated, by comparisons with actual successful surgery, that it is possible to make calculations of the exact amount of strabismus surgery required, based on an individual computer model of the patient's own oculomotor mechanics. We can evaluate the parameters of his model from physical measurements made before and at surgery. However, the necessary calculations cannot be derived from a general model, but the parameters of the patient's own individual model must be evaluated within this framework to formulate a unique model representing only that patient. The necessary measurements and techniques for making these measurements have been outlined.

In simple, uncomplicated cases these calculations agree with the usual formulas in millimeters. However, the complications of difficult cases, including asymmetrical stiffnesses, and particularly re-operations, markedly reduce the probability of success when proceeding by the usual formulas, leading to re-operations in many cases. It has been noted that often these unusual but successful cases fall far from the usual formula. It is in just these difficult and abnormal cases that the technique of physical measurement of tissue stiffnesses and tether locations should provide a pay-off in the ability to calculate the unusual and often unorthodox amount of surgery to do on each muscle, and should permit more accurate surgery the first time.

The techniques and concepts learned in making these objective measurements can permit the surgeon to quantitatively visualize a mechanical frame of reference into which to fit the patient's measured stiffnesses and tether locations. This can be helpful to the surgeon in planning strabismus surgery. In practicing with the length-force forceps, the surgeon can rapidly develop the concept of absolute magnitudes of forces and stiffnesses. He can learn to sense what 30 or 40 grams of force feels like at his fingertips and this may suggest that he back-off one or two millimeters to make sure he has not resected too much muscle and thus avoid a restriction or tightness of the muscle post-operatively .

The quantitative concepts contained in length-force tissue diagrams have been found particularly useful for teaching resident surgeons who are not yet well experienced with strabismus surgery. The use of the forceps can help a surgeon refine his own choice of the amounts of surgery to do based on his own measurements. It is faster and easier to learn to make force and stiffness estimations with the length-force forceps than by feel alone. Trainees having used these forceps in training can now fairly closely call the actual grams of force without the use of forceps. This absolute force estimation could otherwise be difficult for some surgeons to learn. These surgeons now visualize the active force and forced duction characteristics with finger diagnosis and utilize this information in their treatment. One surgeon claims that his ability to train himself using a length-force instrument a few times was probably the equivalent of performing many, perhaps hundreds, of surgeries.

We can determine the amount of active contribution to the strabismus by noting the difference between the awake and anesthetized positions of rest of the eyes. We utilize this technique routinely and find it to be helpful in determining the amount of active contribution to the strabismus. Also, active force measurements in the awake, cooperative patient are necessary for defining disorders such as anomalous innervation which is found in Duane's syndrome.

Whether strabismus cases are predominantly passive in etiology or whether there is an active component resulting in a comitant, stable strabismus, the same techniques for surgical calculation outlined here have been shown to apply. It appears that a comitant and stable tonic (innervational) force component can be successfully balanced by a purely mechanical repositioning of the muscles just as if the deviation had been produced by wholly passive mechanical factors alone.

It is expected that the quantitative information derived in making these clinical length-force measurements on specific individual patients will provide a pool of basic information for better understanding of oculomotion as well as modeling in general.

We are now extending our computer program to make its calculations in real-time in the operating room and to present the surgeon with the recommended amounts of surgery before he is ready to reattach the muscles to the globe. Such a facility would essentially provide the ophthalmologist with a "second opinion".

The primary significance of this research will be to provide a rational approach to the most difficult cases, utilizing physical measurements capable of easy performance by the average clinician, which should allow him to derive the necessary surgery and limits, rather than using purely experiential or judgmental factors.

PATHOLOGICAL PHYSIOLOGY OF BINOCULAR PARALLELISM

G. WESTHEIMER

Department of Physiology-Anatomy, University of California, Berkeley, CA 94720, USA

That the two eyes ordinarily stay parallel is taken so much for granted that deviation from parallelism is regarded as a significant problem. And indeed it is from the clinical standpoint, but here we are making an attempt at tackling it by turning the question on its head: Why is it reasonable to expect the two eyes to remain parallel? The extent and depth of this question is made clear by a reiteration of the litany of conditions in which parallelism of the two eyes is maintained in spite of all counterindications:

1. When one eye is occluded, the occluded eye moves along with the seeing eye though no visual advantage is gained from this.
2. Even in congenital uniocular blindness there is conjugacy.
3. Even when the fixation axes are not parallel, as in concomitant strabismus, the eye movements are parallel.
4. Vestibular nystagmus in the dark is still characterized by parallel eye movements.
5. The two eyes move together within most of the field of fixation even in patients with slight paresis of one muscle.

In case you think this enumeration of surprising situations during which there are conjugate eye movements is novel, let me hasten to state that the above is a verbatim quote from Hering's treatise of 1868. We may add to the list the essential conjugacy of neonatal eye movements, which seems to be perfect in the macaque monkey, and almost so in most human babies.

Just how timely this argument was when brought to the attention of the scientific audience, is shown by the following quotation published a year or so earlier.

"Although each eye has a completely independent muscular mechanism and hence has the facility to execute every kind of movement independently of the other eye, we have learned to make movements that are necessary so that we may see all points clearly and singly with both eyes." This from Helmholtz (1911) the most prestigeous vision scientist of his day.

Hering's law of the yoking of the two eyes in their movement is an essential ingredient of all of our knowledge and procedures concerning binocularity. At the clinical end, every time one performs a cover test it is presupposed.

The extent of the scope of Hering's law has recently been illuminated by two observations, one clinical, the other in primate experimental neurology.

Hering drew attention to the inability of patients with monocular abducens palsy to maintain ocular parallelism; in a mild case the affected eye can assume almost all eye positions, certainly the straight-ahead one. Yet when the good eye looks straight ahead, the affected eye is slightly adducted. When the good eye is occluded and the patient is asked to change fixation to an object in the field of gaze of the affected muscle, the open eye makes a smaller saccade than demanded, followed by a series of corrective ones. Behind the cover, the good eye makes the same sequence of movements, only with larger amplitudes. This is in accord with Hering's law of equal innervation; normal innervation does not get through to bring about a normal eye position where the paretic muscle is needed, hence, in the face of a normal neural input, the affected eye moves less and assumes a less eccentric position than the normal one. Kommerell and his collaborators (1976) patched the good eye in some patients with this condition. They observed that after a few days, the affected eye made much more appropriate saccades - the patients had learned to increase the gain of the signal that relates peripheral retinal stimulation to the corresponding eye movement innervation. But the other eye, behind the cover, continued to make saccades larger than the affected eye. Reprogramming of the peripheral retinal eye position signal left unaffected the ratio of the open loop output to the eye position in the two eyes. That such reprogramming takes place need not surprise us, because it is necessary every time a patient with high refractive error changes from spectacle to contact lenses. The second finding this time from the realm of experimental intervention in the neuro-ocular system of monkeys is quite similar. It arose out of the attempt by Optican and Robinson (1980) to demonstrate that the cerebellum is needed for reprogramming of the gain of the eye movement responses. They did surgery on the muscles of one eye of a monkey reattaching them in such a way that the saccades in that eye were smaller than in the other eye. They now patched the good eye, allowing the monkey to learn to program larger saccades. But when he had done so, the saccadic amplitudes in the two eyes were still unequal.

The two experiments show that the neural channel carrying the signal from the peripheral retinal stimulus to the eye movement command station is capable of modification on the basis of experiential need, but the signal from the eye movement command station to the eye muscles is not, or at least not nearly as readily.

This leads to a reaffirmation of Hering's view that the latter signal is innate, or as we are wont to say these days, hard wired. It is a manifestation of a truly amazing feat of design. There are six muscles in each orbit, each with an individual and rather peculiar direction of action. Because the two orbits are mirror symmetrical, it will not do just to duplicate the wiring to the two eyes. The essence of the yoking of the eyes according to Hering's law is parallel eye movement, not mirror symmetric eye movement. The innervation set to move the right eye up and out has to have a completely different counterpart in the left eye for parallel eye movements to be achieved.

When it is observed that a new-born macaque has beautiful conjugacy of both eyes, one is forced to assign an incredibly exact, genetically programmed neural design to this conjugacy. The features of the underlying circuitry are fascinating and it is appropriate that they are beginning to attract the interest of mathematically sophisticated analysts (Pellionis & Llinas, 1980).

But when the same is said about an adult, uniocularly blind from birth, we have to ask ourselves whether we are willing to accept the proposition that conjugacy is not only innate but also immutable and at the same time exact to, say, a prism diopter. I cannot accept that we are born with a distribution of synaptic connections in our brainstems that permit us to start off with Hering's law of binocular conjugacy at birth, and still retain accurate yoking throughout the period of growth, adulthood and senescence without some mechanism of testing it, reinforcing it, and adjusting for deviations. Fine-tuning of the incoming visual signals with experience is now accepted, and it is time to take it seriously on the oculomotor side.

Let us briefly examine here what, in principle, would have to be involved. Accurate measurements on the neonate would permit us to ascertain just how good is the innate neural connectivity for yoking of the two eyes. Careful tracing of changes in subjects with uniocular sensory defects can tell us how immutable the innate circuitry is, and pointed experimental intervention in monkeys should be able to give insight into the mechanism of possible readjustment. If self-correction of imposed changes in the muscular apparatus takes place when one eye does not see, we have to admit the role of some muscular sensing, or detection of discrepancies in neural outflow. If accurate conjugacy (tested without fusion) is maintained much better over longish periods in people with good binocular fusion than those without it, sensory feedback has to be involved, and we are not talking about the quick disparity-induced convergence loop with latency and time constants of the order of a fraction of a second.

The evidence from Marlow's prolonged occlusion test (1924) is suggestive, but it must be recognized that we are here addressing the wider question of maintained conjugacy over the whole field of fixation, not just a defect of parallelism of the eye in the straight-ahead position.

One hundred and fifteen years later, the old controversy between Helmholtz and Hering has to be taken up again, albeit with the advantage of new insights from other areas of neurobiology. Hering no doubt was right about the innateness of the circuitry for binocular conjugacy, but surely Helmholtz also has to be right about the contribution made by experiential factors to normal functioning. There are obvious consequences of this kind of analysis for our views of the etiology of many kinds of strabismus, concomitant and incomitant. The immediate information mation feedback of diplopia to the maintenance of conjugacy does not need to be stressed, but surely, once this is allowed for, we have not exhausted the possibilities for the utilization of error signals in keeping the eyes statically and dynamically parallel. The problem is that we are unclear about the nature of the signals being used and the level at which they operate. But once we have admitted the existence of homeostatic mechanisms for the maintenance of ocular conjugacy other than diplopia, we can take the next step. Whenever therapeutic procedures like wearing prisms or simple surgery do not lead to expected results, we are probably faced with a malfunctioning of some as yet undiscovered self-correcting apparatus. The search for these should open a chapter in oculomotor physiology that is sure to add depth to our understanding of normal function and eventually lead to benefit patients suffering from abnormalities.

PHARMACOLOGICAL TREATMENT OF STRABISMUS

A. B. SCOTT

Smith-Kettlewell Institute of Visual Sciences, 2232 Webster Street, San Francisco, California 94115, USA

ABSTRACT

"Oculinum" (botulinum A toxin) was injected into extraocular muscles of 63 humans aged 6 1/2 to 81. The effect on horizontal strabismus was uniformly beneficial, and effect lasting over two years was documented. The effect in vertical strabismus, paralytic strabismus, and in lid retraction was beneficial, but less strongly so. No systemic effect or local complications were encountered except for transient effect on adjacent muscles. The drug appears to be a safe and useful therapy for strabismus.

KEY WORDS

Strabismus; Botulinum Toxin; Extraocular Muscle; Endocrine Exophthalmos.

INTRODUCTION

I describe below our experience in humans from injection of Oculinum into extraocular muscles as a therapeutic modality. Preliminary animal studies (1) and preliminary studies in a few patients are already published (2).

HUMAN INJECTIONS

Rationale

If the paralysis of an individual extraocular muscle is mild in extent and brief in duration, recovery can be complete with no residual whatsoever. If the paralysis is more long-lasting, there is often contracture of the medial rectus muscle and stretching of the paralyzed lateral rectus muscle during the period of paralysis; then, although the recovery of the lateral rectus can be quite complete, a nearly concomitant esotropia results. It is just this that we hope to create: controlling intensity of paralysis by varying the injection doses; controlling duration of paralysis by varying the injection dose and by re-injection at intervals. Persistent long-term weakness of extraocular muscles is not the goal: most strabismus is concomitant in nature and non-paralytic concomitant change in deviation is the desired treatment outcome.

To accomplish this, we need drugs which are effective for days to weeks, controllable by dosage variation, devoid of major ocular or systemic side effects, able to be re-injected without allergy or loss of potency from immune response, and which leave the muscle normal after its effects. Oculinum (botulinum A toxin) fulfills these criteria well.

METHODS

Clinical Measurements

Alignment was assessed by prism-cover test in seeing patients, by corneal reflex in others, and by photography of alignment in all patients. Speed of saccades into the field of action on the involved muscle and active force (isometric) testing were done in some cases. The amplitude of rotation into the field of action of the injected muscle was measured in eyes with good vision. In lid retraction, photographic measurement before and after injection was used.

Technic of Injection

One proparacaine drop is followed one minute later by one drop of 1% epinephrine to reduce vascularity of tissues. Five additional proparacaine drops at one minute intervals are then given. The Oculinum was mixed to the appropriate dose for a 0.1 cc volume. About 0.3 cc extra were injected into a waste container to clear the needle of any bubbles, and to test the electromyographic (EMG) needle electrode. The needle is advanced about 15-20 mm along the orbital side of the muscle with the eye looking in the primary position. Then, after moving gaze into the field of action to increase muscle activity, the needle is angled into the muscle and injection made when a high level EMG signal is heard.

Patient Data

We are interested in all forms of strabismus and make little effort to recruit particular types. All patients had stable deviations for 6 months of more, prior to injection (except lid retraction and acute paralysis).

RESULTS AND DISCUSSION

The threshold paralysis effect lies between 1.25×10^{-5} mcg and 6.25×10^{-5} mcg for our preparation with a LD/50 potency of about 3.5×10^{-4}. The more the dose, the greater and better maintained the response; the threshold for permanent alignment changes was about 3×10^{-4} in adults (Fig. 1).

With the exceptions of the small doses early in the series, of paralytic strabismus and of lid retraction, all cases have been helped. The cases followed for over one year are maintaining their deviation at the present level and they are either symptomatically or cosmetically comfortable, and do not wish further treatment (Fig. 2).

Multiple Injections

The drug is a competent antigen in milligram quantities, but at these doses no patient has shown any tendency to tolerance. For example, patient #3 received 9 injections in horizontal muscles in attempt to correct his paralytic strabismus (with only limited success). Thereafter, two injections to the superior rectus to correct vertical deviation were normally effective in creating paralysis and developing a long-term alignment change.

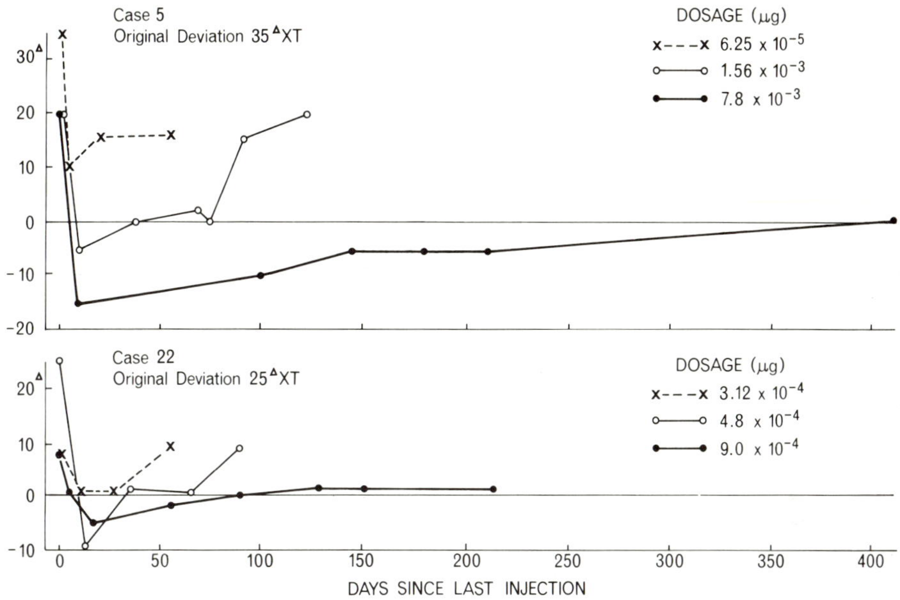

Fig. 1 Ordinate is deviation in prism diopters before injection.

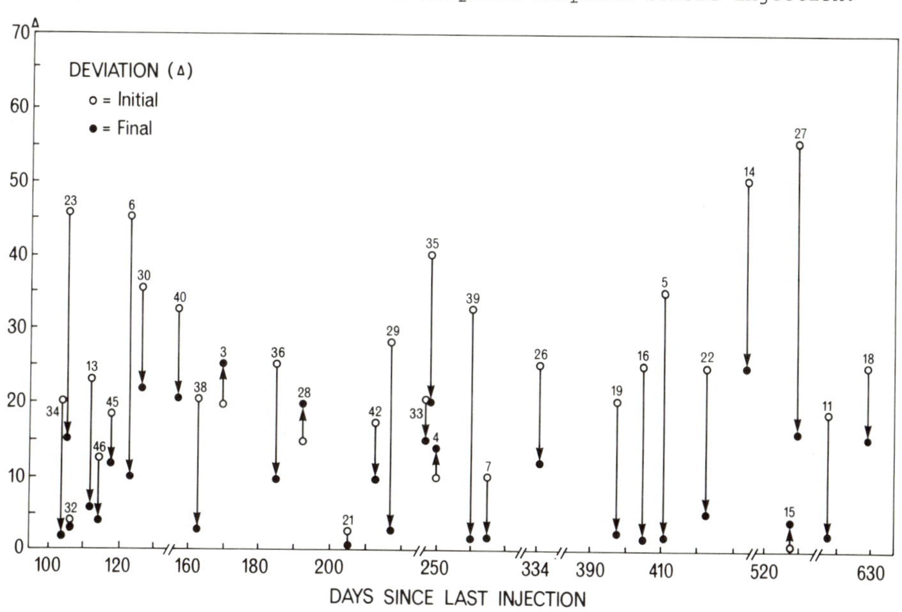

Fig. 2. Injection effects. Ordinate is deviation; Abscissa is days since last injection. Included are patients with concomitant strabismus followed for 100 days or more since the last injection. Beside each arrow is patient indentification number.

Variation in Response

There is a marked variation of toxin effectiveness in various species, and in human botulism epidemics a tremendous variability exists. The basis for these differences is not known. Most adult patients respond in a similar manner but a few unusual responders were found and these fell into two groups: the most sensitive eye muscles were consistently found in young women; the most unresponsive muscles were consistently in husky, tall men. Younger patients, 8 and 12 year-old girls, showed a response equal to the usual adult response.

Patient 21, a young woman, was injected (levator) on the same day with the same dose from the same vial as Patient 19, a tall, robust man (lateral rectus). Effect in Patient 21, a young woman, was a marked weakness of the injected muscle over an extended period of time. Patient 19 got only a mild response which lasted not over 7 to 10 days, and later required a dose ten times larger. Two further low responses in young men and 2 high responses in young women approach these extremes. We tend to make the initial injection at a moderate level for the condition existing, with the recognition that the majority of patients will require a second injection at a later time (Table I). Since a prolonged period of weakness is advantageous, this second injection carries with it some positive value. Ultimately, we estimate that about 40% of patients will be adequately treated by a single injection, perhaps another 40% by the second injection, and further injections will be required as part of the initial treatment series for the remainder.

TABLE I

Suggested beginning dose levels (for lot # 79-11-1, mouse LD/50 $3.5 \times 10^{-4}\ \mu g$).

Horizontal Strabismus

10^{Δ} - 20^{Δ}	-	$5 \times 10^{-4}\ \mu g$
20^{Δ} - 35^{Δ}	-	$1 \times 10^{-3}\ \mu g$
35^{Δ} or more	-	$2 \times 10^{-3}\ \mu g$

For vertical strabismus or young women, reduce dose by 50%.

Subsequent injections to be at dosages up to 5 fold higher or lower depending on initial response.

Injection Where Strabismus Surgery Is Not Indicated

Anterior segment ischemia from a retinal detachment procedure was present in Case #38. Strabismus surgery on the unoperated horizontal muscle was not considered safe. Injection was spectacularly helpful in aligning his eye with regaining of fusion and removal of diplopia. Case #40 had a tension of less than six in a blind eye with an existing retinal detachment and 60 prism diopters of exotropia. He was advised by a glaucoma consultant that a 50% chance of phthisis existed if strabismus surgery were done. He elected an injection which has placed his eye in a satisfactory alignment position. Case #41 has a tension of 60 with no light perception and continuing uveitis in an eye previously operated for cataract.

Bilateral Injection

This has been done in three cases without systemic or other complication, and should carry the same indications as bilateral strabismus surgery. For example, bilateral medial rectus weakening in high AC/A ratios. (Patient #15).

Effect of The Drug on Adjacent Muscles

In doses greater than 1.0×10^{-3} micrograms this is seen almost uniformly. The levator appears to be especially susceptible. These effects on adjacent muscles typically occur only when the injected muscle itself receives a strongly weakening effect. They have gone away entirely in every case. In one case of thyroid myopathy injection was technically misplaced. When surgery was done 3 months later in that case for the persistent vertical deviation, the induced horizontal deviation was also corrected.

Pupilo-motor and accommodation changes have not been encountered. The combination of proparacaine drops and epinephrine drops does cause some pupil enlargement at the time of injection in most patients. No systemic effect has been seen or suspected in any patient.

Effects on Various Muscle Fiber Types

In case 21, injection was made into the levator with secondary diffusion into the superior rectus. About 30 days later the pattern of deviation with mild superior rectus weakness was: upgaze, 2 prism diopters LH; primary position, 10 prism diopters LH; downgaze, 1 prism diopter LH.

In case 34 the levator was secondarily involved after injection of the LMR. At a time 10 days later, there was 1.0 ptosis in the upgaze position, 3 millimeters of ptosis in the primary position,and no ptosis in downgaze. To a smaller degree this pattern of greater deviation in the primary position of gaze has been seen in the recovery stage following other injections. This pattern is explicable for the superior rectus by assuming that the outer layer of small muscle fibers active in the primary position was preferentially influenced by proximity of this outer layer to the levator. The intact inner fibers, much larger in total number and size, then provided the bulk of force for saccades and for supra duction. The levator is not documented to have this same layering, but does have many small singly innervated fibers that may be especially sensitive to the drug. This would be fortunate--influencing the tonic activity with effect on phasic movements and on the amplitude of rotation.

Effect of Contracture

In total lateral rectus palsy from 2 to 12 months old confirmed by force testing and EMG we have injected the medial rectus with marked reduction of contracture and increase in rotation towards the primary position with adduction attempts. These changes are seen within a week following effective injection. This type of contracture seems due to changes within the muscle fiber rather than due to connective tissue shortening.

In cases where multiple operations have occurred, or in long-standing, large angle strabismus with contractures present, there was probably a structural connective tissue limitation and this is not able to be fully influenced by injection (Case 23). However, existence of contracture limiting full rotation may not limit ability to move the eye part way towards the primary position; thus some moderate improvement is possible even in these less favorable settings. Intentionally induced contracture of the antagonist by injection of the agonist probably occurs, but is difficult to measure; more sensitive appartus is just now being employed.

Levator

Injection of the levator in lid retraction was done in Cases 9, 21, and 37 with only mild long-term effect. This is probably due to the relative inactivity of the orbicularis muscle during most of the day--this antagonist muscle is not continuously innervated as are the extra-ocular muscles. Injection of the upper lid as a temporary technique to close the lid for corneal exposure works nicely, with good recovery subsequently. For lid retraction without much muscle thickening and exophthalmos involvement of the subjacent superior rectus may be substantial (Case 21). When thickened levator exists with exophthalmos no effect on superior rectus is seen (Cases 9,38)

Vertical Muscles

It is a practical problem to restrain effect to an individual vertical muscle without effect on adjacent muscles. For the inferior rectus Case #10 and Case #28, no effect on adjacent muscles occurred, and therapeutic levels of effect were obtained in the injected muscle. Particular care, restriction of dosage, and restriction of injected volume to 0.05 ml may be important in injection of these muscle areas.

After the superior rectus injection, partial ptosis lasting 1-2 months (fully recovering, however) was seen in each of the three instances.

Postoperative Injection

A significant over-correction or under-correction following surgery should be especially amenable to alteration before healing and scar tissue have settled the eye into its new position. Thus, in case 50, a large angle exotropia was surgically corrected by recession and resection of horizontal muscles. A week later the eye was 5 prism diopters exotropia and three weeks after surgery it was 15 prism diopters exotropia. Paralyzing injection of the operated lateral rectus moved the eye into an esotropic position for three weeks. Thereafter, adduction was regained and the eye position remained straight (90 day follow-up).

Paralytic Strabismus

Injection of the medial rectus in recent lateral rectus paralysis was spectacularly successful in bringing the eye back toward the primary position and in preventing and actually obliterating contracture. (Cases 3, 12, 17, 60) This approach was used to prevent lateral rectus contracture when a medial rectus muscle had been damaged during nasal sinus surgery (Case #24). However, long term effect does not occur. Without the antagonist to take up the slack created by paralysis, the eye simply drifts back to the original position. Thus, the toxin should not be used as a treatment for chronic paralytic strabismus cases. The effect in moderate vertical palsy, especially superior oblique palsy, has not yet been adequately documented.

Amplitude of Change

It is relatively easy to achieve the first five or ten degrees of strabismus change. Further equal increments of change require progressively longer duration agonist paralysis to allow stretching of the injected muscle, and shortening of the antagonist. Nevertheless, as much as 25 degrees of change can be achieved with four to five months of total paralysis of the agonist muscle (Case 14).

Functional Results

Unexpected binocular fusion has occurred with suprising frequency. In Case #40 there was a history of esotropia since infancy, and an existing deviation of approximately 55 prism diopters without glasses (25 prism diopters with hyperoptic correction). Definite motor fusion was regained. Similar fusion has developed in Cases 11,13, and 29. I speculate that the marked incomitancy which exists during the period of paralysis allows the eyes to be exotropic in one gaze position, esotropic in the opposite gaze position, but usually there is some point where the two eyes are perfectly aligned. Thus during all waking hours constant stimulation of the retina on both sides of the fovea, plus the opportunity to tune the two foveas together by small head movements, apparently provides the opportunity to develop or to regain binocular fusion to a degree not obtainable in the usual surgical correction.

ACKNOWLEDGEMENT

Supported by NIH Grant Nos. 1 R01 EY02106 and 5 P30 EY 01186, and The Smith-Kettlewell Eye Research Foundation.

COMMENTS

H. E. A. BICAS

Departamento de Oftalmologia, Faculdade de Medicina,
Ribeirão Preto, Brazil

THE "FADEN" OPERATION

Fadenoperation seems to be a valuable tool for the treatment of some types of oculomotor imbalances. But some contraditory positions arise from the paper. For instance:

a) The author admits that a Fd increases the mm/degree ratio of an additional recession and even offers some quantitative prediction for that ("the addition of a Fd to a recession roughly will double the effect of the recession to the basic angle"). However, when comparing his own results (235 surgeries of Fd only, and 69 in which it was "essential to add recessions"), he finds that "the results are, in cases with angles up to 25°, about the same..."

b) Conclusion that "11 mm corrects maximum angles about 10° to 15°, 12 mm are adequate for 15° to 20°, and 13 mm give good result up to 25°", can not be supported. For instance, the *only* group of deviations (15°) in which there was a significant difference between success and type of surgery, shows 29% of *under*corrections with a fadenoperation of 13 mm, fewer (19%) with a 12 mm Fd and even less (11%) with the "weakest" (11 mm) surgery. (On the contrary, the corrective and over-corrective effect of the fadenoperations upon the angles,were *inversely* proportional, i.e., to the greater surgery, the smaller effect).

c) If Fd is combined to recessions, the hypothesis that "the rates of success of different fadenoperations, are different",is rejected,even if very tolerant levels of acceptability are considered.

d) Though one could expect that bilateral Fd give more correction than unilateral Fd, this is not supported by the paper. If one takes angles up to 20°, the rate of failures with unilateral Fd (7/46= 15.2%) is about the same than the rate of failures with bilateral Fd (31/161 = = 19.3%; or 21/161= 13.0% if one does not consider overcorrections). The author remarks that "unilateral Fd is not so sucessful", but the rates of success with pure bilateral or unilateral types of such surgery are the same (181/235= 77.0% and 30/39= 76.9%).

Why should such discrepancies appear? A given amount of fadenoperation

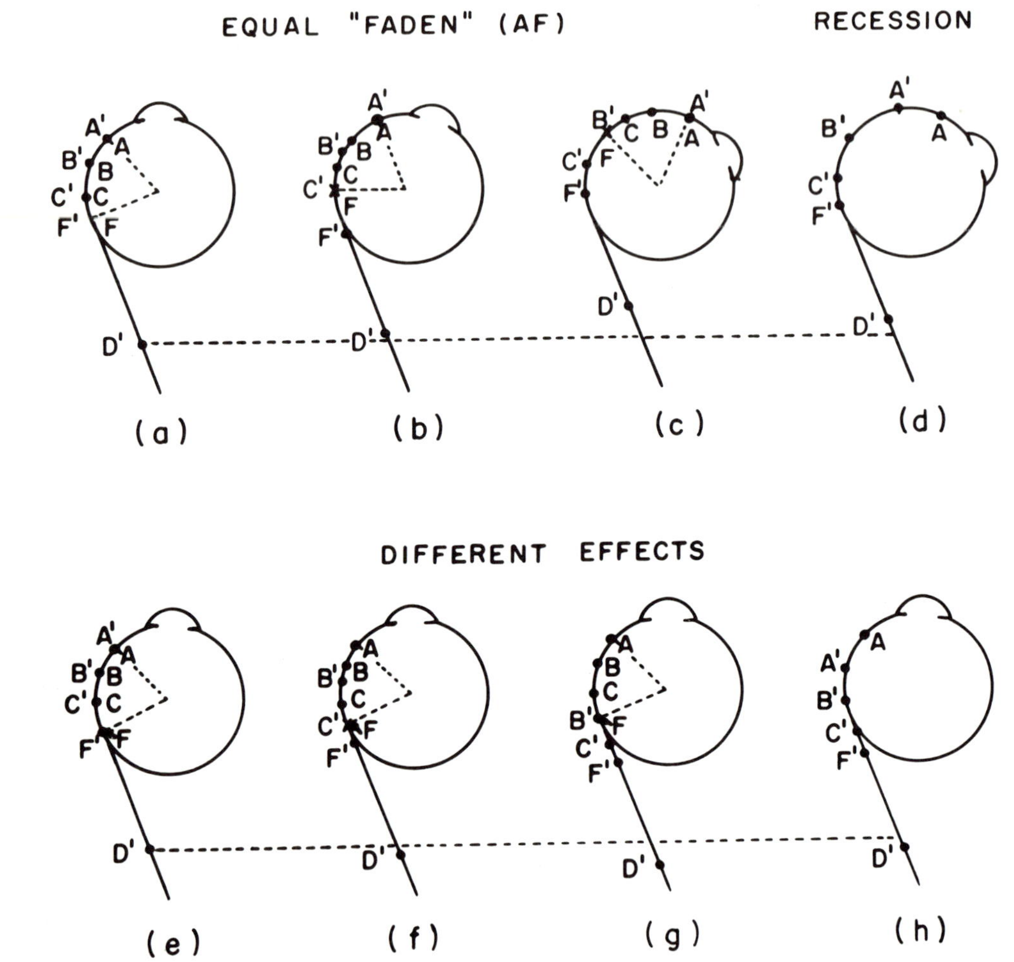

Fig. 1. Schematic relationships between eye and muscle, before (*a* to *c*) and after (*d* to *h*) surgeries. (*a*) The eye in primary position shows points of muscle (A', B', C', F') and respectively corresponding points of the sclera (A, B, C, F). If a suture is made between F and F', all relations remain the same after surgery (*e*). However, if the (intact) eye is rotated, the muscle is proportionally stretched (*b* and *c*) and when a suture is made at the same *scleral* point F, it will coincide with the muscular points C' (in *b*) or B' (in *c*). This cause the fixed part of the muscle to remain stretched, but the "unfixed" (posterior) part of it differently slacked after surgery (*f* and *g*). In a recession (*d*) the new muscular insertion (A') is backward placed to its original position (A). This will also slack the muscle (*h*). The amount of such a slack may be greater ($h > f > e$) os smaller ($h < g$) than that of "equal" fadenoperations (arcs AF in *a*, *e*; *b*, *f*; *c*, *g*).

(arc AF, fig.1 *a* to *c*) will not have the same predictable effect (even for similar eyes) because the part of the muscle which is fixed to the sclera (F' to F in fig. 1 *a*, C' to F in fig. 1 *b*, or B' to F in fig. 1 *c*) depends on the surgical technique, i.e., for reaching such a position (F), the surgeon will rotate the eye, and therefore stretch the muscle, less (fig. 1 *b*) or more (fig. 1*c*). As a consequence, the muscular slack when the eye returns to its original position is smaller in the first case (fig. 1 *f*) than in the second (fig.1 *g*), which cause the surgical effect to be different in each of them. In other words, it is not the *scleral* arc (AF) which counts, but the *muscular elastic* conditions (A'C' in the first case, A'B' in the second) which has to be considered. Then, what limits the success of a fadenoperation, is not the surgeon's inability to reach a *posterior* scleral position, but the difficulty of rotating it to an *anterior* position (i.e., to stretch the muscle). Conversely, a constant amount ocular rotation (i.e., of muscular stretch) may not necessarily be obtained with the same "passive" force in different eyes or, in another way, their elastic (spring back) forces may be different. Note that even when the effect of a recession (AA', fig. 1 *d*, *h*) can be taken as the same, for *similar* eyes (i.e., muscular relationships, A'C', C'D', will only depend on the position of the new insertion, A'), a fixed amount of a recession does not give equal results in *different* cases (Collins and Jampolsky show it beautifully in this Section). It is therefore doubtful to expect reproduction of effects (degress/mm) in faden-operations, or predict some kind of constant relationship between recessions and fadenoperations.

On the other hand when basic preoperative conditions (small angles, "constant angles", sensorial anomalies) are taken into consideration, the rates of success in those groups can not be considered as significantly different, even, again, at very tolerant levels.

For proving the effect of Fd upon nystagmic amblyopia, more consistent criteria of improvement should be taken (not "occlusion tolerated", "alternates freely", or other). Why not to take the stability of the eye, against nystagmus, before and after surgery, as an objetive, easy way of evaluating the treatment?

At last, it is advisable to avoid some conceptual mistakes, e.g., "set the medial rectus back... reduce the lever arm as in a Fd". In fact both, a recession, and a fadenoperation, *do not* reduce the *lever arm*.

OBJECTIVE CALCULATION OF STRABISMUS SURGERY

Fortunately a mechanistic approach to the study of the oculomotor system has been receiving ever increasing attention, since it provides the basis for rational and objective understanding to the diagnosis and treatment of strabismus. This paper deals with a project for determining the *passive* characteristics of the oculomotor system and presents a method by which a correspondence between *force* and *eye position* can be directly appreciated.

The method is quite precise and possible sources of experimental errors are almost negligible:

a) The position of the microphone, very close to the eye, minimizes possible influences of inadequate inclinations of the forceps.

b) From the original inclination proposed for the bars (-20°) variations up to -10° (more horizontal positioning) do not cause any significant error of measurements. However, at each side of this interval, further inclinations of the bars can be falsely interpreted as eye rotations to the *nasal* side (i.e., adductions will be overestimated and abductions underestimated) by a factor f (*).

c) If the eye is grabed by the forceps at the temporal side of the limbus, an almost precise linear variation between eye rotations and ultrasonic measurements can be accepted ($\simeq 4{,}1^{o}$/mm) on the range $+50^{o}$ to -30°. But if the forceps is placed at the nasal side of the limbus, the range where the linearity applies is narrowed (around $+20^{o}$ to -20°).

The present project for objective calculation of strabismus surgery has sound theoretic basis. It is not, however, to be expected that *all* surgeries made under such recomendations will result in a state of eye parallelism. When the patient awakes, the return of "tonic forces" in a different basis to that expected by the method, may, certainly, explain some possible failures of the plane (either after a short or a long time following the surgery). Even then, the project has to be considered as a very important scientific advance, since it will lead investigations to concentrate on the innervational causes of the imbalance.

Above all, the paper contributes to reassure, once more, that surgery can not be looked upon as a pure therapeutic procedure, and that diagnosis does not end before it, but must go through it.

(*): $f \simeq e\,(0.35 + 0.025\,e)$, where *e* is the *excess* of angular error on the positioning of the bars (inclinations above -10° or below -20°). For instance, an error of $e = 20^{o}$ (i.e., inclination of $+10^{o}$ or -40°) will give an overestimate of adduction or an underestimate of abduction (f) around 17.5^{o}.

DISCUSSION:

We have some excellent questions that have been submitted, and in order to maximize the discussion I shall forego my own summary in order to all Dr. deDecker to finish his slide presentations, which unfortunately he was not able to complete earlier.

Dr. deDecker

This is the slide taken from a publication that my co-worker, Dr. Conrad, has published this year. This curve shows the character of the artificial palsy produced by the current operation with increasing adduction. For this reason, in most cases, where we do not like to have the characteristics of a paralysis, we prefer the bilateral Faden operation to both medial recti, as it smooths this characteristic, and distributes it to both sides.

An old question, that I thank Dr. Jampolsky for repeatedly asking, is how does a Faden work? In our hands, the Faden does not work in the way in which Cüppers has stated so frequently. Cüppers said that the Faden operation would not influence the primary position deviation, but in our hands it does. The influence on the primary position is not zero, and there is a change in the angle at 20 degrees adduction, in a Faden operation without recession.

If there is a recession added, for instance of 3 millimeters, and a Faden of 13 millimeters, then the effects of the two aspects have to be divided. The muscle is made stiffer, so that the characteristic of the artificial palsy is flatter, the shape of the curve is not as steep, but the entrance to the position is the same here, nearly the same in adduction, but increases in the primary position, and markedly in adduction. The recession that is added increases the last inputs, or the characteristics of the Faden. Thank you.

Dr. Jampolsky

Relative to the rotatory effect upon the globe of a muscle that has been recessed a considerable amount, can anyone explain the following well known circumstance: In sixth nerve paralysis, one treatment method is to make the medial rectus ineffective by recessing it 16 millimeters from its insertion, and the resection of the dead lateral rectus in order to mechanically align the eye, thus balancing apparently zero effective agonist-antagonist forces. In such a patient, it sometimes happens that ten years later the esotropia recurs, and the eye will adduct very well indeed, even with the medial rectus demonstrably back at the reinsertion site, 16 millimeters recessed from its original insertion. How is this explained, with the usual concepts of lever arm, the importance of the globe equator, etc.? Does anyone on the panel have an explanation for this clinical observation?

Dr. Bicas

I think the superior and inferior rectus muscles could explain some sort of adduction.

Dr. deDecker

This may not be an explanation, but there is another example that works similarly. Children who have congenital unilateral cataracts and strabismus, usually adduct their only good eye in a very marked way. They are difficult to correct. Sometimes we did 6 to 7 millimeter recession, in combination with a 14 or 15 millimeter Faden operation, which is the utmost borderline. And they still could adduct. Then, following Dr. Jampolsky's advice, when this failed, we took the Faden out, then recessed the muscle to 14 millimeters, without an additional Faden which was not possible. And they still could adduct. So, there still is a lever arm. It is taking up the slack in your sense, Dr. Jampolsky, isn't it?

Dr. Jampolsky

Yes, it takes up the slack completely. The vertical muscles do not adduct the eye very much. When the medial rectus has taken up all its slack, then adduction becomes almost normal. So, it does seem probable that it is the medial rectus.

Dr. Scott

Well you can show that, in those eyes, they rotate around a center very far temporally placed, and that adduction is accompanied by substantial retraction, which is almost a uniform characteristic of those cases.

Dr. Jampolsky

So there is a translation of the globe as well, is that correct?

Dr. Scott

Yes, there is a large translation associated with the rotation in all of those situations where it has been very far back.

Dr. Jampolsky

Dr. Bicas, you have done a lot of work, and published extensively, comparing the muscle vector forces of Helmholz, Volkmann, Krusen, and Boeder. I remember your pointing out, in your analysis, that the yolk muscle of the right superior rectus is the left superior rectus. In case that surprises anybody, would you like to elaborate, and perhaps summarize what are some of the non-traditional things that you would like to emphasize in 1981, relative to the past and present analyses of such muscle functions?

Dr. Bicas

Well, I think a lot of mistakes have been made, for many years, because the superior rectus has been related to the inferior oblique, and the inferior rectus to the superior oblique. This is like comparing whiskey and milk, oranges and bananas. These are completely different muscles, and they are not related at all for these movements. So I would like to say that if a simplified view of Hering's Law exists for vertical movements, it should be superior rectus with superior rectus, and inferior rectus with inferior rectus. Now, this is a very simplified view, because Hering's Law is not equal innervation. The eyes did change their positions. One adducts, and the other abducts, so the positions of the muscles are quite different even for horizontal recti.

Let us consider vertical recti. If the superior rectus is related to the superior rectus, they cannot have equal innervation. What is Hering's Law about? It is about movement, of course, conjugate movement. Now, for that to happen, it has to be a modulation of the system, as Dr. Westheimer pointed out in his paper. There is a dynamic difference, in that each part of the rotation requires a different innervation for each of the six muscles. I would say, at least three in each eye to keep horizontal, vertical, and torsional movements on perfect conjugacy. Now, I'm not sure if Hering's Law was only concerned about muscles which contract. Some muscles are contracted. Are they working? If there is some slackness or contraction, are they working? I'm not sure. I think that one point to be investigated should be how much of the innervation each muscle gets in different positions of gaze, and what part of the muscles are innervated. For instance, when the eye goes upward, the inferior part of the medial and lateral rectus muscles, which are stretched, are they equally innervated, compared to the superior fibers which are slack? I don't know.

Dr. Robinson

When I was visiting Volker Henn's lab in Zurich, he had some very interesting data on iso-innervation contours, by recording from motor neurons. I wonder if instead of my giving the results, whether Volker would be interested in describing what he found.

Volker Henn

This is work we did with monkeys trained to look in different directions. For instance, in nasal, temporal, up, down, the firing would be 50 Hz, and whenever there is 50 Hz in specific abducent motor neurons, the eyes might be 5 degrees nasally, for instance. Then if it increases to 100 Hz, we would find eye positions which would be aligned parallel to a vertical. And so on, 200 Hz would be a little farther out. That means for the horizontal movers, the iso-frequency lines are aligned parallel to the vertical, and this is quite clear, and what is to be expected. For the vertical motor neurons, the picture is more complex, and no final word can be given now. That is, for most of the superior or inferior recti muscles, the iso-frequency lines are more or less parallel to the horizontal. And then in further up directions, there might be some curvature towards the nasal quadrant. The important point is that in the same muscle, from neighboring motor neurons, we found neurons which were curved and others which were more or less straight. That means that individual motor neurons have slightly different iso-innervation curves and we do not know why. The iso-innervation curves were usually flat in the nasal quadrant, with more pronounced curvature in the temporal quadrant.

Dr. Jampolsky

Are these tangent screen positions you're talking about?

Volken Henn

Yes. These are tangent screen positions.

Dr. Scott

I think this is a very valuable thing to do. It is not uncommon that one has to operate upon the inferior rectus, say to correct an incommitant deviation, and it is not always a uniform result that one gets. The weakening of one inferior rectus in one patient will be much greater in abduction, and in the next patient it will have an effect all the way across the inferior gaze line. And it pertains exactly to what Dr. Henn has done. We have been measuring this in patients, and also injecting those muscles with Zylocaine, just for a brief paralysis, to perhaps show what the effect of the contribution of that muscle is before it is operated upon. It has been very helpful in some cases, and shown that one inferior rectus weakening will have a very great effect across the whole range of gaze, and the next one will be isolated very much to say the temporal range on that particular side. It's a very useful diagnostic kind of approach that helps to get to this question. It's therapeutically useful.

Dr. deDecker

From the point of view of practical surgery I may add one experience. We sometimes see children with cerebral palsy, with a nystagmus and a vertical deviation, with abnormal head position. We sometimes operate on four muscles, as Kestenbaum suggested, and sometimes by symmetrical Faden operations to both inferior recti. There is a difference when we touch four muscles, according to Kestenbaum's procedure, compared with touching two inferior recti by Faden operation. In a number of such patients we have obtained correction by oblique muscle surgery. When we did not, the patients reset their subjective vertical meridians in about one to two months.

Dr. Jampolsky

Let me carry that one step further, to bring out another point for discussion following on Professor Granit's nice statement at the beginning of this symposium, that we are all programmed for adaptive plasticity. I should like to ask the panel to discuss plasticity on the motor side, less well known perhaps. The four muscle procedure for shifting a minimal point of nystagmus, with compensatory head position, is a frequently done procedure. Kestenbaum (in the French literature), and Anderson (in the Australian literature) independently described similar procedures at about the same time, in order to shift the nystagmus null point to a more straight ahead position, with a beneficial cosmetic and visual result. The point here is that the characteristics of the medial and lateral rectus muscles in such a longstanding case are completely different. And here, one surgically shifts each eye a tremendous amount, 30 to 50 degrees. Patients almost always end up, in my experience, with the same degree of fusion lock (usually a small but very stable angle of deviation). Certainly it is not the skill of the surgeon that operates that successfully and accurately. The fusion lock mechanism obviously commands, and the muscles readjust to the rather indelicate surgery, to end up with the same balance in the newly shifted position. The muscles take up whatever slack they appropriately need to take up, and maintain the fusion lock. Before asking the panelists, I will ask Dr. Dell Osso if he would care to comment, since he has long had an interest in this area. And, to perhaps comment, as to whether or not he feels such cases all belong to the same class, i.e., they are unidirectional, but only insofar as the null point is so far in to the nose that one cannot get the bidirectional characteristic. Postoperatively, with repositioning of the null point, now one gets the fast component to either side of the new null point. So, aren't they really the same class, one is just a degree of the other?

Dr. Dell Osso

In congenital nystagmus that's true, even if you can't reach the null point, but you see that it's going to be out there somewhere. You do a maximal rotation. What you might find is that if the null is way out to the right, postoperatively, you might find that the whole right field of gaze is now a null. Then, in looking in right gaze, you would get some jerk right nystagmus, so you would assume there is a null out there when it goes off the chart. I don't see that there's any difference between that, and the place where you really find the null at 20 or so.

Dr. Jampolsky

Thank you, Dr. Dell Osso. Let me ask the panel a question in referrence to Dr. Westheimer's paper, relative to the motor side hard wiring, and its plasticity. What are some clinical examples where Hering's Law might be abrogated, such as the clinical circumstance of dissociated vertical divergence?

Dr. Scott

Sure, as I understand it. Hering's Law refers to frontal plane conjugate movements, by and large. He didn't comment very much about convergence, and other things like that, in regard to Hering's Law.

Dr. Stark

I disagree with Dr. Scott. Hering did put forth his law about versional movements and vergence movements. He had it translated into English. You could explain the dissociated vertical deviation, with Hering's Law, by summing a version, and a vergence movement at the same time. Now, I'm not saying that that's what happens in this alternating sursumduction, that well may be a violation of Hering's Law, because it is a pathological eye movement. But, one could construct a vergence and a version movement together, a vertical vergence and a vertical version, which would obey Hering's Law, and which could account for that movement. Hering points out that just because eyes move according to Hering's Law, that doesn't mean you can't position the eyes in any particular position.

Dr. deDecker

This so-called dissociated vertical deviation, is not a phenomenon that stands like a foreign body beneath all the other strabismus phenomena. It is part of a congenital strabismus syndrome, and often seen in combination with other system anomalies. Let me say that one of the most well known phenomena is that of the V-syndrome, of the overacting inferior obliques. The phenomenon where the more one eye adducts, the more it is elevated. The esodeviation increases in downgaze. This can look like a very good process, and gives the impression that it follows Hering's Law in principle. On the other hand, you can have a DVD that elevates not only under covering conditions, but sometimes periodically without covering the eye. This looks ugly. These patients from time to time do not look like patients who follow Hering's Law. When both conditions exist, we find combinations, and we see a thing that looks like overacting inferior oblique, but it is more or less a DVD which takes part only in this field of action of the inferior oblique. And, if you follow the old masters and let the dominant eye see through a dark red glass or gray filter, the other eye comes down even in this position. So, there is any combination. It is not easy to say when it follows

Hering's Law, and when the DVD does not.

Dr. Jampolsky

Let us return to some specific audience questions for the panel. Dr. Scott, is binocular sensory feedback necessary for the drug injection therapy of strabismus? And, if so, is amblyopia a contraindication for this technique?

Dr. Scott

Most of our early patients were amblyopic, and like surgically aligned patients, they are less stable than those who have fusion. Some of our patients have fusion, or have gained fusion from the procedure. They are more stable again just as surgically aligned patients are more stable if they happen to have fusion, or gain fusion from the procedure. It's simply a way of moving the eye over, much as surgery does, but with one exception. If you take an eye that is esotropic, and you bring it out now, with a paralysis, then with gaze over toward this side the patient is exotropic, and with gaze over toward the other side, they are usually still somewhat esotropic. That patient then has the opportunity, should he wish to turn his head and tune the eyes together, of doing so. We have seen fusion in several patients in whom we would not have anticipated getting fusion. I think it then represents a sort of orthoptic opportunity for many of these people, and they do indeed tune their head. Interestingly, even those who have monofixation, and a type of phoria, they tune their heads to get the eyes perfect when they have the chance to do so. I think it has the potential to give slightly greater functional results in that particular group.

Dr. Jampolsky

I'll combine a couple of questions here, for Dr. Collins. Do you modify your method for eyes which are not standard, and do you find your predictions to be less accurate in the small angle, as compared with the larger angle deviations?

Dr. Collins

In the small sample of patients we've done, we don't find a real correlation between the small or large angle accuracy of our calculations. There is quite a spread. Yes, we do modify the technique. I guess I did not make it entirely clear, that in cases of restriction, the muscles will be moved up on the diagonal curve that we have put on the screen, to take account of restriction. It is necessary, in special cases, to modify the surgery that is done. Nevertheless, we can calculate the amount of surgery to do for each muscle in these cases.

Dr. Jampolsky

Dr. Robinson, in your original and appropriately changing model, what assumptions in the human model are most in need of testing? What additional data would you like to see the clinician provide you and the computer?

Dr. Robinson

There are two things where the model is really in a lot of trouble. One is that the muscles sideslip across the globe. That is, if the horizontal recti come around from the back of the globe, then when the eye looks up, the horizontal muscles sideslip around the globe. How much are they tethered to their primary position track? We have no physiological data for this. We have thought to try to look at this using a CAT scanner, but I don't think the resolution of CAT scanners is yet sufficient to outline the muscle as it tracks across the surface of the globe. If you limit the amount of sideslipping, or do not limit the effect, the moment arm of a given muscle can change quite a lot. I mean it just is an absurd case if you take the lateral rectus of the left eye. All you have to do is look 24 degrees in that direction and the insertion of the lateral rectus is exactly opposite from its origin. If you go any further, and you ask the muscle to take the shortest path, then it would slip right around the globe, and lie across the cornea and become an adductor. It is clear it doesn't happen. But our lack of knowledge about lateral restraints to sideslipping is a feature where we really need information of an experimental nature, whether one should do this in humans or monkeys, I'm not sure.

The other thing has already been mentioned, and that is, if you ask a muscle that has been living happily at a certain length for ten years, to live at some other length, it doesn't like that. It reacts in some way. As days, weeks, or months go by, muscles do funny things, and they are no longer the muscle that you operated on. Consequently, drifts come and deviations come and go. We have absolutely no way to put this into our model because this phenomenon has never been quantitated at all. I think this is really a hot area, a very important area for some kind of clinical or basic research needs to be done. I'd like to know the reaction to that.

Dr. Jampolsky

I think Dr. Bicus and Dr. Scott have addressed that. Would either of you like to comment?

Dr. Bicas

Well I think that yes, it is important to know how much it slides around the globe. But sometimes, for some muscles, and for most of the clinical positions, it is not so important. You can say, well, let's suppose a complete sliding for great circle allowances, let's suppose another way, a complete fixation of the muscle in its original position. There is not quite a bit of difference in many cases. In some cases, it is a small difference, but in some cases a greater difference. But it is to be stressed to clinicians, that when they cut intermuscular membranes, they do a lot of difference in that. Correct? Because it can allow the muscle to slip a little more, to slide a little more, than before.

Dr. Scott

I don't think the sideslip problem is usually much of a real modelling problem. You can look at the eye and take an alert patient, and have him look in extreme oblique gaze, which gives the greatest sideslip for the lateral rectus. If you cut the membranes on one side, and it moves down a millimeter or two, it's hardly out of place at all if you mark it on the sclera, because the fascia on the front of the eye is just like a cap over the front of it, and holds all those muscles normally right in place. It's only these weird cases of Duane's Syndrome, and abnormal situations, where those muscles flip up. As far as measuring the other things, yes, that's a real problem, David. You have to measure not only the muscles, but you have to measure all those fascial tissues, because they are all put in a different place every time you change the muscles around. Most patients who have had surgery don't want to have the thing done to them that would give the information that you would like to have, and I don't know how to answer that problem. There is just no way to measure those physical characteristics neatly.

Dr. Robinson

I think as a hard shelled basic scientist, I would like to see motion pictures of this lack of sideslipping, and I'd be perfectly happy to put that on my model. But what you just discussed are important results, as far as I'm concerned. You're saying that because it's small, it's negligible. But to know that it's small is a very important finding.

Dr. deDecker

The practice of doing a Faden operation shows that about 13 millimeters behind the muscle insertion, there is something existing like a mouth, where the muscles come out from the surrounding tissue. Sometimes, if we have larger amounts of Faden fixation, we have to make a destruction of this mouth in order to reach the edges of the muscles. In these cases, we have the danger that the orbital fat comes out. My opinion is that the tissue surrounding the muscle, where it comes out, is more or less a thing that acts functionally like a true offspring of the muscle. The muscle in a functional way does not slide between its insertion and its offspring, but it is more or less constant in direction between the tip of the orbit and this mouth. I agree with Dr. Robinson, that we do not know how much freedom there is, and we'll have to wait for a better scan in order to know what the freedom is in an untouched patient.

Dr. Jampolsky

Dr. Campos has a question: "I would like to ask Dr. Collins and Dr. Robinson -- how do they take into account for ocular motility modelling, the sensory-motor aspects, or if you want to call it a vergence movement, of the calculation of the effect of surgery. And also, how do they take into account the fact that Dr. Bicus showed, and it is our clinical experience, the effect of surgery does change in time."

Dr. Collins

Addressing the last question first, my primary goal has been to place the eyes straight after surgery. And, we do not yet have a satisfactory method for predicting the drift after surgery. This drift is due to a number of other factors, not necessarily related to the factors of importance in attaining the desired alignment at the time, or after, surgery. Perhaps Dr. Jampolsky would like to address the problem of postoperative drift, or change of deviation with time.

Dr. Jampolsky

I think that one must separate that question completely from the question and problem of where you wish to place an eye by surgery upon the ocular muscles and surrounding tissues. What happens to it from that time on, composes a different set of questions and problems. A surgical technique that predicts where one puts the eye is one thing. The sensory factor that Dr. Campos just mentioned --amblyopia, uncorrected refractive errors, poor fusion lock -- all of these things are overwhelmingly germane in answering the question of whether or not that eye stays put. And there are still anatomical factors that subsequently affect the eye position, one way or another, such as lost or slipped muscles, cicatrizing tissue changes, etc.

Dr. Robinson, would you also like to respond to Dr. Campos's question?

Dr. Robinson

Well, only to reiterate that postoperative drift is one of the things I was complaining about; that we don't have quantitative knowledge of what muscles do, and so that is a problem in the model. As far as the innervation is concerned, we have to confess that our models only deal with the mechanics of the orbit, and not with the central nervous system. We would have to make a model of the entire oculomotor system in order to bring all of that into play.

Dr. Jampolsky

There has been some mention of animal models and human models. There has been a recent challenge, stating that the monkey model, on the input side of things, is a good model for comparison to the human. But, that the output systems are really not comparable at all, especially in our problem of strabismus management. It is apples and bananas. The uniquely characterizing thing about the human neonatal visual system is its instability of alignment. Anything will upset it. Unequal inputs, sensory disturbances, motor disturbances -- practically anything. In the monkey, you really have to try hard to give a strabismus during this period of time. The monkey is very hyperopic, has a lot of anisometropia, and orbital anatomy considerably different from the human. If all human infants had the refractive errors that monkeys have, they all would have strabismus. In the monkey, you simply don't see the natural occurence of accommodative esotropia, intermittant exotropia, dissociated vertical deviation, and the rest of the all too common strabismic states seen in humans. In fact, you see almost none of the human type of strabismus, in monkeys. A strabismic monkey is a rare thing indeed, unlike strabismic humans. It has been said (and I guess that I said it) that it would be helpful and productive to admit this difference, in the strabismic motor model comparison of monkeys and humans. If we focused on the important differences, the stability of the monkey's motor apparatus, and the instability of the human neonatal motor apparatus, we would advance our knowledge by a study of the differences. We should get on with it, rather than try to pretend that the monkey is a good motor strabismic model. Would you like to comment on that flat-footed, provocative statement, Dr. Robinson?

Dr. Robinson

Well, as you know from previous conversations, I am still not convinced. I think we don't know whether there is an incidence of strabismus in normal monkey colonies, simply because very few people have gone and looked with the right techniques to determine if it's there or not. Sticking eye coils in monkeys is a very good way to make them strabismic, incidentally. But before we just give up totally on the monkeys, or assume that it's immune to strabismus somehow or another, I think a good investigation is still needed to make sure that it does not occur as a natural disease in subhuman primates.

Dr. Jampolsky

I think that one can fairly state, that one does not see infant monkeys with the huge amounts of esotropia that are obvious to anyone, that so characterizes human congenital or infantile esotropia.

Dr. Robinson

One of the problems is that monkeys have no sclera, or it's almost impossible to see sclera. So, you look at a monkey looking out of a cage, and it could have a 10 diopter deviation, and you wouldn't know it, since it looks like it's perfectly straight-eyed. There could be all kinds of cross-eyed monkeys living in cages, and we just don't know it.

Dr. Jampolsky

It's hard to confuse or miss a 60 prism diopter esotropic infant, human or monkey, with a questionably straight-eyed monkey, I think.

I would like to ask Dr. Berard to comment. You have published a considerable amount of work relative to the vergence responses to prism introduction in a variety of strabismic subjects. Would you care to comment about the presence or absence of prism-induced vergence movements, their characteristics, etc.?

Dr. Berard

Thank you, Dr. Jampolsky, for asking me to give my opinion about this topic. Yes, I have been using prisms for many years in strabismus. There is no discussion, in strabismus, mainly esotropia, a vergence is frequent under prisms. But I would like to stress three points:

1. You observe vergence mainly in small angles of esotropia. It is, in my opinion, because the vergence is symptomatic of some form of fusion at the angle of anomaly. This type of fusion is impossible in large angles of deviation because of suppression. It is the reason why you observe vergence under prisms mainly after surgery.

2. To observe vergence, you have not to be in a hurry. The adaptations to the prisms needs a few minutes, to several hours. So in a rush, the phenomenon is not seen.

3. The measurement of the vergences under prisms is easy. The amount of vergence equals the power of the prisms put in front of both eyes. But keep in mind that at the same time, you measure the amplitudes of fusion at the angle of anomaly too.

   High prism power equals strong amplitude.
   Small prism power equals weak amplitude.

   And, in this last case, if you operate on residual angle, the result of surgery is more promising.

Dr. Stark

I thank Dr. Berard for his comments on the possible occurrence of vergence in small angle strabismics. He has had much more experience, of course, than I or my colleagues have at this particular time. But I think even he suggested that he really wasn't getting a vergence, which is to change the position of the eyes, which may or may not be a pure vergence. That depends partly on semantics, and partly on more complete studies. But I think, following our discussion, that there really isn't any disparity vergence in patients with strabismus. Of course, with further studies, we might even find it ourselves. I'm not making that a blanket statement. I think we're the first group to really look for it with careful methods.

Dr. Jampolsky

Are there any comments that the panelists would care to make at this time?

Dr. Collins

I would like to respond to some comments relative to our technique, if there is time. Our technique attempts to provide a rational basis, using physical measurements capable of easy performance by the average clinician, allowing him to calculate the amount of surgery, and limits, rather than using purely experiential or judgmental factors.

Dr. Robinson

One of the fun things you can do with this mathematical model in strabismus is to do lousy surgery on it. You can, for example, do the accepted amount of surgery on one eye, and then change the eye by making its muscles very stiff, and the orbital fascia very loose. Or, you can make the orbital fascia very stiff, and you can make the muscles very loose. And then you can make the medial rectus stiff, and the lateral rectus loose. It's incredible, the amount of overcorrection, and undercorrection, that you can get by not accounting for the individual variability and stiffness of muscles. So I would like to reiterate, that to me the beautiful thing that you are doing, is to tailor the surgery to the individual eye that you are operating upon. There is an enormous range or variability from one eye to another, and to do a standard number of millimeter resect or recession, for a standard deviation, I think is just not the way to go.

Dr. Jampolsky

I quite agree. Dr. Collins and I had two recent examples that are relevant. We had what appeared to be a routine, 30 prism diopter intermittent exotrope, never before operated upon. While making the orbital and muscle measurements with Dr. Collins, we disinserted the lateral rectus muscle, and it made not one iota of difference in the spring-back, or anatomical eye position, during the surgical anesthesia. This indicated that more than the anticipated amount of resection of the medial rectus was indicated at the time. Without paying attention to the ineffectual lateral rectus muscle, I think the patient would have had an unexpectedly poor result.

In another instance, that same surgical day, we had a patient with intermittent exotropia, who clinically exhibited what is called lateral incommitancy. That is, less exodeviation in right and left gaze, than in the primary position. This is a well known warning flag for surgeons, which clinically portends overcorrection of the exodeviation with the usual amount of surgery. For this patient during surgical anesthesia, recessing one lateral rectus muscle only 4 millimeters, caused a shift in the eye position of some 35 prism diopters. Comparing this patient with the previous one, shows in the first example the almost zero effect from detaching the lateral rectus completely, compared with the second instance, of a tremendous effect from recessing the lateral rectus only 4 millimeters. In the latter instance, the opposing medial rectus muscle's unusual stiffness, would have resulted in a disastrous effect had it been resected and made still stiffer. Unless one knows these muscle and orbital tissue stiffnesses at the time of surgery, and alters one's surgery accordingly, one can certainly have a sorry result.

There is an old and outworn surgical adage, that one should not change horses in the middle of the stream (during surgery). This may be a fine statement for someone riding a horse in the middle of the stream, but it is certainly very bad advice for the strabismus surgeon and his judgment during the middle of surgery.

Dr. deDecker

I would like to make a short comment relative to Dr. Bicus's criticisms. The material I sent him, was complex material, and contained the data from a previous small study, which represented our very first year of experience. This was based on only 35 patients. So, for the paper presented here, having all the same experience with the hundreds later, I came indeed to the complete conclusion that he is right. The difference between the obviously changed conditions, and those who looked constant in the office, indeed is a small one. And that is the reason why I told you that even the blind procedures, against constant looking, was not significant, but only showed trends. I think that is how to understand that.

Dr. Jampolsky

I will combine several questions into one remaining question for Dr. Scott. What are the functional results from muscle injection? How many patients have you done? What about the availability?

Dr. Scott

I commented on function already. We've done 63 patients, and there are another more or less 20 done by others. The drug is available to qualified investigators, typically in university settings, who have the equipment, and are willing to keep and report the data in accord with the usual Food and Drug Administration requirements. There are several foreign investigators, and there is not such a restriction on them.

Dr. Jampolsky

I think that our time is up. I wish to thank the participants, the panelists, and the questioners, for the fine discussion.

SECTION V

Coordinator: G. Lennerstrand

FREE PAPERS: STRABISMUS AND RELATED DISORDERS

THE INCIDENCE OF PARALYTIC SQUINT IN MENINGITIS

L. S. HANNA*, N. I. GIRGIS*, M. W. YASSIN**, R. H. WATTEN* and J. E. SIPPEL*

*U.S. Naval Medical Research Unit No. 3, Cairo, Egypt
**Abbassia Fever Hospital, Cairo, Egypt

ABSTRACT

The incidence of paralytic squint was studied in the different types of meningitis in Egypt during the period from 1971-1981. Of a total of 2049 patients studied, ocular paralysis occurred in 524 patients (25.5%). The 6th cranial nerve showed the highest incidence (17.9%) of affection, followed by the 3rd cranial nerve (3.8%), the 7th cranial nerve (3.6%), and lastly the 4th and 5th cranial nerves (each 0.04%). Clinical recovery of the paralysed muscles occurred following standard treatment, while 2% of patients showed residual paralysis.

KEYWORDS

Paralytic squint; meningococcal meningitis; pneumococcal meningitis; influenzal meningitis; tuberculous meningitis.

INTRODUCTION

Paralysis of the ocular muscles is a frequent complication in meningitis (Duke-Elder 1971). The 6th cranial nerve is usually the first to be affected, followed by the 3rd and 7th cranial nerves. The 4th and 5th cranial nerves are very rarely affected. Paralytic squint has been reported to occur secondary to meningococcal meningitis (4.28% by Lewis, 1940; 20% by McLean and Gaffy, 1928; and 31.2% by Smithburn et al. 1930). In tuberculous meningitis the 6th cranial nerve affection may be the first sign of the disease (Moorey, 1956; Mishra and Gupta, 1962). An incidence of 10% of abducent palsy, and 18% of oculomotor palsy was reported by Kyrieleis, 1931.

The purpose of this study was to document the incidence of paralytic squint in the various types of meningitis, whether meningococcal, pneumococcal, influenzal, tuberculous, or purulent meningitis of unknown etiology. It was carried out at the Abbassia Fever Hospital and the United States Naval Medical Research Unit No.3 (NAMRU-3), Meningitis Ward, Cairo, Egypt, during the period from 1971 to 1981.

MATERIAL AND METHOD

A total of 2049 cases were included in this study. There were 1216 males and 833

This work was sponsored by NMRDC, NNMC, Bethesda, MD 20014, Work Unit No.MR00001-01-3038 females, and their ages ranged from 1 1/2 months to 65 years, with a mean age of 13.2 years (Table 1).

TABLE 1 Age and Sex Distribution in the Different Types of Meningitis

Age Years	No. of Pts.	Sex M	Sex F	Meningo-coccal	Pneumo-coccal	Influ-enzal	Tuber-culous	Purulent of Unknown Etiology
0-5	802	480	322	134	107	86	299	176
6-10	378	213	165	124	28	1	96	129
11-15	274	152	122	81	21	1	73	98
16-20	207	130	77	45	17	4	73	68
> 20	388	241	147	85	39	4	152	108
TOTAL	2049	1216	833	469	212	96	693	579

The highest group of meningitis patients (802) were within the first 5 years of age, and males were more than females.

On admission to hospital a diagnostic lumbar puncture (LP) was performed and the cerebrospinal fluid (CSF) collected was examined microscopically for total and differential leucocytic count, chemically for glucose and protein content, and bacteriologically by stain and culture. Blood was also drawn for complete blood count, glucose, urea nitrogen content, liver function tests, and bacteriological culture.

Neisseria meningitidis was isolated from the CSF of 469 patients, Streptococcus pneumonia from 212 patients, Haemophilus influenza from 96 patients, and no organisms could be isolated from 579 patients (Pyogenic meningitis of unknown etiology). The 693 patients initially diagnosed as having tuberculous meningitis, 346 were confirmed by culture, 10 by acid fast stain, and the remaining 337 patients were diagnosed on clinical grounds and the CSF picture (low glucose, high protein content and a moderate pleocytosis lymphocytic in nature and failure to respond to broad spectrum antibacterial chemotherapy.

An ophthalmological examination was performed for all patients on admission to hospital for muscle functions, pupillary reaction, and fundus changes. Visual field, visual acuity, and colour vision tests were performed once patients were alert. Repeated eye examinations were carried out twice weekly until patients recovered, and were discharged from hospital. In cases of tuberculous meningitis the examinations were carried out for a period of two years.

Therapeutic regimens consisted of either ampicillin (160 mg/kg/day divided 4 hourly I.M. or I.V.) or a combination of penicillin (120,000 I.U./kg/day divided 4 hourly I.M. or I.V.) and chloramphenicol (100 mg/kg/day divided 4 hourly I.M. or I.V.). Once sensitivity results were available, therapy was changed accordingly. Patients with tuberculous meningitis received streptomycin (25 mg/kg once daily), ethambutol (25 mg/kg maximum 1200 mg daily for 60 days then reduced to 15 mg/kg daily) and isonicotinic acid hydrazide (10 mg/kg/day maximum 600 mg/day). Streptomycin was withdrawn after 42 days and the other 2 drugs were continued for 2 years

RESULTS

As seen in Table 2, out of 2049 patients examined, 524 (25.5%) manifested signs of cranial nerve affection. The predominant cranial nerve involved appeared to be the 6th cranial nerve. 368 (17.9%) patients showed 6th cranial nerve paralysis, of which 206 (10%) showed a unilateral 6th nerve paralysis, and 162 (7.9%) showed a bilateral 6th nerve paralysis. 79 (3.8%) patients showed 3rd cranial nerve affection, 75(3.6%) patients showed 7th cranial nerve affection, 1 (0.04%) patient showed affection of the ophthalmic division of the 5th cranial nerve, and 1 (0.04%) patient showed affection of the 4th cranial nerve (Table 2). More than one cranial nerve affection was seen in some patients, depending on the specific type and severity of meningitis. The onset and duration of cranial nerve paralysis varied in the different types of meningitis. The paralytic squint was noticed usually either at the onset of meningitis or within the first week. The 7th cranial nerve usually developed late in the course.

TABLE 2 Incidence of Cranial Nerve Affection in the Different Types of Meningitis

Cranial Nerve Affection	Total No.	Meningo-coccal	Pneumo-coccal	Influ-enzal	Tuber-culous	Purulent of Unknown Etiology
Sixth	368(17.9%)	35(7.5%)	35(16.5%)	15(15.6%)	244(35.2%)	39(6.7%)
Third	79(3.8%)	6(1.2%)	8(3.7%)	1	55(7.9%)	9(1.5%)
Seventh	75(3.6%)	7(1.4%)	10(4.7%)	0	44(6.3%)	14(2.4%)
Fourth	1(0.04%)	0	0	0	1(0.1%)	0
Fifth	1(0.04%)	0	0	0	1(0.1%)	0
TOTAL 2049	524(25.5%)	48(10.2%)	53(25.0%)	16(16.6%)	345(49.7%)	62(10.7%)

of the disease, and with few patients lagophthalmos was even seen in the follow up examination after discharge from hospital.

DISCUSSION

The 6th cranial nerve showed the highest incidence of affection in meningitis (17.9%). Unilateral nerve affection appeared to be more prevelantly affected (10%) than a bilateral affection (7.9%). The 3rd cranial nerve was next affected (3.8%), followed by the 7th cranial nerve (3.6%), then the 4th and 5th cranial nerves (each 0.04%).

From this study we noticed that tuberculous meningitis showed the highest incidence of cranial nerve affection (49.7%), followed in decreasing frequency by pneumococcal meningitis (25%), influenzal meningitis (16.6%), purulent meningitis of unknown etiology (10.7%) and lastly meningococcal meningitis (10.2%) (Table 2).

Patients presenting with more than one cranial nerve affection usually occurred in severe prolonged infections as tuberculous meningitis. Recovery from paralytic squint also depended on the type and severity of meningitis. As tuberculous meningitis runs a less acute course compared to other types of meningitis, the cranial nerves are subjected for prolonged periods of time to fever, intracellular oedema due to rise of intracranial pressure and fibrous tissue formation, all of which might be the etiological cause for the high incidence of ocular motor nerve paralysis noticed in tuberculous meningitis.

AKNOWLEDGEMENT

The authors thank Mrs. Magda Erian for data compilation and technical assistance.

BINOCULAR OCULOMOTOR ADAPTATION TO INDUCED INCOMITANT DEVIATIONS

D. B. HENSON and B. G. DHARAMSHI

Laboratory of Experimental Optometry, University of Wales Institute of Science and Technology, Cardiff, Wales, UK

ABSTRACT

We have measured how normal subjects binocularly adapt their oculomotor systems to induced incomitant deviations. We have also measured the spread of adaptation from the direction in which a fusion stimulus was given.

INTRODUCTION

Several researchers have reported on the way the oculomotor system adapts to an induced heterophoria (Carter, 1965; Henson and North, 1980; Ogle, Martens and Dyer, 1967; Schor, 1979b).Their results show that while an ophthalmic prism placed before one eye initially induces a 'phoria and fixation disparity in a formally orthophoric subject, continued fusion through the prism results in an adaptation of the oculomotor system and a loss of the 'phoria and fixation disparity. We have performed two experiments that extend this work. In the first, we demonstrate that the oculomotor system can also adapt to an induced incomitant deviation of the type found in ocularmotor paresis. In the second, we show that the type of adaptation reported by the researchers cited above to an induced 'phoria occurs over limited motor fields when the fusion stimulus is confined to a single visual direction.

EXPERIMENT 1

We have induced incomitant deviations in normal subjects by making them ametropic with a soft contact lens and then correcting the induced ametropia with a spectacle lens. Because the contact lens moves with the eye, the combined contact/spectacle lens system induces a prismatic effect whose magnitude is dependent upon eye position. The further the subject's line of sight is from the optical centre of the spectacle lens, the greater will be the prismatic effect. When a subject first puts this contact/spectacle lens system on, he exhibits a 'phoria whose magnitude is dependent upon eye position. By measuring the amplitude of the 'phorias at specific positions of gaze, we are able to monitor any adaptation to the incomitance. In this experiment, we measured the 'phoria at 12 positions of gaze, 7.6, 14.9 and 21.8 deg up, down, to the right and to the left. Fig. 1 shows the results of one

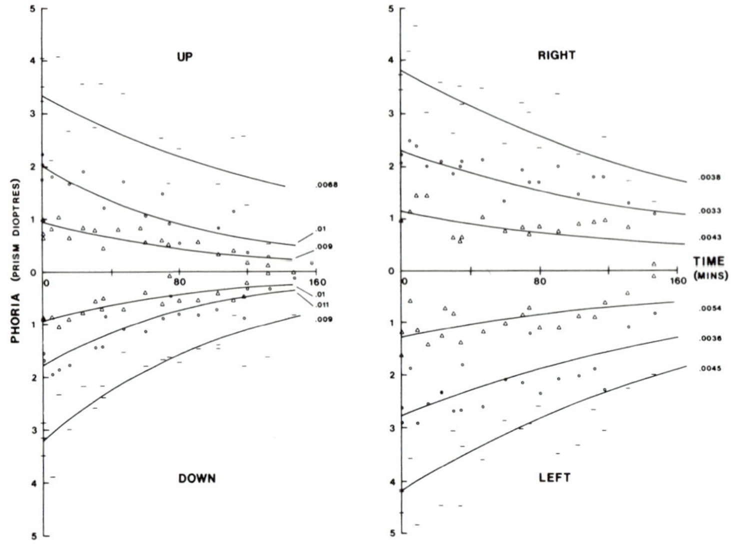

Fig. 1. Oculomotor adaptation to -3.00D of induced anisometropia

subject to such an induced incomitance. The lines drawn through the data are the best fitting ones (least squares) of the equation $y = P.\exp^{-Bx}$. The value of B is given at the end of each line. It can be seen that at the beginning of the experiment the subject exhibited a 'phoria whose magnitude was dependent upon eye position. However, during the course of the next two hours, during which time the subject performed normal office/lab type functions, the 'phorias gradually reduced to their base line values. This experiment has been repeated on 3 other subjects, all of whom gave similar results. The results of this experiment quite clearly show that subjects can binocularly adapt to incomitant deviations when the magnitude of the incomitance is approximately equal to 0.11 deg/deg. When the incomitance is increased to approximately 0.24 deg/deg by increasing the power of the contact/spectacle lens system, we find that the rate of adaptation decreases to practically zero, a result which suggests that the oculomotor system is only capable of adapting to a limited degree of incomitance.

An unwanted side effect of the contact/spectacle lens system is an induced anisokonia which increases with the power of the contact lens. Because of this, it is impossible to categorically state that binocular adaptation is only capable of dealing with a small amount of incomitance as the anisokonia may be indirectly restricting the adaptive system. The results do, however, clearly show that binocular adaptation to incomitant deviations is possible and that the failure of paretic patients to obtain normal binocular coordination may be the result of their incomitance exceeding the limits of this adaptive system.

EXPERIMENT 2

Adaptation to incomitant deviations requires the oculomotor system to adapt each position of gaze by a different amount. To enable this type of adaptation, the oculomotor system must be capable of binocularly adapting over limited motor fields.

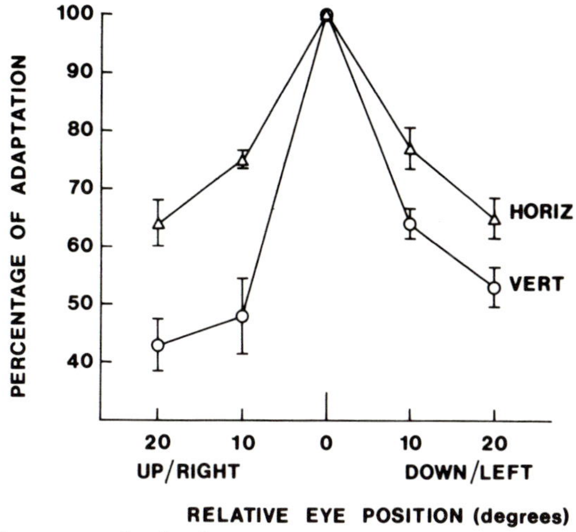

Fig. 2. The spread of adaptation

In the second experiment, we have demonstrated this by presenting the oculomotor system with an adaptation task (a 2.00D prism base down before one eye) while confining any fusion stimulus to one specific visual direction. After 3.75 mins of fusion, during which time the eyes remained stationary, the subject's 'phoria had reduced by about 1.50D. At the end of this adaptation period, the 'phoria was measured at points both 10 and 20 degrees away from the direction in which fusion was allowed, in both the vertical and horizontal meridians. Our results are shown in Fig. 2. The maximum amount of adaptation occurred in the direction in which fusion was allowed. When the eyes were turned away from this direction, adaptation still occurred but to a lesser extent.

The spread of adaptation shown in this experiment obviously aids the oculomotor system in adapting its whole motor field. Without it, visual experience would have to be gained in every visual direction before adaptation would be complete. However, the spread also acts to limit the amount of incomitance with which the oculomotor system is capable of dealing. When the incomitance exceeds a certain value, then the spread of adaptation from one direction of gaze will produce inappropriate adaptation in the neighbouring positions of gaze. Everytime the eye moves to a new direction, the adaptation that occurs spreads to interfere with the adaptation gained in neighbouring visual directions. This results in the oculomotor system perpetually trying to adapt and never succeeding.

CONCLUSIONS

Firstly, the oculomotor system is capable of adapting to incomitant deviations of 0.11 deg/deg. This finding explains why certain patients who suffer a paresis eventually gain normal binocular oculomotor coordination. Secondly, the limitation of binocular adaptation to incomitance is produced by the spread of adaptation from one visual direction to the neighbouring ones. This spread, while aiding total adaptation to small, relatively comitant deviations, limits the degree of incomitance to which the oculomotor system can adapt.

FOVEAL FIXATION COMPETING WITH BINOCULAR FUSION? A DEVELOPMENTAL HYPOTHESIS

A. I. COGAN

Smith-Kettlewell Institute of Visual Sciences, San Francisco, California, USA

ABSTRACT

It is proposed that fusion and foveal fixation normally compete during binocular-visual development. Alternating strabismus ensues when foveal fixation is precocious while fusion is weak. Bilateral optical blurring of the retinal images (soft focus) would reduce the impetus to monocular fixation and promote fusion.

KEYWORDS

Binocular development; competition in development; strabismus etiology; soft-focus blurring.

INTRODUCTION

In the traditional view (e.g., Duke-Elder and Wybar, 1973), binocular fusion develops on the basis of monocular fixation reflexes; comitant strabismus is caused by failures of bifixation resulting from optical, neural, or muscular defects in one or in both monocular systems. In particular, subnormal visual acuity as an obstacle to precise foveal fixation is held responsible for preventing bifoveal fixation and thus fusion. Originally, Worth (1903) had proposed that fusion was a faculty separate from foveal fixation, and Cogan (1967a) suggested that maturation of foveal vision, on a sharp upturn until age 2 to 4, increased the strain upon fusion, and provoked strabismus in children with insufficient fusion reserves.
The traditional view is probably based on the fact that stereoamblyopia and strabismus are frequently found in combination with subnormal acuity. At an age when binocular development is already complete, a direct correlation between reduced binocularity and subnormal acuity is indeed present (Fig. 1). Thus among 47 hyperopes with manifest refraction error and subnormal corrected acuity, there were 16 individuals with strabismus and/or deficient stereopsis (34%), while among 283 emmetropes with normal bilateral acuity there were only 23 such individuals (8.1%).
Yet, it is not clear why the majority of ametropes and anisometropes have normal fusion and stereopsis, nor why some emmetropes do not have it.
Very little is known about concurrent dynamics of acuity, foveal fixation and binocularity during early postnatal development, but the notion which attributes strabismus to subnormal acuity and poor fixation has little support in strabismus epidemiology. Incidence of strabismus with age (Fig. 2) shows two maxima: one, prior to age 1, and another, between 2 to 4 years of age. Typically, the early

onset group has an alternating pattern of squint, and high visual acuity in both eyes; in the late onset group, strabismus is largely monolateral, amblyopia is frequent, and refraction anomalies are common (Crone and Velzboer, 1956).

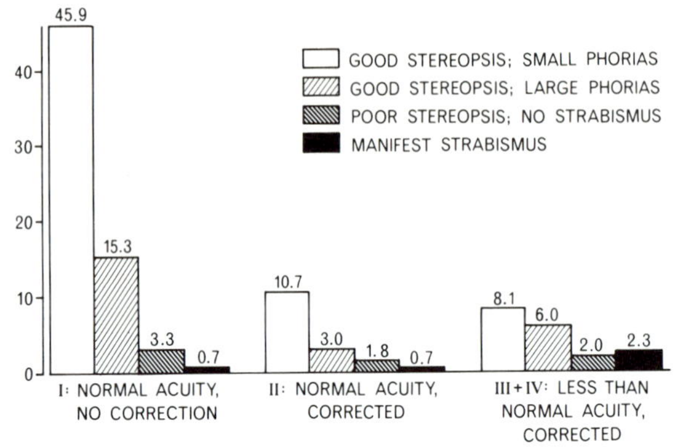

Fig. 1 Incidence (<u>ordinate</u>, %) of normal and subnormal binocularity and acuity in an unbiased sample of school population (13-year-olds; sample size 566). Acuity less than 0.9 in at least one eye assumed "less than normal"; stereothresholds in excess of 2 arc min signify "poor stereopsis". Reduced binocularity is correlated with subnormal acuity (chi-square criterion; $p<0.001$; $r=0.3$). (Cogan, 1967b).

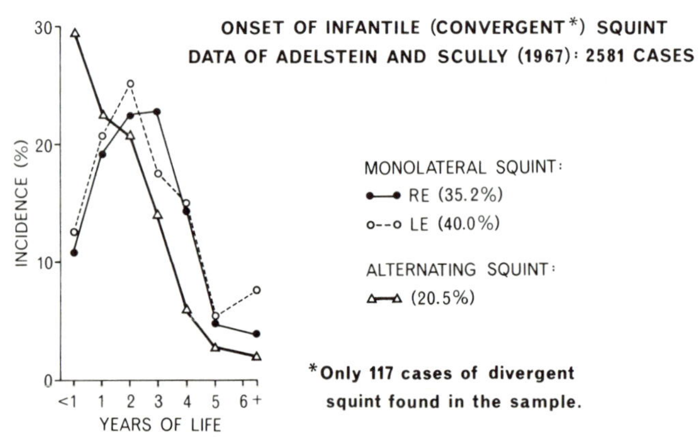

Fig. 2 Onset of convergent concomitant strabismus with age. I plotted the data of Adelstein and Scully (1967): theirs seems the least biased sample to be found.

Available data do not show an increase in the incidence of defects affecting foveal vision during the time periods typical for strabismus onset. Generally, the opposite is true: during the first months and years of human visual development, acuity and fixation are improving (Teller, 1978), and astigmatism is decreasing

(Atkinson, Braddick, French, 1980). We also know that fusional vergence is normally present by 6 months of age (Worth, 1903), if not earlier. Recently, proximal vergence was demonstrated in one-month-olds (Aslin, 1977), and the binocular response to retinal disparity has been obtained in some two-months-olds (Atkinson and Braddick, 1976). In the emerging pattern, fusion and foveal fixation develop independently at first, and then interact, eventually forming a complex unified system. This proposition is presented in the following hypothesis.

HYPOTHESIS

(i) Fusional movements are innately binocular, symmetric. Fixation movements are initially monocular, independent. (Fusion is driven towards minimization of global disparity in the field, while foveal fixation is prompted by selection of form and orientation. The foveae are presumed to have dual representation: together, they form the cyclopean fovea which serves as origin of the symmetrical binocular response; and each fovea serves also as origin of monocular fixation movements, with alternating monocular fixation as the limiting case of fusion failure).
(ii) The fusion response normally matures earlier than the foveal response. Relatively strong fusion is necessary to establish bifoveal fixation.
(iii) Interocular competition for dominance goes through several stages. At first, the competition involves different sensory-motor responses; in effect, the fusion response competes with the (alternating) fixation response. If the latter has matured precociously, while fusion is weak, then alternating strabismus ensues. Otherwise, the system goes through the next stage: sensory competition for eye dominance. (By this time, the motor component of the competition has been abrogated due to integration of responses in fusion and bifixation.) If harmonious bifoveal vision is not achieved, then secondary modifications of the binocular-visual system may occur, such as amblyopia, stereoblindness, and monolateral strabismus.
(iiii) Neural plasticity serves to accommodate competition between the various subsystems during development and then to perpetuate the outcome.

Plasticity of the visual cortex abunduntly demonstrated during an early postnatal period in cat and monkey appears to be a general phenomenon (superbly reviewed by Mitchell, 1980) and thus must serve a basic developmental purpose. But the often suggested goal of "adaptation to environment" does not provide a clear reason for the existence of plasticity. Generally, the salient environmental features: light, contrast, movement, form, are ubiquitous. Therefore, barring influences such as starvation, disease, trauma, etc, environment is unlikely to play a formative role in visual development. In the context of the present hypothesis, neural plasticity serves to accomodate the interplay of internal forces which dominate sequentially in the developing system. Given normal visual environment, the "countdown" for each event in the genetically programmed sequence of development starts at the moment of conception, rather than birth (cf., Dobson, Mayer, Lee, 1980). Accordingly, "the period of susceptibility" probably starts at different ages for neural substrata serving different visual functions. Thus meridional amblyopia is not found in infants who got rid of their astigmatism prior to 3 years of age (Mohindra, Held, Gwiazda, Brill, 1978). The period during which various interocular imbalances can lead to amblyopia, probably starts early in the first year of life, and stretches until at least age four (von Noorden, 1973). Generally, it seems likely that each visual subsystem is initially built at a predetermined time by a largely autonomous process, and later it is refined or even strongly modified through interaction with related subsystems. The whole process must be directed towards adequate visual guidance of behavior; plasticity, then, serves to achieve the best overall, **individual** functional result.

A direct test of the hypothesis is possible using techniques such as preferential looking, to evaluate eye movements in response to foveal acuity targets (Teller, 1979), and to binocular disparity (Shea, Fox, Aslin and Dumais, 1980). Infants with familial history of alternating strabismus should form the test group. Precocious development of bilateral foveal vision in incipient alternators, is the crucial prediction of the present hypothesis. Prior to developing manifest cross-fixation, these subjects will be behind the controls in their oculomotor responses to disparity stimulation, but they will match or even exceed the controls in their (bilateral) acuity as determined by fixation responses. If this prediction is borne out, the test will identify the relationship between motor fusion and foveal fixation which will be specific to incipient alternators, with important clinical as well as theoretical implications.

Medical-orthoptic treatment is one "environmental influence" which obviously **can** affect the outcome of visual development. But our understanding of the process being treated is incomplete, even a posteriori. Thus, the question of when to operate for "congenital" strabismus (cf., Costenbader, 1961; Jampolsky, 1977; Parks, 1977) has not been settled by the results of surgery. Assuming that incompatibility of the foveal images in the two eyes is a common cause of strabismus (cf., Duke-Elder and Wybar, 1973), without answer is also a more general question: if the system goes strabismic to avoid confusion, in the first place, then why does not strabismus recur after surgery more often? In the context of the present hypothesis, the eyes remain straight after surgical re-alignement, if interocular competition has abated before surgery is performed. Conversely, early surgery may be counterproductive if undertaken before the interocular competition has been resolved through neural plasticity. Another implication of the hypothesis presented in this paper is that early correction of refractive errors may exacerbate interocular competition for dominance and thus discourage binocularity, if fusion is weak.

A clinical trial based on the present hypothesis is aimed at alleviating interocular competition for dominance. To weaken bilateral fixation stimuli yet preserve binocular disparity, lenses (goggles, or contacs) would be given such that optically degrade edges (high contrast borders) by using "cloudy" material producing a mild scatter of light and thus a slight overall blurring of the retinal images: a "soft focus" effect. Note that by varying the amount of light scatter in the material used to produce the lenses, visual acuity can be reduced (in theory) to any desired level, and acuity will remain roughly the same at all viewing distances (which would not be the case if, say, plus lenses were used to blur retinal images). Unlike atropine, which also produces blurring of all retinal images except those in the conjugate plane (reviewed by Guibor, 1950), soft focus lenses leave accomodation and pupil size unaffected. With optically degraded edges, binocular disparity is preserved in the lower contrast and lower spatial frequency domain. The expected effect is that foveal fixation will be made less active, while fusion is promoted.

Free alternators will be treated by equal optical blurring. In treating monocular strabismus, acuity in the amblyopic eye will be restored by occluding the fixing eye, before equal blurring is introduced. Maximum effect of soft-focus blurring might be expected in incipient alternators, treated before the pattern of cross-fixation has become established.

ACKNOWLEDGEMENT

I thank Alan B. Scott for discussion. Financial support by the National Eye Institute grant EYO 1558 and by the Smith-Kettlewell Eye Research Foundation is sincerely appreciated.

CENTRAL OCULAR MOTOR DISORDERS

SECTION VI

Coordinator: R. B. Daroff

DISORDERS OF HORIZONTAL AND VERTICAL GAZE

DISORDERS OF HORIZONTAL GAZE

V. HENN and U. BÜTTNER

Department of Neurology, University of Zürich, Zürich, Switzerland

ABSTRACT

A one-sided horizontal gaze palsy is the result of a lesion of the ipsilateral paramedian pontine reticular formation (PPRF) or the ipsilateral abducens nucleus. A PPRF lesion leads to a loss of all rapid eye movements towards the ipsilateral side. In experimental lesions with selective cell loss in the PPRF the vestibulo--ocular reflex remains intact. A bilateral PPRF lesion leads to a loss of all rapid eye movements, also in the vertical plane. The clinical syndromes have experimentally been reproduced in monkeys.

KEY WORDS

Paramedian pontine reticular formation (PPRF); eye movements, rapid; abducens nucleus, lesion; gaze palsy, horizontal; gaze palsy, global.

INTRODUCTION

Gaze palsies occur either in a horizontal or vertical direction. Horizontal gaze palsies towards the ipsilateral side occur with lesions of the paramedian pontine reticular formation (PPRF) or lesions of the abducens nucleus. The lesions which lead to gaze palsies in the vertical plane are located in the mesencephalon. The effect of lesions are the same in man and monkey. Because more extensive recordings are available from monkeys, they will be shown instead of less complete, but qualitatively similar recordings from humans.

ANATOMY

The medial portions of the nucleus reticularis magnocellularis (or nucleus centralis pontis oralis and caudalis) have been designated as PPRF (Cohen and others, 1968; Goebel and others, 1971). The region extends from the abducens nucleus in a rostral direction towards the brachium conjunctivum and trochlear nucleus. The PPRF has been first defined functionally, as there are no distinct histological boundaries. There are two major oculomotor pathways originating from the PPRF: one pathway ascending rostrally, close to but outside of the MLF, to the rostral mesencephalon that appears to be important for coordination of horizontal and vertical gaze; the other pathway descends caudally and sends off a projection to the abducens nucleus (Büttner-Ennever and Henn, 1976; Büttner-Ennever, 1977; Graybiel, 1977a, 1977b). This pathway directs horizontal gaze to the ipsilateral side by contacting abducens motoneurons and internuclear neurons within the abducens nucleus which project via the MLF to the medial rectus motoneurons of the contralateral oculomotor nucleus (Büttner-Ennever, 1979). Afferent pathways to the PPRF are largely unexplored. Functionally, one would expect connections from the vestibular nuclei, from visual areas like the superior colliculi, frontal eye fields and prestriate cortex, and from the cerebellum.

ACQUIRED PPRF LESIONS IN PATIENTS

Numerous reports have described the deficits after unilateral PPRF lesions (Bender, 1980; Bleuler, 1885; Crosby, 1953; Freeman, 1922; Freeman and others, 1943; Halsey and others, 1967; Holmes, 1921, 1931; Hoyt and Daroff, 1971; Jung and Kornhuber, 1964; Pierrot-Deseilligny and others, 1978, 1979; Reese and Yaskin, 1941). As the extent of pathology and its temporal development differed, as well as the availability or feasability of formal testing, the authors' own interpretations vary. However, the following symptoms, compiled from the literature and our own observations, seem to be characteristic of a chronic PPRF lesion.

1. At rest the eyes can be held in the primary position.
2. There is a total gaze palsy towards the ipsilateral side.
3. No saccades or fast nystagmus phases can be elicited towards the ipsilateral side, even not in the contralateral hemifield.
4. Vestibular stimulation leads to normal nystagmus towards the contralateral side, and during slow phases the eyes can move across midline into the ipsilateral hemifield. During attempted nystagmus towards the ipsilateral side, the eyes are tonically deviated towards the contralateral side and held there (Fig. 1).

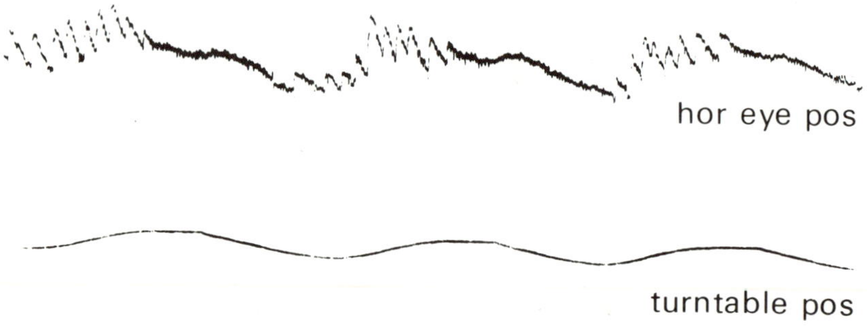

Fig. 1. Horizontal eye movement recordings from a patient with the clinical diagnosis of a vascular left-sided PPRF lesion. The recording was made 10 days after the infarction. The patient was rotated over an angle of about 90° and asked to look at the face of the examiner in front of her. There is normal nystagmus to the right, and only a tonic eye deviation during rotation to the left. As is often the case with such patients, more formal testing like rotation in the dark gave unsatisfying results, because vigilance could not be maintained.

5. Optokinetic nystagmus cannot be elicited towards the ipsilateral side; in all other directions it can be elicited.
6. Convergence is present.

Acute lesions present with the following additional symptoms:
7. At rest the eyes are in a paramedian contralateral position.
8. There is spontaneous horizontal nystagmus toward the contralateral side, which increases with more lateral gaze positions or in the dark.

In partial lesions the main symptoms include:
1. Gaze preference towards the contralateral side.
2. Saccades towards the ipsilateral side are infrequent, small in amplitude and prolonged in duration.

Often encountered clinical signs with invasion of neighboring structures are:
1. Damage of vestibulo-abducens fibers in the immediate surrounding of the VIth nucleus lead to deficits or abolishment of the VOR.
2. An MLF lesion leads to an additional supranuclear medial rectus paresis on the same side (Fisher, 1967; Newman and others, 1978; Sharpe and others, 1974).
3. With an invasion of the abducens nucleus on the same side both eyes cannot move across midline during vestibular stimulation.
4. With a lesion of the facial genu, a "peripheral" type palsy develops with sparing of gustatory fibers.
5. With extensive lesions of the reticular formation patients are drowsy, but can be alerted.

The etiology includes:
1. Vascular lesions are often incomplete and show a tendency towards recovery.
2. Tumors can be primary or metastatic. Besides neoplasmas, tuberculomas have been encountered.
3. With other lesions, because of their large extension, patients are frequently comatose and cannot be appropriately tested (central pontine myelinolysis, etc.).
4. Degenerative or diseases of unkown etiology include progressive supranuclear palsy or some forms of pontocerebellar degeneration. Particularly in progressive supranuclear palsy the PPRF is commonly affected and in the late stage of the disease often all rapid eye movements are absent. Because of the widespread cell loss in other brainstem structures in this and other degenerative diseases, clinico-pathological correlations can usually not be made.

Bilateral lesions have infrequently been reported and with different findings. Such patients are usually severely ill and exhibit decreased vigilance. In accordance with results of experimental lesions in monkeys, a total loss of all rapid eye movements, also in the vertical plane, has been reported (Hoyt and Daroff, 1971; Christoff, 1974).

Experimental lesions in monkeys show phenomena which are identical to those seen in humans (Bender and Shanzer, 1964; Cohen and others, 1968; Cohen and Henn, 1972). Earlier experiments applied electrolytic lesions which destroy all cells and fibers. More recently, chemical lesions have been done with kainic acid (Jäger and others, 1981). It selectively destroys cells, but leaves fibers en passage intact. These experiments together with single neuron recordings prove that the cells in the PPRF are the elements responsible for generating rapid eye movements towards the ipsilateral side (review: Hepp and Henn, this volume). Figure 2 shows a recording from a monkey with a unilateral PPRF lesion on the right side (details Jäger and others, 1981).

Bilateral experimental PPRF lesions have first been described by Bender and Shanzer (1964). The most striking feature is a loss of all rapid eye movements,

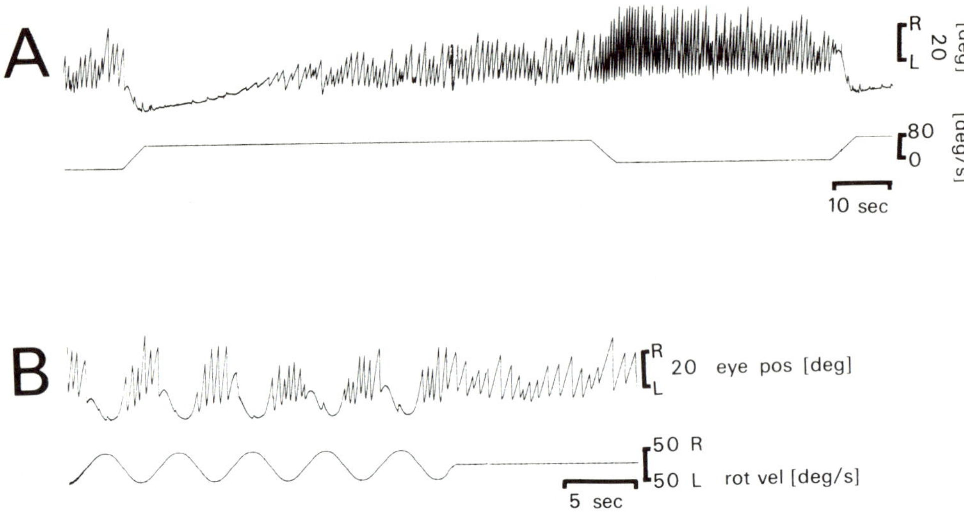

Fig. 2. Monkey with a two week old PPRF lesion on the right side. At rest, in the dark (far left in A, or right in B) there is spontaneous nystagmus to the left. In A the monkey was rotated about a vertical axis in total darkness with constant velocity to the right, and in B with a sinusoidal velocity as indicated below. Note that there is normal nystagmus to the left which declines with a time constant of about 15 sec. Although calibration for primary position in this untrained monkey could not be given, direct visual inspection clearly showed that during slow phases the eyes often crossed into the right hemifield. During rotation towards the right in A, the eyes are caught in an extreme left position, from which they return with a time constant of about 15 sec to exhibit spontaneous nystagmus.

also in the vertical plane. Monkeys exhibit a staring expression. They can move their eyes slowly towards a visual target. During vestibular or optokinetic stimulation there is a slow movement into the expected direction. If the stimulus continues, the eyes stay eccentrically, and they drift towards midposition when the stimulus cedes. Figure 3 shows these deficits in a monkey with a bilateral PPRF lesion brought about by local injection of kainic acid (Lang and Henn, in preparation).

ACQUIRED ABDUCENS NUCLEUS LESIONS IN PATIENTS

The patient will present the following symptoms (Gorel, 1882; Bennett and Savill, 1890; Blocq and Guison, 1891: Wernicke, 1877):
1. Complete gaze palsy towards the ipsilateral side.
2. Also during nystagmus, the eyes cannot move into the ipsilateral hemifield.
3. Convergence is intact.
4. Because of the immediate neighborhood of the facial nerve genu, a facial nerve palsy can be considered to be an almost obligatory symptom.

The above described symptoms are understandable because abducens motoneurons are damaged in addition to internuclear neurons, the main excitatory input for contralateral medial rectus motoneurons during conjugate gaze. This differentiates it from a pure PPRF lesion. Metastatic tumors have most frequently been the cause of

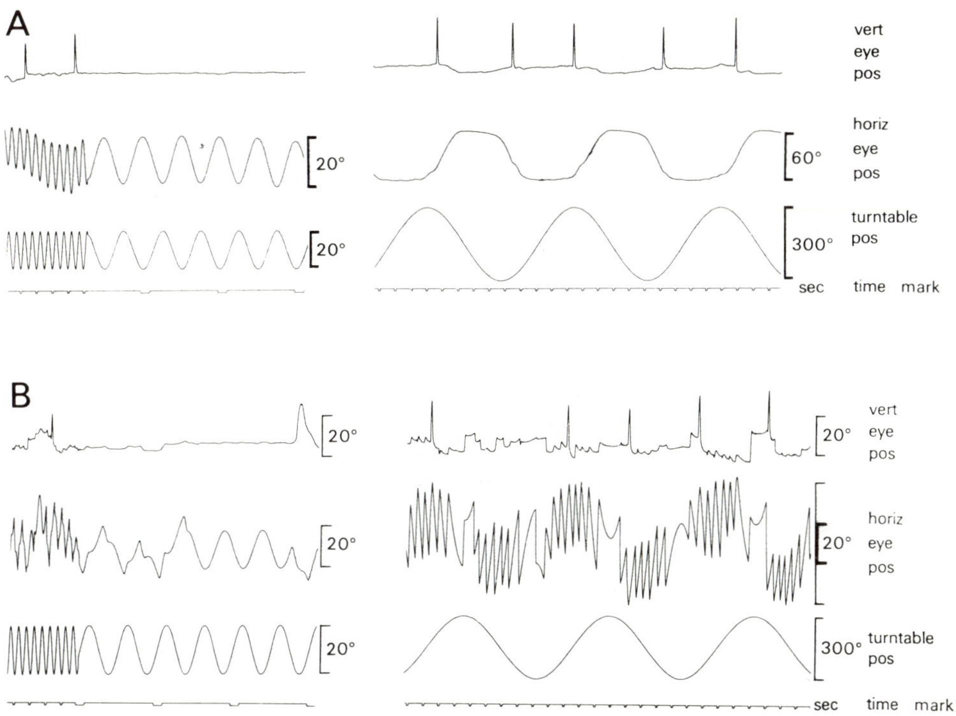

Fig. 3. A, eye movement recording from a monkey with a bilateral PPRF lesion. B, for comparison a recording from a normal monkey using the same stimulus parameters. At left, the monkey was rotated about a vertical axis in darkness at a frequency of 2 Hz. The eyes move in a compensatory fashion. For much higher amplitudes of rotation, shown on the right side, the eyes move into an extreme lateral eye position and stay there. The normal monkey exhibits fast eye movements superimposed on the compensatory movements on the left, and vigorous direction changing nystagmus at a stimulus frequency of 0.1 Hz on the right.

such lesions. In acute lesions confined to the abducens nucleus one would not expect spontaneous nystagmus towards the contralateral side which would differentiate it from a PPRF lesion. However, from the vascularization pattern one would expect such vascular lesion to occur infrequently.
Experimental lesions in monkeys exhibit the same symptomatology (Carpenter and others, 1963; Carpenter, 1971).

CONGENITAL HORIZONTAL GAZE PALSY

A familial disorder has been described with total absence of horizontal gaze, but normal range of vertical gaze and intact convergence. This disorder often goes together with abnormalities of the boney spine (fusion of vertebrae, kyphoscoliosis). The neuro-pathology is not known, but a bilateral aplasia of the abducens nuclei and MLF would be the most likely explanation (recent review Vetterli and Henn, 1981).

EXTRAPONTINE LESIONS

a, Paresis of voluntary gaze can occur with lesions of the mesencephalic reticular formation. The syndrome has first been fully described in monkeys (Komatsuzaki and others, 1972). Without a conjugate deviation of the eyes, the monkeys display an asymmetry in moving their eyes: they make infrequent movements into the ipsilateral hemifield, while movements in the contralateral field are normal. With strong stimuli they have a normal range of gaze. Vestibular nystagmus is symmetrical which differentiates it from a partial PPRF lesion.

b, Paresis with déviation conjugée is a prominent feature of precentral cortical lesions. With the resolution of the tonic eye deviation, the normal range of gaze returns. Occasionally, a déviation conjugée also occurs with an acute cerebellar space occupying lesion like a hemorrhage or abscess (Fisher and others, 1965).

COMMENT

This survey of disorders in horizontal gaze has focused on immediate premotor structures located in the pons. These disorders can be diagnosed at the bedside without any further laboratory investigations. Symptoms have been listed which in patients rarely occur in isolation. The vestibulo-ocular reflex, for instance, can often not be elicited in patients with a PPRF lesion. Such a deficit is brought about by concomitant lesions of fibers and not by local cell damage, as has been shown in experimental lesions. Therefore, the clinically often encountered syndrome with more diffuse pathology shall not be confused with the rarely observed case of an isolated lesion.

A wider interpretation of "horizontal gaze disorders" should include discussion of deficits in pursuit movement, optokinetic nystagmus, and the impairment to suppress vestibular or optokinetic nystagmus by visual fixation. These topics are discussed elsewhere at this symposium. Only if respective tests are normal, can disorders be excluded which affect the parieto-occipital lobe, the corticopontine pathways, or the cerebellum. One also has to take into account parallel pathways and parallel information processing. For example, a chronic lesion of the frontal eye field or superior colliculus alone does not lead to clinical deficits, but a combined lesion leads to a severe disorder of gaze as recently demonstrated in the monkey (Schiller and others, 1980).

OPEN QUESTIONS

Despite considerable progress in understanding how input signals are transformed in the pons to generate motor signals to move the eyes, there are still many questions the clinician would like to ask the physiologist. We will concentrate on a few questions, answers to which would be helpful in topical diagnosis of brainstem lesions.

Concerning the normal function of supranuclear organization, how is normal coordination between horizontal and vertical gaze achieved? Most eye movements are oblique, but there are two premotor centers for horizontal and vertical gaze which are anatomically widely separate. To what extent can the vertical premotor center for vertical gaze in the mesencephalon function independently without appropriate input from the PPRF? Rapid eye movements are normally spaced at least 160 msec apart. What are the mechanisms to block rapid movements once a saccade has been executed?

With a unilateral PPRF lesion, nystagmus towards the contralateral side is normal. This includes normal slow phases towards the ipsilateral side frequently crossing the midline. If these reflexive slow movements are possible into the "paretic" hemifield, why are pursuit movement or fixation not possible? Would that imply separate velocity-to-position integrators for rapid and slow movements?

Bilateral PPRF lesions lead to more deficits than the sum of two unilateral lesions, as all rapid eye movements in the vertical plane are also abolished. However, some movements are better possible than with a unilateral lesion: monkeys can visually follow a target with low velocity, and the eyes can be held in eccentric gaze positions. This would point towards an intact velocity-to-position integrator for slow movements. There are no comparable data from the very few human cases.

With a unilateral nuclear abducens lesion, gaze palsies towards the ipsilateral side are described. However, if the lesion is restricted to the nuclear region, abortive saccades towards the ipsilateral side should still be possible in the contralateral hemifield, because inhibition of antagonists should not be impaired. It seems that this question has not been discussed in clinical cases nor had it been addressed experimentally.

At the symposium, a short film was shown to demonstrate the typical clinical symptoms of an experimental PPRF lesion in a monkey.

PHYSIOLOGY OF HORIZONTAL GAZE

K. HEPP* and V. HENN**

*Physics Department, ETH, CH-8093 Zürich, Switzerland
**Neurology Department, University Hospital, CH-8091 Zürich, Switzerland

ABSTRACT

Single unit studies have been made in the paramedian pontine reticular formation (PPRF) of alert monkeys. Saccade related neurons can be classified as medium- and long lead bursters and pause cells. The analysis of their firing patterns together with results from lesion studies lead to the formulation of a hypothetical premotor circuit responsible for generating rapid eye movements in the horizontal as well as in vertical directions. The main characteristic is a central eye displacement signal which can be followed through the different neuronal populations.

KEY WORDS

Paramedian pontine reticular formation (PPRF); saccade; integrator; burst generator; lesion; neuron, long lead burst; neuron, medium lead burst; neuron, pause; command; control; model.

INTRODUCTION

In eye movements all extraocular muscles work together in a synergistic action. Thus a separation of horizontal and vertical gaze would seem artificial to the physiologist. In the saccadic system, however, such a separation appears more meaningful, since horizontal gaze palsies toward the ipsilateral side occur with lesions in the paramedian pontine reticular formation (PPRF) (Henn and Büttner, preceding contribution).

Neurophysiological studies by Cohen and Henn (1972), Luschei and Fuchs (1972), Keller (1974) and Henn and Cohen (1976) have isolated different neuronal populations in the PPRF and periabducens region, e.g., long lead burst-, medium lead burst-, follow burst-, burst-tonic-, and pause neurons. The firing patterns of these putative premotor neurons during a horizontal saccade to the right are summarized in Fig. 1, together with a hypothetical premotor circuit proposed by Robinson (1975 a).

Horizontal motoneurons display a tonic activity which increases linearly with horizontal eye position (above a threshold). In addition, they burst for saccades in the on-direction with an on-latency of about 5 ms prior to the onset of the saccade. The number of spikes during the burst (additional to the tonic activity) increases linearly with eye displacement. During saccades in the off-direction their firing rate is reduced. Medium lead burst neurons fire with an on-latency of 5 to 10 ms. The number of spikes during the burst increases linearly with change of eye position in the on-direction. During movements in the off-direction there are often some late spikes which are not observed in motoneuron activity except in instances of a saccadic overshoot. Pause neurons have an unmodulated frequency of 150 to 200 Hz except for a pause during every saccade beginning at - 15 to - 5 ms before saccadic onset.

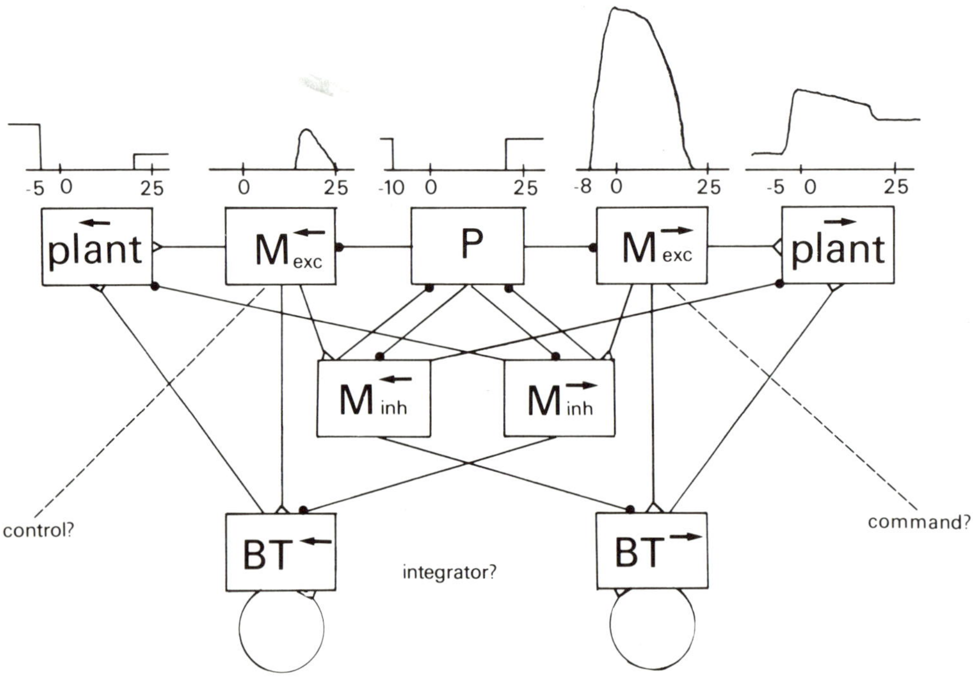

Fig. 1. Hypothetical premotor organization of horizontal gaze. Top line: typical firing patterns (instantaneous frequency) and on-latencies of motoneurons ("plant"), medium lead bursters (M) and pausers (P) during a rightward saccade with onset at 0 and 25 ms duration. BT: burst tonic neurons. Arrows: on-direction, exc<u>itatory</u> (-◁) or inhibitory (-•).

The strength of the proposed scheme in Fig. 1 stems from the fact that the destruction of the right PPRF containing the excitatory medium lead burst neurons, $M_{exc}^{\rightarrow}$, with on-direction to the right will completely abolish rapid eye movements to the right. The $M_{exc}^{\rightarrow}$ not only provide the saccadic burst to the right oculomotor plant (motoneurons with on-directions to the right and internuclear neurons) and the phasic inhibition of the left oculomotor plant, but they also provide the changes in tonic activation of all motoneurons through two reverberatory networks of burst-tonic neurons, i.e., the "horizontal integrator".

By combined morphological and electrophysiological methods Baker and others (this symposium) have partially established the excitatory and inhibitory connections of the premotor circuit in the cat (Fig. 1). Since all premotor pathways are expected to be polysynaptic, further detailed extracellular microelectrode studies in awake monkeys under controlled stimulus conditions are necessary, in order to gain additional insight into the relative strengths of the many parallel channels of the system. We shall address three topics in this presentation:

- the organization of gaze in oblique directions;
- the coding properties of long lead burst neurons, which are possible candidates for the command input to the immediate premotor network;
- the structure of the integrator as revealed by lesions of the PPRF.

ORGANIZATION OF GAZE DURING HORIZONTAL AND OBLIQUE SACCADES

Neglecting torsional movements, eye positions can be plotted in a two-dimensional frame with horizontal and vertical eye positions as Cartesian coordinates. If curves of equal discharge frequency during fixation are determined in such a scheme, then one finds that motoneurons for horizontal and vertical extraocular muscles can have oblique iso-frequency curves and therefore oblique on-directions depending on the position of the eye (Hepp and Henn, 1981). For example, in synergy with all other extraocular muscles, the trochlear muscle pulls downward in adduction and down-outward in abduction. It is an open question how the appropriate horizontal gaze command enters into the vertical gaze system.

Figure 2 shows the quantitative analysis of a medium lead burster in the PPRF, which is "ideal" in the sense that the coding of rapid eye movement parameters is precise and representative for a large population of similar neurons. As one sees from the non-linear relation (B) between number of spikes in the burst and the horizontal saccadic component, Δh, for small movements and from the increase of fluctuations with saccade size, perifoveal saccades are more precisely encoded than large saccades. The iso-burst curves (A) for small and large saccades are parallel to the vertical axis. Hence the on-direction of this neuron is unambiguously horizontal. In D one sees the differential form of A and B: From the instantaneous frequency f(t) of this single burster one can predict the saccadic velocity 10 ms later for all saccades to the right, by one function for large or small, oblique or purely horizontal movements. This is physiological evidence that the medium lead burster can drive the horizontal motoneurons. In C another function is shown, which has been discovered by van Gisbergen and others (1981). For all horizontal saccades, f(t) is a universal function of the horizontal motor error e(t + 5 ms). For oblique saccades, this striking correlation is lost, and f(t) could be matched with $a(t + 5 \text{ ms})\cos\alpha$, where a is the error amplitude and α the direction of the saccade. This is the differential form of the saccade vector relation used by Henn and Cohen (1976).

There are many different subpopulations of horizontal medium lead bursters in the PPRF, which indicates that the saccadic system uses many different channels. The most frequent deviations from the pattern for the medium lead burster in Fig. 2 are

- late latency discharge in the off-direction of different strength up to complete isotropy of the burst;
- wide range of saccadic gain (spikes per eye displacement), which can be constant for saccades of all sizes, or smaller or larger for small saccades (similar to the large and small saccade long lead bursters in Figs. 3 and 4);
- various degree of convexity of the iso-burst curves;
- angular distributions ranging from constant firing to a $\cos\alpha$-distribution in a sector of $\pm$ 60 deg around the on-direction.

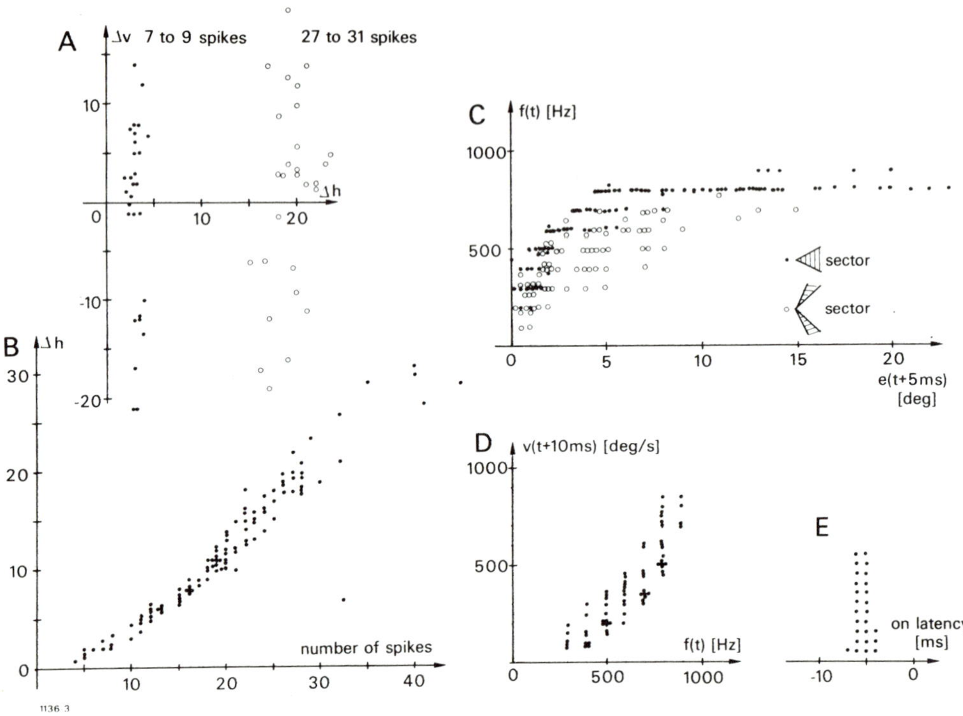

Fig. 2. Quantitative analysis of a medium lead burster with rightward on-direction. E: sharp onset of the high frequency burst preceding the saccade by 5 to 6 ms. In B the number of spikes during the burst is related to the horizontal eye-displacement component Δh for all saccades with Δh exceeding the vertical eye-displacement component ($\Delta h \geq |\Delta v|$), i.e. saccades with a larger horizontal than vertical movement component. This neuron does not fire for leftward saccades. In A all saccadic eye-displacement vectors are shown for a given number of spikes in the burst, either in the bin 7 to 9 spikes (filled dots) or 27 to 31 spikes (open dots). In D the 10 ms averaged instantaneous firing frequency f(t) of the burst at time t is related to the 10 ms averaged horizontal eye velocity component, v(t+10 ms), 10 ms later for all rightward saccades. In C f(t) is related to the horizontal motor error, e(t+5 ms), 5 ms later (e(t): difference between horizontal eye position at saccade offset and h(t)). Black dots are saccades into the sector $\Delta h > 2\,|\Delta v|$, light dots for $|\Delta v| > \Delta h > 1/2\,|\Delta v|$.

It is interesting that the PPRF, the "horizontal gaze center", also contains a smaller proportion of vertical medium lead bursters of identical characteristics, with iso-burst curves which can be off-vertical by up to 20 degrees. In close vicinity the PPRF contains medium lead burst neurons with ipsilateral on-directions of all eye muscles. The characteristics of these neurons do not differ from units found in the mesencephalic reticular formation (MRF).

Summary: In the PPRF at the level of medium lead burst neurons there is a clear functional, but not anatomical, separation into subpopulations for horizontal and vertical saccades. There are indications for different channels responsible for small and large saccades, which are members of a continuous distribution (similar to the distribution of high and low threshold motoneurons).

LONG LEAD BURST NEURONS

A theoretical prediction about the nature of the command for driving the medium lead bursters in Fig. 1 has been made by van Gisbergen and others (1981), in close agreement with the fact that visually-evoked saccades can be strongly perturbed in midflight and still reach their target position in head (Keller, 1974; Mays and Sparks, 1980). Since in Fig. 2C f(t) (and therefore horizontal eye velocity) and e(t+5 ms) are tightly coupled for horizontal saccades, Robinson's "bang-bang" model proposes that the medium lead bursters are driven by the difference between two inputs, of an excitatory desired eye position signal (which encodes the new eye position about 10 ms before the eyes have moved) and an inhibitory internal feedback signal coding present eye position (possibly from the integrator). This model relies only on few parameters and leads to many interesting predictions. However, for slow or oblique saccades, horizontal motor error does not predict the firing pattern of the horizontal medium lead burst neurons. Furthermore, ten years of microelectrode search in the awake monkey have failed to identify a neuronal signal of desired eye position. We shall therefore turn to the analysis of horizontal eye movement parameters in long lead bursters in the PPRF, as possible alternative candidates for driving the premotor circuit of Fig. 1.

Long lead burst neurons coding saccadic displacement independent of eye position are found in the PPRF in numbers almost equal to those of medium lead bursters. We shall restrict ourselves to describing neurons with saccade-related bursts of maximal frequency $>$ 400 Hz, in which the metrics of individual saccades can still be predicted from the firing patterns of single neurons. Long lead bursters have an onset (defined by the time at which the instantaneous frequency reaches half the maximal frequency) preceding saccadic onset by more than 10 ms. They have a highly variable early activity which is often related to metric properties of the saccade.

With long lead bursters in the PPRF a strict functional separation of horizontal and vertical gaze can no longer be found. While horizontal medium lead bursters can have ipsi- or contralateral on-directions, the on-directions of long lead bursters vary over the whole ipsilateral hemifield.

The coding of saccades in a long lead burster can be either directed (also called temporal) or by a movement field. In a directed long lead burster the number of spikes in the burst increases in fairly tight correlation with eye displacement up to the limit of the oculomotor range in the on-direction, as in medium lead bursters, but in general with a better encoding of either small or large eye displacement components.

We shall discuss the quantitative analysis of two typical and rather illustrative directed long lead bursters. Large saccades to the right with amplitude larger than 10 deg are represented in the long lead burster of Fig. 3 almost as well as in a medium lead burster. Within the sector $\Delta h \geq |\Delta v|$ the 10 ms-averaged firing frequency, f(t), is a universal function of the horizontal motor error. Figure 4 depicts an extreme case of a long lead burster representing small saccade components into the right hemifield by high gain. These neurons appear to trigger the ipsilateral saccadic burst generator.

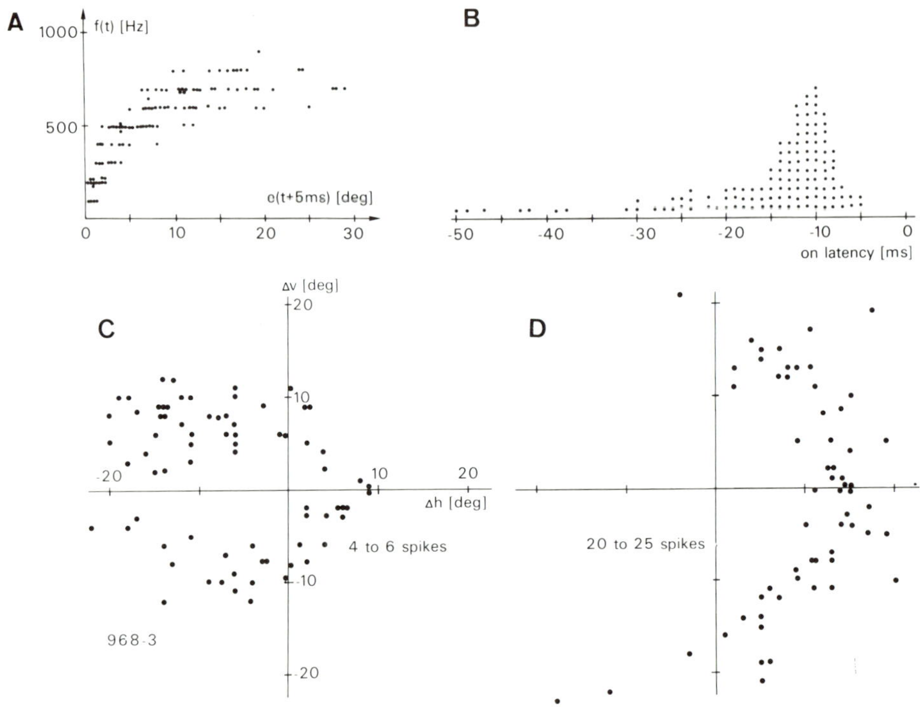

Fig. 3. Quantitative analysis for a directed large saccade long lead burster. The on-latency t_{on} is the time of occurrence of the first high frequency spike (inverse interspike interval larger than 1/2 the maximal value) and its distribution is shown in B. In C and D the eye displacement is shown for the bins of 4 to 6 spikes and 20 to 25 spikes (between t_{on} and the last high frequency spike at t_{off}). In A the instantaneous 10 ms-averaged frequency f(t) is plotted against the motor error e(t+5 ms) for all saccades with $\Delta h > 1/2\ |\Delta v|$ and amplitude $> 10^0$.

Long lead burst neurons with movement fields discharge maximally for all saccades close to a saccadic vector. The burst strength can be defined by the total number of spikes in the burst, or (less precisely) by the early presaccadic activity, or by the average frequency at saccadic onset. Two typical examples from the rostral PPRF are given in Fig. 5. If one defines the movement field by the region of half-maximal burst events, then its diameter has about the size of the desired saccadic amplitude, and this could give a reasonably precise "spatial" encoding of saccades by a family of such neurons. It is conceivable that these neurons provide an important input to the directed long lead bursters in the PPRF.

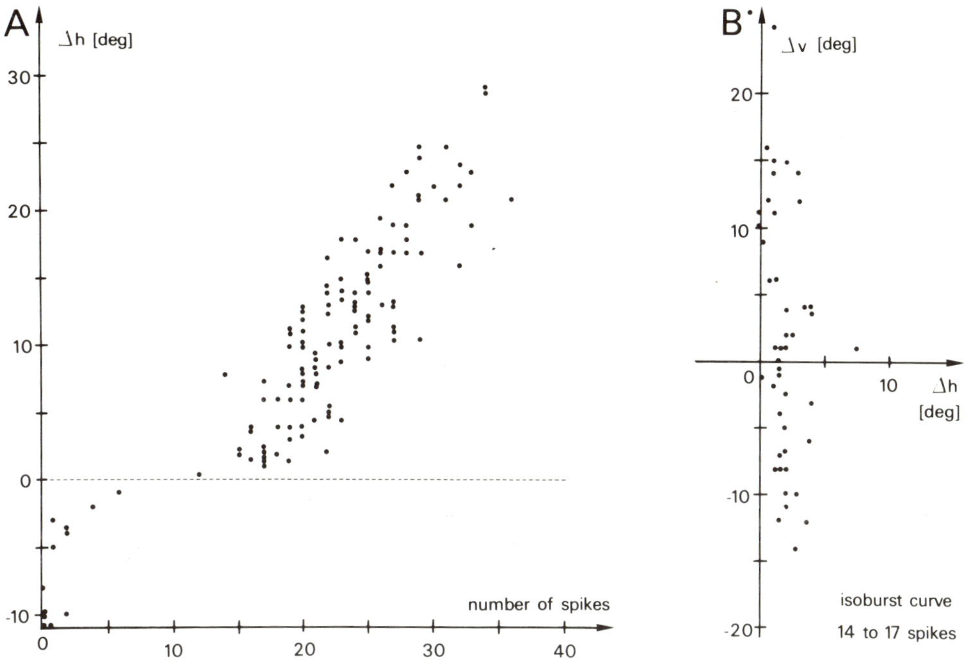

Fig. 4. Quantitative analysis of a directed small saccade long lead burster with right on-direction. In A the number of spikes in the burst is related to horizontal eye displacement for $|\Delta h| \geq |\Delta v|$. In B the iso-burst curve shows the (Δh, Δv) coordinates for all saccades with 14 to 17 spikes in the burst.

Summary: It is possible that long lead burst neurons provide the dominant eye displacement input to the medium lead burster during normal saccades. By superposition of the patterns of directed long lead bursters of the type of Figs. 3 and 4 one can reproduce the patterns of medium lead bursters, using the pause neurons as a triggered gate. Within the PPRF there is a rostro-caudal gradation from the preponderance of long lead burst neurons in the rostral part to the dominance of medium lead and burst tonic neurons in the periabducens area. If the long lead bursters provide the "desired maximal velocity signal" to the generator of rapid eye movements, then lesions in the rostral PPRF should selectively impair the stereotyped high velocity pattern of visually evoked saccades.

INTEGRATOR

Bilateral PPRF lesions in otherwise perfectly healthy Rhesus monkeys have given important new information about the integrator as well as about the saccadic burst generator. In collaboration with W. Lang experimental lesions were made in two monkeys, in which the pause region (Keller, 1974) was also affected; there were no longer any periods of fixation in the strict sense. Slow involuntary eye movements occurred in all directions, in particular vertically. The horizontal and the vertical burst generators were strongly affected, although when recording

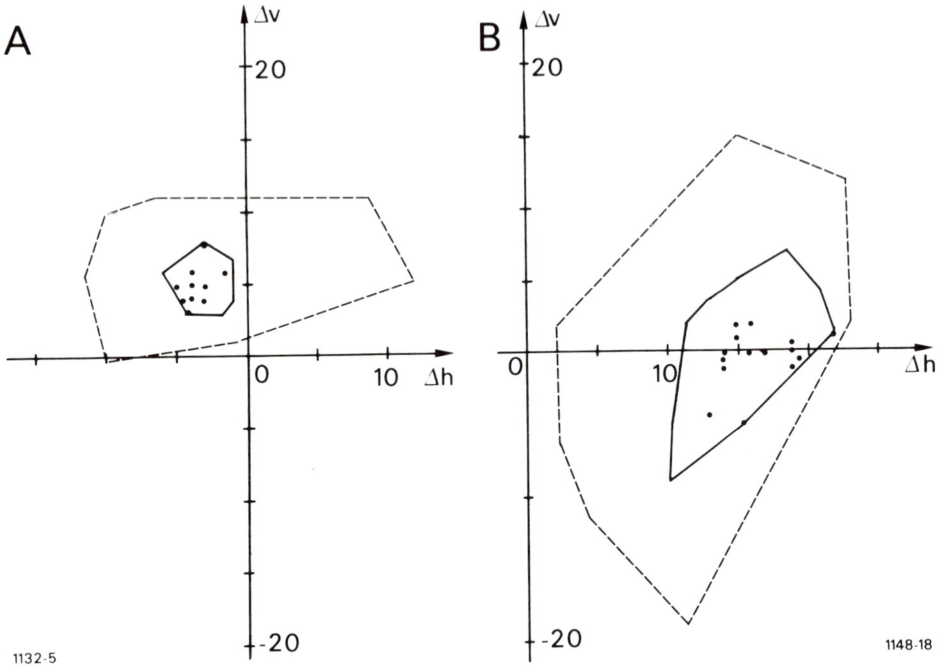

Fig. 5. Quantitative analysis of two long lead bursters with small and large saccade movement fields. In A and B the black dots correspond to saccades, where the number of spikes exceeds 3/4 of the maximal value, the black line encircles the half-maximal burst events while the broken line shows the just-visible events, where the instantaneous firing rate reaches half of the maximal value.

in the rostral iMLF one could still find burst neurons, which behaved like medium lead bursters in the drowsy monkey, with strongest discharge related to slow vertical pendular movements. One of the functions of the integrator is to provide the appropriate tonic input to the motoneurons during fixation. One sees from Fig. 6C that this function is not completely abolished: The eyes can be held in eccentric positions after a turn-table position step. They do not drift backwards towards midposition with anything near the time constant of about 0.2 sec typical for the oculomotor plant (Skavenski and Robinson, 1973). A second function of the (same or different) integrator is to produce from the velocity signal in the vestibular nuclei the appropriate combination of eye position and eye velocity signals for essentially compensatory eye movements in the frequency range of 0.1 to 5 Hz. The phase shift to be produced by the integrator in the range of 0.5 to 5 Hz has been estimated to decrease from about 40 to 20 degrees (Skavenski and Robinson, 1973). Figure 6 shows that for sinusoidal rotations with 3 deg amplitude the eye movements after a bilateral PPRF lesion are almost compensatory.

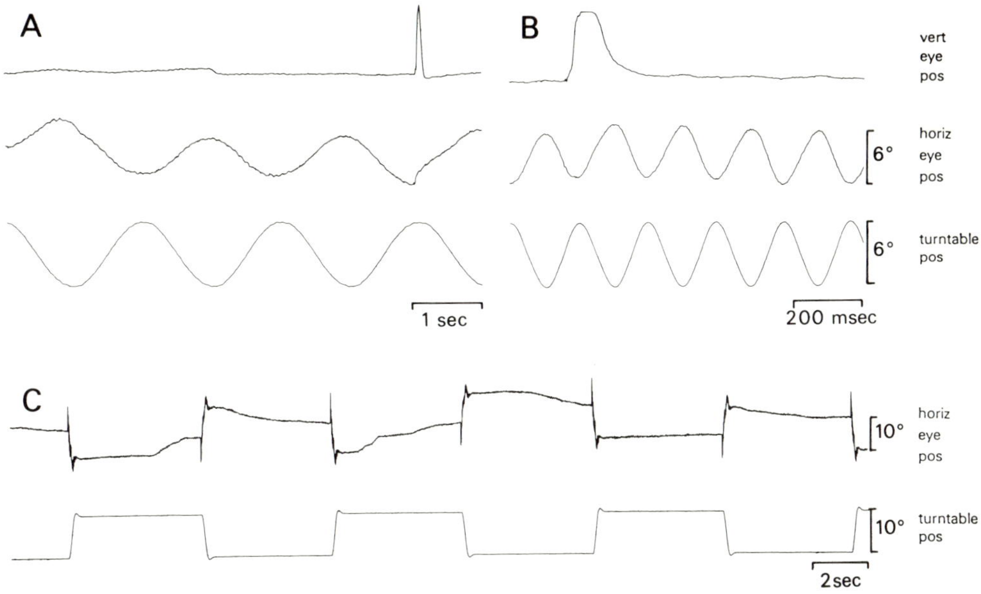

Fig. 6. Compensatory eye movements in a monkey with bilateral PPRF lesion which led to a loss of all rapid eye movements. The monkey was sinusoidally rotated about a vertical axis in complete darkness at 0.5 Hz (A) and 5 Hz (B) with 3 deg amplitude. In C the monkey was subjected to abrupt position changes of ± 10 deg, in the dark. The high head acceleration has produced transient artefacts in the EOG recording.

Summary: We expect the horizontal integrator to be a polysynaptic network of burst- (and/or pause-) tonic cells extending over most of the caudal oculomotor regions of the brainstem and the lateral cerebellar nuclei. Even with a larger bilateral lesion leading to a loss of all rapid eye movements the VOR can be close to compensatory over a wide range.

CONCLUSION

In the immediate premotor structures many parallel and recurrent pathways converge to produce the appropriate extraocular muscle innervation. Our results show that single unit recordings in the awake monkey and controlled lesions can help to estimate the importance of different oculomotor channels.

VERTICAL GAZE DISORDERS

R. J. LEIGH, S. A. NEWMAN and W. M. KING

Departments of Ophthalmology and Neurology, Johns Hopkins University, School of Medicine, Baltimore, Maryland, USA

ABSTRACT

We quantitatively studied the deficits of different functional classes of eye movements in selected patients with vertical gaze disorders. (1) Slow vertical saccades may be the only ocular motor abnormality early in the course of certain metabolic and degenerative diseases. This suggests that mesencephalic medium-lead burst cells may have properties that make them selectively vulnerable to these conditions. (2) Asymmetrical deficits of the vertical vestibulo-ocular reflex and vertical smooth pursuit may occur in patients with bilateral internuclear ophthalmoplegia. These findings suggest that ascending pathways besides the medial longitudinal fasciculus are important for upward vestibular and pursuit eye movements. (3) A patient with downgaze palsy had deficits that differed from those reported with experimental bilateral lesions of the pre-rubral fields and which suggested a total inability to modulate the activity of depressor ocular motor neurons. (4) A patient with vertical and horizontal saccadic oscillations (opsoclonus) showed relative independence of oscillations in the vertical and horizontal planes.

KEYWORDS

Vertical gaze palsy; slow saccades; progressive supranuclear palsy; Huntington's disease; vestibulo-ocular reflex; internuclear ophthalmoplegia; opsoclonus.

INTRODUCTION

Our first understanding of how the brain controls vertical eye movements came from clinical observation and clinico-pathological correlations. Disturbances of conjugate vertical gaze have been recognized for over a century (e.g. Henoch, 1864; Parinaud, 1883; Smith, 1876). It was apparent to these early investigators that when an inability to look up or down was unaccompanied by diplopia, nuclear oculomotor lesions could not be held responsible. As Holmes (1921) commented: "We are consequently, in my opinion, forced to the conclusion that, as in the case of the lateral conjugate rotators of the eyes, there are supranuclear mechanisms for upward and downward movements....".

Many aspects of these "supranuclear mechanisms" remain unknown. However, Henoch's report of a patient with a tuberculoma of the quadrigeminal plate directed attention to the midbrain. Spiller (1905) suggested that it was not the colliculi but rather the adjacent periaqueductal region that was important. A further insight into the organization of vertical gaze was given by Bender's (1960) observation that such eye movements appear to depend on bilateral innervation and that consequently vertical gaze palsies result from bilateral or midline lesions.

More recent advances in our understanding of vertical gaze mechanisms are mainly the result of basic research techniques. Studies of the effects of discrete lesions in the monkey have shown the posterior commissure and its interstitial nuclei to be important for upward gaze (Pasik, Pasik and Bender, 1969) and the region of the pre-rubral fields to be important for downward movements, particular saccades (Kompf and coworkers, 1979). Modern anatomical tracer techniques were used to define a cell group in the pre-rubral fields that has direct connections with ocular motor neurons -- the rostral interstitial nucleus of the medial longitudinal fasciculus, riMLF (Büttner-Ennever and Büttner, 1978). Electrophysiologic studies in the alert monkey showed cells in the region of the riMLF to be medium-lead burst neurons for vertical saccades (Büttner and coworkers, 1977; King and Fuchs, 1979). Another class of neurons that discharge in relation to vertical eye position and velocity were shown to be located in the mesencephalic reticular formation in and around the interstitial nucleus of Cajal (King, Fuchs and Magnin, 1981). The neural signals for vertical smooth pursuit and the vertical vestibulo-ocular reflex (VVOR) were shown to ascend from the caudal brain stem, at least in part, in the medial longitudinal fasciculus (King, Lisberger and Fuchs, 1976; Pola and Robinson, 1978). These findings are discussed further in the accompanying paper by King and Leigh.

Lacking a reliable method[1] for recording vertical eye movements, the clinician may seem hard-pressed to keep pace with these advances. Nevertheless, the effects of disease are remarkable in presenting insights into the neural control of eye movements. This paper presents the results of our study of selected patients showing vertical gaze disorders and reviews clinical reports by others. The approach will be to discuss the effects of certain conditions upon each of the various functional classes of eye movement, relating the findings to the known neural substrate.

Clinical Material and Methods

Eye movements were recorded from patients showing a variety of vertical gaze disorders and from seven healthy male volunteers (age range 23-73 years). A scleral search coil method was used to measure both eye and head movements (Collewijn, Van Der Mark and Jansen, 1974; Robinson, 1963). Data were recorded onto magnetic tape and displayed by a pen recorder for analysis. The bandwidth of this sytem was 0-70 Hz[2] and maximum sensitivity was 5 min of arc.

---

[1]Although photographic, infrared and electro-oculographic methods have been used to study vertical eye movements, technical difficults have prevented them from becoming popular for clinical studies. We have used the scleral search coil method (see methods) in over 50 patients and have found it generally well-tolerated and have encountered no complications.

[2]We checked our measurement of saccadic velocity, in selective instances, by photographing the oscilloscope image of eye movements (system bandwidth 0-160 Hz) and found no significant difference in the two sets of results.

Blinks were monitored by direct current electrooculography. Subjects and patients attempted fixation of an array of small light-emitting diodes. Pursuit eye movements were tested by asking the patient to track a small laser spot rear-projected onto a semi-translucent screen. This target was driven in a triangular waveform with velocities of up to 40 deg/sec and an amplitude of 10-30 degrees. For some patients, sine wave pursuit stimuli were also used. During pursuit eye movements, the head was held still. During combined eye-head tracking, the patient was encouraged to follow the target with the head. The magnetic coil system enabled measurement of eye in space (gaze) and head rotation during free head tracking. Vertical and horizontal vestibular responses were obtained by asking the patient to actively shake the head in either plane at a number of frequencies, while in darkness.

Saccades from normal subjects were analyzed for peak velocity/amplitude relationships. A linear regression analysis was performed after logarithmic transformation of both variables; 95% confidence limits were computed by standard methods (Fig. 1). Smooth pursuit gain (eye velocity/target velocity) was measured as the eye passed through the primary position.

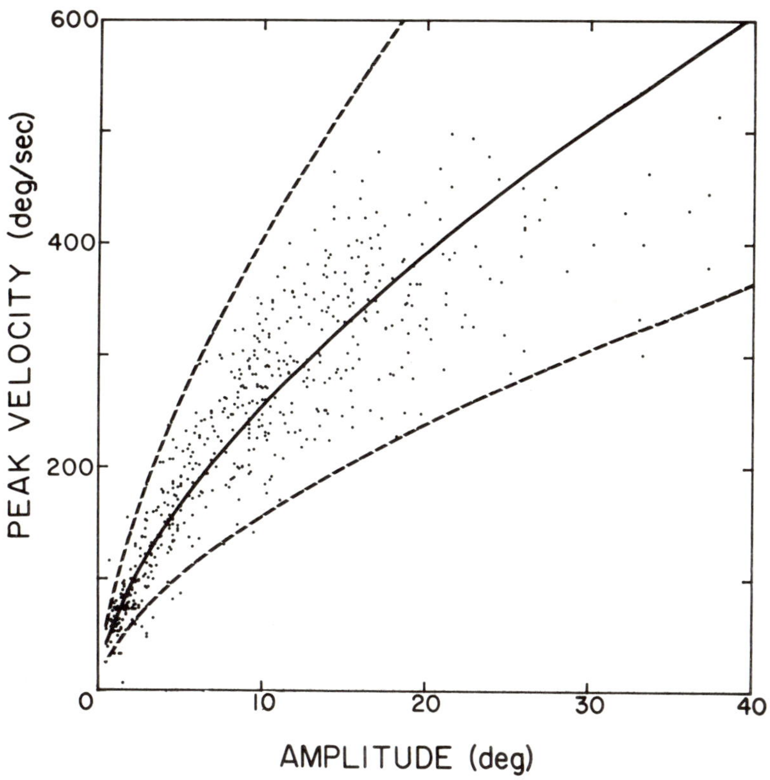

Fig. 1. Peak velocity/amplitude relationships of 609 vertical saccades from 7 normal subjects. The regression line and 95% confidence limits (broken lines) are shown. (A similar analysis was also performed for 274 horizontal saccades, pooled from the same subjects. The slopes of the regression lines from the two sets of data did not differ significantly, though the vertical saccades showed a greater scatter.)

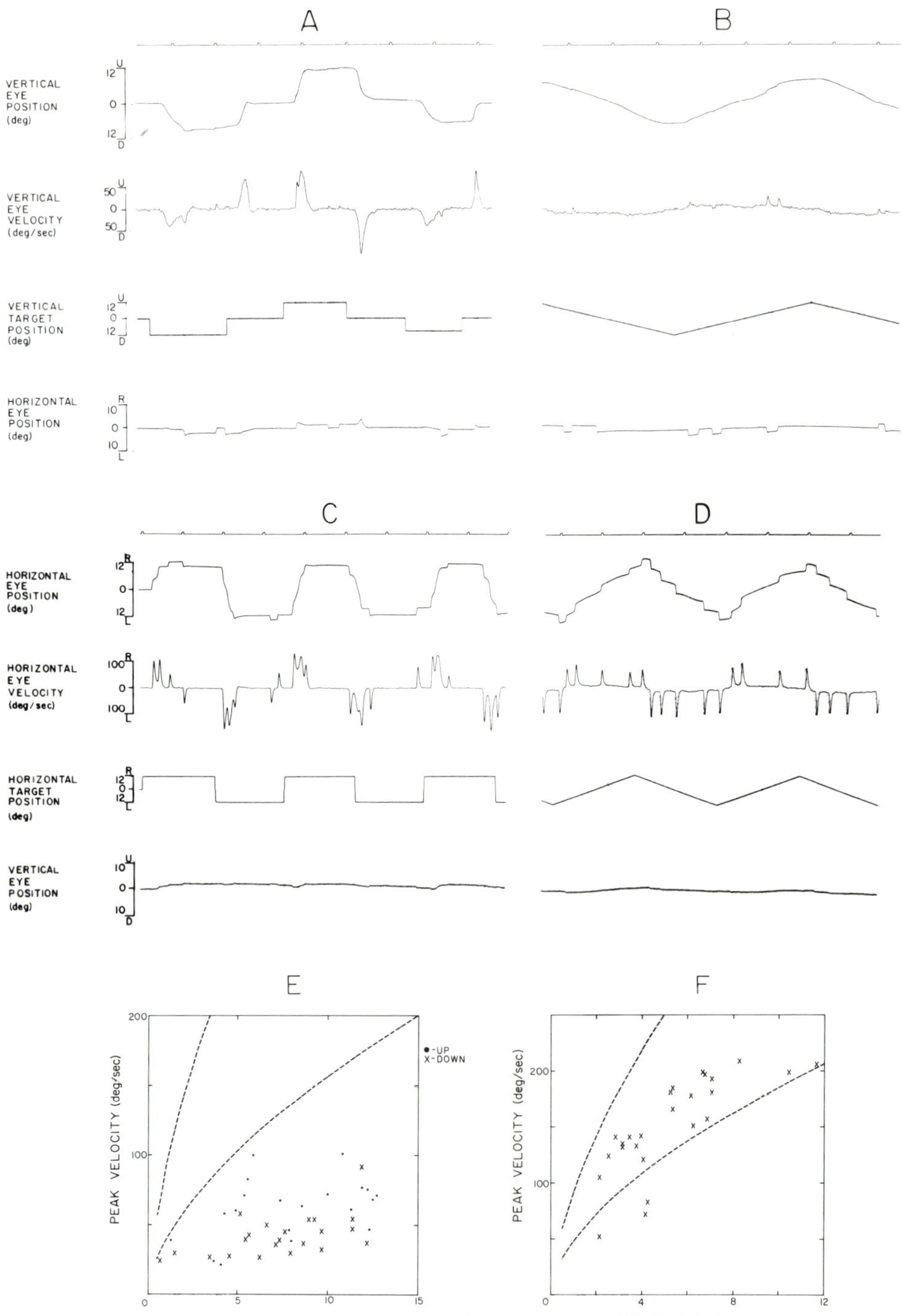

Fig. 2. The eye movements of a patient with progressive supranuclear palsy (see text).

Selective Abnormalities of Vertical Saccades

While destructive brain lesions (e.g. infarction) usually causes a combination of ocular motor deficits, certain metabolic and degenerative diseases of the nervous system are known to selectively impair "willed" eye movements. Certain such conditions -- for example, variants of Niemann-Pick disease (Neville and coworkers, 1973) and progressive supranuclear palsy (Steele, Richardson and Olszewski, 1964) -- principally affect vertical movements. An early sign of progressive supranuclear palsy may be a selective slowing of vertical saccades even when the range of movement is still full. Smooth pursuit may be preserved and the vestibulo-ocular reflex usually remains intact until late in the course of the disease.

Figure 2 shows the eye movements of a patient with progressive supranuclear palsy. Her vertical saccades are slow (Fig. 2A and E) but generally, orthometric. Eccentric gaze holding is not impaired. She is able to smoothly track a vertically-moving target (Fig. 2B) with only occasional small slow saccades evident on the velocity trace. During vertical smooth pursuit, horizontal square wave jerks occur -- "Gegenrücke" (Troost and Daroff, 1977). Horizontal saccades (Fig. 2C and F) are hypometric but are not slower than those of our control subjects. Horizontal smooth pursuit is deficient (Fig. 2D).

The earliest ocular motor deficit in progressive supranuclear palsy was originally described as a selective deficit in downward willed movements (Steele, Richardson and Olszewski, 1964). In fact, such patients may present with selective deficits of up or down saccades, though as the disease progresses, all vertical movements become affected. We have encountered a similar unidirectional vertical saccadic deficit in patients with early Huntington's chorea (Leigh and colleagues, 1981). Figure 3 shows peak velocity/amplitude analysis of vertical saccades from one such patient. His down saccades are slow while up saccades fall within our normal range. His horizontal saccades were also normal.

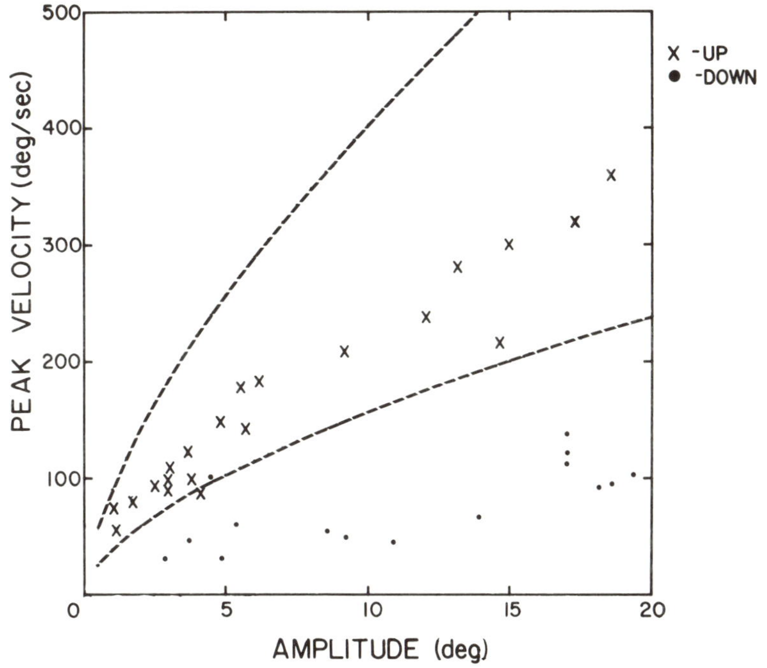

Fig. 3. See text.

What is the significance of such findings? To the basic scientist, the presence of slow vertical saccades but otherwise normal eye movements suggests a selective impairment of the substrate for saccades -- presumably mesencephalic medium-lead burst cells. Progressive supranuclear palsy is known to affect the brain stem reticulum (David, Mackey and Smith, 1968; Steele, Richardson and Olszewski, 1964) but similar involvement in Huntington's disease has yet to be clearly documented. The pathophysiology of the saccadic deficit is also unclear; perhaps the vigorous discharge rate that characterizes burst cells is paralleled by metabolic demands that cannot be met in these diseases. Another possibility is that the saccadic deficit reflects distinctive pharmacologic properties of burst cells. In any case, it is intriguing that subpopulations of neurons responsible for just vertical saccades, or even unidirectional (up or down) saccades may be impaired.[3] Another issue that might be studied is whether excitatory and inhibitory burst neurons are both affected by such processes. Electromyographic studies suggest that the inhibition of the antagonist muscle that occurs during normal saccades is faulty in progressive supranuclear palsy (Newman and coworkers, 1970; Pinhas and coworkers, 1978).

The explanation for the vertical saccadic hypometria in degenerative and metabolic diseases of the nervous system is unclear. Vertical saccadic hypometria also occurs in cerebellar degenerations (Zee and coworkers, 1976a and in Parkinson's disease (Corin, Elizan and Bender, 1972).

To clinicians, selective saccadic deficits may be of great importance. For example, it is possible that patients at risk for developing Huntington's chorea might be identified by careful analysis of saccadic velocity. This matter is currently under study at a number of centers.

Selective Abnormalities of the Vertical Vestibulo-Ocular Reflex (VVOR) and Vertical Smooth Tracking

Since the medial longitudinal fasciculus (MLF) conveys neural signals related to vertical head velocity, smooth pursuit eye velocity and eye position (King, Lisberger and Fuchs, 1976; Pola and Robinson, 1978) bilateral lesions of this fiber tract would be expected to produce corresponding ocular motor deficits. Experimental lesions of the MLF in monkeys (Evinger, Fuchs and Baker, 1977) and study of the deficits due to bilateral internuclear ophthalmoplegia in patients (Baloh, Yee and Honrubia, 1978a, 1978b) have shown decreased gain of the VVOR, impaired vertical smooth pursuit and vertical gaze holding but normal vertical saccades. However, the MLF is not the only ascending pathway conveying vertical eye movement signals. Study of the up-down symmetry of such deficits might suggest the role of other pathways such as the brachium conjunctivum (Chubb and Fuchs, 1981; Ghelarducci, Highstein and Ito, 1977; King and Leigh, this symposium; Stanton, 1980).

We have studied the VVOR in two patients with partial bilateral internuclear ophthalmoplegia, due to multiple sclerosis. We measured the gain of the reflex during active head shaking, at about 1 Hz in darkness. Our normal subjects showed symmetrical up/down responses with typical gain values of 0.95. In one patient, precise quantitation was confounded by the presence of a resting downbeating nystagmus; it was on the order of 0.5. In the other patient, the gain could be

---

[3] Certain other diseases (e.g. Gaucher's disease and olivopontocerebellar atrophy typically disturb horizontal before vertical eye movements (Leigh and Zee, 1982).

accurately quantitated and was 0.75 for upward compensatory eye movements, but 0.64 for downward compensatory eye movements, the difference being statistically significant ($p < 0.05$). Of course, it is possible that demyelinative lesions disseminated in other neural pathways were responsible for this asymmetry of the VVOR. However, Jenkyn, Margolis and Reeves (1978) studied a patient with autopsy-verified bilateral MLF lesions due to infarction and found a similar asymmetry of vestibular responses.

We also studied the vertical smooth pursuit gains for a range of target velocities in our patient and compared results with our control subjects (Fig. 4).

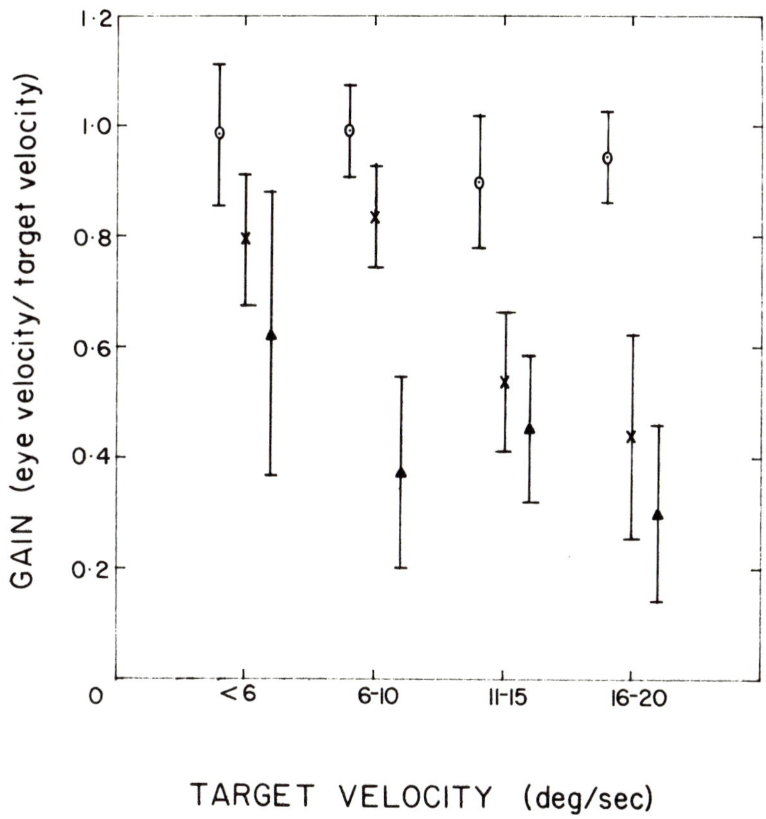

Fig. 4. Comparison of vertical smooth pursuit in a patient with bilateral internuclear ophthalmoplegia and our control subjects. Mean gain (± S.D.) for several ranges of target velocity are shown. Control subjects pursuit gains (⊙), for the range of testing, was similar for tracking up and down. The patients pursuit gains for tracking up (X) and down (▲) are shown.

Especially for slower target velocities, pursuit gains during tracking of targets moving down were lower than corresponding values during tracking up; both were deficient compared with controls.

During combined eye-head tracking (during which subjects and patients were encouraged to follow the target with head movements) our patient with bilateral MLF lesions tracked much better and gain values (gaze velocity/target velocity) were not greatly different from some of our control subjects. This might be because the deficient VVOR was more easily cancelled or suppressed by the pursuit command. Additional findings in our two patients were impaired vertical gaze holding, but normal saccadic peak velocity/amplitude relationships.

In summary, these results and those of others suggest that the MLF may be more concerned with downward VVOR and vertical smooth pursuit than corresponding upward movements. Alternate pathways such as the brachium conjunctivum may be relatively concerned with upward movements (King and Leigh, this symposium). Further quantitative studies are required to confirmed these findings.

Total Paralysis of Up or Down Gaze

Total inability to move the eyes above the horizontal meridian is not uncommon. It is perhaps most frequently caused by tumors of the pineal region or acute hydrocephalus. Selective paralysis of downgaze is rare but has been documented by a number of authors (e.g. Cogan, 1974; Halmagyi, Evans and Hallinan, 1978; Jacobs, Anderson and Bender, 1973; Thomas, Schaefer and Bertrans, 1933; Trojanowski and Wray, 1980). The usual cause is bilateral infarction at the mesencephalic-diencephalic junction.

We have studied . 20 year old male with a low grade thalamic glioma who, following radiation therapy, developed a vasculitic reaction that lead to a hemorrhage affecting the thalamus and adjacent midbrain. After treatment of hydrocephalus, he made a slow recovery, but was left with total loss of eye movements below the horizontal meridian. Vergence movements and pupillary responses were absent. He also had a short-term memory deficit and somnolence and therefore showed similarities to the patients described by Segarra (1970) and Mills and Swanson (1978). His eye movements are shown in Fig. 5.

Upward saccades were slow (Fig. 5A and C) and he had difficulty in maintaining upward gaze with his eyes drifting back to the horizontal meridian. Down saccades were small and very slow. By contrast, his horizontal saccades showed normal peak velocity/amplitude relationships. Smooth pursuit within the intact upper field of gaze was partially preserved for tracking of slow targets (Fig. 5B). His VVOR gain (during active head pitch in darkness) was 0.8 within the persisting range of eye movement.

What might the findings in this patient tell us about the organization of up and down gaze? One tentative explanation is that the slow upward saccades and drift towards primary position were due to lack of any modulation in the antagonist (depressor) muscles. In any case, the deficit of our patient and that of others (e.g. Halmagyi, Evans and Hallinan, 1978; Jacobs, Anderson and Bender, 1973; Trojanowski and Wray, 1980), i.e. total downgaze palsy, is not that produced by experimental bilateral lesions of the riMLF in the monkey (Kompf and coworkers, 1979). In that case, the downward deficit was mainly saccadic with preservation of some downward movement on vertical head rotation and, in some monkeys, some preservation of downward pursuit. The inability of vestibular stimuli to drive our patients eyes below the horizontal meridian need not necessarily imply that the "elementary" disynaptic vestibular reflex arc was disrupted. An alternate explanation is that this deficit was due to impairment of indirect reticular pathways -- as was emphasised by Lorente de No (1933).

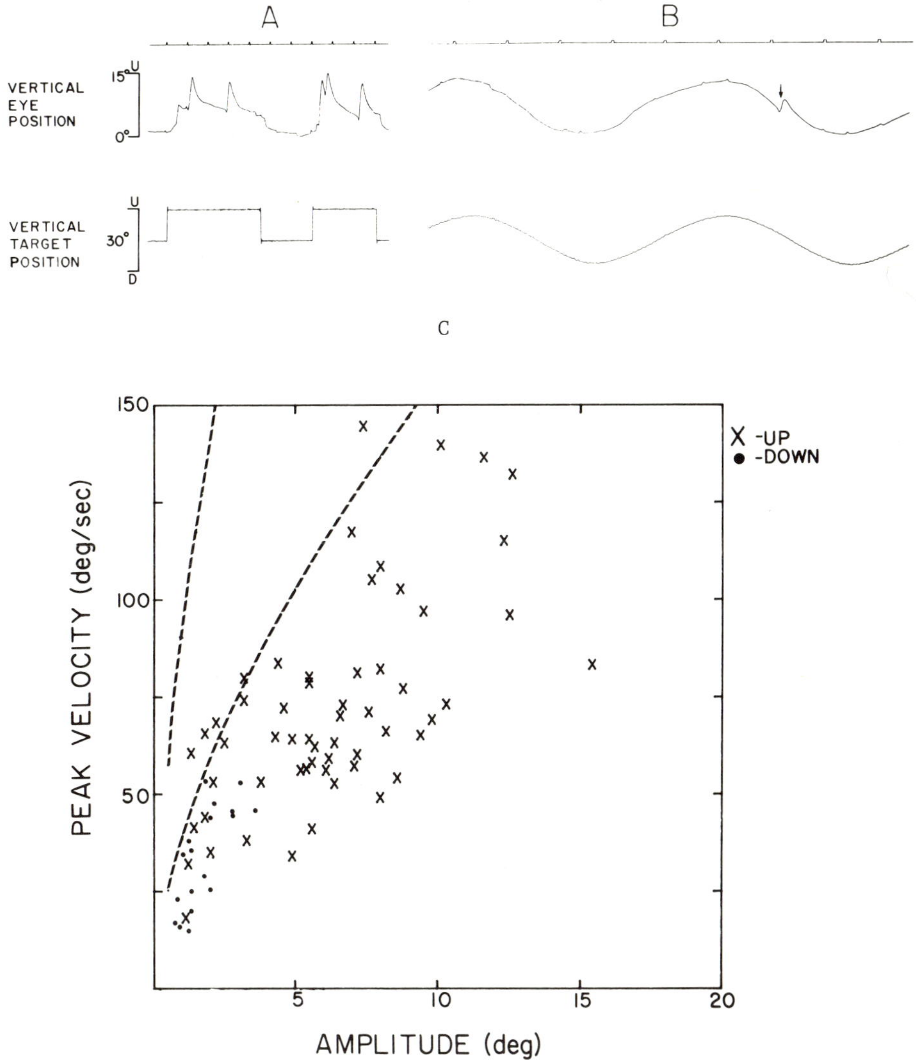

Fig. 5. The eye movements of a patient with a total downgaze palsy -- see text (arrow in B indicates blink artifact).

<u>Horizontal Eye Movement Abnormalities That Frequently Co-Exist with Vertical Gaze Disorders: The Interaction of Vertical and Horizontal Eye Movements</u>

Commonly, vertical gaze disorders are accompanied by abnormalities of horizontal eye movements. Some of these (e.g. square wave jerks) are unexplained, but others give us insight into certain interactions between eye movements in the horizontal and vertical planes. Vergence eye movements are frequently impaired with vertical gaze palsy. They are to be differentiated from convergence or convergence-retraction nystagmus which has recently been shown, in one patient, to consist of slightly asynchronous, opposed adducting saccades (Ochs and coworkers, 1979).

The majority of saccades in normal individuals are oblique (i.e.) have both horizontal and vertical components. What do disease states tell us about this interaction? Firstly, the observation that bilateral pontine lesions may cause disturbance of vertical eye movements, particularly saccades (Hennerici and Fromm, 1981) has received a possible anatomic substrate with the demonstration of a pathway from the paramedian pontine reticular formation to the riMLF (Büttner-Ennever and Büttner, 1978). Secondly, oblique saccades in a patient with slow horizontal but relatively normal vertical saccades due to spinocerebellar degeneration have been studied (Zee and coworkers, 1976 a). The trajectory of these movements was notable in that the vertical component finished before the horizontal and thus the final part of the movement was purely horizontal. Finally, we have studied a 55 year old woman who showed saccadic oscillations, without an intersaccadic interval, in all three planes (horizontal, vertical and torsional -- although we could not measure the last of these). Her "opsoclonus" (Cogan, 1956; Gresty, Findley and Wade, 1980; Zangemeister, Muller-Jensen and Zschocke, 1979) was presumed to be a remote effect of an occult neoplasm. The rapid oscillations (Fig. 6) had peak velocity/amplitude relationships which were similar to normal horizontal and vertical saccades.

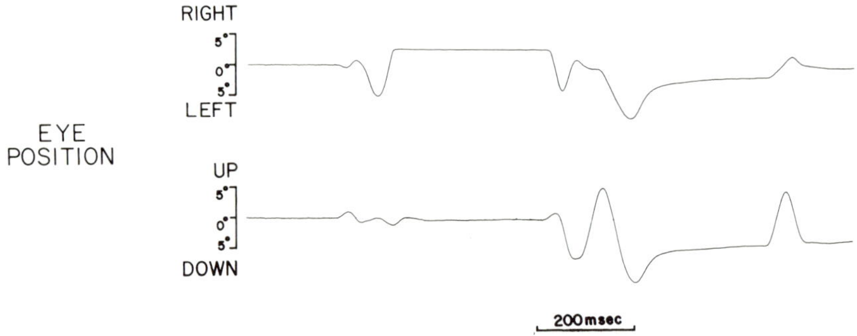

Fig. 6. Record of saccadic oscillations.

The horizontal and vertical components of her oscillations seemed relatively -- but not completely -- independent of each other. The result was apparent clinically as rapid eye movements that took crescentic or circuitous trajectories. Taken together, these results indicate that although the horizontal and vertical saccadic systems are (and have to be) closely anatomically and physiologically linked, each has separate properties that became evident in certain disease states.

ACKNOWLEDGEMENTS

We are grateful to M. Marvin Newhouse and Argye I. Hillis of the Biostatistical Center for help with our saccadic analyses, to Adrian G. Lasker for technical support and to Vendetta Matthews for editorial assistance. Supported by National Institutes of Health Grants AG00061 and 1 P01-NS-16375 (Dr. Leigh) EY07047 (Dr. Newman), EY02717 (Dr. King) and a core grant to the Wilmer Institute (EY01765).

PHYSIOLOGY OF VERTICAL GAZE

W. M. KING and R. J. LEIGH

The Wilmer Institute and the Department of Neurology, The Johns Hopkins University, School of Medicine, Baltimore, Maryland, USA

ABSTRACT

The rostral interstitial nucleus of the medial longitudinal fasciculus (riMLF) is thought to be part of a vertical saccade generating network. Consistent with this suggestion, unilateral riMLF lesions, made with kainic acid, caused a reduction in the frequency of occurrence of vertical saccades or vestibular quick phases.

The interstitial nucleus of Cajal (INC) is thought to be part of a neural integrating network for the vertical vestibulo-ocular reflex (VOR). Consistent with this suggestion, downward post rotatory nystagmus was abolished by unilateral kainic acid lesions of the INC.

KEYWORDS

Vertical eye movements; vestibulo-ocular reflex; nystagmus; vertical saccades; kainic acid lesions; interstitial nucleus of Cajal; rostral interstitial nucleus of the medial longitudinal fasciculus; cat eye movements.

INTRODUCTION

In the clinic, vertical gaze disorders may be as common as horizontal gaze disorders, but their diagnostic usefulness is limited because of the relative difficulty in recording vertical eye movements, and because the underlying physiology is less well understood. In recent years, however, three technical advances have vastly increased our understanding of the physiology of vertical gaze: 1) the scleral search coil method has increased the accuracy of our recordings of vertical eye movements (Robinson, 1963), 2) single neuron recordings from alert animals have provided supportive evidence for premotor vertical gaze centers in the midbrain (Buettner and co-workers, 1977; King and Fuchs, 1979; King and co-workers, 1981), and 3) the neural pathways linking these centers to each other and to the various oculomotor nuclei can now be mapped using highly sensitive anatomical tracer substances (Buettner-Ennever and Buettner, 1978; Graybiel, 1977; Steiger and Buettner-Ennever, 1979). Using these techniques, researchers have produced new evidence leading to specific hypotheses about the neural circuitry underlying vertical gaze. In this report, the evidence implicating two midbrain structures, the rostral interstitial nucleus of the medial longitudinal fasciculus (riMLF) and the interstitial nucleus of Cajal (INC) in vertical gaze control will be critically reviewed in conjunction with new experimental findings from our laboratory. Impairment of normal activity in these nuclei may partially account for the vertical gaze deficits discussed in the accompanying paper (Leigh and co-workers, this volume).

PHYSIOLOGY OF VERTICAL SACCADES

The high velocities characteristic of saccadic eye movements are produced by a high frequency burst of spikes in agonist motoneurons, and a pause or cessation of activity in antagonist motoneurons. For horizontal saccades the required excitatory or inhibitory inputs are produced in the paramedian pontine reticular formation (PPRF) and medulla respectively by excitatory or inhibitory burst neurons that have monosynaptic connections with motor and internuclear neurons in the abducens nucleus (Hepp and Henn, this volume). For vertical saccades, the evidence suggests that the excitatory and inhibitory inputs are produced by another population of burst neurons located in the midbrain rostral to the oculomotor nucleus. Cell loss or lowered discharge rates caused by various degenerative diseases may underlie the selective slowing of vertical saccades described in the accompanying paper (Leigh and co-workers, this volume).

The evidence for this hypothesis is suggestive but not yet conclusive. Burst cells with discharge patterns related to up or downward components of saccades were recorded in the monkey's riMLF, in the mesencephalic reticular formation, and in the rostral periaqueductal gray (Buettner and co-workers, 1977; King and Fuchs, 1979). Retrograde tracers injected into the oculomotor or trochlear nuclei labelled cells in the riMLF (Graybiel, 1977; Steiger and Buettner-Ennever, 1979), but these experiments did not demonstrate that the labelled cells were burst neurons or that they synapsed on oculomotor neurons. It is disconcerting that the reported locations of labelled cells were not coextensive with the recording sites of burst neurons. Few burst neurons, for example, were reported in the INC which was heavily labelled, and few labelled cells were reported in the mesencephalic reticular formation or periaqueductal gray where many burst cells were recorded. Lesion experiments help to correlate these anatomical and physiological data. Koempf and co-workers (1979) showed that bilateral electrolytic lesions of the monkey's midbrain, centered in the riMLF, led to downward gaze deficits characterized by an apparent inability to produce downward saccades or quick phases. This finding is consistent with the notion that riMLF burst neurons produce downward saccades and quick phases. Unilateral lesions, however, were reported not to cause any observable deficit in saccadic eye movements. This finding is somewhat strange, since one would expect that destruction of about 50% of the burst neurons in a burst generator would at least noticeably decrease the velocity of vertical saccades and quick phases. Slow saccades would, however, be difficult to detect from heavily filtered EOG records. The interpretation of these data was also confounded by the fact that an electrolytic lesion necessarily destroys en passage axons as well as cell somata, so that any deficit might be due to loss of fibers as well as cells. In fact, Leichnetz (1981) has suggested that some of the deficits be attributed to destruction of frontal cortical axons en route to the superior colliculus, the midbrain oculomotor centers, and the oculomotor nucleus itself. In order to resolve some of these problems, we recently conducted our own midbrain lesion study, but with two significant technical improvements: first, our experimental subjects were cats equipped with scleral search coils for accurate recording of vertical eye movements; and second, our lesions were made with a neurotoxin, kainic acid, believed to be highly toxic to cell somata but not to en passage fibers (Coyle and co-workers, 1978; Masterton and co-workers, 1979; Peterson and Moore, 1980; Wuerthele and co-workers, 1978). Our injection sites were unilateral and centered in the INC. In early experiments, however, extensive cell losses occurred in the riMLF as well. Immediately after a unilateral midbrain lesion, the cats presented a consistent clinical picture: head tilt opposite the lesion, paucity of vertical saccades and quick phases up or down, and an impaired vertical VOR. Figure 1 illustrates the typical pattern of the saccade deficit in a cat with a unilateral midbrain lesion. Saccades and quick phases were shown in the figure as vectors in polar coordinates. The saccade data were obtained with the animal looking about the room, the quick phase data were obtained during pitch in the dark. Before the lesion (Fig. 1, left) the eye movement vectors were more or less radially symmetric, showing that the animal made eye movements of about the same size in any direction. One week after the lesion (Fig. 1, right), most of the eye movements were horizontal, but when vertical components did occur, they were rather small. Cats were followed up to 5 weeks after the lesion. There was partial recovery of spontaneous vertical saccades and quick phases so that on clinical examination the animals appeared to be normal. However, during comparison of spontaneous eye movement records or periods

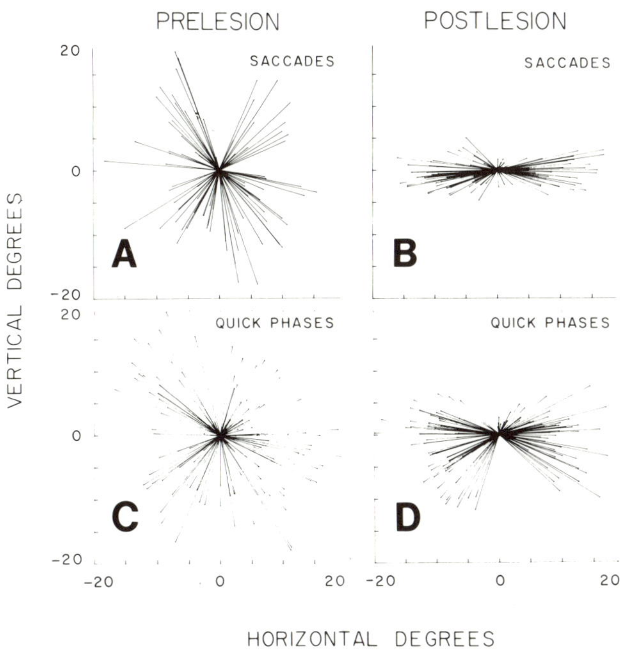

Fig. 1. Vertical saccade deficit following midbrain lesion. Details in text.

of vestibular nystagmus (see Fig. 5 below), it was evident that the frequency of occurrence of rapid vertical eye movements was reduced. Visual inspection of eye movement records also suggested that vertical saccades were slowed following the lesion as would be expected if the midbrain burst neurons produced the innervation pulse for vertical saccades. A similar saccade deficit in cats with midbrain lesions was described 40 years ago by Szentágothai (1943). These preliminary results suggest that the deficits described by earlier studies were in fact due to cell losses thereby supporting the notion that the midbrain, especially the portion containing the riMLF, contains burst generators for vertical saccades. There remain, however, two unresolved but significant questions. First, if the riMLF contains only down gaze cells, where then are the up gaze cells and why were they not labelled by the tracer studies? Second, are excitatory and inhibitory burst cells mixed together, or are they anatomically separated as in the horizontal system?

PHYSIOLOGY OF THE VERTICAL VESTIBULO-OCULAR REFLEX (VVOR)

The VVOR is an oculomotor response to angular accelerations of the head in the sagittal plane. When the head pitches forward, anterior canal receptors are bilaterally excited and posterior canal receptors disfacilitated, producing compensatory upward eye movements (up VOR). When the head pitches backward, posterior canal receptors are excited and anterior canal receptors disfacilitated, producing compensatory downward eye movements (down VOR). Head rotations in the sagittal plane also excite otolith receptors giving rise to an otolith-ocular reflex that is synergistic with the canal reflex. In the light, the optokinetic reflex complements canal and otolith reflexes.

Although the horizontal VOR is symmetric to the left or right of the midline, there are reports in the literature suggesting that the vertical VOR may be asymmetric (Collins and co-workers, 1970; Money and Scott, 1962; Matsuo and co-workers, 1979). Preliminary to our midbrain lesion study, we examined the VVOR in normal cats. We attempted to isolate the separate contributions of the canal, otolith-ocular, and optokinetic reflexes. Canal induced eye movements were isolated by placing the cats on their sides and rotating them about an earth vertical axis in the dark. In this position, the canals were stimulated as in pitch, but the otoliths were not since the direction of gravity acting on the maculae was constant.

The cats were subjected to constant velocity steps ranging from 15 to 120 deg/sec. Figure 2 shows representative post rotatory responses to velocity steps in the dark. On the left, up VOR slow phase velocities were plotted as a function of time. For the largest step (120 deg/sec), the slow phase velocity decayed over more than 30 seconds implying a time constant of about 10 seconds. A 10 second time constant is about twice the cupula time constant for the cat as estimated from primary afferent data (Anderson and co-workers, 1978). In contrast, for the down VOR plotted on the right, the entire post rotatory response was over within 17 seconds for the 120 deg/sec step implying a time constant less than 6 seconds, only slightly more than the estimated cupula time constant. The VOR gain, estimated from the initial slow phase velocity, was about 0.5 in either direction. These results show a two to one difference between the time constants governing the up and down VORs evoked by exciting anterior or posterior canal receptors. This asymmetry was previously observed in cat (Darlot and co-workers, 1981), in monkey (Matsuo and co-workers, 1979) and man (King and Leigh, unpublished results).

The time constant governing the horizontal VOR is also much larger than the cupula time constant. To account for the extended time constant, Raphan and co-workers

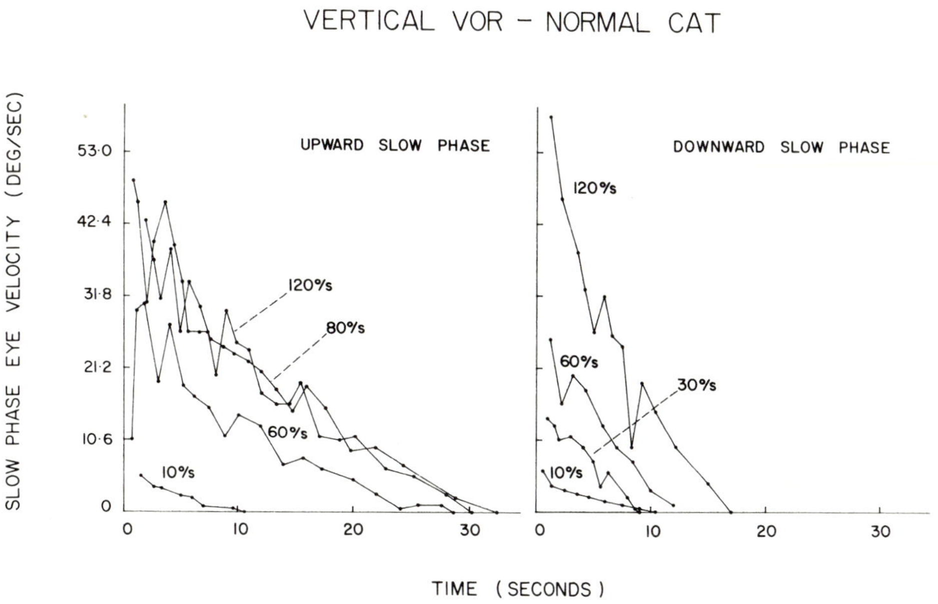

Fig. 2. Post rotatory vertical vestibular nystagmus. Details in text.

(1979) proposed the existence of a velocity storage mechanism internal to the VOR. Robinson (1977) had previously achieved the same result with a model employing a positive feedback loop. Whatever the actual neural mechanism, the extended time constant governing the up VOR is likely to be produced by neural circuitry analogous to that postulated for the horizontal VOR. In contrast, there appears to be little or no velocity storage in the down VOR.

The horizontal velocity storage element is shared by the VOR and the optokinetic reflex. Optokinetic after nystagmus (OKAN) and post rotatory vestibular nystagmus are both produced by the discharge of the same velocity storage mechanism and have, therefore, the same time constant of decay (but see Skavenski and Westheimer, 1981). To determine if the vertical VOR (at least in the up direction) is organized in a similar fashion, we tested vertical OKN and OKAN responses with the cats on their sides by rotating an OKN drum about a vertical axis around them. OKN velocity steps were simulated by rotating the drum in darkness to constant velocity, and then switching the light on or off. Figure 3 shows representative responses to up or down OKN steps. As with the VVOR, the cat's vertical OKN responses were clearly asymmetrical; in the up direction eye velocity followed drum velocity up to about 30 degrees/sec, but in the down direction, the response saturated at less than 5 degrees/sec and may have been entirely smooth pursuit. Up OKAN decayed with about the same time constant as the up VOR, but down OKAN in this cat was too small to estimate a time constant. Data from other cats, however, suggest that OKAN and VOR time constants were about equal in either direction. In summary, the time constant of the up VOR, like the horizontal VOR, is extended, and the prolonged time constant is associated with strong OKN and OKAN responses,

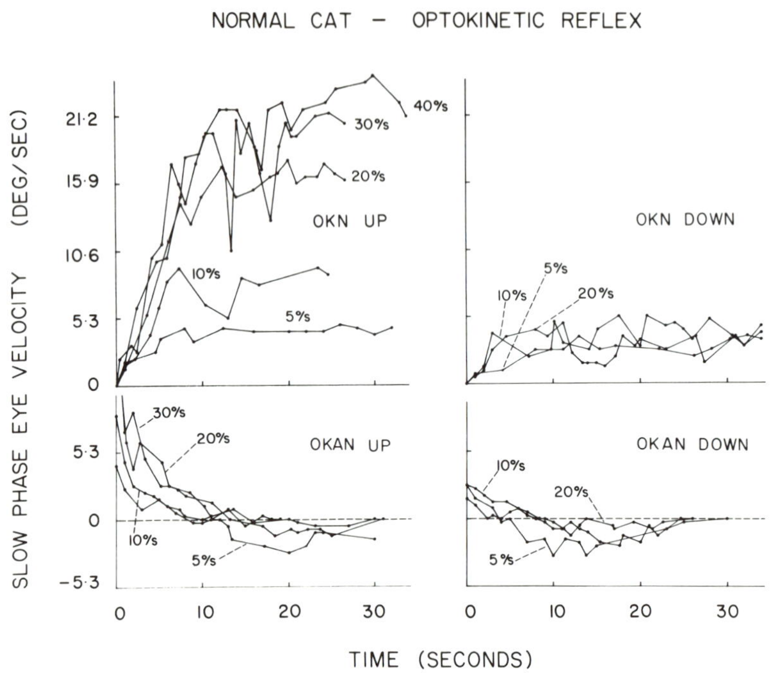

Fig. 3. Vertical OKN and OKAN. Details in text.

suggesting a velocity storage mechanism for up gaze involving shared visual-vestibular pathways. On the other hand, the time constant of the down VOR is only slightly larger than the cupula time constant, and this short time constant is associated with weak OKN and OKAN responses, suggesting much less velocity storage for down gaze.

Figure 4 shows that there are significant differences in the central pathways used by the up and down VORs that might account for the physiological differences. For either reflex, there is a 3-neuron pathway from the peripheral receptor cell via the vestibular nuclei to the extraocular motoneuron. From the vestibular nuclei, there are excitatory and inhibitory ascending branches for each reflex but the pathways are different. For the up VOR, the vestibular relay cells are located in the superior vestibular nucleus (SVN), but the excitatory ascending projection is via the brachium conjunctivum (BC), and the inhibitory projection is via the MLF. For the down VOR, the inhibitory relay cells are in the SVN, but the excitatory cells are located in the medial vestibular nucleus, and all the ascending projections are in the MLF. Most of the evidence for these pathways has been gathered in the rabbit. However, single unit recordings from monkey SVN reveal a preponderance of up gaze cells (Tomlinson and Robinson, unpublished data) and recordings from MLF fibers (King and co-workers, 1976; Pola and Robinson, 1978) reveal a preponderance of down gaze cells consistent with Fig. 4. The single unit recordings from MLF fibers or from vestibular nucleus neurons suggest that the relay cells transmit a complex signal related to eye position and velocity and to head velocity. These cells are called tonic-vestibular-pause (TVP)

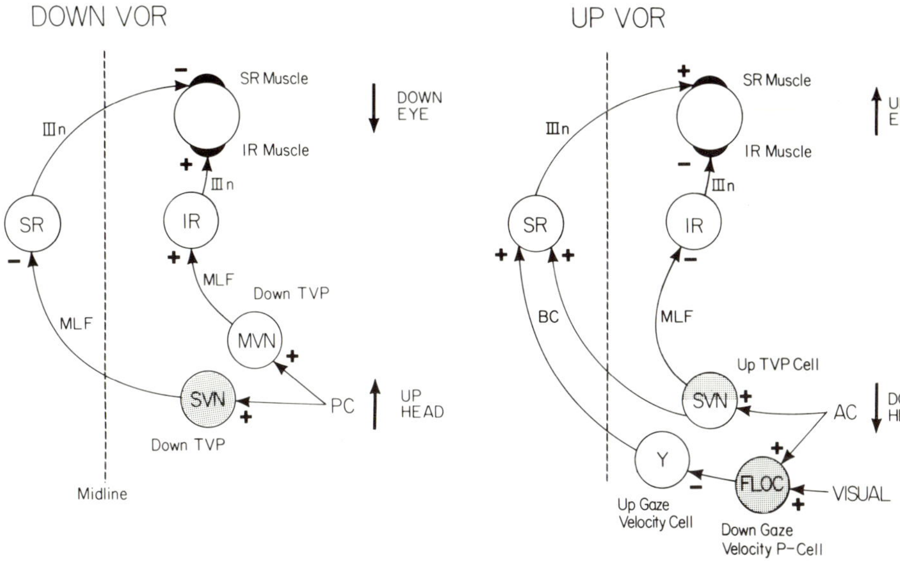

Fig. 4. Vertical VOR pathways. Details in text.

cells. Bilateral MLF lesions cause severe vertical gaze deficits consistent with the loss of this signal -- an inability to maintain eccentric vertical gaze positions, loss of the VVOR, and impaired smooth pursuit. Figure 4 suggests that the deficit should be more severe for down gaze, as discussed by Leigh and co-workers (this volume).

The up VOR has also an additional excitatory pathway from Y-group cells to the superior rectus muscle (Ghelarducci and co-workers, 1977; Yamamoto and co-workers, 1978). Recordings from the Y-group in alert monkeys have shown that it contains a population of cells that encode up gaze velocity (Chubb and Fuchs, 1981; Tomlinson and Robinson, unpublished data). Since the BC is believed to carry only excitatory fibers (Ito and co-workers, 1976), up gaze cells could feed forward an upward eye velocity signal to the superior rectus muscle that would add to the signal carried by the TVP cell. The flocculus, which receives both visual and vestibular inputs, also projects heavily to the Y-group, and contains a population of down gaze, but not up gaze, Purkinje cells (Miles and co-workers, 1980). Since these cells are inhibitory, they are functionally part of the up gaze system, and this pathway may account for the selective depression of the up VOR observed when the flocculus is electrically stimulated (Ito and co-workers, 1977). Comparable pathways for the down VOR have not been demonstrated. It is tempting to speculate that this additional pathway in the up gaze system, involving the Y-group, may be part of the velocity storage mechanism that accounts for the extended time constant of the up VOR. Although such a system may exist for the down VOR, the anatomical and physiological evidence suggest it is not very important.

Figure 4 is incomplete in a rather significant way because it does not include any midbrain pathways in the VVOR. Neither the TVP signal carried by MLF fibers (or by BC fibers for the up VOR), nor the gaze velocity signal carried by the BC would produce a normal VOR if applied in isolation to oculomotoneurons. Either of these signals encode head or eye velocity, and must be integrated to produce an eye position signal. In accord with earlier ideas of Lorente de Nó (1933), Robinson (1975a)proposed that the integration occur in a parallel reticular pathway linking the vestibular nuclei with the oculomotor nuclei. In the horizontal gaze system the so called neural integrator is presumed to lie in the PPRF or in the nucleus prepositus hypoglossus (Hepp and Henn, this volume). In the vertical system, we suggest that the neural integrator is located, at least in part, in the INC. The evidence for this assumption is mostly anatomical. Retrograde tracers injected into the oculomotor complex label cells in the INC, confirming earlier degeneration studies (Graybiel, 1977; Graybiel and Hartweig, 1974; Steiger and Buettner-Ennever, 1979). Electrical stimulation centered in the INC evokes monosynaptic EPSP-IPSPs in trochlear motoneurons (Schwindt and co-workers, 1974), although this result could be attributed to stimulation of en passage axons from other parts of the brain (e.g., the riMLF). The INC also has efferent connections with the spinal cord (Fukushima and co-workers, 1978; Mabuchi and Kusama, 1970; Pompeiano and Walberg, 1958; Walberg, 1974), the vestibular nucleus (Mabuchi and Kusama, 1970; Markham and co-workers, 1966; Pompeiano and Walberg, 1958), the perihypoglossal nucleus (Mabuchi and Kusama, 1970; Pompeiano and Walberg, 1958), the PPRF (Mabuchi and Kusama, 1970; Schwindt and co-workers, 1974), and the inferior olive (Mabuchi and Kusama, 1970; Walberg, 1974), and receives afferents from the frontal eye fields (King and co-workers, 1980 b; Leichnetz, 1981; Szentágothai, 1943), vestibular nuclei (Gacek, 1971; King and co-workers, 1980b;Szentágothai, 1943), and the prepositus nucleus (Hikosaka and Igusa, 1980). In the alert monkey, single unit studies have shown that the INC contains burst tonic eye movement neurons with vertical preferred directions that carry an integrated eye position signal (King and co-workers, 1981). Taken together, this evidence strongly suggests a major role for the INC in the control of vertical gaze, and the extensive anatomical connections are certainly consistent with those expected of a neural integrating network. However, as with the riMLF, there is a problem of relating anatomy to function. Although there is suggestive evidence that INC burst tonic cells receive vestibular inputs (King and co-workers, 1980), there is as yet no demonstration that these cells project to vertical oculomotor neurons and are, therefore, the output elements of a neural integrator. In fact, in seeming contradiction to this idea, the oculomotor and postural deficits attributed to lesions of the INC in primates have been reported as inconsequential. Carpenter and co-workers' (1970) excellent anatomical study in the monkey has been particularly influential, and is cited as evidence that the INC only plays a minor role in vertical gaze control (e.g. Trojanowski and Wray, 1980). However, this study was primarily an anatomical investigation, and the oculomotor observations were based entirely on qualitative clinical examinations. Eye movements were not recorded, nor were vestibular function tests other than calorics employed. Without quantitative evidence, it is quite possible that physiologically significant eye movement deficits escaped detection. For example, the monkeys were observed to make vertical saccades after the lesion, but were the frequency of occurrence, latency, accuracy, and temporal characteristics of these saccades normal? Evidently, the animals responded to caloric tests, but were the gain and phase of the separate up and down VORs normal? If the INC were part of a vertical eye velocity to position integrator, one would expect gaze holding deficits in the dark, and significantly increased VOR phase leads. Either of these deficits would be easily overlooked in clinical examinations.

Our midbrain lesion study using kainic acid was designed to test the idea that the INC was part of a neural integrator for vertical eye movements. Our results show that unilateral INC lesions do cause gaze defects partially consistent with the

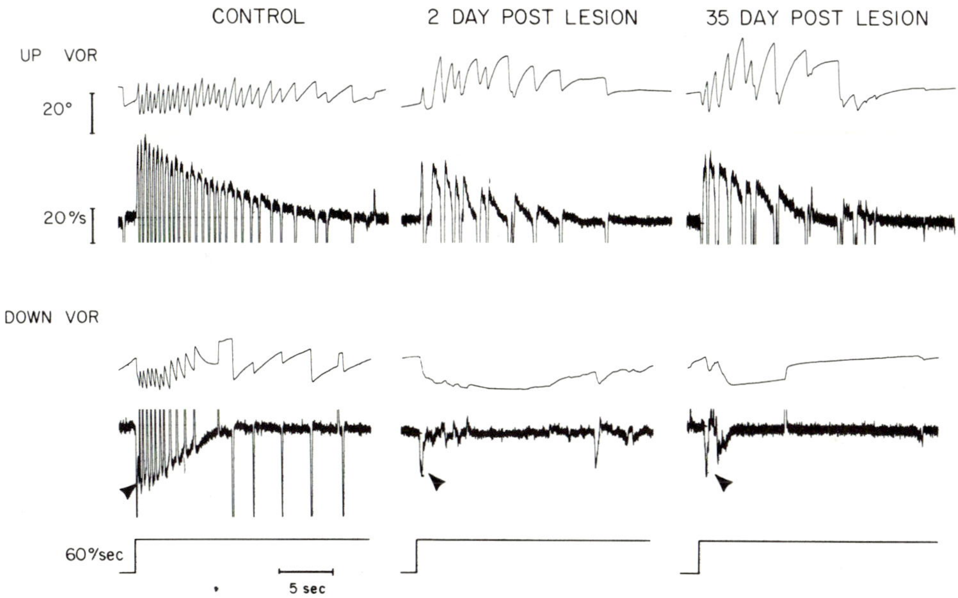

Fig. 5. Vertical VOR deficit following unilateral midbrain lesion. Details in text.

proposed role for the INC, but the up and down VORs are differentially affected. Figure 5 shows data from a cat with a unilateral lesion that destroyed the INC and a small portion of the caudal riMLF. The nucleus of the posterior commissure periaqueductal gray, and nucleus of Darkeschewitsch were intact. The lesion was made on the left side and the data were collected with the animal lying on his right side. The control data show the up and down post rotatory VORs to velocity steps of 60 deg/sec. As in Fig 2 (data from a different cat), the up VOR lasts about twice as long as the down VOR. Two days after the unilateral lesion, the down VOR was abolished, except for the initial deflection of the eye indicated by the black arrowhead. Initial eye velocity and deflection were about the same as in the control record, but there were no upward quick phases to reset the eye position. After an extended time, the eye slowly returned to its original position in the orbit. In contrast, there was an up VOR, but the gain was slightly reduced, and the response was shorter than the control record. Notice that the upward slow phases traversed markedly curved trajectories after the lesion so that the final velocity of each slow phase was less than the initial velocity. Five weeks after the lesion, the down VOR had only slightly recovered, but the up VOR was normal except for a decrease in the number of quick phases and the curved slow phase trajectories.

Unilateral INC lesions were made in 7 cats. When the lesions were restricted to the INC, there were two consistent deficits. First, the number of vertical saccades in either direction was reduced. Up quick phases were more affected than down quick phases, but Fig. 5 shows a 50% reduction in the beat frequency of downward saccades 5 weeks after the lesion. Second, the down VOR was more impaired than the up VOR. In either direction, the initial slow phase or beat was preserved in velocity and direction, suggesting that the direct oculomotor pathways were intact and that oculomotor neuron excitability had not been substantially altered by the lesion. For the down VOR, however, there was little or no sustained response after the first beat for up to 5 weeks following the lesion. For the up VOR, slow phase trajectories were curved in a direction consistent with a leaky down integrator (Zee and co-workers,in press). These data suggest that unilateral INC lesions make the down integrator leaky or inoperative. The apparent loss of upward quick phases, however, complicates this interpretation, since without quick phases to reset it, the integrator may merely be saturated. Additional data analysis and experiments will be needed to resolve this question.

In most cats, there were differences in the VVORs produced by positioning the cat on its left (lesioned side) or right side. If the lesioned side were down, the VVOR was more impaired than if the lesioned side were up. This position dependency suggests the involvement of an otolith-ocular reflex. It should also be remembered that lesioned animals always had a significant rightward head tilt, so that the right side down position was closer to the head position normally held by the animal after the lesion.

Anderson and his colleagues made bilateral kainic acid lesions of the cat's INC. They reported significant phase leads in the VVOR consistent with deficits in the integrator or in the otolith-ocular reflex (Anderson and co-workers, 1979). After unilateral lesions, they reported maintained ocular torsion to the side contralateral to the lesion (and we confirm their data), a defect that also suggests impairment of otolith-ocular pathways (Anderson and Pappas, 1981). Although still preliminary, these new findings certainly establish a central role for the INC in vertical gaze control consistent with its extensive connectivity within the oculomotor system.

ACKNOWLEDGEMENTS

We are grateful to Mr. James Maxwell for his excellent technical assistance at all stages of this work, and to Wendy Keck for preparing the final manuscript. Supported by National Institutes of Health Grants EY 02717 (Dr. King) and AL-00061 and 1 P01-NS-16375 (Dr. Leigh).

STRUCTURE-FUNCTION STUDY IN THE OCULOMOTOR SYSTEM

R. BAKER*, R. SPENCER** and C. EVINGER*

**Department of Physiology & Biophysics, New York University Medical Center, New York, NY 10016, USA*
***Department of Anatomy, Medical College of Virginia, Richmond, VA 23298, USA*

The papers in this symposium offer ample evidence that the neurons, nuclei and circuitry underlying vertical and horizontal eye movement are nearing their final stage of elucidation. Given the more extensive experimental analysis of the abducens nucleus, conjugate horizontal eye movement is still a little better understood than vertical. Even so, information on synaptic organization will accumulate rapidly in the next few years due to the increasing use of intracellular HRP in alert animals. Utilizing the latter technique 'function' can be simultaneously correlated with 'structure'. This powerful new approach permits on one hand, remarkably clear insight into certain morphological problems related to the generation of neuronal activity but at the same time it raises new problems and questions at a different level. The above view is briefly discussed below.

Since their discovery a few years ago, the inhibitory reticular neurons projecting to the contralateral abducens nucleus (see Hikosaka et al 1977, 1980; Maciewicz et al 1977) have been intensively studied and the definitive 'structure-function' is presented in Yoshida et al (1979, 1981 and in press). Two such neurons identified during eye movement in the alert cat and located in the same coronal section 1 mm posterior to the abducens nucleus are shown in Fig. 1. Their dorsal to ventral organization in the medulla points to the importance of a unique cellular distribution for producing the burst of impulses inhibiting contralateral abducens motoneurons and internuclear neurons. One notable characteristic of these inhibitory reticular neurons is that in addition to their major target site (i.e. the abducens nucleus) there is extensive collateralization to the vestibular, reticular and prepositus nuclei (Fig. 2). This multiple arborization pattern is shared by all posterior brainstem neurons projecting to the abducens nucleus and immediately raises the question of how each of the unique eye movement related signals described in the above neurons may be interpreted at the different target sites. Some of these signals (e.g. the saccadic signal on second order vestibular neurons) may be more significant for secondary or tertiary target sites than primary. Thus, it certainly is too early to assume that a particular discharge pattern is equally important at all target sites. To a large extent, the above surmise depends on both a) the synaptic innervation (i.e. density) and b) the arborization pattern in target nuclei. For example compare one terminal arborization pattern of the inhibitory reticular neuron shown in Figure 1 and that of an inhibitory vestibular neuron in the oculomotor nucleus in Figure 3. When the terminal arborization is defined as the final collateral containing boutons en passant and terminaux (as shown via electron microscopy; Figure 3 and Evinger et al, this volume) then it can be seen that extremely fine collaterals

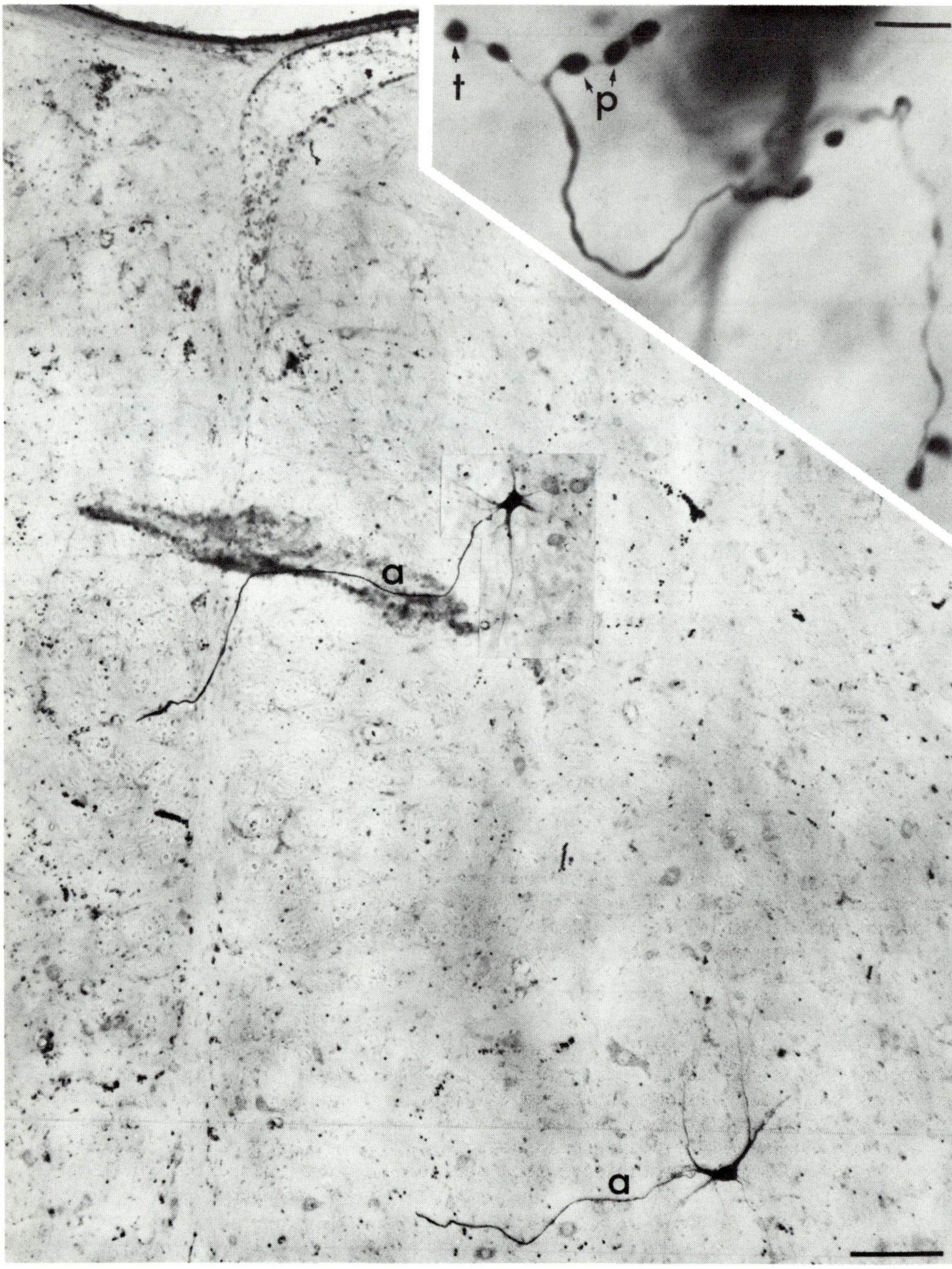

Fig. 1. Microphotograph of two inhibitory reticular neurons recorded intra-axonally in the contralateral abducens nucleus with an intracellular HRP microelectrode. The axonal (a) trajectory is illustrated in the 100 μm coronal section. The inset in the upper right shows two terminal arborization patterns in the contralateral abducens nucleus. The dark counter-stained structure is a neuronal soma. Boutons en passant (p) and terminaux (t) are indicated. Calibrations are 100 μm and 10 μm. (See Yoshida et al, in press)

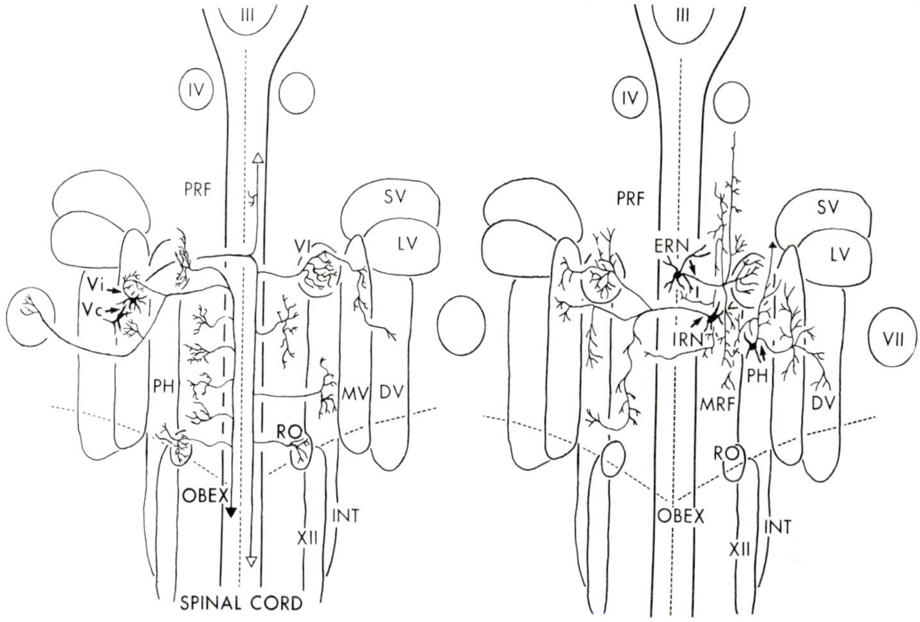

Fig. 2. Morphological reconstruction of vestibular and reticular neurons functionally identified in the alert cat and injected with HRP. On the left typical inhibitory (Vi) and excitatory (Vc) vestibular neurons are illustrated in horizontal section. On the right representative inhibitory (IRN) and excitatory (ERN) reticular neurons are shown. The axonal distribution of a typical principal neuron in the prepositus nucleus (PH) is also illustrated. Rostral and caudal extensions of the vestibular and prepositus neurons are not included. (See Baker et al 1981; Berthoz et al 1981; McCrea et al 1980, 1981 and Yoshida et al 1981).

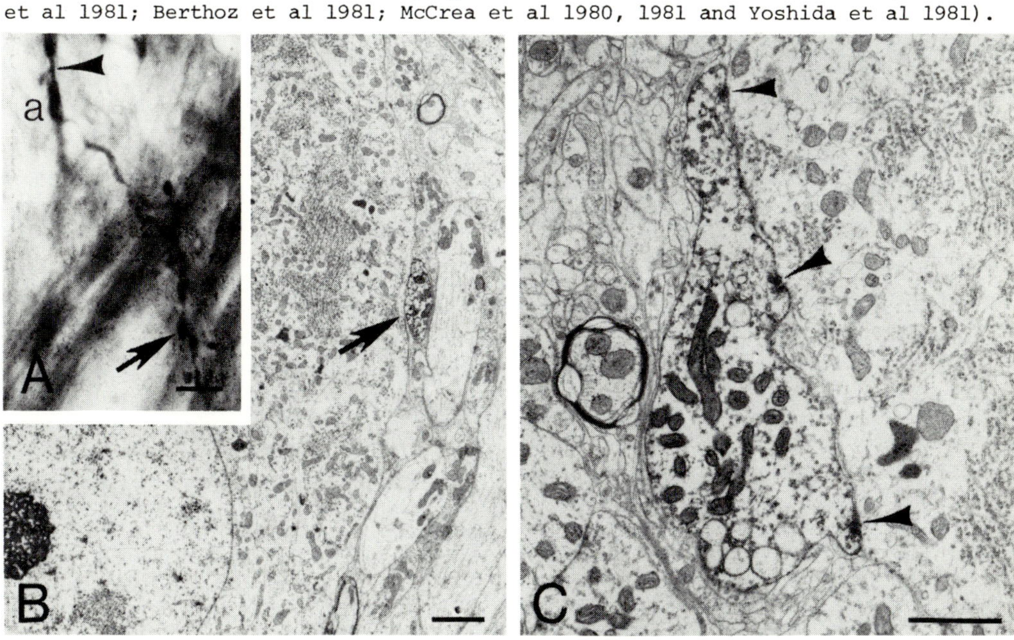

Fig. 3. Electron microscopy of an intracellular HRP labeled inhibitory Vi axonal arborization in the inferior rectus subdivisions of the oculomotor nucleus.

A, Light micrograph of the arborization showing the branch to arise from the parent axon (a) at node of Ranvier (arrowhead) and give rise to several boutons (arrow). B, Electron micrograph of axosomatic synaptic endings (arrow) formed by bouton indicated in A. C, Another axosomatic synaptic ending from the same Vi axon branch showing 3 separate synaptic contact zones (arrowheads). Calibrations: A, 10 μm; B, 2 μm; C, 1 μm.

from .1 - .5 μm connect larger, distended 2 - 5 μm synaptic boutons (Fig. 1). Since action potentials are not likely to pass the branch point then the question becomes one of attaining sufficient depolarization throughout the collateral. Since the length of the terminals range from 20 - 100 μm and often include up to 8 boutons en passant, they, undoubtedly, are several space constants removed from the branch point. More than one action potential at relatively short interval (i.e. high frequency) would be required to produce equivalent and simultaneous transmitter release from all the synaptic boutons. Such frequency potentiation and presynaptic control of axonal branch points (Spencer et al 1981) are ultra-structural features that need further investigation before the transfer function at any target neuron or nuclei is fully appreciated. Recent studies employing electron microscopy with the intracellular HRP technique has indeed demonstrated another level of complexity as illustrated in Fig. 3 wherein a synaptic bouton identified by light microscopy exhibits multiple (up to 9) active zones with the target motoneuron. This morphological feature raises the question of whether one identified synaptic bouton acts as a single or multiple transmitter release site. Since this finding is rather ubiquitous for many of the en passant synapses in the oculomotor system a satisfactory answer will require a quantal synaptic analysis. In conclusion, although the physiological signal(s) and the morphological profile of neurons may be identified via intracellular HRP several important questions remain to be addressed before a neuron's behavior in the circuit is well under-stood. Fortunately the oculomotor system is uniquely organized to permit the above technical questions to be studied and, in fact, these steps may be necessary.

DISCUSSION:

Robert Daroff, Coordinator of the Session, began the formal discussion with comments on the paper by Henn and Büttner. Daroff reminded the audience that in the first of these symposia, sponsored by the Smith-Kettlewell Eye Research Foundation in San Francisco in 1969, there was only one clinical paper dealing with central eye movement disturbances. This was co-authored by Daroff and Hoyt (1971) who, after reviewing all the clinical and experimental literature, as well as their own experiences, made a distinction between the manifestations of gaze palsies in lesions of the PPRF in the upper pons from those of the PPRF in the lower pons at the level of the abducens nucleus. The human pons is approximately 2.5 cm long and the abducens nucleus is situated in the rostral portion of the caudal third of the pons; approximately two-thirds of the PPRF is rostral to the level of the nucleus. The authors contended that with PPRF lesions rostral to the abducens there was ipsilateral paralysis of saccades and pursuit but the eyes could be driven to the side of gaze palsy with vestibular stimulation. However, at the level of the abducens nucleus, lesions of the PPRF were associated with loss of reflex vestibular (and tonic neck) movements. They presumed that there was a critical synapse within the caudal PPRF for the vestibulo-ocular pathways or, at the very least, the functional integrity of the PPRF at that level was necessary for vestibulo-ocular eye movements.

Daroff stated that, since the 1969 symposium, the published literature on the subject and his own clinical experience have not changed his opinion concerning rostral and caudal PPRF lesions. It was on this point that he differed, perhaps only semantically, with Henn and Büttner. These latter authors did not distinguish between rostral and caudal PPRF lesions. In their kainic acid experiments, which selectively destroyed PPRF neurons, vestibulo-ocular movements to the ipsilateral side were intact. They inferred that clinical lesions which abolish vestibular induced ipsilateral movements did so because of interference with axons, in addition to neurons, in the PPRF. While this may be true, Daroff reemphasized that the rostral-caudal dichotomy remains valid for the clinician since the common pathological conditions involving the pons (infarctions, hemorrhage, and tumors) affect both axons and neurons. He agreed with Henn and Büttner that a facial nerve palsy must coexist with an abducens nuclear lesion. The fact that some patients have gaze palsies, absent caloric deviation, and intact seventh nerve function supports his argument. The case report found elsewhere in this volume by Meienberg, Büttner-Ennevar, and Kraus-Ruppert did not resolve the issue. Many authors feel that the paper of Pierrot-Deseilligny and associates (1979) proved that PPRF lesions are associated with intact vestibular movements. Daroff reviewed the paper which reported two cases, the first of which being relevant to the controversy. The pathology of that case was a tumor of considerable rostral-caudal extent within the pons. Rostrally it involved the PPRF but caudally, at the level of the abducens nucleus, it was ventral to the tegmentum. Daroff restated his conviction that a lesion of the PPRF at the level of the abducens nucleus, of sufficient density to paralyze ipsilateral saccades and pursuit, is also associated with paralysis of reflex eye movements. He admitted being unable to distinguish, clinically, a lesion of the PPRF at the level of the abducens nucleus from a lesion of the nucleus itself on the basis of the eye movement disorder. Absence of a facial paralysis would rule out the nuclear lesion but the presence of a paralysis could not confirm such a lesion.

Henn and Büttner mentioned a total paralysis of vertical saccades with bilateral PPRF lesions and the finding of vertical bursters in the PPRF by Hepp and Henn would provide the anatomical basis for this. In their clinical paper on vertical gaze disorders, Leigh, Newman, and King did not mention any saccadic deficits consequent to pontine lesions. Daroff stated his impression that with pontine lesions, there were problems with vertical pursuit, vertical VOR, and gaze-evoked vertical nystagmus. However, a vertical saccadic paralysis has not been described with isolated pontine lesions, except acutely; the paralysis is only transient.

He then discussed the paper by Hepp and Henn which described the firing pattern of the PPRF neurons related to horizontal saccades. He queried whether the failure to find "purely tonic" cells (reflecting the output of the integrator) represented a sampling error. This is distinctly possible with single cell recording; witness the number of years before cells in the frontal eye fields were found which fired before a saccade. Until, or if, a tonic cell is found, their hypothesis that many of the burst-tonic cells in the brain stem and lateral cerebellar nuclei function as reverberating networks, and are therefore the horizontal integrators, has appeal but must be contrasted with Baker's (Baker, Evinger, and McCrea, in press) that the nucleus prepositus is the probable site for integration since it has the proper location, input, output, and firing patterns.

Daroff then discussed ocular electromyography (EMG). He felt that Hepp and Henn's postulate that selective destruction of the midline population of pause and follow-burst neurons could theoretically lead to decomposition of movements through inappropriate antagonist firing could be resolved with ocular EMG. Unfortunately, the era of ocular EMG preceded that of quantitative oculography. During the 1960's, there were many clinical papers on ocular EMG but rarely with simultaneous oculography. There was only a presumption of what the eyes were doing based upon clinical observations and the EMG findings. Without simultaneous oculography, precise relationships between muscle activity and the eye movements cannot be made. At least in the United States, the potential risks have virtually eliminated ocular EMG studies. He urged researchers in countries where EMG clinical research is still feasible to conduct such studies with simultaneous quantitative oculography since this would yield considerable information about the mechanism of many eye movement disturbances.

He reminded basic scientists of the problems with clinico-pathological correlations. In the autopsied examples of patients who have had oculography shortly prior to death, either the oculography or the pathological examination has been incomplete. Often, the disease progresses between the time of the eye movement recording and post-mortem examination. Moreover, there are only a few centers throughout the world where good eye movement recordings are being done. This is particularly relevant with vertical gaze disorders. As mentioned by Leigh and colleagues, most eye movement recording techniques are not suited for quantitative vertical oculography. Thus, the bulk of our clinical literature contains mere descriptions of the eye movement disturbance or, at best, non-quantitative ENG. The well-studied case reports presented by Leigh and colleagues represent the beginning of a systematic attempt to fill the void. Leigh's mention of progressive supranuclear palsy spurred Daroff to admit to a long-standing intrigue with this disease which involves neurons (sparing axons) in the thalamus, basal ganglia, and midbrain. The pons is generally not affected. The disease characteristically affects vertical eye movements but then ultimately results in a total horizontal saccadic and pursuit palsy with preservation of the vestibulo-ocular reflexes in all directions. Thus, a neuronal disease, rostral to the pons, paralyzes horizontal saccades and pursuit, suggesting a polysynaptic saccadic and pursuit pathway from cortex to the pons.

Daroff regarded the paper by King and Leigh as interposing a welcome sense of restraint. Whereas our tendency is to put bits of experimental pieces together to form a plausible hypothesis, they have reminded us of the contradictory evidence surrounding the anatomy and physiology of vertical gaze, particularly concerning the role of the rostral interstitial nucleus of the medial longitudinal fasciculus (iMLF).

Ulrich Büttner and Bernard Cohen were then invited to make brief separate presentations of recent experiments related to the topic of the Session. Büttner summarized the findings in a recent paper (Büttner-Ennever et al., in press) concerning the role of the iMLF in monkey and man. After carefully combining the results of all previous experiments and clinico-pathologic correlations, they concluded that lateral lesions of both rostral iMLF resulted in isolated downgaze palsy whereas medial lesions produced both up and down palsies. Büttner regards the lateral iMLF as the downward gaze center and the medial iMLF as the center for upward gaze. Pathways from the lateral iMLF must pass through the medial lesions. He recognized isolated upward gaze palsies with lesions in or about the posterior commissure but could not explain the mechanism.

Cohen presented data concerning a striking asymmetry between upward and downward nystagmus in both the monkey and cat (Matsuo and co-workers, 1979). With animals on their sides receiving stimulation about a vertical axis, upward OKN had a lower gain than downward OKN; it was also more irregular and lower in frequency. Moreover, there was little or no upward OKAN. In contrast, downward OKAN was much stronger, and was similar to horizontal OKAN. The differences between upward and downward OKN and OKAN seemed related to two factors: a reduced gain in direct visual-ocular motor pathways responsible for ocular pursuit in the downward direction, and an inability to store activity related to slow phase velocity during upward nystagmus. The weaker storage for upward than downward nystagmus was also manifest during vestibular nystagmus induced by steps of velocity about a vertical axis. The initial gain of the vertical VOR was symmetrical and close to unity. However, the time constant of upward nystagmus was 5-7 seconds, whereas the time constant of downward nystagmus was 12-20 seconds, similar to that of horizontal nystagmus. This indicated that upward nystagmus did not last much beyond the change in activity coming in over the nerves from the vertical canals. Downward and horizontal nystagmus, however, were prolonged well beyond the end of vestibular nerve activation due to action of the velocity storage mechanism. A consequence of this was that when animals were in the lateral position, the low frequency characteristics of the vertical VOR were asymmetrical for movements in the upward and downward direction; there would be better ocular compensation for slow downward than for slow upward head movements. A second consequence was little or no stored velocity available after rotation in the upward direction to counteract the post-rotatory nystagmus that occurred at the end of the velocity step. Downward post-rotatory nystagmus, recorded in darkness after rotation in light, was as strong as if the animal had been rotating only in darkness. Upward post-rotatory nystagmus, however, was much weaker after downward rotation about a vertical axis in light than after rotation in darkness. These findings all occurred when animals were on their sides. Cohen recently found that when animals were upright and received optokinetic stimulation in the pitch plane, downward OKAN disappeared (Matsuo and Cohen, 1981). That is, velocity storage for downward nystagmus was markedly attenuated when animals were erect. As a result, the saturation velocity for downward OKN falls, and the nystagmus was frequently more irregular when erect than in the lateral position. This change in velocity storage between the lateral and upright positions was presumably due to activity that arose in the otolith organs. Previous workers showed that the gain of downward OKN increased after the saccules were ablated. If the same was true in man, Cohen felt there might be a strong asymmetry in the vertical VOR when the otolith organs were inactivated, as for example, in space. This may relate to the motion sickness that has been a problem in many space flights.

The discussion was then opened to the panelists and audience. Larry Stark had several criticisms. He felt that horizontal and vertical saccadic generation should be independent because of the independence of horizontal and vertical channels as demonstrated in his study of oblique eye movements. Hepp responded that the behavior of oblique saccades proves that the horizontal and vertical vectors can not be independent but must be coordinated. Stark felt that the velocities for vertical saccades shown by Leigh and colleagues were too slow for normal subjects. Leigh responded that the velocites of his group were more compatible with others in the literature as distinct from those reported by Bahill and Stark who, Leigh felt, arbitrarily selected out all but the fastest saccades and therefore constructed an artificial main sequence for normal subjects.

The moderator encouraged David Robinson to comment on Hepp's paper which could be interpreted as being critical of Robinson's model. Robinson allowed that models are made to be discarded and substituted with new and better models. He has not seen one better than his that he could accept and cited the recent paper by Mays and Sparks (1980) as supporting his notion that planned eye position in the orbit was the key saccadic signal rather than a retinotopic drive. Louis Dell'Osso volunteered that Robinson's model would be improved by the addition of a second neural integrator which he and co-workers had proposed (Abel et al., 1978). This was determined while modeling gaze-evoked nystagmus where the position command was defective but not the characteristics of the saccadic fast phases. The same integrator could not be responsible for both since a single leaky neural integrator would result in distorted saccades as well as the observed slow phase exponential drift. Therefore the leaky neural integrator causing gaze-evoked nystagmus was distinct from the neural integrator contained in the bootstrap circuit of the pulse generator. Such a model, Dell'Osso contended, is also consistent with the apparent existence of neural integrators (tonic cells) in both the PPRF and nucleus prepositus. He proposed that the bootstrap neural integrator was in the PPRF and the eye position neural integrator in the nucleus prepositus.

Hepp mentioned that Robinson's model does not explain the behavior of horizontal bursters during either oblique saccades or slow saccades (such as seen in drowsy monkeys). He felt that two signals, an internal feedback as well as a ballistic signal from long-lead bursters, were necessary for saccadic generation.

In response to Daroff's comment that vertical saccadic paresis was transient following acute bilateral PPRF lesions, Henn described two monkeys with chronic lesions, one more than eight weeks in duration, who still could not generate vertical saccades.

King felt that the Hepp and Stark disagreement regarding oblique saccades and the relative independence of the horizontal and vertical vectors related to saccadic amplitude. With small oblique saccades the horizontal and vertical components are independent but with larger saccades the two vectors are linked to each other.

King went on to discuss Cohen's presentation and the significance of whether the animal was on its side or upright. He restated that lesions of the interstitial nucleus of Cajal (INC) produced fewer vertical saccades and affected the vertical VOR by abolition or impairment of post-rotary nystagmus. Only the VOR deficit was obviously influenced by the animal's head position, being severe when the animal was placed on his lesioned side. All animals exhibited a head tilt to the side opposite the lesion. Presumably the unilateral lesion caused an imbalance in the vertical vestibulo-ocular system. He suggested that the head tilt might be a response to the imbalance (mediated by direct INC-cervical motor neuron projections) or an adopted position to compensate the perceived imbalance by altering otolith inflow. It seemed reasonable to him that the animal's compensatory adaptation would be dependent upon head position (a given pattern of otolith inflow) and would be upset if the animal's head was rotated into another plane, as when placed lesion-side down. He felt that the reduced frequency of saccades might be secondary to reductions in VOR gains but there were also fewer voluntary saccades as if the animal had difficulty triggering or initiating any rapid vertical eye movement. This finding was regarded as consistent with a functional distinction between the INC and prerubral neurons. INC neurons may process signals used to initiate or sustain vertical saccades or quick phases. Burst-tonic cells in the INC might provide the efference copy eye position signal postulated by Robinson's bang-bang model. On the other hand, prerubral medium lead burst neurons are probably output elements of the burst generator itself and contribute directly to producing saccades. If these ideas were correct, we would expect partial prerubral lesions to slow vertical saccades whereas INC lesions would interfere with the initiation or accuracy of the saccades. Preliminary data from King's laboratory were consistent with this hypothesis. Large lesions that included the prerubral field were associated with slow saccades whereas small lesions centered in the INC reduced the number but not the velocity of vertical saccades.

Neil Barmack commented that when an animal is lying on its side, one is maximally activating, through linear acceleration, one macula of a utricle and maximally inhibiting the opposite side. When the animal is then rotated around, there may be centripetal forces acting upon both saccula which creates a complicated situation further confounded by gravitational effects upon the ampulla of the semicircular canals. Thus, he proposed that we postpone judgement on whether there is in fact an asymmetry of the VOR and OKN reflexes until an experiment is devised where the animal can be oriented to assure that gravity was not changing or differentially acting on the otoliths. Henn asked how this could be accomplished, and Barmack responded that in the rabbit is it easy with the animal's nose up but for the cat one would have to look at vertical OKN with the animal prone. After a brief pause, Barmack reasoned that, with a cat in the supine position, gravity would be orthogonal to both saccula and macula. When the cat was then rotated, the only force would be angular acceleration and with no effect of gravity on the system when measuring the OKN reflex. The experiment may be feasible but the results incomprehensible.

A discussion ensued among participants concerning the relative symmetry and asymmetry of VOR and OKN in the vertical direction, without general agreement. G. R. Barnes commented that he and his colleague, Allen Benson, some years previously obtained modified responses of the horizontal VOR related to the assumed influence of otolithic stimulation which may have some bearing upon the asymmetry of responses obtained by King for the vertical VOR (Benson, 1970). After the sudden cessation of rotation about the vertical axis with the subject in the upright position, the subject was quickly repositioned so as to be either prone, supine, or side down. In these conditions, the decay of the nystagmus was more rapid in the upright position and because of the nature of the reverse secondary nystagmus, the effect was interpreted as a change in the adaptation time constant of the VOR. He did not think that this explains the asymmetry of the vertical VOR response but it does serve to illustrate the rather non-specific effect which static stimulation of the otoliths can exert on the VOR. Thus, Barnes felt it can <u>not</u> be assumed that the observed response was purely of vertical canal origin when the animal was side-down, particularly as the utricles may well have played an important part in the normal response when the animal was upright.

Robert Baloh commented that, in humans, the otolith macula are orthogonal, unlike the situation in the cat.

King recognized that placing an animal on its side was not an ideal way to test the vertical VOR but was one of the most practical. He felt that Cohen's data clearly showed that otolith inflow can alter the apparent time constant of the vertical VOR but did not believe it explains the asymmetry between up and down VORs as suggested by Barmack. The inflow can affect the time constant, but why should it influence down more than up, regardless of whether the animal is on the right or left side?

Baker commented that the MLF organization for vertical eye movements was more complex than generally recognized. Data from the rabbit indicated that all vertical canal vestibulo-ocular pathways (except the anterior canal pathway via the brachium conjunctivum to the contralateral inferior oblique and superior rectus motor neurons) lie in the MLF. Recent unpublished studies in the cat, however, suggested all vertical canal pathways lie in the MLF. Prior work by a number of investigators suggested that the dorsal subdivision of the Y group (called the infracerebellar nucleus) did not receive saccula input, but projected via the brachium to the oculomotor complex. Chubb and Fuchs have shown that these neurons exhibit vertical vestibular gaze velocity signals; it is likely this pathway may function solely for connecting the cerebellum to the vertical oculomotor nuclei in the midbrain. Since horizontal conjugate eye movements were probably synthesized entirely in the abducens nucleus, comparable cerebellar actions could be implemented locally via the prepositus and/or subdivisions of the vestibular nucleus. Thus, Baker concluded, it is primarily because of the different brain stem location of motor centers that the brachium pathway became unique for vertical movements.

Johannes Dichgans asked Henn about the nature of smooth pursuit and full field OKN with bilateral PPRF lesions. Henn responded that the animals were able to slowly move their eyes toward points of interest but since they were untrained it was not possible to formally test pursuit. The animals could direct their gaze which seemed remarkable given the fact that with unilateral lesions animals cannot move their eyes across the midline into the paretic field. He surmised that the latter situation might relate to the strong spontaneous nystagmus seen with unilateral lesions. During full field OKN or acceleration in the dark, the eyes were driven into the direction of the expected slow phase and stayed in this eccentric position until the stimulus was over.

King returned to the discussion of the up-and-down organization in the rostral iMLF, stating there were too many vertical medium lead burst neurons in the rostral iMLF, PPRF, and other midbrain areas. Furthermore, there was a disparity between physiological and anatomical studies. Tracer studies showed a clean projection from rostral iMLF to the oculomotor nucleus but there are burst cells outside of that projection pattern which shouldn't be there if they played the same role as with horizontal saccades. Also, these burst cells encoded for both up and down saccadic components. Indeed, all the rostral iMLF, periaqueductal gray, and midbrain paramedian reticular formation neurons fired for both up and down saccades. The only place that projected to the oculomotor nucleus where saccades cannot be recorded was the INC.

Hepp stated that Baker's contention that the horizontal integrator was in the nucleus prepositus was primarily by exclusion. Hepp felt there was evidence for horizontal integration in the propositus, medial vestibular nucleus, PPRF, and lateral cerebellar nuclei; they all may function as a highly interconnected network working together to achieve integration with each part possibly having a more dominant role in different situations. For example, the lateral cerebellar nuclei may be more dominant in eccentric horizontal gaze. Hepp then asked Baker whether there was strong morphological evidence that the prepositus was the integrator. Baker responded by stating that the morphological and physiological evidence indicated that the integrator "should be" in the nucleus prepositus. There are at least ten unique neurons in the nucleus and they have fantastic intraprepositus collateralization. Each of the neurons is "unique" because of efferent connections; some go to the cerebellum, some to the abducens, and some project only to other neurons in the prepositus. Physiologically, within the nucleus there exists a "purely tonic" cell which carries only position and very little velocity information. Although Baker admitted that more investigation was needed before being absolutely certain, the prepositus is the only nucleus in the posterior brain stem with both the afferent and efferent connections as well as appropriate cyto-architectonic organization of neurons necessary to function as the integrator. Thus, the prepositus is the only nucleus that can do the job that the modelers tell us is required of the integrator.

Cohen then admonished the group not to fall into the trap of regarding certain areas of the brain stem as "centers." Speaking as a well-trained disciple of Dr. Morris Bender, Cohen warned of the dangers of regarding complex neural networks as centers for anything. With this, the Discussion ended.

SECTION VII

Coordinator: J. Dichgans

DISORDERS OF OPTOKINETIC AND VESTIBULAR NYSTAGMUS

ANATOMICAL AND FUNCTIONAL ORGANISATION OF OPTOKINETIC PATHWAYS

W. PRECHT

Institute for Brain Research, University of Zürich, August Forel-Strasse 1, Postfach CH-8029 Zürich, Switzerland

ABSTRACT

The paper gives a brief review of the experimental work that has been devoted to the anatomy and physiology of the pathways and relay nuclei responsible for the optokinetic eye reflexes. The emphasis is on the mammalian optokinetic system but reference will be made to those in submammalian species as well.

KEYWORDS

Optokinetic pathways; optokinetic nystagmus; foveal pursuit; visual-vestibular interaction.

When the visual world surrounding an animal is moved the head and/or the eyes move in the direction of the surround motion. Typically these slow compensatory movements are regularly interrupted by fast anticompensatory movements (quick phases) leading to the pattern of response known as optokinetic nystagmus (OKN). Within a range typical for a given species the velocity of the slow phase is close to surround velocity so that the image of the world on the retina remains stable i.e. the retinal slip is close to zero. The stimulus-response behavior of this velocity control system, particularly that evoked from the eyes in the head-fixed condition by horizontal stimulus movement, has been studied extensively in fish (Easter, 1972), frog (Birukow, 1937; Dieringer, Blight and Precht, 1980), birds (Conley and Fite, 1980), rabbit (Collewijn, 1969), cat (Evinger and Fuchs, 1979; Honrubia, Scott and Ward, 1967; Keller and Precht, 1979a; Montarolo, Precht and Strata, 1981; Precht, Montarolo and Strata, 1980), monkey (Cohen, Matsuo and Raphan, 1977) and man (see Baloh, this vol.), however, the neuronal circuitry responsible for producing OKN is still poorly understood. In recent years several investigators have attempted to study the morphological and functional pathway- and neuronal organization of the optokinetic system and it is the purpose of this brief review to summarize the main findings obtained with anatomical and physiological techniques in a variety of species.

1. Responses of Retinal Ganglion Cells to Optokinetic Stimulation

Oyster, Takahashi and Collewijn (1972) were the first to demonstrate that direction-selective retinal ganglion cells of the rabbit responded vigorously to optokinetic stimuli that cover large areas of the visual field and are frequently used to elicit OKN. Two classes were noted: 1) on-off units were maximally sensitive to four directions of movement (forward, upward, backward, downward), reached their peak firing at stimulus velocities of ca. 10°/sec and had their receptive fields mainly outside the visual streak; 2) on units were sensitive to three directions only (forward, upward, downward), reached maximal firing near 1°/sec stimulus velocity and had their receptive fields more commonly within the visual streak. Later it was shown by retrograde labelling techniques that ganglion cells projecting to OKN relay nuclei (see below) were among the 20% largest cells in the visual streak (Oyster and co-workers, 1980). The question then arose which of the two classes of ganglion cells were mainly responsible for OKN. To answer this question the tuning curves of the direction-selective ganglion cell classes were compared to the open-loop gain of OKN, and it was found that on-type ganglion cell responses corresponded very well with the velocity tuning curves of the slow phase OKN, whereas on-off units played only a secondary role in this reflex.

In the cat W-ganglion cells appear to carry the visual input to optokinetic relay cells (Hoffmann and Schoppmann, 1975), however, only a small fraction (ca. 1%) of them is direction-selective (on-off and on) and they do not seem to have preferred axes of sensitivity (for ref. see Rodieck, 1979). Since the on-type ganglion cells of the rabbit which presumably are responsible for mediating OKN comprise only 5% of the 25% direction-selective ganglion cells, it is not impossible that in the cat the ca. 1% direction-selective W-cells also represent an important specific retinal input source for OKN. This point, however, needs to be studied further. Finally, it should be mentioned that almost all of the direction-selective units send their axons into the contralateral optic tract. Since uncrossed fibers alone (see below) are capable of mediating OKN the identification of the specific retinal input fibers becomes even more difficult in the ipsilateral system.

In the frog some class-3 retinal ganglion cells show directional selectivity (Lettvin and co-workers, 1959). Since they terminate in the pretectum and nBON both of which are crucial structures for OKN (see below) they may well represent a specific retinal input source to the OKN system.

2. Primary Optokinetic Relay Nuclei in the Midbrain

In recent years several studies performed in various species have shown that the nuclei of the accessory optic system (AOS) and the nucleus of the optic tract (NOT) are the major primary relay nuclei of the optokinetic system in lower forms. In higher vertebrates the path via the lateral geniculate nucleus to the visual cortex gains more importance (see below).

2.1 Anatomy of the AOS and NOT. Before describing the response properties of neurons in these nuclei a brief account of their anatomy will be given. The AOS proper is present in all mammals, and a similar system is also found in lower vertebrates. The readers interested in details are referred to some original papers (amphibia: (Riss, Knapp and Scalia, 1963); birds: (Cowan, Adamson and Powell, 1961); rabbit: (Giolli, 1961); cat: (Hayhow, 1959); rat: (Hayhow, Webb and Jervie, 1960); primates: (Giolli, 1963; Tigges and Tigges, 1969; Tigges, Bos and Tigges, 1977), and reviews: (Marg, 1964, 1973).

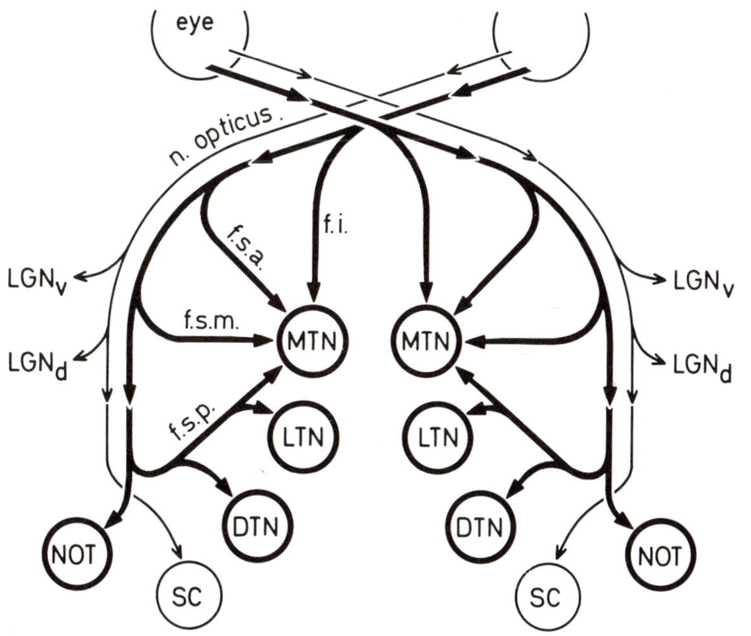

Fig. 1. Schematic representation of the accessory optic/n. of the optic tract (NOT) system. Abreviations not defined in text: f.i, fasciculus inferior; f.s.a, f.s.m, f.s.p, fasciculus superior, pars anterior, medialis, posterior.

In most mammals the AOS consists of three nuclei: dorsal (DTN), lateral (LTN) and medial (MTN) terminal nuclei (Fig. 1). On functional grounds (see below) the DTN and the NOT may be considered an entity although the NOT is generally considered a pretectal nucleus. The MTN is located at the ventral midbrain, the LTN lies ventral to the posterior edge of the medial geniculate body at the dorsal edge of the cerebral peduncle and the DTN and NOT lie near the surface along the ventral part of the anterior border of the tectum. DTN, MTN, LTN and probably also NOT receive retinal afferents via the accessory optic tract predominantly from the contralateral eye.

In lower vertebrates the subdivisions of the AOS are less distinct; it appears, however, that the homologue of the MTN is the nucleus of the basal optic root (nBON) whereas the DTN/NOT complex appears to correspond to a small group of cells in the pretectum at least in amphibia (see below). The AOS in primates is of greatly reduced dimensions and differs from other mammals in that the MTN is not found in its typical location; its place is taken by the n. of the transpeduncular tract which probably receives fibers from other nuclei of the AOS.

The efferent connections of the AON/NOT will be described in section 3 together with their functional organisation. Here it should only be mentioned that the AON/NOT are interconnected, e.g. NOT projects to MTN and vice versa (Giolli, Blanks and Sang Pham, 1981).

2.2 Physiology of the AOS and NOT. The horizontal OKN of the rabbit was the first optokinetic reflex system in which one of the above described nuclei, the NOT, was shown to represent an essential relay station (Collewijn, 1975a, 1975b). Unilateral lesion of this area abolished OKN evoked in intact animals by stimulation of the contralateral eye, and electrical stimulation of this area generated OKN even in animals in which the optic nerve projection had degenerated prior to stimulation. Subsequently it was shown that most units in the NOT were excited by an optokinetic pattern moving in a temporonasal or anterior direction in front of the contralateral eye, and resting discharge (25 - 50 Hz) was inhibited by motion in the opposite direction, the decrease in firing being smaller than the increase. Many units responded to a large range of retinal slip velocities (0.01-20°/sec) indicating that both on and on-off type of ganglion cells projected on NOT cells (Collewijn, 1975b). Their receptive fields seemed to be restricted to the visual streak. Electrical stimulation of the optic nerve and optokinetic stimuli evoked units with latencies of ca. 2.0 msec and 60 msec, respectively. From these latencies conduction velocities of ganglion cells were calculated to measure ca. 13 m/sec which is similar to that of W-cells in cat. Given that OKN latency is ca. 75 msec and that of NOT units 60 msec, 15 msec are available for central processing along the sensorimotor chain.

Similar studies performed in the NOT of the cat showed that lesion likewise abolished OKN (Precht and Strata, 1980), and units coded velocity and were direction selective (Hoffmann and Schoppmann, 1975). A full account of the NOT responses in the cat is given by Hoffmann's article in this volume. In the rat the majority of NOT units showed an increased discharge when stimuli were moving temporonasally in front of the contralateral eye; all other stimuli were essentially ineffective in these units (Cazin, Precht and Lannou, 1980c). The mean peak of the tuning curve of these units occurred at 1°/sec retinal slip velocity and was thus lower than that measured in cat and rabbit. Typically, pretectal or NOT units gave a step output in firing to a velocity step input. Some cells showed an initial phasic component.

No signs of sensory vestibular and/or motor signals, e.g. eye velocity convergence were observed.

Since it has also been shown in rat that in monocular condition horizontal OKN can only be evoked by forward motion of the surround (Cazin, Precht and Lannou, 1980b) the directional response pattern of the majority of units in the pretectum is in good agreement with the directional preference of the OKN. As in rabbit and cat unilateral lesion of the pretectum abolished OKN evoked from the contralateral eye (Cazin, Precht and Lannou, 1980b). Furthermore in albino rats in which OKN is missing (Precht and Cazin, 1979) pretectal units did not respond to surround motion in a direction-selective manner but showed only brief on-or off-responses (Lannou and co-workers, 1981).

In the frog a small group of cells located in the pretectum (Cochran, Precht and Dieringer, 1980, 1981) was found that showed direction-selective responses to horizontally moving patterns. An increase of resting rate occurred on temporonasal and a decrease on nasotemporal pattern movements in front of the contralateral eye. The small range available for a decrease of discharge may explain the very small gain of the OKN on nasotemporal pattern movement. The peaks of the velocity tuning curves occurred at ca. 10°/sec retinal slip velocity. Pretectal units were monosynaptically driven by the contralateral optic nerve (Cochran and Precht, 1980). Lesion of the pretectal area impaired horizontal optokinetic reflexes.

Now let us turn to the relay nuclei mediating vertical optokinetic reflexes. They are best studied in rabbits (Simpson, Soodak and Hess, 1979; Walley, 1967), frogs (Cochran, Precht and Dieringer, 1980, 1981) and birds (Burns and Wallman, 1981; Morgan and Frost, 1981).

In the rabbit MTN and LTN units typically show a resting discharge (25-50 Hz) and exhibit direction- and velocity sensitivity (peak ca. 0.1 - 1.0°/sec retinal slip velocity). Preferred directions are vertical with a posterior component. There are twice as many cells preferring upward rather than downward motion in MTN, whereas in the LTN almost all cells preferred down and posterior. Receptive fields of the units are large and small stimuli (spots or bars) have little effect on cell activity. Latencies for electrical activation are ca. 2 msec which is compatible with a monosynaptic input.

In the cat MTN units also have large receptive fields located predominantly in the contralateral visual field. They prefer vertical-downward motion and respond best at velocities between 0.5-10°/sec (Grasse and Cynader, 1980). In the chicken (Burns and Wallman, 1981) and pigeon (Morgan and Frost, 1981) very similar unit responses were found in the nBOR which corresponds to the MTN of mammals (see section 1). As in the rabbit, preferred and null directions were not exactly opposite to each other. This asymmetry as well as other response properties are interpreted as physiological evidence for the AOS being arranged in the coordinate system of the semicircular canals (Simpson, Soodak and Hess, 1979).

In amphibia the nBOR units likewise code upward or downward retinal slip velocity (peak of tuning curves ca. 1°/sec); in addition, some units responded to nasotemporal stimulus directions (Cochran, Precht and Dieringer, 1980, 1981) and most of them were monosynaptically driven from the contralateral optic nerve (Cochran and Precht, 1980). Contrary to pretectal cells most units showed no resting discharge.

In the monkey very little work has been done in this area. It has been reported that neurons in the n. of the transpeduncular tract (see section 1) responded to contralateral, vertical, whole field motion in a direction-selective, velocity-related mode (Westheimer and Blair, 1974).

In summary physiological studies performed in the nuclei of the AOS proper and NOT in a wide variety of species show remarkable similarities of their response properties such as direction-selectivity, velocity-coding, topographical localisation of preferred directions in certain subdivisions and monosynaptic, contralateral retinal inputs. In addition, lesion of these nuclei abolished irreversibly OKN. These findings then suggest that these nuclei are primary relay nuclei for horizontal and vertical optokinetic reflexes.

3. Pathways to the Motor System

The next problem to be discussed will be how the primary relay nuclei convey their information to the motoneurons. Most of the work in this field has been done on horizontal OKN. Based on studies of the exact time course of the OKN generated by velocity steps of surround motion of long duration the existence of direct and indirect pathways has been postulated (Cohen, Matsuo and Raphan, 1977). The terms direct and indirect are functional terms and do not imply anatomical connections of direct or indirect nature. The direct path very rapidly brings OKN slow-phase velocity to a species-dependent fraction of the final steady-state velocity, whereas the indirect path provides the additional slower rise of the eye velocity to the steady-state value observed during prolonged stimulation. From studies performed in man and monkey (see Baloh, this volume) the direct path has been postulated to consist of the foveal-LGN-visual cortex path or the pursuit system which reaches motoneurons through corticofucal paths probably also involving the parietal cortex, cerebellar flocculus, pons and paramedian reticular formation (PPRF). Impairment of this path abolished the fast rise of OKN velocity leaving only the slowly rising part intact (Fig. 2B). The indirect path is believed to be entirely restricted to the brainstem involving the AOS and its connections through the vestibular nuclei and velocity storage integrator to the motoneurons (Fig. 2C).

In the following a brief account will be given of the anatomy and functional organisation of these pathways. Rather than speaking of direct and indirect paths, I'll use in this context the terms short- and long latency paths and assign some possible function to them later.

3.1 Short latency paths. It has been demonstrated both anatomically and physiologically that in amphibia (Cochran and Precht, 1980; Montgomery, Fite and Bengston, 1979) the nBOR projects directly to oculomotor neurons (Fig. 2A); similarly the pretectal cells described above seem to project to abducens motoneurons directly (Cochran, Precht and Dieringer, 1981). Short latency connections have also been described from nBOR to the motoneurons of the IIIrd and IVth nuclei in the pigeon (Brecha and Karten, 1979). In mammals, however, such connections so far have not been reported.

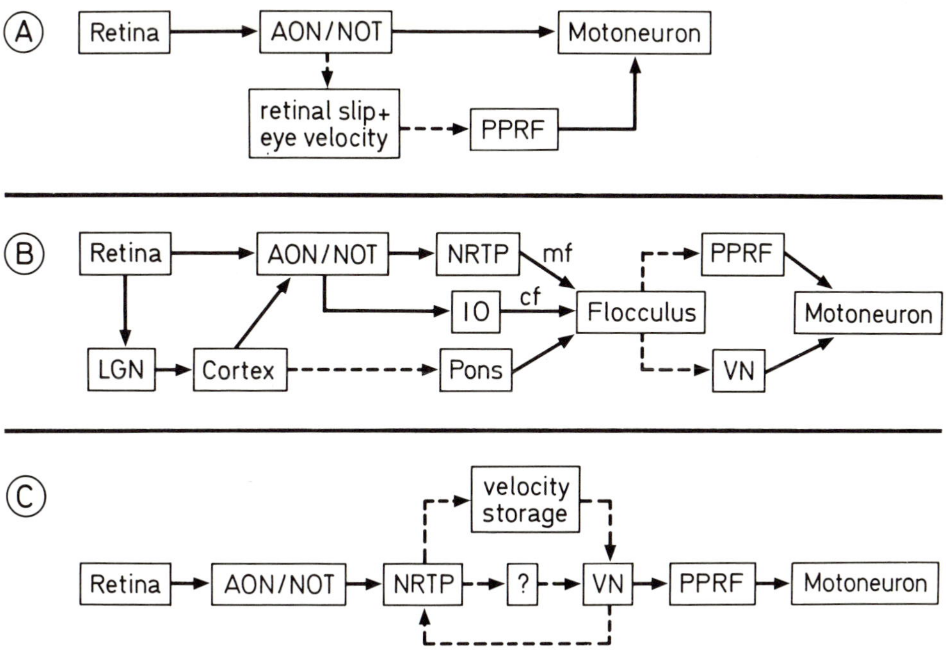

Fig. 2. Diagrammatic representation of possible optokinetic pathways. Abreviations not defined in text: cf, mf, climbing and mossy fiber afferents to cerebellum; IO, inf. olive.

What is the functional role of this short path? It is somewhat reminiscent of the three neuronal arcs connecting semicircular canal receptors and ocular motoneurons. This vestibular path carries a head/eye velocity signal to motoneurons. From the available data we may postulate that the three-neuronal optokinetic path carries a retinal slip velocity signal to motoneurons. Of course, as it is the case for the three-neuronal VOR paths, the velocity inputs can not by themselves produce the proper reflexive eye movements, since motoneurons not only require a step signal but rather a ramp-step signal produced by the position integrator to produce a change in eye position (Robinson, 1976). This could be achieved by feeding the nBOR or pretectal retinal slip signals, in addition, through the position integrator (Fig. 2A). Also we may assume that before the retinal slip signal reaches the integrator it converges with an eye velocity signal somewhere in the brain (see below) to generate a signal that represents target velocity in space (Robinson, 1977). The function of the short latency path could be to rapidly increase initial eye velocity. Thus it would be a 'direct' path in the above discussed sense. In fact, OKN in the frog rapidly reaches final velocity (Dieringer, Blight and Precht, 1980). Apparently, higher vertebrates have abandoned this direct path through short connections and, instead, use the pursuit system for this purpose.

3.2 Long - latency paths

3.2.1 Pretectal-vestibular nuclei path. As mentioned above the functionally defined indirect path associated with the velocity storage integrator has been postulated to involve the vestibular nuclei (VN). The evidence has been fully reviewed in a recent paper (Precht, 1981) and a monograph (Henn, Cohen and Young, 1980) and, therefore, only a brief account will be given here: 1. Vestibular neurons (Vn) respond to pure optokinetic stimulation in a wide variety of vertebrates except in the frog, their response characteristics (slow rise and fall of firing in response to optokinetic velocity steps) show evidence of velocity storage and their velocity tuning curves are similar to those of pretectal neurons (Cazin, Precht and Lannou, 1980c); 2. bilateral labyrinthectomy abolished the storage mechanism presumably by changing the resting level of Vn.

Here we are concerned with the problem of how the optokinetic signal gets to the vestibular nuclei. Since no direct connections exist between AOS/NOT and VN we must search for intermediate links. Projections have been described with anatomical methods from the pretectum (NOT) to the n.reticularis tegmenti pontis (NRTP) in the rat (Terasawa, Otani and Yamada, 1979) and both anatomically and physiologically in the rabbit (Maekawa and Kimura, 1981). NRTP neurons were activated in the rabbit with short latencies compatible with a disynaptic path from the optic nerve to this nucleus, and NOT neurons were antidromically driven from NRTP (Maekawa and Kimura, 1981; Maekawa, Takeda and Kimura, 1981). In the rat NRTP units responded to optokinetic stimuli with the same directional selectivity and similar velocity tuning curves (Cazin, Precht and Lannou, 1980c) as did pretectal and vestibular units. Lesion of the NRTP abolished optokinetic responses in the Vn and OKN in both rat (Cochran and Precht, 1980) and cat (Precht and Strata, 1980).

Is there a direct connection from the presumed relay nucleus NRTP to VN? NRTP projections to all main vestibular nuclei have been reported in the cat (Hellstrøm-Hoddevik, Brodal and Walberg, 1975) but were not found with the HRP method (Pompeiano, Mergner and Corvaja, 1978) and anterograde labelling techniques (Blanks, pers. comm.).

Stimulation data in the rat also do not seem to indicate a strong monosynaptic input from NRTP to Vn but rather suggest oligosynaptic connections. It is not known where the additional and crucial links are located. Certainly they are not in the cerebellum (Keller and Precht, 1979) or inferior olive (Barmack and Pettorossi, 1978) since after placing lesions in either one of them Vn optokinetic responses are still present. On theoretical grounds (see below) one might speculate that part of the NRTP output goes to the velocity integrator network thereby reaching indirectly the Vn (Fig. 2C). One possible candidate for such an integrator might be the n. prepositus hypoglossi (Blanks and co-workers, 1977). There is recent anatomical evidence for NRTP-prepositus hypoglossi (Cazin, pers. comm.) as well as prepositus-VN projections in the rat.

What type of Vn is reached by the optokinetic signal? Our studies in the rat (Cazin, 1980b) suggest that type II Vn are reached first by the input. These neurons, in turn, inhibit type I and influence - via the vestibular commissure - type II and type I Vn on the other side of the brainstem which show mirror image responses to optokinetic stimuli: Effective crossing rostral to the Vn does not occur.

The NRTP deserves interest for another reason: in the rat its units respond to head rotation in the dark showing mainly type II responses (Cazin, Precht and Lannou, 1980c). Thus, contrary to NOT these neurons show visual-vestibular convergence. The vestibular-evoked response may, however, also be viewed as an eye velocity signal which reaches NRTP via vestibular or reticular projections. If so, the NRTP may be the site at which retinal slip and eye velocity are believed to converge to represent the velocity of the environment relative to the head (Robinson, 1977). This signal after passing through the velocity storage integrator network, could be fed into Vn yielding the sluggish time course of their responses to velocity steps.

Finally, it should be mentioned that in the cat there exists a class of Vn which rather rapidly reaches maximum firing during optokinetic stimulation and shows less of a phase lag when tested in the frequency domain (Keller and Precht, 1979a; these units may contribute to the so-called direct path.

3.2.2 Pretecto-NRTP-flocculus path. That the flocculus is involved in OKN has been first deduced from lesion experiments in which impairment of smooth pursuit to the ipsilateral side and loss of fixation suppression of VOR were found together with slowing of OKN at higher stimulus velocities and absence of the immediate fast rise in OKN slow phase velocity on velocity step presentation (Keller and Precht, 1979a; Takemori and Cohen, 1974). These findings would indicate that the flocculus is a crucial link in the direct OKN path (see above). Further support for this notion was obtained by single unit recordings from the flocculus in the monkey (Waespe and Henn, 1981; Waespe, Büttner and Henn, 1981, rat (Blanks and Precht, 1981) and rabbit (Ghelarducci, Ito and Yagi, 1975). Rat Purkinje cells responded both to vestibular (type I and II) and optokinetic stimuli. The latter responses were bidirectional and synergistic to the vestibular ones. Velocity steps of optokinetic stimuli produced in the paralyzed animal a fast rise of P-cell simple spike firing (time constant 0.3 - 1 sec). This phasic component often was followed by a smaller tonic one. Peaks of tuning curves of P-cells were higher (2°/sec) than those of Vn and NRTP units in the same animal (see above). In the monkey, a set of P-cells responded to ipsilaterally directed optokinetic stimulus velocities in excess of 60°/sec with a fast rise in firing and rapidly ceased to fire once the lights were turned off, i.e.

there was no activity related to OKAN. Firing could be related but not directly equated to retinal slip velocity over a wide range. The signal may represent an eye velocity control signal (Lisberger and Fuchs, 1978). P-cell activity during OKN is thus distinctly different from that of Vn (Waespe and Henn, 1981) which saturate just about at stimulus levels when P-cells start to respond and show a distinctly different time course.

How does the optokinetic response reach the flocculus? It has recently been shown that in the rabbit (Maekawa and Takeda, 1978), rat (Blanks and Precht, 1981, unpublished observations) and cat (Hoddevik, 1978) the NRTP - known to receive pretectal afferents and respond to horizontal optokinetic stimuli (see section 3.2.1) - projects strongly to the flocculus bilaterally, and that NRTP neurons were antidromically driven from the flocculus (Maekawa, Takeda and Kimura, 1981). P-cell optokinetic responses and visual-vestibular interactions in the VOR were strongly reduced following lesions in the NRTP (Miyashita, 1981). Thus the Pt-NRTP-Floc projection system may be part of the functionally defined direct pathway, at least in some species. At present it is not known, however, which of the several functional classes of NRTP neurons (Cazin, Precht and Lannou, 1980c) project to the flocculus. Also unknown is how the P-cells reach the motor system. It is probably not through the Vn since their optokinetic response characteristics are different except for one class of eye movement related Vn described in the monkey (Keller and Kamath, 1975). Other candidates may be a group of units related to eye velocity found just caudal to the abducens nucleus (Eckmiller and Mackeben, 1980).

3.2.3 LGN-transcortical-flocculus path. In higher vertebrates particularly primates the contribution of the foveal LGN-cortical flocculus system becomes very important for OKN and it probably represents the major direct path as evidenced from lesion studies (see above and Baloh, this volume). Presently available evidence does not favor the NRTP as a major brainstem relay of the foveal pursuit path to the flocculus in primates (Keller, 1981), and other nuclei, e.g. pontine nuclei may be more likely candidates (Fig. 2). There is, however, evidence that in the cat the visual cortex exerts an influence on NOT (see Hoffmann, this vol.) and thereby gains indirect access to the NRTP and flocculus as well (Fig. 2). That in the cat and monkey the visual cortex is of great importance for OKN will be documented below. It should also be noted that 'optokinetic' neurons have been recorded in area 7 of the monkey; these units fire in a direction-selective mode to optokinetic stimuli even when OKN is suppressed by fixation (Kawano and Sasaki, 1981). Area 7 has access to the pretectum, and lesion of this area impaires OKN (see Baloh, this vol.). In rabbit and rat the contribution of the cortex is apparently of negligible importance. Accordingly, the direct path is of minor importance.

3.2.4 Pretecto-olivary-floccular path. It has been well-established that both NOT and AOS project to the dorsal cap of the inferior olive in the cat (Berman, 1977; Hoffmann, Behrend and Schoppmann, 1976; Itoh, 1977; Walberg and co-workers, 1981), rabbit (Maekawa and Simpson, 1973) and rat (Terasawa, Otani and Yamada, 1979) and from there, via climbing fibers, to the contralateral flocculus and via climbing fiber collaterals to the vestibular nuclei (Balaban and co-workers, 1981). Stimulation of the dorsal cap produced nystagmus (Barmack and Hess, 1980b), lesions modified it (Barmack and Simpson, 1980) and units were shown to be sensitive to retinal slip velocity in a range similar to that of Purkinje cell complex spikes (Barmack and Hess, 1980a). When the dorsal cap was lesioned Vn optokinetic and OKN responses were not abolished though somewhat modified (Barmack and Pettorossi, 1978; Precht and Strata, 1980). This shows that climbing fibers may carry an optokinetic signal to Vn both directly (via collaterals) and indirectly (via Purkinje cells) but that there exist other more powerful routes, e.g. via NRTP (see above). Recently, some experimental evidence has been provided showing that the long-term alteration of the VOR gain in the rabbit introduced by optokinetic stimulation may be mediated by the pretecto-olivo-floccular path (Miyashita, 1981).

4. Relative Importance of Crossed and Uncrossed Retinofugal Pathways

Monocular optokinetic stimulation evokes in some species such as rat (Cazin, Precht and Lannou, 1980a), rabbit (Collewijn, 1969) and frog (Birukow, 1937) asymmetric OKN such that the temporonasal pattern movements are more effective than nasotemporal ones whereas in cat (Montarolo, Precht and Strata, 1981; Precht, Montarolo and Strata, 1980) and monkey monocularly evoked OKN is quite symmetric. It has been postulated that symmetry is caused by the advent of uncrossed projections (Fukuda, 1959) mediating the responses to nasotemporal stimuli. Alternatively, data have been presented suggesting that the uncrossed path is related to the presence of a fovea (Tauber and Atkin, 1968) and frontal eyes. In support of this notion is the finding that both in monkeys (Pasik and Pasik, 1964b; and cat (Montarolo, Precht and Strata, 1981; Precht, Montarolo and Strata, 1980) crossed and uncrossed systems, when stimulated separately, are able to evoke OKN in monocular condition. There existed some small directional preponderances such that the crossed system responded slightly better to temporonasal, and the uncrossed path better to nasotemporal stimuli. Removal of either the crossed or uncrossed paths resulted in a gain decrease.

In other species (rat, rabbit, frog) the uncrossed system is so poorly developed that selective stimulation (optic chiasma split) fails to evoke OKN, so that the reason for asymmetric responses lies in the fact that the nasotemporal sensitivity of the crossed system is very much reduced or absent.

5. Role of the Transcortical Path

When the bilateral visual cortices are removed in animals showing strong asymmetric OKN in the monocular condition, no change in OKN responses is observed (Cazin, Precht and Lannou, 1980b; Hobbelen and Collewijn, 1971). However, when such a lesion is performed in animals with symmetric OKN a large asymmetry is generated due to very poor responses to nasotemporal stimulation (Montarolo, Precht and Strata,

1981; Wood, Spear and Braun, 1973). It is also important to emphasize that the gain of the OKN to temporonasal stimuli is strongly reduced in this condition (Montarolo, Precht and Strata, 1981). This reduction in gain shows that transcortical or geniculo-striate routes (the direct pathways as defined above), are important for OKN evoked by nasotemporal but also temporonasal directions in foveate animals having binocular vision.

Given that nasotemporal and temporonasal systems show a differential sensitivity to cortical lesions the next question would be to assess the relative role of the transcortical path on crossed and uncrossed retinofugal systems. When one optic tract is sectioned in cortically lesioned animals monocular stimulation allows selective stimulation of the two systems depending on which eye is covered (Montarolo, Precht and Strata, 1981). It was shown that OKN could only be elicited by temporonasal stimuli of the crossed path, i.e. the weak nasotemporal response observed in cortically lesioned animals was no longer observed because the uncrossed system was eliminated by optic tract lesion. This and other findings indicate that both crossed and uncrossed fibers act on subcortical centers directly as well as through the LGN-visual cortex path. Anatomical findings in the cat (Berman, 1977) showing crossed and uncrossed retinofugal projections to AOS and pretectal nuclei are in agreement with this conclusion.

ACKNOWLEDGEMENT

Supported by grants nos 3.505.79 and 3.616.80 of the Swiss National Foundation for Scientific Research and the Dr Eric Slack-Gyr Foundation.

CORTICAL VERSUS SUBCORTICAL CONTRIBUTIONS TO THE OPTOKINETIC REFLEX IN THE CAT

K. P. HOFFMANN

Abteilung für Vergleichende Neurobiologie, Universität Ulm, D-7900 Ulm, Federal Republic of Germany

ABSTRACT

A model is presented which relates neural activity differences in the left and right nucleus of the optic tract (NOT) to the gain of optokinetic nystagmus in the cat. With stimuli presented to one eye only, it can be shown, that the direct retinal and the indirect cortical visual pathways play a different role for activating the contra and ipsilateral NOT. Cortical lesions reveal a retinal dominance for the slow phase of OKN during temporo-nasal stimulus movement, which activates the contralateral NOT and a cortical dominance during naso-temporal stimulus movement, which normally activates the ipsilateral NOT.

KEYWORDS

Visual cortex; nucleus of the optic tract; optokinetic nystagmus; cat.

INTRODUCTION

A way to demonstrate the contribution of the cortical and subcortical visual pathways to optokinetic nystagmus (OKN) is to change OKN by cortical lesions or developmental manipulations and to see whether or not these changes can be explained by changes in the response properties of those neurons on which these two pathways converge. The nucleus of the optic tract in the pretectum (NOT) has been identified as this side of convergence and as a sensory motor link between retina and premotor structures in the pathway mediating OKN in mammals (see Precht's chapter in this book). In the cat the NOT is a diffuse cell aggregation in the pretectum, with most of the cells embedded in fibers from retina and from visual cortex as they pass through the brachium of the superior colliculus. NOT cells are thus optimally located in the mid-brain to integrate both strong direct retinal and extensive diffuse cortical projections (Berman, 1977; Updyke, 1977). Our results presented below suggest, that the cortical projection provides a binocular input, whereas the retinal input is mainly from the contralateral eye. One target area of the NOT output fibers in the cat is the dorsal cap of the inferior olive (Hoffmann and co-workers, 1976; Walberg and co-workers, 1981). In this paper we want to present quantitative data on the response properties of direction selective cells in the NOT of normal adult cats and of cats with cortical lesions and we wish to discuss the possible role of the output of these cells for the control of optokinetic nystagmus.

In the normal cat, OKN to horizontal stimulus movement is slightly asymmetric. This asymmetry of OKN is such, that for each eye, the temporo-nasal direction of the stimulus elicits a better OKN. This monocular response can be rendered more and more asymmetric by lesions of visual cortex. Temporo-nasal stimulus movement, i.e. from left to right through the left eye and from right to left through the right eye, is then much more effective in eliciting the slow phase of OKN (Wood, Spear and Brown, 1973). This clear behavioural effect can be explained completely by equivalent changes in response properties of NOT cells.

Methods for recording from units in the NOT and for visual stimulation were the same as described previously (Hoffmann and Schoppmann, 1981). Large random noise patterns projected onto a tangent screen by a slide projector via a double mirror system served as visual stimuli. These patterns were moved along a circular path without changing their orientation. The cells' responses were analysed by on-line computation of average response histograms, which were then displayed in polar coordinates. The responses of cells could be pooled to receive the response characteristics of the total population of one nucleus. One pair of stimulating electrodes was stereotaxically inserted into the inferior olive, ipsilateral to the NOT in which recordings were to be made. A second pair of stimulating electrodes was placed in the optic chiasma to measure the conduction velocity of retinal fibers to the NOT. Our main criterion, which we assume to be unaffected by experimental manipulations like cortex lesions or visual deprivation, to identify the cells, was that patterns rich in contour and covering a large area of the visual field are significantly more effective stimuli than single spots or bars. As expected from the anatomical experiment, these cells can be antidromically activated from electrical stimulation at the inferior olive and secondly, these cells received direct retinal input from the contralateral eye. The conduction velocity of the retinal fibers to NOT cells measured between the optic chiasma and the optic tract near the lateral geniculate nucleus indicate that W-cells from the retina supply the input to NOT cells.

NEUROPHYSIOLOGICAL PROPERTIES OF NOT-CELLS

The outstanding property of the NOT cells is their direction specificity. All cells studied were direction specific in such a way, that cells in the right nucleus prefer movements from left to right and cells in the left nucleus from right to left. In the visual field contralateral to the recording site, the preferred movements are from the periphery towards the vertical zero meridian. In binocular cells the preferred direction was identical in visual space through both eyes.

All units can be influenced by the contralateral eye and only about half of them by the ipsilateral one as well. The response elicited from both eyes in binocular cells was not significantly stronger than that from the contralateral eye alone.

In 7 cats, large lesions of the visual cortex were performed several months before recording in the NOT ipsilateral to the lesion. The response properties of NOT cells remained unaltered except that binocularity was lost. Only one out of 40 units could be activated from both eyes. Normal direction specific responses could be elicited, however, only at low velocities through the contralateral eye in all units. Therefore, the main difference between normal and decorticated animals was the loss of the ipsilateral input to the NOT and a decreased sensitivity to visual stimuli moving at velocities above 10 deg / sec. These properties seem to require an intact cortico-pretectal projection. Direction specificity of the units' responses was tested by continuously moving a large pattern on a circular path over a receptive field. The average activity of the population of 49 cells analysed in

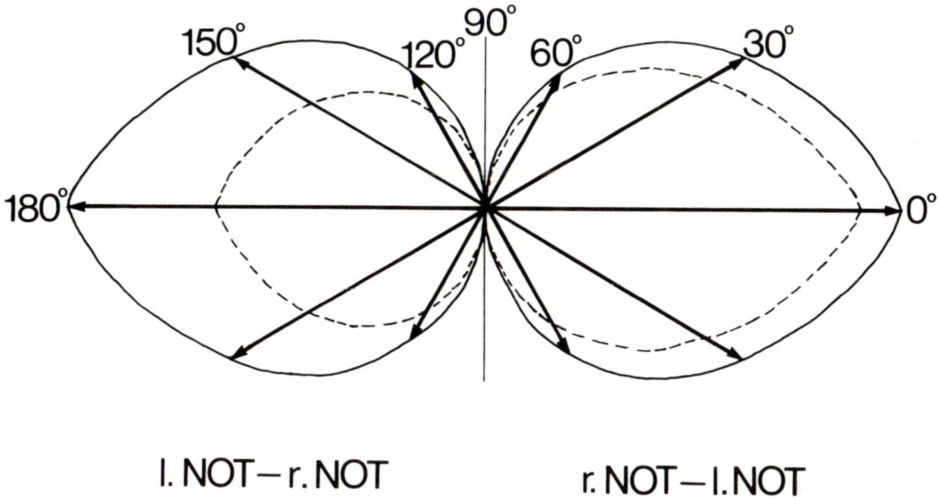

Fig. 1. NOT output signal defined as the difference between the activity of the left and right nucleus of the optic tract plotted in polar coordinates. Full line gives the values for binocular stimulation, broken line for stimulation of the left eye alone. Movements from left to right (0°) increase the activity maximally in the right NOT and decrease it in the left NOT. The difference in activity between both NOTs is maximal. This difference is zero with vertical movements and maximal again with movements from right to left. But now the activity in the left nucleus is increased and decreased in the right.

relation to different directions is given by the equation

$$f\alpha = A - M \sin \alpha/2$$

where $f\alpha$ is the discharge rate as a function of α the angle of deviation from the horizon, A is the response in the preferred direction and M is the difference between the response in the preferred and null directions. Binocular stimulation as in natural conditions leads to a direction specific difference signal between the two nuclei as presented in Fig. 1 in polar coordinates for all stimulus directions. We assume, that stimulus movement in a particular direction in visual space is coded by the activity in one NOT minus the activity in the other NOT. For vertical directions, the NOT output is zero because vertical movements do not influence the NOT cells; for horizontal movement the NOT output is maximum. This signal will be called the NOT output and it is this signal which we want to relate to OKN.

SOME PROPERTIES OF OPTOKINETIC NYSTAGMUS

Optokinetic nystagmus was measured by implanting a magnetic search coil to one eye, according to the technique as described by Judge, Richmond and Chu (1980). In addition, head restraining bolts were attached to the skull by means of dental acrylic. Some days after surgery the animals were put into a horizontal and vertical alter-

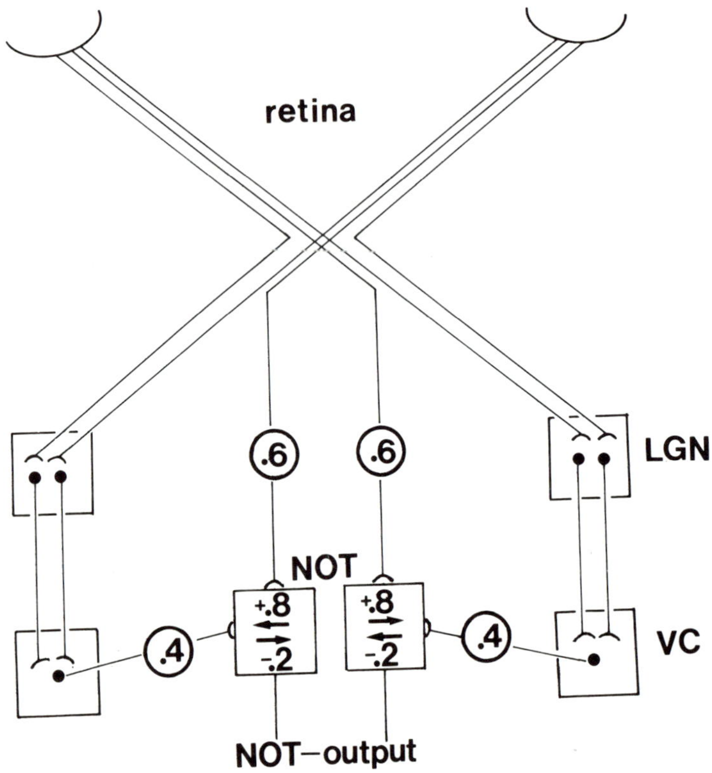

Fig. 2. Input - output model for the NOT. LGN: lateral geniculate nucleus; VC: visual cortex; NOT: nucleus of the optic tract. Each NOT is reached by direct retinal fibers from the contralateral eye (.6) and by binocularly driven axons from the ipsilateral visual cortex (.4). The activity of NOT can increase (+.8) with temporo-nasal movement or decrease (-.2) with naso-temporal movement presented to the contralateral eye. From this model tables I and II are calculated. For further explanation see text.

nating magnetic field and eye movements were elicited by the movement of a random dot pattern across a 90° by 90° screen 40 cm in front of the animal. This stimulus is different from the more commonly used optokinetic drum, providing full field stimulation. We chose our condition for several reasons. Firstly and most importantly, we wanted to test OKN with stimuli more or less identical to those used to test the neuronal responses in the NOT. Secondly, it was easy to test OKN in directions other than horizontal. Thirdly, being a possibly less powerful stimulus more subtle changes in the central pathways mediating OKN could be revealed because the contrast of the pattern could be easily varied. Of course, comparison of normal and experimental conditions were always carried out using the same stimulus parameters. For a comparison of OKN with responses of NOT cells we investigated the eye velocity in relation to stimulus velocity for the two eyes separately and binocularly. Eye velocity was calculated from the eye position signal by on-line computer analysis.

Normal cats

The most striking result in testing the optokinetic nystagmus of normal adult cats is the asymmetry between responses to temporo-nasal movement and to naso-temporal movement when only one eye is stimulated. This means, that the left to right movements are more effective for the left eye and vice versa (see Fig. 3).

From our neurophysiological analysis a straight forward explanation can be provided. As was explained in the previous chapter, each eye alone strongly activates all units in the contralateral NOT when the visual stimulus moves temporo-nasally, but only about 40 % of the units are activated in the ipsilateral nucleus when the stimulus moves naso-temporally. This different amount of activation by number of units and response strength in the contra and in the ipsilateral NOT could lead to the different quality of OKN (frequency and gain) elicited monocularly in the naso-temporal and in the temporo-nasal directions, respectively. Our quantitative neurophysiological results, included in what is known about the anatomy of the input to NOT, form the basis for the model proposed in Fig. 2. Two components normally contribute to the NOT activity, a strongly contralateral dominated retinal input and binocular input from the visual cortex. By this model each eye reaches the ipsilateral NOT only via the binocular cells in the cortex, whereas the contralateral eye has two ways to influence NOT cells, one by direct retinal fibers and the other one through binocular cells in the visual cortex. We assume, that in monocular units the retinal input is dominant and in binocular units the cortical input is dominant. The ratio of monocular to binocular units is 0.6 : 0.4. This is taken as the relative strength of retinal versus cortical input. With horizontal movement, 80 % of the NOT output is supplied by the activation of one nucleus and 20 % by the inhibition of the other nucleus. Thus, the weighting factor for the contribution to the NOT output made up by excitation is 0.5 (0.8 x 0.6) for the retinal and 0.3 (0.8 x 0.4) for the cortical input from each eye. The weighting factor for the contribution from inhibition is 0.1 (0.2 x 0.6) retinal and 0.1 (0.2 x 0.4) cortical for each eye. To keep the model simple, we do not introduce changing weighting factors as a function of stimulus velocity. For a more complete description of the system, however, this will be necessary. The maximal NOT output of 1.0 is reached with binocular stimulation only. Then one NOT is fully activated and the other fully inhibited by the retinal and cortical inputs. With monocular stimulation the NOT output is dependent on the stimulus direction and becomes asymmetric. With temporonasal stimulus direction the contralateral NOT is fully activated (0.8) and the ipsilateral NOT inhibited via the cortex (0.1). With naso-temporal stimulus direction the contralateral NOT is fully inhibited (0.2) and the ipsilateral NOT only activated via the cortex (0.3). These values of the NOT output are matched more or less by the gain of OKN in the same stimulus conditions (Table I).

Animals with Cortical Lesions

This model can now be used to predict the effect of cortical lesions. Lesions of the visual cortex were performed in 6 adult cats. With aseptic precautions all of areas 17, 18, 19, Clare Bishop and the suprasylvian gyrus were removed. Gain of OKN as a function of stimulus velocity is presented for one animal in Fig. 3. In this animal the OKN was tested before and after the lesion and finally the animal was used for neurophysiological analysis of the NOT responses. With the lesion of the left cortex, leftward stimulus movement is not as effective in eliciting OKN as in the normal cat. This direction in visual space normally activates the NOT ipsilateral to the lesion. The clearest effect is seen for leftward movement presented to the eye ipsilateral to the lesion (left eye), but also through the right eye, which has a direct retinal projection to the left NOT, a decreased effectiveness can be observed. Table II summarizes the NOT output values from our model and compares them to the OKN gains measured after left cortex lesion. They correspond

TABLE 1

NORMAL		left NOT cort.	ret.	right NOT cort.	ret.	l - r NOT output	OKN gain
bin	←	0.3	0.5	-0.1	-0.1	1.0	1.0
	→	-0.1	-0.1	0.3	0.5	-1.0	1.0
r. eye	←	0.3	0.5	-0.1	---	0.9	0.9
	→	-0.1	-0.1	0.3	---	-0.5	0.6
l. eye	←	0.3	---	-0.1	-0.1	0.5	0.6
	→	-0.1	---	0.3	0.5	-0.9	0.9

TABLE 2

CORTICAL LESION LEFT		left NOT cort.	ret.	right NOT cort.	ret.	l - r NOT output	OKN gain
bin	←	---	0.5	-0.1	-0.1	0.7	0.7
	→	---	-0.1	0.3	0.5	-0.9	0.8
r. eye	←	---	0.5	-0.1	---	0.6	0.7
	→	---	-0.1	0.3	---	-0.4	0.5
l. eye	←	---	---	-0.1	-0.1	0.2	0.3
	→	---	---	0.3	0.5	-0.8	0.8
LESION BILATERAL							
bin	←	---	0.5	---	-0.1	0.6	0.4
	→	---	-0.1	---	0.5	-0.6	0.5
r. eye	←	---	0.5	---	---	0.5	0.4
	→	---	-0.1	---	---	-0.1	0.2
l. eye	←	---	---	---	-0.1	0.1	0.2
	→	---	---	---	0.5	-0.5	0.5

bin: binocular stimulation; r., l.: monocular stimulation of the right or left eye; cort.: cortical contribution; ret.: retinal contribution; l - r: discharge rate in the left NOT minus discharge rate in the right NOT; arrows indicate direction of stimulus movement.

at least qualitatively very well. The right cortex was then also removed. After such a bilateral lesion the results are shown in Fig. 3 by the crosses. There is a further reduction in OKN gain with an OKN being practically absent at higher velocities with naso-temporal stimulus movement. As with the unilateral lesion, the additional lesion of the right cortex has a global effect on both directions tested through each eye. Again, the values predicted from our model for this preparation are given in Table II. In summary, decortication strongly reduces the naso-temporal direction of monocularly elicited OKN which coincides with the preferred direction of cells in the ipsilateral NOT. The pathway activating the ipsilateral NOT from each eye seems almost entirely dependent on a relay through the cortex.

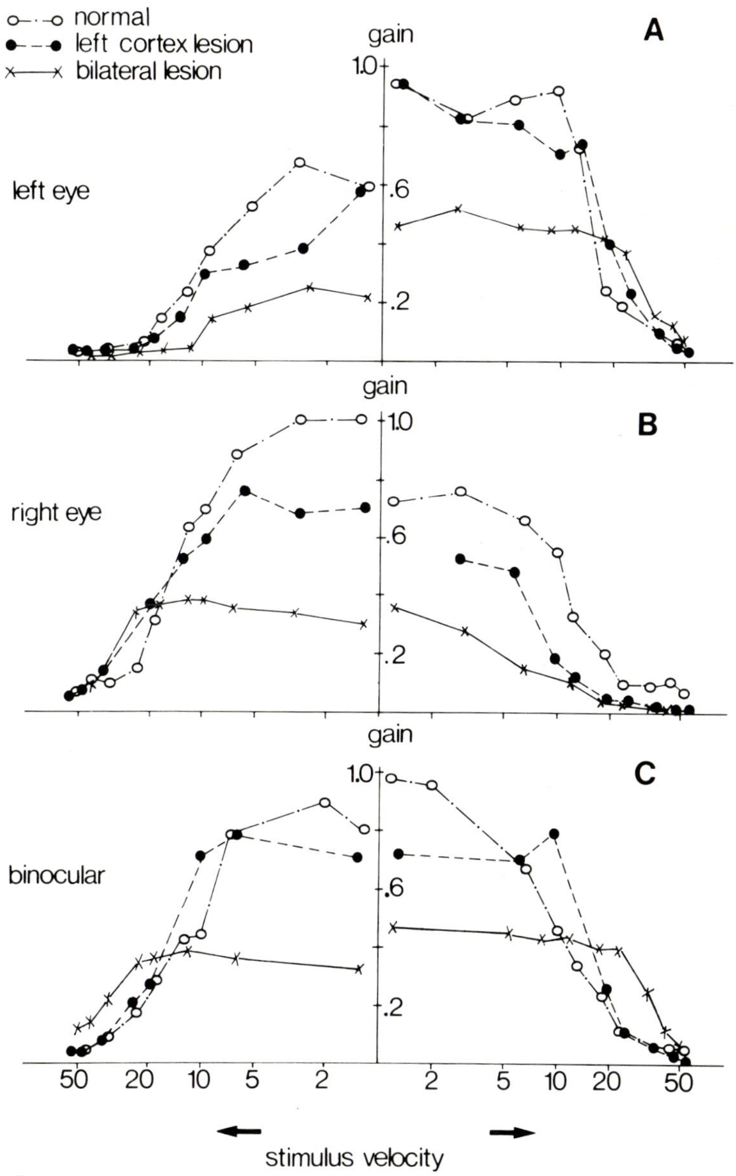

Fig. 3. Gain of OKN in normal, unilateral or bilateral decorticated cats. Stimulus velocity is plotted along the X-axis, OKN gain (eye velocity/stimulus velocity) along the Y-axis. Movement of the pattern from right to left is plotted to the left and pattern movement from left to right is presented on the right. A: stimulus presented to the left eye; B: stimulus presented to the right eye; C: binocular stimulation.

CONCLUSION

We have presented a model in which the activity difference in the left and the right NOT is related to the gain of OKN. The activity difference between the two nuclei is always made up by an increase in the activity in one nucleus and a decrease in activity in the opposite nucleus, when compared to spontaneous activity. A decrease of activity in one nucleus compared to the spontaneous activity in the other seems to be sufficient to elicit OKN at very low gains. We have tested this model with binocular and monocular stimulation in the normal animal and in animals with unilateral and bilateral large cortical lesions. Characteristic modifications of OKN can be observed, which have their counterparts in the changes of activity differences between left and right NOT. Retinal and cortical contributions play a different role in temporo-nasal and naso-temporal directions of stimulus movement when presented to one eye. Cortical lesions as well as visual deprivation (Hoffmann, 1979) reveal a retinal dominance during temporo-nasal stimulus movement and a cortical dominance for the slow phase of OKN during naso-temporal stimulus movement.

ACKNOWLEDGEMENT

I should like to thank Ms. C. Markner and Dr. A. Meier-Koll who recorded and analysed most of the data in the eye movement experiments and Mr. H.P. Huber who wrote the computer programmes. I am thankful to Ms. L. Harrison for secretarial assistance. The research was supported by DFG grants Ho 450/7 and 12 to K.P. Hoffmann.

CLINICAL ABNORMALITIES OF OPTOKINETIC NYSTAGMUS

R. W. BALOH*, R. D. YEE** and V. HONRUBIA***

*Department of Neurology, Reed Neurological Research Center, University of California, Los Angeles, California 90024, USA
**Department of Ophthalmology, Jules Stein Eye Institute, University of California, Los Angeles, California 90024, USA
***Department of Surgery/Division of Head and Neck, School of Medicine, University of California, Los Angeles, California 90024, USA

ABSTRACT

Clinical disorders of optokinetic nystagmus are divided into those affecting the fast component and those affecting the slow component. The optokinetic slow phase in humans appears to represent the combined output of a foveal pursuit pathway and a full field pursuit pathway. The former normally dominates the latter, however, by using interaction tests such as those described in this report the contribution of each pathway can be quantitatively assessed. Since small changes in foveal pursuit gain lead to large changes in interaction, interaction tests may detect otherwise subclinical impairment of pursuit in patients. Earlier diagnosis and localization of clinical lesions could result.

KEYWORDS

Optokinetic nystagmus; pursuit; interaction.

INTRODUCTION

Optokinetic nystagmus (OKN) is a rhythmic oscillation of the eyes induced by movement of the visual surround or a series of targets in the surround. Slow following movements (slow components) are regularly interrupted by fast movements (fast components) in the opposite direction. Clinicians have traditionally tested OKN by moving a series of vertical stripes directly in front of the patient (usually on a hand-held drum or strip of cloth). Gross asymmetries in OKN amplitude and frequency are visually identified. Although this method has provided useful information in selected cases (e.g. separating parietal from occipital lobe lesions) it suffers from an imprecise stimulus and a poorly defined response. Only a small part of the visual field is stimulated and the velocity of the stripe movement is not controlled. Furthermore, since OKN consists of a slow and fast component, abnormalities in either or both can account for any observed asymmetry. Not surprisingly, the clinical literature on optokinetic testing contains many opposing views concerning its anatomical localizing value (Baloh, Yee and Honrubia, 1980a).

In this report we describe our experience in testing OKN using full-field controlled stimulation in over 500 patients with localized neurologic lesions. The induced nystagmus was recorded with electro-oculography (EOG) and quantitatively analyzed using digital computer techniques previously described (Baloh and co-workers, 1980). Based on this data and recent animal studies we propose a model that includes two parallel OKN systems in humans.

OKN IN NORMAL SUBJECTS

The subject is seated within a 1.5 meter diameter, black cloth drum whose interior is lined with 2.5 cm. wide white vertical stripes placed every 15 degrees. Rotation of the drum stimulates the entire visual field. The subject is instructed to stare at, but not follow, the stripes directly in front of him. After a small initial slow phase in the direction of drum rotation the eyes deviate in the direction of the fast phase and remain on that side of the orbit until stimulus velocity returns to zero or changes direction (Lau, Honrubia and Baloh, 1978). After a step change in drum velocity the OKN slow phase velocity reaches a steady state within one nystagmus beat. This normal pattern of OKN is so consistent that alterations in the pattern can provide clinically useful information (as described later).

OKN slow phase velocity approximates the drum velocity for low stimulus velocities but progressively decreases at higher drum velocities (Fig. 1) (Honrubia and co-workers, 1968; Sills and co-workers, 1975). Step, ramp and sinusoidal changes in drum velocity can be used with each having advantages and disadvantages. A step stimulus allows one to identify a build-up in OKN slow phase velocity and optokinetic after nystagmus (OKAN) but a lengthy test session is required to assess multiple drum velocities in each direction. The ramp and sinusoidal stimuli rapidly screen multiple stimulus velocities but do not permit evaluation of OKN build-up and OKAN. As a compromise we routinely use steps of 30 and 60 degrees/second in each direction and a sinusoidal stimulus of 0.05 Hz and peak velocity of 60 degrees/second.

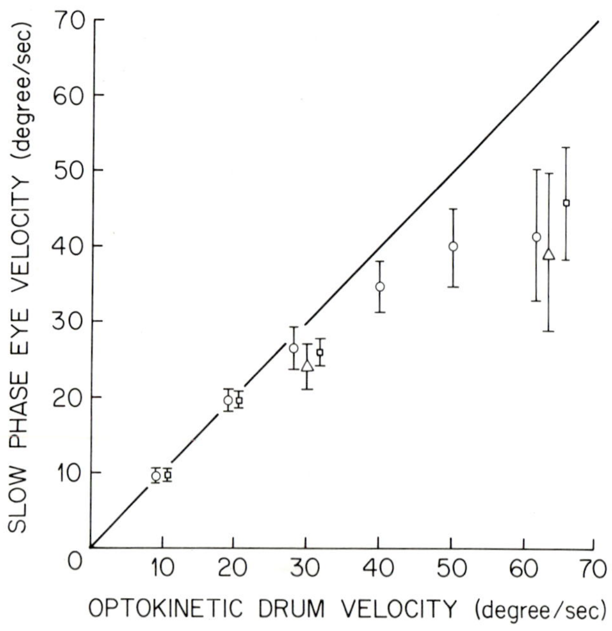

Fig. 1 Normal mean ± 1 standard deviation for horizontal OKN slow phase velocity at different drum velocities o - ramp optokinetic stimulus, ▫ - constant velocity optokinetic stimulus, Δ - sinusoidal optokinetic stimulus (0.05 Hz).

OKAN is induced by shutting off the lights after 1 minute of constant velocity OKN stimulation. OKAN is much more variable than OKN in normal subjects. For example, in a series of 30 normal subjects tested in our laboratory 3 had no detectable OKAN in either direction after the 30 or 60 degree/second constant velocity stimulation despite the fact that each had normal OKN. In the remaining subjects the duration ranged from 2 to 85 seconds and asymmetric responses were not uncommon.

FAST COMPONENT PRODUCTION

Fast components of OKN have a similar peak velocity-amplitude relationship as voluntary refixation saccades and are probably generated by the same burst neurons in the pontine paramedian reticular formation (PPRF) (Ron, Robinson and Skavenski, 1972). How the OKN stimulus controls the initiation of fast components is unknown. However, there is evidence that during OKN the initiation of fast components is correlated with the position of the eyes in the orbit and with the velocity of the slow component (Honrubia, Baloh and Lau, 1977, Lau, Honrubia and Baloh, 1978). The fast component is not a "resetting" movement that carries the eyes back to the center of the orbit but rather an "anticipatory" movement carrying the eyes eccentrically in the orbit.

FAST COMPONENT ABNORMALITIES

Abnormalities of OKN fast components can be divided into those that decrease peak velocity, those that alter amplitude and those that impair initiation (Table 1). Fast component peak velocities are decreased with lesions involving the PPRF, medial longitudinal fasciculus (MLF),oculomotor nuclei and nerves,and the extraocular muscles (Baloh and Honrubia, 1979). Fast component slowing is also seen with several diffuse degenerative disorders (e.g. Huntington disease, olivopontocerebellar atrophy and progressive supranuclear palsy) in which the focus producing the saccade abnormalities is unknown. A typical example of the effect of fast component slowing on OKN is shown in Fig. 2a (right side). The nystagmus waveform is rounded with the slow fast component ending subtracting from the initial segment of the slow phase. In this case adducting

TABLE 1 Summary of OKN Abnormalities

Abnormality	Anatomical Localization
Decreased fast component velocity	Paramedian pontine, MLF, oculomotor nuclei and nerves, extraocular muscles
Fast component amplitude dysmetria or asymmetry	Cerebellum
Impaired initiation of fast components	Basal ganglia ?
Symmetrical decreased slow component velocity	Not localizing
Unilateral decreased slow component velocity	Ipsilateral parietal lobe, brain stem or cerebellum
Slow component velocity build-up	Retina, parietal lobe, vestibulocerebellum
Monocular asymmetry slow component velocity	Foveal dysfunction

fast component slowing resulted from an MLF lesion in a patient with multiple sclerosis. The high pulse rate of firing generated by the PPRF could not reach the medial rectus subnucleus because of demylination in the MLF but did pass unaffected to the lateral rectus nucleus resulting in disconjugate fast components (Baloh, Yee and Honrubia, 1978 a). The slow phase velocity remained symmetrical despite the fast component disorder.

Abnormalities of fast component amplitude are usually associated with lesions of the cerebellum. Unilateral lesions produce asymmetric amplitude (e.g. Fig. 2b) while diffuse lesions produce fast components with large variability in beat-to-beat amplitude (e.g. Fig. 2c). In the patient illustrated in Fig. 2b (left cerebellar infarction) voluntary saccades to the left overshot the target while those to the right undershot the target. By contrast in the patient with diffuse cerebellar atrophy illustrated in Fig. 2c, voluntary saccades under and overshot the target in both directions.

In several neurologic disorders fast component initiation is impaired and the eyes deviate in the direction of the slow phase often becoming pinned in an extreme orbital position (Fig. 2d). The disorders producing this phenomena include: congenital ocular motor apraxia, ataxia-telangiectasia, Huntington disease, progressive supranuclear palsy and olivopontocerebellar atrophy. Each of these conditions is associated with diffuse neuronal loss although involvement of the basal ganglia may be a common thread. These patients have impaired initiation of voluntary refixation saccades as well and often have decreased peak velocity or amplitude of voluntary saccades. Of note in the patient with progressive supranuclear palsy

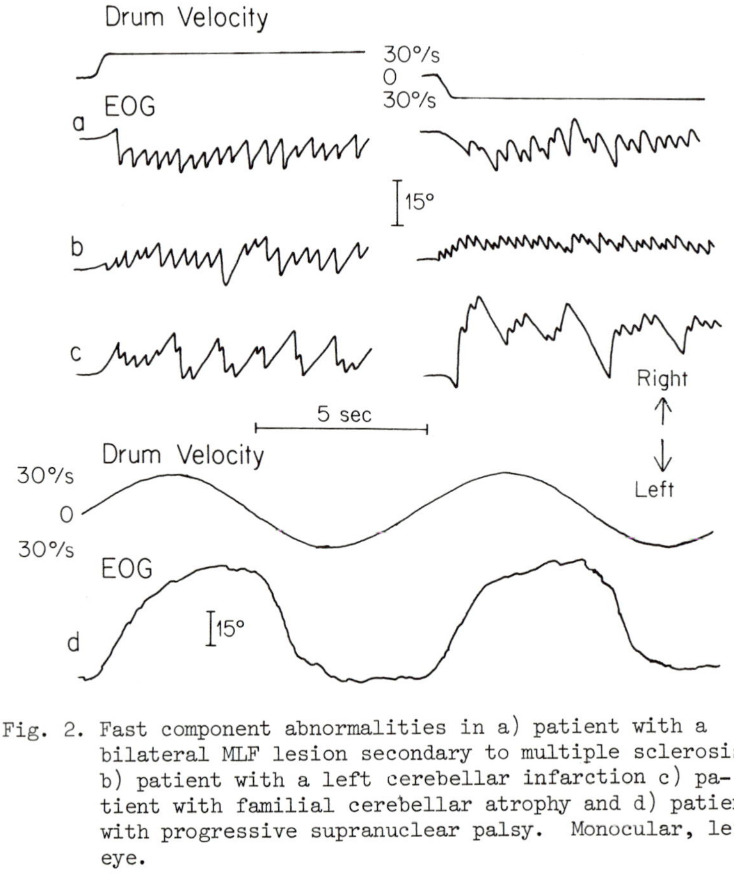

Fig. 2. Fast component abnormalities in a) patient with a bilateral MLF lesion secondary to multiple sclerosis, b) patient with a left cerebellar infarction c) patient with familial cerebellar atrophy and d) patient with progressive supranuclear palsy. Monocular, left eye.

illustrated in Fig. 2d despite the inability to produce fast components, the OKN slow phase velocity was normal during the period when the eyes were moving from one side of the orbit to the other (i.e. before they became pinned).

SLOW COMPONENT PRODUCTION

Ter Braak first provided evidence for separate cortical and subcortical optokinetic slow phase pathways in several animal species (ter Braak, 1936). Cortical OKN was elicited by movement of a series of small objects that attracted the animal's attention (so-called active nystagmus) while subcortical OKN was produced by movement of the entire visual surround (passive nystagmus). In animals without a fovea such as the rabbit, only passive OKN can be induced and bilateral occipital lobectomy produces minimal effect on induced OKN (Collewijn, 1969, Hobbelen and Collewijn, 1971). In afoveate animals the velocity of OKN slow components slowly builds to a maximum value after 20 to 30 seconds of constant velocity stimulation and during monocular stimulation targets moving from temporal to nasal on the retina induce greater OKN slow phase velocity than those moving nasal-temporal (Collewijn, 1969). The production of OKAN may also be a unique feature of the subcortical OKN system. Recent animal studies suggest that at least part of this subcortical slow phase pathway includes the accessory optic system (Hoffman and Schoppman, 1975, Maekawa and Takeda, 1975, Brandth and Karten, 1977).

Apparently with the development of the fovea a more sensitive tracking system without slow phase build-up or directional asymmetry developed - the cortical pursuit pathway. This system receives afferent signals from the retino-geniculo-calcarine projections and sends motor commands to the brain stem via the occipito-mesencephalic projections. In humans both slow phase systems participate in the production of OKN but the phylogenetically newer cortical system overshadows the older subcortical system.

CLINICAL SLOW COMPONENT ABNORMALITIES

Moderate symmetrical slowing of OKN slow phase velocity is a common nonspecific finding seen with lesions throughout the neuroaxis. It often results from sedating drugs such as diazepam or alcohol or endogenous metabolic disorders (e.g. renal or hepatic encephalopathy).

Lesions of the afferent visual pathways not surprisingly decrease OKN slow phase velocity. Several studies that have artificially restricted the peripheral visual fields in normal subjects have demonstrated decreased OKN slow phase velocity as the size of the remaining visual field decreased (Dichgans, Nauck and Wolpert, 1973, Cheng and Outerbridge, 1975, Duboid and Collewijn, 1979). We studied OKN in 14 patients with severe loss of peripheral vision (tunnel vision) due to chronic open-angle glaucoma (Yee and co-workers, In press). Each patient had monocular loss of peripheral vision so that the intact eye acted as a control for the abnormal eye. Central visual acuity was normal bilaterally and pursuit of a 1° diameter red laser light was the same when tracking with either eye. OKN slow phase velocity, however, was decreased in the eye with tunnel vision compared to the normal eye in each patient. Furthermore, the degree of slow phase velocity impairment correlated with the degree of peripheral visual field loss (Fig. 3).

On the other hand we found normal symmetrical OKN slow phase velocity in 6 patients with unilateral central scotomas from senile macular degeneration. Visual acuity in the affected eye ranged from 20/70 to 20/400, and the central scotomas varied from 5 to 15° in diameter. As expected, pursuit of a small target was markedly impaired in the affected eye compared to the normal eye. These studies document partial

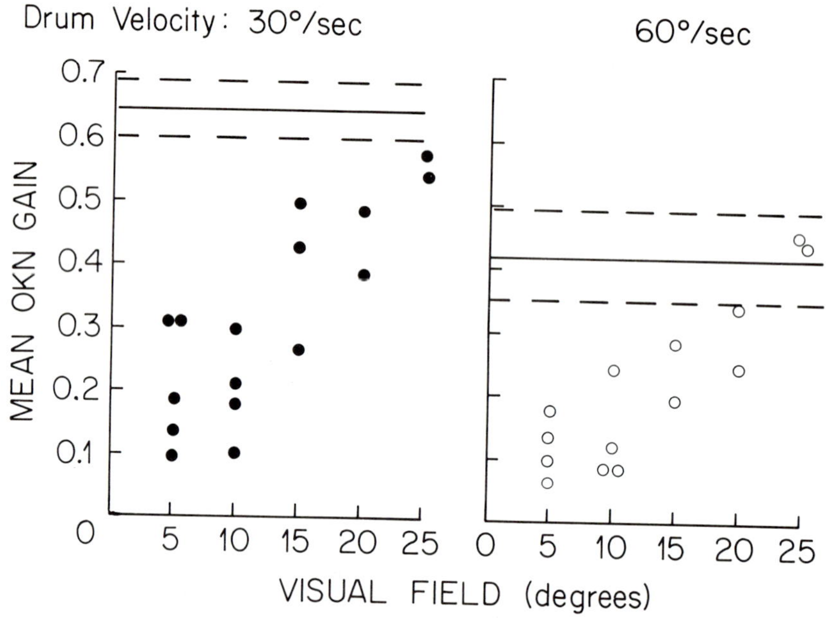

Fig. 3 OKN gain (mean slow phase velocity/drum velocity) vs. size of remaining central visual field in patients with monocular tunnel vision. Solid and dash lines indicate mean ± 1 standard deviation for stimulation of the normal eye.

separation for the afferent signals for foveal pursuit and full field pursuit at the level of the retina.

Unilateral decreased OKN slow phase velocity is a useful clinical sign since it is localizing to the ipsilateral parietal lobe, brain stem or cerebellum (Baloh, Sills and Honrubia, 1977). When present in isolation or with an ipsilateral homonymous hemianopsia it is highly localizing to the parietal lobe (Baloh, Yee and Honrubia, 1980a). Asymmetric OKN slow phase velocity in a patient with signs of a cerebello-pontine angle tumor indicates that the tumor is compressing the brain stem and/or cerebellum (Baloh and co-workers, 1976). Patients with acute unilateral peripheral vestibular lesions may also have asymmetric OKN but the decreased slow phase velocity occurs with drum rotation away from the side of the lesion, i.e. in the direction of their spontaneous nystagmus. This OKN asymmetry rapidly disappears within a few days as compensation occurs.

Some patients exhibit a gradual build-up of OKN slow phase velocity after the step onset of a constant velocity stimulus. For example, patients with localized lesions involving the vestibulocerebellum (flocculus, nodulus, uvula and paraflocculus) exhibit almost total absence of smooth pursuit and sinusoidal optokinetic responses in either direction yet develop normal or near normal OKN slow phase velocity with prolonged constant velocity stimulation (Yee and co-workers, 1979, Baloh and co-workers 1981). In addition to this unusual OKN build-up these patients have spontaneous downbeat nystagmus and severely impaired visual-vestibular interaction. Patients with congenital achromatopsia (a disorder in which severe loss of visual acuity and complete loss of color vision results from maldevelopment of the cone photoreceptors of the retina) exhibit not only a gradual build-up of OKN slow phase velocity but also monocular directional asymmetry (Baloh, Yee and Honrubia, 1980b). With monocul

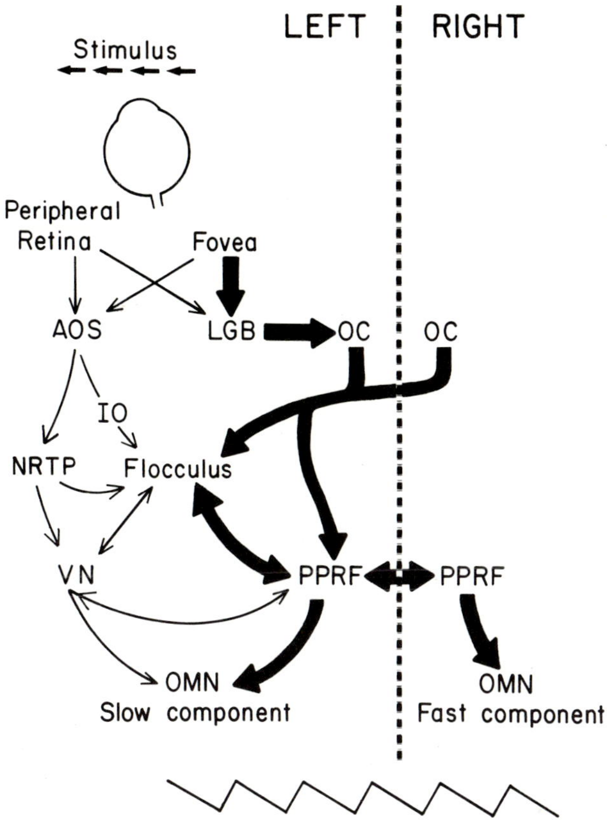

Fig. 4 Schematic illustration of cortical and subcortical OKN pathways. Thick lines - cortical pathway, thin lines - subcortical pathway. LGB - lateral geniculate body, OC - occipital lobe cortex, PPRF - pontine paramedian reticular formation, OMN - ocular motor neurons, AOS - accessory optic system, IO - inferior olive, NRTP - nucleus reticularis tegmenti pontis, VN - vestibular nuclei. Crossing pathways within the accessor optic system are not included.

stimulation temporal-nasal drum movement induces much greater slow phase velocity than nasal-temporal movement. Such OKN responses are remarkably similar to those seen in afoveate animals and suggest that certain neural lesions may uncover OKN characteristics of the subcortical pathway that are normally overshadowed by those of the foveal pursuit pathway.

So far clinical assessment of OKAN has been of limited use. Not surprisingly, patients with spontaneous vestibular nystagmus have prolonged OKAN when the OKAN slow phases are in the same direction as the spontaneous nystagmus slow phases. Patients with bilateral peripheral vestibular lesions have decreased or absent OKAN in both directions (Zee, Yee and Robinson, 1976c but since approximately 10% of normal subjects have minimal OKAN the finding of bilateral decreased OKAN is not a reliable diagnostic indicator.

NEUROANATOMICAL CORRELATES

A neuroanatomical model of parallel OKN slow phase pathways in humans is schematically illustrated in Fig. 4. The proposed connections of the subcortical pathway via the assessory optic system are based on a series of neuroanatomical and physiologic studies in animals, primarily afoveate animals (Hoffman and Schoppman, 1975, Maekowa and Takeda, 1975, Brandth and Karten, 1977, Miyoshita and co-workers, 1980, Precht and Strata, 1980). Crossing pathways within this system are not included for illustrative purposes. The connections of the cortical pathways are less well defined by animal studies and here we rely more on clinical data. The cortical pathway is designated by thick lines to indicate its normal dominance of the subcortical pathway.

Consistent with our findings in patients with retinal lesions the model assumes that the major input to the cortical pathway is via the fovea while that to the subcortical pathway is via the peripheral retina. However, overlap in afferent signals to both systems probably occurs since central and peripheral retinal lesions are not entirely selective in their effect on either pathway.

Patients with unilateral occipital lobe lesions have normal OKN and smooth pursuit indicating that each occipital lobe is capable of generating motor commands for tracking in both directions (Baloh, Yee and Honrubia, 1980a). For tracking a stimulus to the left (as in Fig. 4), the motor command from the right occipital lobe (probably from association cortex) decussates in the splenium of the corpus callosum to join the motor command from the left occipital lobe in the left parietal lobe. From here the motor command descends near the posterior limb of the internal capsule and continues to the ipsilateral PPRF and flocculus via incompletely delineated pathways in the brain stem tegmentum. The joining of pursuit motor commands from both occipital lobes in the parietal lobe accounts for why ipsilateral pursuit and OKN abnormalities occur in patients with unilateral parietal lobe lesions. The flocculus is considered a major relay nucleus for the cortical pathway since lesions involving this structure profoundly impair smooth pursuit and OKN. As indicated earlier,patients with lesions involving this and other centers of the cortical system produce OKN with features characteristic of the subcortical system (e.g. slow build-up in OKN slow phase velocity).

The model assumes that fast components are reflexly initiated in the PPRF based on certain features of the slow component, e.g. orbital position and velocity. This is consistent with the clinical observation that chronic cortical lesions do not impair OKN fast components. After an acute frontal lobe lesion, contralateral voluntary saccades and fast components are transiently impaired but this abnormality is rapidly reversed within a few days. Subcortical centers such as the basal ganglia may play a role in the initiation of OKN fast components but the neuroanatomical and physiologic basis of this role is currently unknown.

A MODEL FOR PARALLEL OKN SLOW PHASE PATHWAYS

A block diagram for the 2 parallel OKN slow phase pathways is shown in Fig. 5. This model is based on the following assumptions: 1. the foveal pursuit pathway (SP) receives its afferent input entirely from the fovea and the full field pursuit pathway (OK) receives its input entirely from the peripheral retina, 2. each pathway is anatomically distinct and 3. the resulting output ($\dot{\theta}_e$) is a linear addition of the output from each pathway. Clearly all 3 assumptions are oversimplifications but as a first approximation this model does provide a useful framework for studying foveal and full field pursuit in normal subjects and patients.

By application of control system theory (Lau, Honrubia and Baloh, 1981) the output

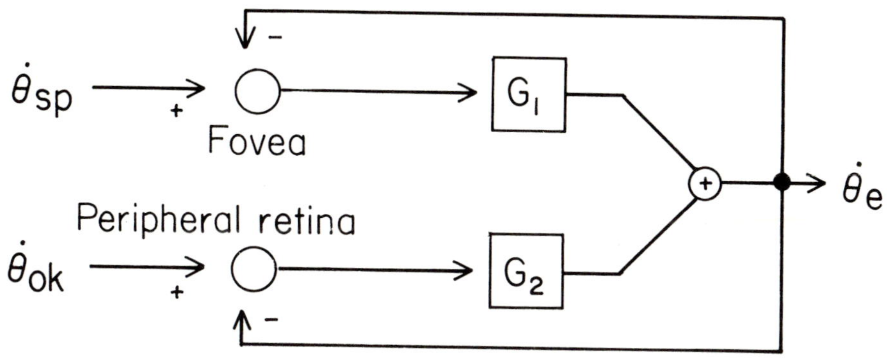

Fig. 5 Block diagram of the parallel closed-loop visual pursuit systems.

of the combined systems ($\dot{\theta}_e$) to separate foveal and peripheral retinal stimuli can be mathematically described by the following equation:

$$\frac{G_1}{1 + G_1 + G_2}\dot{\theta}_{sp} + \frac{G_2}{1 + G_2 + G_1}\dot{\theta}_{ok} = \dot{\theta}_e \qquad \text{Equation 1}$$

Where G_1 = open-loop transfer function of the sp system; G_2 = open-loop transfer function of the ok system; $\dot{\theta}_{sp}$ = velocity of foveal pursuit target; $\dot{\theta}_{ok}$ = velocity of visual surround.

Since there is no simple way of removing retinal feedback we routinely evaluate the closed-loop transfer functions of foveal and full field pursuit. The closed-loop transfer functions (H) are related to the open-loop transfer functions (G) by the following equation:

$$G = \frac{H}{1 - H} \qquad \text{Equation 2}$$

In normal subjects G_1 is an order of magnitude greater than G_2 and thus the velocity of the foveal target dominates the eye velocity output. For example the normal closed-loop foveal pursuit gain for a 30°/second constant velocity target is 0.97. With constant velocity stimuli the transfer function of the system is equal to the gain. From equation 2 the open-loop gain G_1 is approximately 32. The normal full field pursuit gain is more difficult to measure because of the foveal pursuit contribution but an average gain of 0.8 for full field OKN stimulation (30 degrees/second constant velocity) in normal subjects provides a reasonable upper limit estimate for the closed-loop gain. From equation 2 the open-loop gain G_2 for full field pursuit would then be 4. Thus in normal humans the first term in equation 1 is much larger than the second and the resulting eye velocity ($\dot{\theta}_e$) is determined mainly by the velocity of the pursuit target ($\dot{\theta}_{sp}$). However, in patients with impaired foveal pursuit the second term in equation 1 becomes much more important in determining the resultant eye velocity ($\dot{\theta}_e$).

To test these predictions we studied foveal and full field pursuit interaction in normal subjects and patients by having them track a 1° laser target on a featureless white screen, on a still OKN drum and on an OKN drum moving at a constant velocity clockwise or counterclockwise. Subjects were instructed to attend to the laser target and to track its motion carefully during all tests. The interaction tests of 2 normal subjects and a patient with asymmetric foveal pursuit due to a parietal lobe lesion are illustrated in Fig. 6. As predicted by the linear interaction model, since the first normal subject had a foveal pursuit gain of 0.98 on a featureless background, he showed little interaction when tracking the laser target on the still or moving

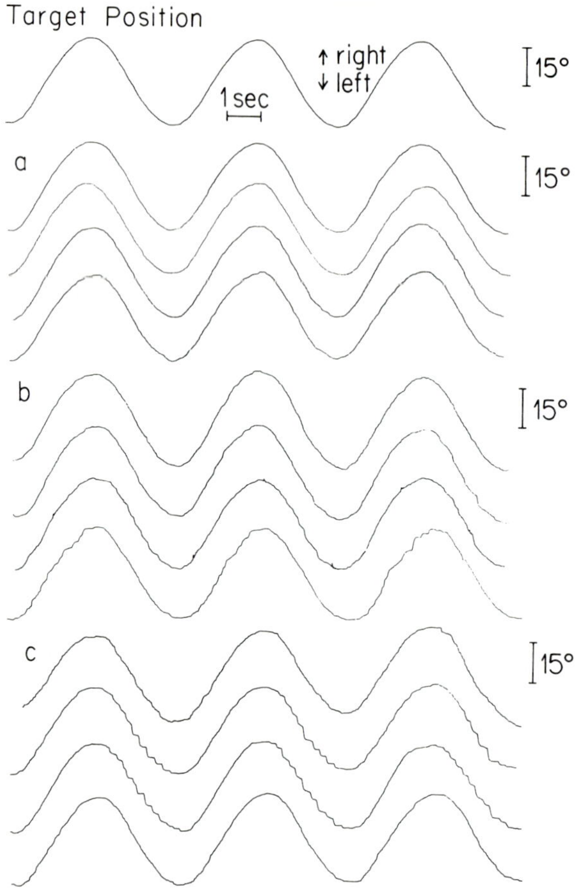

Fig. 6 Foveal - full field pursuit interaction in a) a normal subject with high normal foveal pursuit gain b) a normal subject with low normal foveal pursuit gain and c) a patient with a left parietal lobe glioma. In each case the subject tracked a 1° laser target moving on a featureless background (top trace), on a still optokinetic drum (second trace) and on an optokinetic drum moving at a constant velocity of 30 degrees/second to the right(third trace) and to the left (fourth trace).

OKN drum. By contrast the second normal subject had a lower foveal pursuit gain on a featureless background (0.93) and exhibited much greater interaction during combined stimulation. The patient with a left parietal lobe lesion showed marked interaction between foveal and full field pursuit only when tracking the laser target to the left (the direction of his impaired foveal pursuit). His foveal pursuit deficit to the left was completely reversed when the pursuit target moved in the same direction as the constant velocity optokinetic stimulus. Apparently the parietal lobe selectively damaged the ipsilateral foveal pursuit pathway leaving the full field pursuit pathway intact. These interaction studies support the proposed model of 2 parallel pursuit systems in humans and suggest that linear interaction is a reasonable first approximation of the combined systems.

NASAL-TEMPORAL ASYMMETRY OF THE OPTOKINETIC NYSTAGMUS AFTER BILATERAL OCCIPITAL INFARCTION IN MAN

E. MEHDORN

University Eye Clinic Freiburg, Department of Neuro-Ophthalmology and Strabismus, D-78 Freiburg, Federal Republic of Germany

ABSTRACT

A nasal-temporal asymmetry of the monocularly elicited optokinetic nystagmus (OKN) was observed in two non-strabismic patients who had suffered from a bilateral occipital infarction. This finding suggests two OKN systems in man, a cortical system which is essential for a normal nasal-temporal response, and a subcortical system which mainly mediates the temporal-nasal response.

Optokinetic nystagmus; smooth pursuit; cortical blindness.

INTRODUCTION

Ablation experiments have demonstrated that in the rabbit and other lower vertebrates OKN originates exclusively in subcortical structures as opposed to the cat in which OKN is generated by the visual cortex in cooperation with subcortical structures (see Montarolo and others, 1981, and Wood and others, 1973, for ref.). A very striking feature of the rabbit's OKN as well as of the cat's subcortical OKN after ablation of the visual cortex is a nasal-temporal asymmetry, i.e. monocularly presented patterns moving from temporal to nasal provoke a stronger OKN than patterns moving from nasal to temporal. The present paper describes for the first time an acquired nasal-temporal OKN asymmetry in patients with bilateral occipital infarcts.

PATIENTS AND METHODS

Case 1: 6o-year-old woman. Incomplete bilateral homonymous hemianopia (Fig. 1). CT scan: small infarcts in the supply area of the right medial cerebral artery and large infarcts in the supply area of the left medial and posterior cerebral artery extending to the white matter on both sides. Visual acuity 1.o in both eyes. No ocular anomalies, no strabismus, no anisometropia. Stereoacuity 12o".

Case 2: 47-year-old man.Bilateral homonymous hemianopia with sparing of a small central field rest (Fig. 1). CT scan: large infarcts in both occipital lobes and in the right parietal lobe extending to the white matter on both sides. Visual acuity o.4 in both eyes. No ocular anomalies, no strabismus, no anisometropia. Stereoacuity 33'. Case 3: 48-year-old woman. Gunbarrel visual fields of less than 1o° diameter (Fig. 1). CT scan: large bilateral occipital infarcts extending to the white matter on both sides. Visual acuity o.6 in the right and o.7 in the left eye. No ocular anomalies, no strabismus, no anisometropia. Stereoacuity 12o". - None of the patients had ever had spontaneous, gaze evoked or latent nystagmus. Pupillary reactions had been normal in all three patients.

Eye movements were recorded by means of DC-EOG (see Mehdorn and others, 1979, for details) 6 months, 8 months, and 6 years after the infarctions in the first, second, and third patient respectively. Optokinetic stimulation was provided by projection of 7° wide black-and-white stripes onto a curved screen 18o° large and 6o° high. In order to provoke optokinetic after nystagmus (OKAN), a stimulation of 6o s duration was applied. Slow phase velocities were measured by a semiautomatic x-y-plotter (Pedersen and Schmidt, 1978).

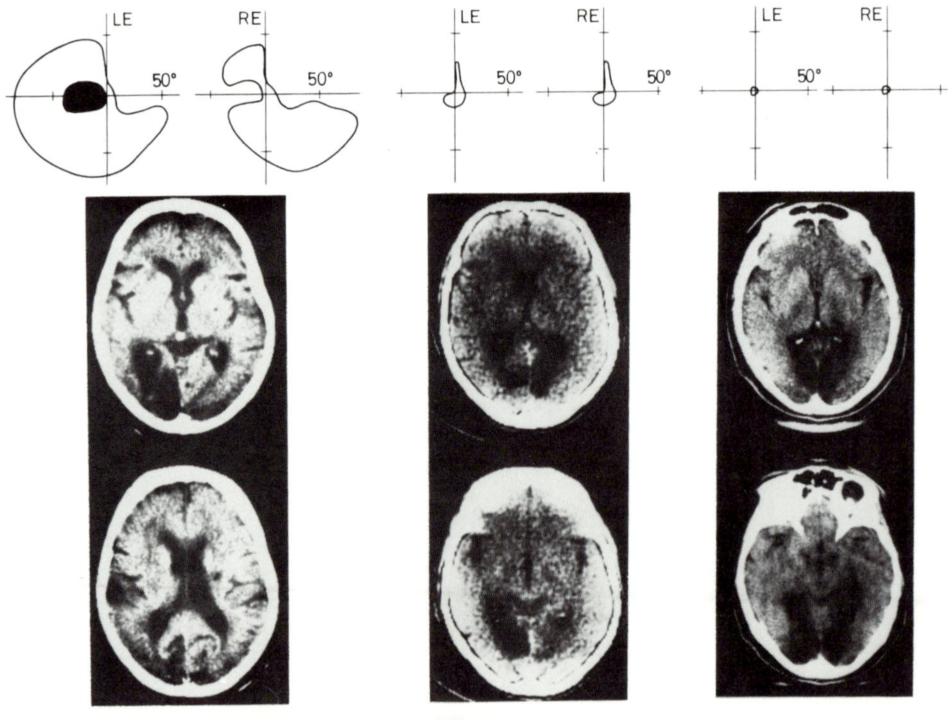

Fig. 1. Visual fields (Goldmann target V4e) and CT scans (courtesy of Dr.Chr.Ostertag and Dr.R.Fürmaier, Dept. of Neurosurgery, University Clinics Freiburg). Case 1 (SS-o8o621), case 2 (BH-29o933), and case 3 (MV-261133) from left to right.

RESULTS

Case 1: OKN was asymmetric upon monocular stimulation of the right eye. The nasal-temporal slow phase velocity was significantly lower ($p \leq 0.001$, Wilcoxon test) than the temporal-nasal slow phase velocity for stimulus velocities above 15°/s (Fig. 2). This asymmetry represented a true nasal-temporal OKN asymmetry since OKN was symmetric upon binocular stimulation. No significant nasal-temporal asymmetry could be observed upon stimulation of the left eye, except after an artificial constriction of its visual field by means of a hand held tube (Fig. 3). Case 2: Visual acuity and visual fields of both eyes did not differ significantly but OKN was asymmetric upon binocular stimulation (Fig. 2) due to the deep parietal lobe lesion on the right side. In order to discover an additional nasal-temporal asymmetry in this case, the OKN elicited via the right eye had to be compared with the OKN of the same direction elicited via the left eye. At 3o°/s and 6o°/s stimulus velocities the nasal-temporal slow phase velocities were significantly lower ($p < 0.001$, Wilcoxon test) than the temporal-nasal slow phase velocities. Case 3: OKN slow phase velocity approached zero at 3o°/s stimulus velocity but even at 15°/s stimulus velocity no nasal-temporal asymmetry could be found (Fig. 2). - None of the cases showed a slow buildup of the slow phase velocity, and only case 1 had a weak OKAN and circular vection (CV). Foveal tracking of a sinusoidally moving light spot (2o° amplitude, peak velocities 15°/s and 3o°/s) as well as fixation suppression of the vestibulo-ocular reflex were only slightly impaired in all three cases, and no nasal-temporal asymmetry was detectable.

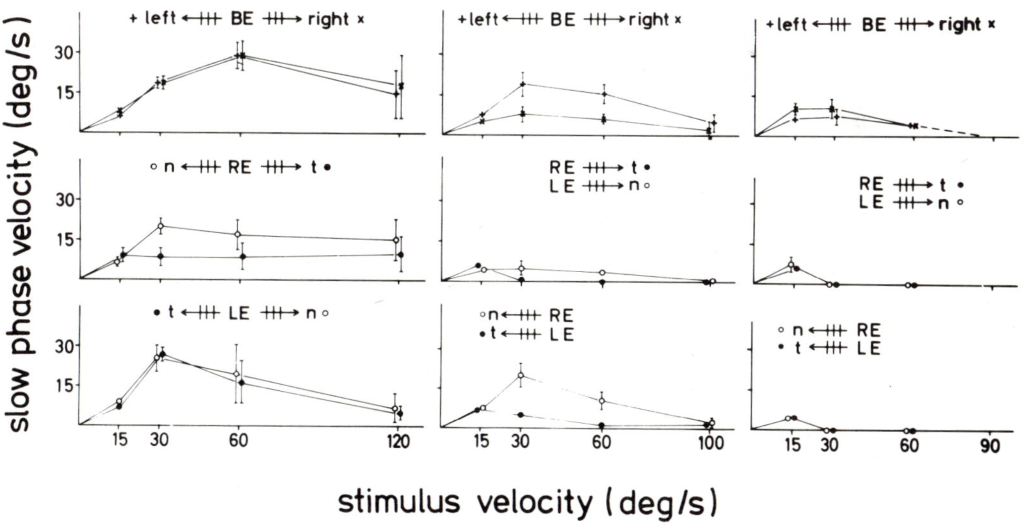

Fig. 2. Stimulus / **response** diagrams for horizontal OKN. Stimulation of both eyes (BE), right eye (RE), and left eye (LE) by patterns moving from nasal to temporal (⟶ t) or from temporal to nasal (⟶ n). Means and ± S.D. are based on three identical stimulations each of which lasted 2o-3o s. Case 1, 2, and 3 from left to right.

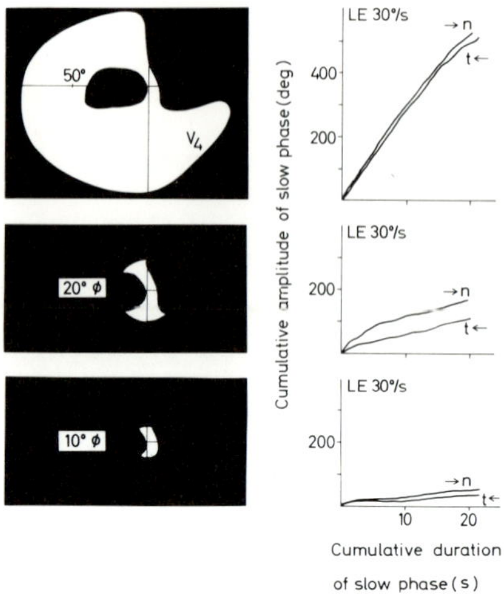

Fig. 3. Nasal-temporal OKN asymmetry revealed by artificial constriction of the visual field (left eye of case 1).

DISCUSSION

The first two cases demonstrate that the destruction of a great part of the visual cortex and of corticofugal pathways can uncover the phylogenetically old nasal-temporal OKN asymmetry even in man.The different impairment of the nasal-temporal and of the temporal-nasal slow phases indicates a different anatomical origin. Obviously, the visual cortex is concerned with an adequate generation of the nasal-temporal slow phase. The better preservation of the temporal-nasal slow phase suggests that it is mainly, although not exclusively, generated by subcortical structures. This conclusion is not at variance with the observation that other signs of subcortical OKN as a slow buildup of the slow phase velocity, OKAN, and CV were absent except in case 1, who had some OKAN and CV. The absence of these phenomena is readily explained by the considerable constriction of the visual fields (Brandt and others, 1973).The present investigation thus indicates a striking similarity of the functional organization of the OKN systems in man and cat. However, the visual cortex had not been completely destroyed in the three cases.They do not prove therefore, that the temporal-nasal slow phase can be generated exclusively by subcortical structures in man.The weak OKN of the third case and the rudimentary or absent OKN of cortically blind patients (TerBraak and others, 1971; VanVliet, 1978) rather indicate that in man, as opposed to the cat, the subcortical OKN system largely depends on a cortical input.

Supported by the Deutsche Forschungsgemeinschaft, SFB 7o, B4.

ADAPTIVE GAIN CONTROL IN THE VESTIBULO-OCULAR REFLEX

F. A. MILES

Laboratory of Sensorimotor Research, National Eye Institute, Bethesda, MD, USA

ABSTRACT

The VOR is an open-loop control system that functions to protect gaze velocity against disturbances due to head movements. Optical devices such as telescopic spectacles that disrupt the visual input associated with head turns have been used to show that the input-output relationship (gain) of the VOR is subject to long-term regulation: Adaptive Gain Control. The information used to compute errors in the gain varies with the species. Earlier models of the adaptive mechanism that invoked directionally-selective visual inputs operating directly on vestibular inputs cannot explain much of the recently acquired data and these new developments are reviewed. Concerning the neural structures involved in this process, adaptation is severely compromised by lesions of the floccular lobes of the cerebellum or its climbing fiber input from the inferior olive. However, attempts to locate the site of the modifiable elements presumed to underlie this adaptive capability are as yet inconclusive and the exact role of the cerebellum is still a matter of speculation. Some current ideas are reviewed.

KEYWORDS

Vestibulo-ocular reflex; adaptive gain control; flocculus; inferior olive; pursuit tracking; optokinetic reflex.

INTRODUCTION

The vestibulo-ocular reflex (VOR) is an open-loop control system that functions to generate compensatory eye movements which offset head rotations. It is now more than a decade since Gonshor and Melvill Jones first demonstrated that the human VOR undergoes extensive changes when subjects wear left-right, reversing-prism spectacles (Gonshor and Melvill Jones, 1971). Since that time, various optical means have been used in a variety of animal species to demonstrate that the VOR is subject to long-term regulation by some visually-mediated adaptive process whose normal function is to keep the system appropriately calibrated. While several different performance parameters appear to be regulated, our major concern will be with the "gain" of the system, usually defined as the ratio of the peak-to-peak compensatory eye velocity (output) to the peak-to-peak head velocity (input) during passive sinusoidal oscillations in the dark. The reflex is said to possess adaptive gain control because it undergoes appropriate increases or decreases in gain when challenged with magnifying or reducing telescopic spectacles (or equivalent optical conditions), respectively. Adaptive gain control has now been demonstrated in the VOR of humans (Gauthier and Robinson, 1975; Gonshor and Melvill Jones, 1971, 1976a, 1976b), monkeys (Miles and Eighmy, 1980; Miles and Fuller, 1974), cats (Keller and Precht, 1979b, Melvill Jones and Davies, 1976; Robinson, 1976), rabbits (Collewijn and Grootendorst, 1978, 1979; Ito, Jastreboff, and Miyashita, 1979), birds (Green and Wallman, 1978), and fish (Schairer and Bennett, 1977, 1978, 1980).

THE FUNCTION OF THE VOR

Recently, investigators using high-resolution techniques to record eye movements have made much of the long-known fact that the gain of the VOR is very rarely exactly 1, and have even gone so far as to suggest that "the VOR serves not simply to stabilize the retinal image of a fixated object during movement, but rather, to produce and maintain retinal image motion" (Collewijn, Martins, and Steinman, 1981a). The crucial dependence of visual acuity on retinal image motion has been particularly evident since the introduction of the technique of stabilizing retinal images and most studies find human acuity optimal (i.e., threshold elevation <10%) when image slip speeds are within the range 0.25-2.00^{o}/sec, with "fading" limiting the lower end and "smearing" the upper (King-Smith and Riggs, 1978; Murphy, 1978; Westheimer and McKee, 1975). When head movements are virtually eliminated with a bite board, retinal image velocities are often below this optimal range for vision. However, when human subjects restrict their head movements more naturally, as when they sit or stand as still as possible, retinal image drift rates are kept within this optimal range for most of the time, in part because the gain of the VOR is quite low for the small amplitude head movements involved here (Skavenski, Hansen, Steinman, and Winterson, 1979). These findings led to the suggestion that "the degree of compensatory oculomotor response is actively adjusted downwards so as to guarantee sufficient retinal image motion to prevent perceptual fading when the body is relatively stationary" (Skavenski, Hansen, Steinman, and Winterson, 1979). I think it more likely that the low VOR gain in these reduced circumstances merely reflects inherent limitations of the reflex, there having been no selective pressure to evolve the ability to eliminate such small retinal image drift "errors". Moreover, these authors have probably exaggerated the likelihood of "fading" due to image stabilization under normal, unrestrained viewing conditions when subjects are constantly shifting their gaze from one object of interest to another and even indulging in head movements that affect retinal images yet are not within the purview of the VOR e.g., lateral, translational movements. I submit that the problem of image "fading" during periods of quiescence is not nearly as great as the problem of "smearing" during periods of activity, and it is this latter problem that the VOR functions to prevent.[1]

If the purpose of the compensatory sub-systems is to maintain retinal slip speeds within the "optimal" range during head turns then ideally the total gain should approach unity, e.g., with only moderately vigorous head rotations of, say, 50°/sec, the gain should be between 0.96 and 1.04 if retinal slip speeds in excess of 2°/sec are to be avoided. Given the inherent variability in the performance of such biological systems (standard deviations typically >5%), it would seem that the optimum adaptive strategy for the system would be to seek unity gain. That moderately vigorous head rotations are often associated with retinal slip speeds well above the range "optimal" for acuity would seem once more to reflect only

1 There are other mechanisms that may be involved in generating compensatory eye movements under normal conditions--neck proprioception, preprogramming and visual tracking--and the degree of dependence on the VOR may vary from one species to another and, perhaps, from one situation to another.

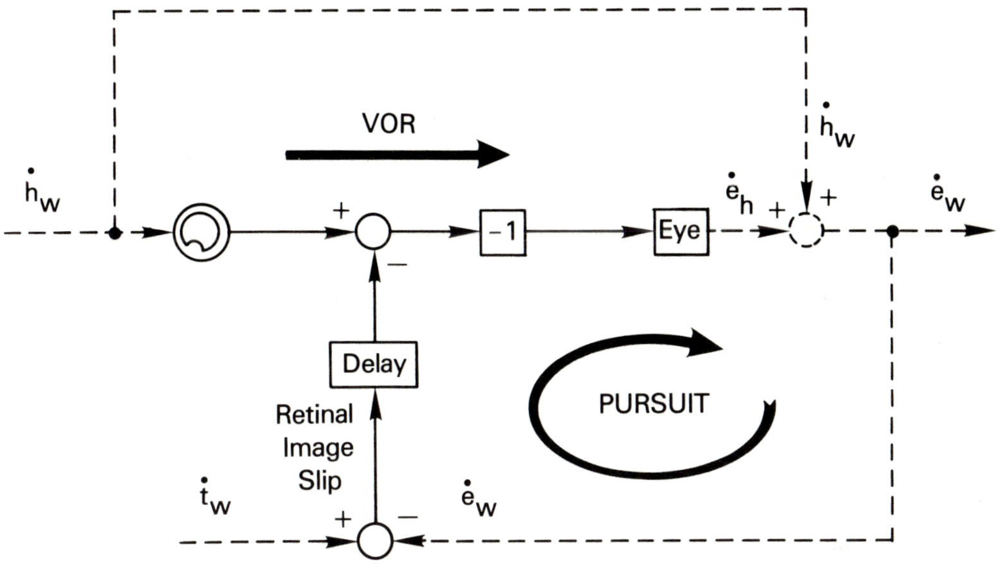

Figure 1. A block diagram of the open-loop VOR and the negative-feedback, pursuit tracking system. Continuous lines represent signal flow channels within the nervous system; discontinuous lines represent external, physical links denoting head velocity with respect to the world ($\dot{h}_w$), eye velocity with respect to the head ($\dot{e}_h$), eye velocity with respect to the world ($\dot{e}_w$, gaze velocity), and target velocity with respect to the world ($\dot{t}_w$). From Miles and Lisberger (1981a).

system limitations rather than deliberate design. However, because some human subjects apparently over-compensated to magnifying spectacles (in the light), Collewijn and co-workers were led to "conclude that the compensatory sub-systems seek some appreciable non-zero retinal image speed rather than virtually perfect image stability" (Collewijn, Martins, and Steinman, 1981a). Setting aside the straw man, "perfect image stability," if adaptation were operating simply to achieve "appreciable non-zero retinal image speed" then it would have settled for an equivalent degree of under-compensation--an option clearly rejected by the system. In my view, such apparently anomalous compensation is entirely consistent with the recently developed idea that the computation of VOR gain errors involves a whole chain of secondary events that are merely set in motion by the primary, visual ones (Miles and Lisberger, 1981a, 1981b). I shall postpone any further consideration of this issue until later in my review when considering current models of the adaptive mechanism.

In foveate animals, such as monkeys or ourselves, we may assume that the paramount need is for stabilization of the foveal retinal image of the fixation target (albeit "stabilization" that falls short of perfection). In fact, the telescopic spectacles often used to demonstrate adaptive gain control (Miles and Eighmy, 1980; Miles and Fuller, 1974) provide only a very restricted field of view and a recent study on monkeys has shown that it is possible to elicit adaptive VOR gain changes when visual inputs are restricted to the fovea (Miles and Lisberger, 1981b). [2] Yet a further characteristic of foveate animals is their ability to

2 Actually, the VOR gain required to stabilize the image of the fixation target will vary slightly with the target's viewing distance due to the translational movement of the eyes during head turns; it is not known what, if anything, the system does about this problem.

track small moving targets--even those viewed against a stationary background--using their negative-feedback, pursuit system. While the pursuit system functions to match the animal's gaze velocity (eye velocity with respect to the world) to the velocity of the (foveal) fixation target--be it stationary or moving--it is the VOR's function to protect that gaze velocity--be it zero or otherwise--against disturbances due to head movements (Lanman, Bizzi, and Allum, 1978; Miles, Fuller, Braitman, and Dow, 1980; Miles and Lisberger, 1981a, 1981b). Thus, in operating to preserve the prevailing gaze velocity, the open-loop VOR works in harmony with the closed-loop pursuit system to "stabilize" the retinal image of the fixation target (see Fig. 1 and also Robinson's article in this volume).

LONG-TERM MODIFICATION vs SHORT TERM MODULATION

Much of the initial interest in adaptive gain control in the VOR arose from its seemingly long-term nature, based on the finding that the changes induced by optical devices were very gradual, often taking several days to achieve asymptote (Gauthier and Robinson, 1975; Gonshor and Melvill Jones, 1976b; Melvill Jones and Davies, 1976; Miles and Eighmy, 1980; Miles and Fuller, 1974; Robinson, 1976). This encouraged the belief that the synaptic linkages in the reflex were undergoing some major, perhaps even structural, "modification". This view received further support when it was found that the system had the ability to retain the modified state during prolonged periods (days) of darkness (Robinson, 1976) or head immobilization (Miles and Eighmy, 1980; Miles and Fuller, 1974), when the usual visuo-vestibular interactions that ordinarily might reinforce that modified state were entirely absent: The system has memory. However, this retention was not permanent, and there is some evidence that a consolidation process might be involved since the tendency to recover decreased somewhat after longer periods of exposure to the adapting conditions (Miles and Eighmy, 1980; Robinson, 1976). While some workers began to hope that this system might eventually yield insights into some of the cellular mechanisms underlying memory and learning, others were more skeptical and in particular questioned the need to invoke any long-term synaptic modifications in the fundamental reflex--might not the experimental subjects simply be learning some strategy by which to exert an immediate influence on eye movements, say, by modulating transmission in the vestibulo-ocular pathways or by injecting additional signals into the system to counteract or reinforce the reflex as the need arose? Such "behavioral" influences clearly would not involve any synaptic modifications in the reflex.[3]

There are several pieces of evidence which suggest that in the monkey the adaptive gain changes associated with telescopic spectacle experience reflect "semi-permanent" changes in the fundamental reflex (Miles and Eighmy, 1980): 1) Neither the rate of adaptation to telescopic spectacles nor the rate of recovery following their removal speeds up with repeated exposures, as might have been expected if the animals had merely been learning some strategy that could then be used at any time to adjust the magnitude of their compensatory eye movements. 2) Standard caloric tests of vestibulo-ocular function in the adapted animals reveal changes in responsiveness that closely parallel the gain changes seen with the usual passive oscillation tests; given the vastly different contextual information available to the animal in these two test situations, one might have expected very different results if strategy-specific parametric adjustments had been involved. 3) In the head-immobilization experiments mentioned earlier to test for retention, several days may have elapsed since the animal last wore the adapting spectacles, yet its VOR gain still retained the adapted state; it seems doubtful that the animal would have continued to employ a strategy for which there was no

3 See also Robinson's article in this volume for a comprehensive discussion of the concept of "VOR cancellation."

longer any apparent, continuing need. 4) The magnitude of the short-latency compensatory eye movements generated by the VOR in response to sudden, unexpected disturbances of the head is simply a function of the measured gain of the reflex, even in contrived situations where the VOR "impedes" fixation (Miles, Braitman, and Dow, 1980); in the short-term, the gain of the VOR seems to be fixed and immutable.

Of course, long-term, plastic alterations on the one hand and short-term, transient adjustments on the other are not mutually exclusive, and in order to determine whether a particular adaptation paradigm elicits one or both of them it is necessary to undertake the kind of experimental scrutiny outlined above. Even so, the issue may remain very difficult to resolve. Unfortunately, such tests have not yet been attempted in any species other than monkey, and the situation in man, in particular, is far from clear. The magnitude of the compensatory eye movements generated by human subjects in the usual VOR test situation is known to depend on the instructions given to them (Barr, Schultheis, and Robinson, 1976; Collewijn, Martins, and Steinman, 1981a), making it very difficult to estimate the gain of their "basic" reflex and rendering the interpretation of human adaptation data highly problematical. When human subjects adapted to 5D spectacles using metronome-paced voluntary head oscillations, their compensatory eye movements (of presumed vestibular origin) underwent alterations in magnitude that were more than half complete within a few minutes (Collewijn, Martins, and Steinman, 1981a, 1981b). On the other hand, their adaptation to 2x telescopic spectacles while undertaking normal physical activities (as far as possible) took days to achieve a similar degree of completion (Gauthier and Robinson, 1975). Clearly, there are substantial differences in these two adaptation paradigms and it is reasonable to ask whether the same mechanisms mediate both adaptive responses. So far, little attempt has been made to characterize the fundamental nature of the adaptive process(es) in the human VOR. It seems safe to assume that the system is extraordinarily resourceful.

THE ERROR SIGNALS SUBSERVING ADAPTIVE GAIN CONTROL

The purpose of this section is to discuss the mechanisms by which the nervous system might compute VOR gain errors. The simplest scheme assumes that any shortcomings in the gain of the VOR will result in persistent retinal image slip during head turns and that the associated visual inputs then automatically elicit an appropriate gain adjustment. Of course, the system cannot diagnose gain errors from retinal slip alone, and must relate it in some way to the ongoing head movement. The directional relationship between the slip and the head movement is assumed to provide a reliable indication of the direction in which the VOR gain needs to be changed to improve image "stabilization", and most models of the adaptive mechanism invoke directionally-selective visual inputs operating on transmission in vestibulo-ocular pathways (Gonshor and Melvill Jones, 1976b; Ito, 1972a;Robinson, 1976). However, the system need not necessarily derive its gain-error information from visual and vestibular signals per se. Theoretically, any reliable central correlates of the same might serve equally well.

Substitutes for Vestibular (Head Velocity) Signals?

Collewijn and Grootendorst (1979) observed that, when the rabbit was passively oscillated in optical situations producing left-right, mirror reversal of the visual input, its VOR gain decreased for the first hour or so, but thereafter, showed a gradual and consistent increase. Moreover, for the first hour or so the animal's compensatory eye movements in the light were attenuated and normally-directed but, thereafter, showed reversal. Thus, while retinal image slip was always in the same direction as head movement, its relationship to eye movement underwent a reversal at about the same time that the VOR gain stopped falling and began to increase. When retinal image slip and eye movements were in opposing directions, VOR gain decreased and when the two movements were in the same direction, VOR gain increased. The clear suggestion here is that, in the rabbit, the adaptive mechanism utilizes the relationship between retinal slip and eye velocity--rather than that between slip and head velocity--to decipher VOR gain errors.[4] Further evidence that the velocity of the eyes (rather than of the head) is the relevant parameter is the finding that the gain of the rabbit's VOR can be increased merely by exposing the animal to sinusoidal optokinetic stimulation with its head fixed in position (Collewijn and Grootendorst, 1979; Collewijn and Kleinschmidt, 1975). In this situation, the animal experiences retinal image slip that is always in the same direction as its smooth eye movements; the fact that in these very artificial circumstances those eye movements are elicited by tracking rather than the VOR seems to be unimportant. Thus, in the rabbit, VOR gain changes can be elicited in the absence of head movements. Similar mechanisms probably operate in the goldfish since prolonged sinusoidal optokinetic stimulation is also known to increase the gain of the VOR in this species (Schairer and Bennett, 1978). By contrast, when similar experiments were carried out in the rhesus monkey the direction of the animal's eye movements was clearly irrelevant and the adaptive mechanism appears to utilize some direct internal measure of the head velocity--presumably the vestibular signal itself--in order to compute errors in VOR gain (Miles and Lisberger, 1981b).

Substitutes for Retinal Slip Signals?

It has been reported recently that human subjects who don magnifying spectacles can achieve full compensation in the light in a matter of minutes--even on occasion, over-compensating--long before adaptation of the VOR gain was even near completion (Collewijn, Martins, and Steinman, 1981a). In this situation, VOR gain was increasing while the associated retinal slip inputs were calling for either no-change or a decrease. Clearly, retinal slip per se was not dictating the observed VOR gain changes here, and the short-term compensation that was quickly achieved in the light was presumably due to the pursuit system. It has already been argued that the VOR works to protect gaze velocity--in primates, the output of the pursuit system--from disturbances due to head movement, but there is another side to this coin: When VOR gain is inappropriate for the conditions, the same retinal slip signals that ultimately underlie adaptive gain control and recalibration also activate the pursuit tracking system, which, in operating to "stabilize" the shifting foveal images, will tend to make up for any shortcomings in the VOR. So long as the VOR gain is inappropriate, pursuit tracking will be invoked to improve retinal image stability. As the VOR gain adapts to the new conditions, the dependence on pursuit decreases. Clearly, the extent to which pursuit is deployed consistently during head turns is itself a highly reliable index of the "error" in the VOR and some central correlate of this pursuit involvement might conceivably substitute for frank visual signals in the adaptive process. Paradoxically, as we have seen, the operation of the pursuit system can undermine the utility of retinal slip per se as a source of VOR gain error information, the reason being that the pursuit system is much more than the simple velocity servo depicted in Fig. 1. It is known, for example, that the pursuit tracking system is able to utilize position information as well as velocity (Pola and Wyatt, 1980) and even displays some predictive capabilities when confronted with recurring patterns of target motion (Michael and Melvill Jones, 1966; Stark, Vossius, and Young, 1962). Both of these factors would seem likely to be

4 Note that unlike ourselves and monkeys, the rabbit never tracks moving targets under normal circumstances and so, outside the laboratory, uses smooth eye movements solely to compensate for head rotations.

potentially important in the short-term compensation for an inappropriate VOR, especially during voluntary head turns. Thus, the over-compensation that can occur rapidly in the light--rendering retinal slip per se unreliable as a source of VOR gain error information--is probably a form of pursuit over-shoot.

In suggesting that adaptive gain control in effect functions to reduce dependence on pursuit during head turns, I am again assuming that the primary need is to "stabilize" the image of the fixation target (Miles and Lisberger, 1981b). Even if this is achieved, images outside the plane of fixation will be seen to move during head turns because of the lateral translation of the eyes and parallax: Those images of objects nearer than the fixation point will be seen to move in a direction contrary to that of the head, while images of more distant objects will be seen to move with the head. Once more, retinal slip patterns during head turns do not necessarily bear any simple relationship to the VOR gain. Furthermore, there is clearly an image selection problem: How does the system distinguish the fixation target's image from the background/foreground images? We know that the pursuit system regularly solves this selection problem (though we do not know how) and the adaptive gain control mechanism would, of course, benefit from this solution if it were to use a central correlate of pursuit to deduce gain errors. In effect, I am suggesting that the pursuit response during head turns is the best estimate of VOR gain error available to the system. Later, I shall suggest that the crucial parameter of pursuit performance that is actually used is a neural correlate of gaze velocity (Miles and Lisberger, 1981a, 1981b).

SITE OF THE MODIFIABLE ELEMENTS

Investigations concerning the possible site of the modifiable synapses that are presumed to underlie adaptive gain control in the VOR have tended to center on the floccular lobes of the cerebellum, largely because of the work and writings of Ito (Dufossé, Ito, and Miyashita, 1978; Ito, 1972a, 1977; Ito, Jastreboff, and Miyashita, 1979; Ito and Miyashita, 1975; Ito, Shiida, Yagi, and Yamamoto, 1974a). He conceived the flocculus as a side-path of the VOR that relayed vestibular signals (borne by mossy fiber inputs) through cortical networks containing modifiable synapses whose long-term efficacy was regulated by climbing fiber inputs. The finding that, in the rabbit at least, the climbing fibers received visual inputs (Maekawa and Simpson, 1973), which were directionally selective (Simpson and Alley, 1974), was nicely consistent with the idea that these fibers might convey retinal slip error signals to guide recalibration of the reflex. However, though a decade has passed since this simple hypothesis was first mooted, it remains the subject of controversy.

In reviewing the current status of work in this area, I shall begin by considering the situation in the rabbit since Ito appears to have based his original ideas largely on his knowledge of the anatomical arrangements in this species, and all of his subsequent studies, which are often cited in support of his hypothesis, have been carried out on these same animals. Unfortunately, Ito and his coworkers chose to work on the albino form, which is now known to have anomalous visual projections in the nasal visual field: When visual inputs are restricted to this region, optokinetic responses are reversed (Collewijn and Grootendorst, 1978; Collewijn, Winterson, and Dubois, 1978) and the gain of the VOR undergoes "maladaptive" decreases (Collewijn, Verhagen, and Grootendorst, 1980). As subjects for the study of adaptive gain control, these albino rabbits seem to present major problems, which may or may not be linked to the above-mentioned anomalies: Their VOR typically has a very low gain (Collewijn and Grootendorst, 1978), shows considerable variation--both from one animal to another and, in individual animals, over time--and so far has shown only very modest adaptive changes (Ito, Jastreboff, and Miyashita, 1979; Ito, Shiida, Yagi, and Yamamoto, 1974a). The failure to demonstrate appreciable adaptation may reflect deficiencies in the optical arrangements used in these experiments rather than in the animals themselves. Whatever the reason, it renders the subsequent claims that lesions of the flocculus (Ito, Shiida, Yagi, and Yamamoto, 1974a) or its sole source of climbing fibers, the inferior olive (Ito and Miyashita, 1975), cause deficits in adaptation less than compelling. Ito and his coworkers have also reported that the modulations of Purkinje cell (P-cell) simple spike discharges in the albino rabbit's flocculus during oscillation in the dark undergo changes in association with VOR gain changes that are appropriate for their postulated causal role in the adaptive process (Dufossé, Ito, Jastreboff, and Miyashita, 1978; Ito, 1977). In view of the above discussion, it is perhaps not surprising that these apparent changes in P-cell discharge modulation were very small. However, even if one were to concede the functional significance claimed for these findings--altered P-cell discharge modulation contributing to altered compensatory eye movements--the etiology of the recorded changes would still remain uncertain because the signal content of the P-cells' discharge modulations has yet to be determined. The view that the observed changes in P-cell discharges and VOR gain both emanate from synaptic modifications in the floccular cortex is predicated upon several assumptions, one of which is that only vestibular inputs are involved. It is known, for instance, that this is not so in the monkey's flocculus (Lisberger and Fuchs, 1978; Miles and Fuller, 1975; Miles, Fuller, Braitman, and Dow, 1980), where most P-cells also discharge in relation to eye movements. Clearly, if this were so in the rabbit, then the alleged changes in P-cell discharges associated with adaptation could be a simple consequence of their discharging in relation to motor events (eye movements) that are themselves subject to adaptation: No alterations in synaptic efficacy need be invoked in the floccular cortex to explain them. In summary, it is clear that the evidence for the flocculus as the site of the modifiable elements in the rabbit is not compelling. Furthermore, it should not be forgotten that the system computing VOR gain errors (in the pigmented rabbit) uses eye velocity signals and not, as featured in the Ito model, vestibular, head velocity signals (Collewijn and Grootendorst, 1978, 1979).

Unequivocal deficits in adaptive gain control have been shown to result from cerebellar lesions in cats (Robinson, 1976), fish (Schairer and Bennett, 1980), and monkeys (Optican, Zee, Miles, and Lisberger, 1980)--findings that continue to sustain interest in the possibility that the modifiable elements reside in the vestibular lobes of the cerebellum. Furthermore, a similar deficit has been shown to follow lesions of the dorsal cap of the inferior olive (which normally supplies the climbing fiber inputs to the flocculus) in the cat (Haddad, Demer, and Robinson, 1980). If, as has been claimed recently in the rat and albino rabbit, destruction of the climbing fibers causes P-cells to lose their customary inhibitory action on the vestibular relay cells in the brainstem (Dufossé, Ito, and Miyashita, 1978; Ito, Orlov, and Shimoyama, 1978; Ito, Nisimaru, and Shibuki, 1979), then in the long term, lesions of the inferior olive should merely mimic lesions of the flocculus. However, the nature of the effects of unilateral microlesions in the dorsal cap on eye movements in pigmented and albino rabbits (Barmack and Simpson, 1980) are not consistent with this "trophic" effect. Also, a recent attempt to replicate the original finding failed to eliminate P-cell inhibition with olivary lesions in rats (Montarolo, Raschi, and Strata, 1981). Demer and Robinson (1981) have reported that in the cat, regardless of its initial value, VOR gain increased immediately after the microinjection of lidocaine into the inferior olive (before any alleged "trophic" effects could have had time to develop) and declined back to control values as the anesthetic wore off. Since climbing fibers are unlikely to participate directly in the VOR because of their extremely low discharge rates, this rise in VOR gain during pharmacological silencing of the climbing fibers would seem to infer that the latter exert some modulatory influence on the transmission of mossy-fiber, vestibular signals through the floccular cortex. For the present, these new observations raise more problems than they solve and, though extremely interesting, their relevance to adaptive gain control is not yet clear. In summary, while it is evident that olivary lesions eliminate adaptive gain control in the cat, the mechanism remains obscure.

Recent studies on the monkey suggest that in this species the flocculus does indeed perform a vital role in the adaptive process but one that may be different from that assigned to it in the Ito hypothesis. In addition to eliminating adaptive gain control (Optican, Zee, Miles, and Lisberger, 1980), floccular lesions also result in major deficits in the monkey's performance on various ocular pursuit tasks (Zee, Yamazaki, and Gucer, 1978).[5] Single unit recordings in the primate flocculus (Lisberger and Fuchs, 1978; Miles, Fuller, Braitman, and Dow, 1980; Noda and Suzuki, 1978) have shown that the activity of the most common type of output P-cell modulates during pursuit tracking and effectively encodes gaze velocity (eye velocity relative to the world). These data raise two further possible explanations for the deficits in VOR adaptation following floccular lesions in the monkey (Miles, Fuller, Braitman, and Dow, 1980; Miles and Lisberger, 1981a, 1981b). One is that the pursuit deficits, which presumably follow from the loss of the gaze-velocity, signal support, disrupt the adaptive process indirectly, by undermining the animal's ability to track--and thereby stabilize--the retinal images seen through the optical devices employed to evoke gain changes; retinal slip speeds are then simply too high for the adaptive mechanism to utilize. Another possibility is that the gaze velocity output signals from the flocculus that are so important for pursuit might also be directly involved in the induction of the modifications underlying adaptive gain control in the VOR pathways: As a "central correlate of pursuit", the discharge modulation of gaze velocity P-cells might provide all or part of the error signal guiding re-calibration of the reflex (Miles, Braitman, and Dow, 1980; Miles and Lisberger, 1981a, 1981b). Significantly, the discharge characteristics of these P-cells undergo changes in association with adaptation that are consistent with this postulated role in signalling VOR gain errors but are not consistent with the idea that they function as part of the modifiable gain element. This point has been argued at some length elsewhere (Miles, Braitman, and Dow, 1980). A perennial criticism that can be levelled at such unit studies, and one that is extremely difficult to refute, is that they considered the "wrong cells": The gaze-velocity P-cells might have nothing to do with adaptive gain control and the much-sought-after modifiable synapses might be associated with one of the other, less common P-cell types that were not studied, e.g., the miscellaneous 10% of P-cells that discharge variously in relation to vestibular and oculomotor events (Miles, Fuller, Braitman, and Dow, 1980). Pursuing this line of argument further, the alterations in gaze-velocity P-cell discharges with VOR gain would be dismissed as irrelevant so far as adaptive gain control is concerned, and related only to their role in pursuit and to the need for them to be regulated in harmony with VOR gain (Miles, Braitman, and Dow, 1980). The only evidence which suggests that this criticism may not be valid is very indirect and comes from the differential effects of floccular lesions and VOR gain changes on the two components of the monkey's optokinetic response (OKR).

The monkey's slow-phase tracking responses following sudden exposure to a continuously-moving visual field consist of, 1) an initial rapid rise in eye velocity that lasts for a few hundred milliseconds and is thought to be due mainly to the operation of the pursuit system, followed by 2) a much more gradual increase in eye velocity that may take 15-30 sec to reach asymptote and is thought to be due to a velocity storage mechanism (Cohen, Matsuo, and Raphan, 1977; Raphan, Matsuo, and Cohen, 1979) that represents the optokinetic system proper (Lisberger, Miles, Optican, and Eighmy, 1981; Zee, Yee, and Robinson, 1976c. If

5 A cautionary note: It should not be forgotten that these lesions also invariably damage the paraflocculus, some of whose P-cells are known to discharge in relation to eye movements (Mikami, Noda, and Suzumura, 1981.)

the lights are extinguished after this build-up has started, the nystagmus persists as optokinetic afternystagmus (OKAN), the initial intensity of which is assumed to be a direct index of the final intensity achieved by the "optokinetic" component of the prior response (Lisberger, Miles, Optican, and Eighmy, 1981; Raphan, Matsuo, and Cohen, 1979). Ablation of the flocculi results in a major deficit in the fast "pursuit" component but leaves the slow "optokinetic" build-up essentially unaltered (Optican, Zee, Miles, and Lisberger, 1980). By contrast, changes in VOR gain are associated with almost proportional changes in the (maximum) intensity of the slow component--as indicated by the initial OKAN--but no significant change in the fast component (Lisberger, Miles, Optican, and Eighmy, 1981); that the changes in the "optokinetic" component of the OKR so nearly mirrored those in the gain of the VOR is consistent with the view that they are a secondary consequence of the latter, and that the modifiable elements are for the most part located in the later stages of the vestibular pathway that are shared with the slow optokinetic system (Lisberger, Miles, Optican and Eighmy, 1981; Waespe and Henn, 1977a). Single unit studies in monkeys have failed to find evidence for significant changes in either semicircular canal primary afferents (Miles and Braitman, 1980) or cells in the medial vestibular nuclei that receive inputs from these afferents (Lisberger and Miles, 1980) in association with large changes in VOR gain. Since other unit studies (Waespe and Henn, 1977a suggest that the slow optokinetic system joins the vestibulo-ocular pathways at the level of the second-order neurons, both systems ought to share the modifiable elements. If the modifiable elements had been located in the flocculus, then lesions of the latter would also have been expected to compromise the slow component of the OKR. That floccular lesions did not have this effect is consistent with the view that the modifiable elements subserving adaptive gain control are located outside the flocculus, presumably in the brainstem.

The situation in other species seems to be rather different from that in the monkey. In the cat, for instance, VOR gain changes are associated with changes in the time constant of the slow component of the OKR (Demer, 1981) and with changes in the vestibular sensitivity of cells in the medial vestibular nuclei (Keller and Precht, 1979). In the rabbit, the optokinetic system always shows a significant increase in gain in association with VOR adaptation regardless of whether the VOR gain increases or decreases (Collewijn and Grootendorst, 1979). Since the optokinetic system operates as a negative-feedback mechanism, such increases in its gain would always work to improve the system's performance and so could be regarded as "adaptive".[6]

ADAPTIVE GAIN CONTROL IN THE PRIMATE: A NEW HYPOTHESIS

I shall close with a brief summary of our current concept of the adaptive gain control mechanism in the monkey, in the hope that it may have some relevance to man, surely a major concern in a meeting such as this designed to bring together clinicians and basic scientists. Figure 2 incorporates the gaze velocity P-cells in the flocculus into a simple model of the open-loop VOR together with its adaptive gain control mechanism and the negative-feedback pursuit system (Miles, Fuller, Braitman, and Dow, 1980; Miles and Lisberger, 1981a). The gaze velocity signal configuration ($\dot{e}'_w$) is achieved by summing together two independent signals separately encoding the velocity of the eyes with respect to the head ($\dot{e}'_h$) and the velocity of the head with respect to the surroundings ($\dot{h}'_w$). The head velocity component is assumed to be vestibular in origin and is configured in the model as

6 In the primate studies, optokinetic responses were assessed using prolonged, unidirectional stimulation, while the rabbit studies used sinusoids; the rabbit showed a somewhat different picture when prolonged unidirectional stimulation was used, hence, some of these differences may be methodological.

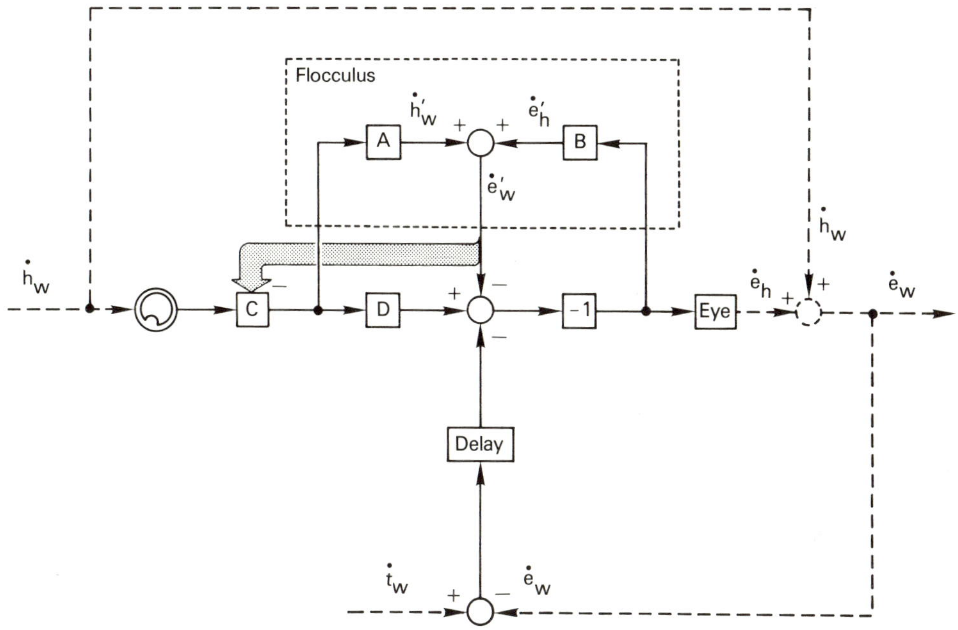

Figure 2. A block diagram of the monkey's VOR and pursuit system, indicating the hypothesized long-term, regulatory influence of the gaze-velocity P-cells (broad stippled arrow) on the postulated modifiable gain elements in the vestibular pathway. Continuous lines represent signal flow channels within the nervous system; discontinuous lines represent external, physical links denoting head velocity with respect to the world ($\dot{h}_w$), eye velocity with respect to the head ($\dot{e}_h$), eye velocity with respect to the world ($\dot{e}_w$, gaze velocity), and target velocity with respect to the world ($\dot{t}_w$). A, B, C and D represent gain elements, with C presumed to be modifiable; $\dot{h}'_w$ and $\dot{e}'_h$ denote the head velocity and eye velocity inputs, respectively, to the P-cells in the flocculus whose discharge modulations effectively encode gaze velocity ($\dot{e}'_w$). From Miles and Lisberger (1981b).

part of an inhibitory side-loop of the vestibulo-ocular pathway. The eye velocity component is assumed to be derived from the motor command to move the eyes (though it might equally well originate from proprioceptive input) and is configured in the model as part of a positive-feedback loop that functions to boost the gain of the negative-feedback pursuit system. Since the monkey's VOR gain is normally close to unity, its gaze velocity during head turns (when not tracking) is close to zero and the gaze velocity P-cells in the flocculus show little or no modulation of their activity (Lisberger and Fuchs, 1978; Miles, Fuller, Braitman, and Dow, 1980). Thus, these P-cells normally make little or no contribution to the VOR. However, when the normal monkey first wears the optical devices used to elicit VOR adaptation, he is confronted with a tracking task every time he turns his head, and uses his pursuit system to supplement the compensatory eye movements generated by the VOR. These tracking efforts will mean that gaze velocities will no longer be zero during head turns and the activity of the floccular P-cells will modulate accordingly in support of the pursuit. In fact, the discharges of the gaze-velocity P-cells will modulate during head turns whenever the monkey uses pursuit to supplement a VOR whose gain is inappropriate for the visual conditions. Such discharge behavior is in keeping with experimental findings (Lisberger and

Fuchs, 1978; Miles, Fuller, Braitman, and Dow, 1980) and is exactly that expected of neurons supposedly signalling VOR gain errors. Thus, in this scheme, the gaze-velocity P-cells have been assigned two quite separate functions. As a part of the pursuit system, their discharge modulation is assumed to have an immediate influence upon their target neurons through conventional (inhibitory) synaptic mechanisms. As a part of the system regulating VOR gain, their persistent discharge modulation during head turns is assumed to indicate errors in the VOR and have a long-term influence on the efficacy of synaptic transmission in the vestibulo-ocular (brainstem) pathway.

When an animal has adapted to, say, magnifying spectacles, the increased magnitude of the compensatory eye movements coupled to head turns (now generated by the VOR and not pursuit) means that the eye velocity input to the P-cells associated with a given head turn will be proportionately higher than normal; however, this increased eye-velocity input is known to be almost exactly counter-balanced by a proportional change (increase) in the strength of the head-velocity input signal, a change presumed to reflect an alteration in synaptic efficacy in the vestibular pathway at gain element C in Fig. 2 (Miles, Braitman, and Dow, 1980). The net result of this is to restore balanced inputs to the P-cells so that their discharges cease modulation during head turns when adaptation is complete (and dependence on pursuit is again minimal). Once more, this is exactly the behavior expected of neurons signalling VOR gain error.

SELECTIVE LABYRINTHINE LESIONS AND NYSTAGMUS INDUCED BY ROTATION ABOUT OFF-VERTICAL AXES

B. COHEN*, J. SUZUKI***, T. RAPHAN*, V. MATSUO* and V. DEJONG**

**Department of Neurology, Mount Sinai School of Medicine, Israel*
***Department of Neurology, University of Amsterdam, The Netherlands*
****Department of Otolaryngology, Teiko University, Tokyo, Japan*

ABSTRACT:

1. Selective labyrinthine lesions were made in monkeys to determine the origin and nature of activity responsible for the continuous horizontal nystagmus that occurs during yaw rotation about off-vertical axes (OVAR). Lesions were of two types: the semicircular canals were inactivated by plugging, and the nerves of the lateral semicircular canals were cut. Eye movements were recorded by electrooculography.

2. After the semicircular canals had been inactivated by plugging, the response to steps of velocity about a vertical axis was lost, but the sustained nystgmus induced by off-vertical axis rotation (OVAR) was maintained. Optokinetic nystagmus (OKN) and optokinetic after-nystagmus (OKAN) were also intact. This supports the theory that labyrinthine activity responsible for the response to OVAR arises largely in the otolith organs.

3. After cutting the nerves of the lateral semicircular canals, horizontal OKAN was abolished, and characteristics of OKN that depend on velocity storage were lost. Sustained nystagmus could no longer be produced by yaw rotation about off-vertical axes. This indicates that otolith activity responsible for nystagmus during OVAR couples to the oculomotor system through the same velocity storage integrator that is responsible for OKAN and for the prolongation of nystagmus induced by angular rotation that activates the semicircular canals.

4. Although horizontal OKN and OKAN were affected by section of the lateral semicircular canal nerves, characteristics of vertical OKN and OKAN dependent on velocity storage were maintained. This indicates that the storage mechanism for horizontal nystagmus depends on activity from the lateral semicircular canals. It suggests that storage mechanisms for horizontal or vertical eye movements are dependent on activity from the semicircular canals that lie in or close to the plane of the movements.

Keywords: Nystagmus, vestibular, optokinetic, otolith organs, semicircular canals, utricle, saccule, gravity, velocity storage, slow phase eye velocity, monkeys.

INTRODUCTION:

The peripheral vestibular system responds to rotational stimuli and to linear accelerations or forces of gravity. Rotation about an axis tilted from the vertical (off-vertical axis rotation, OVAR) induces a rotating gravity vector that generates nystagmus and a sense of movement that persist for the duration of stimulation (Guedry, 1965; Benson and Bodin, 1966; Young and Henn, 1975; Raphan, Cohen and Henn, 1981). At the end of rotation post-rotatory nystagmus is weaker and lasts for a shorter time than after comparable rotation about a vertical axis in darkness. There are two possible sources for the labyrinthine activity that induces the ongoing nystagmus during OVAR: a canal-induced response via a "roller pump" action (Benson and Bodin, 1966; Steer, 1967), and an otolith induced response (Guedry, 1965; Correia and Money, 1970; Raphan, Cohen and Henn, 1981). Recordings from canal afferents in the vestibular nerve do not show a direction specific response that would be necessary to induce continuous nystagmus (Goldberg and Fernandez, 1981; Raphan, Waespe and Cohen, 1981). Therefore, such activity probably arises mainly in the otolith organs.

Recent studies on the dynamics of the nystagmus during off-vertical axis rotation have shown that a velocity storage mechanism is intimately involved in processing signals that originate in the otolith organs (Raphan, Cohen and Henn, 1981). This velocity storage mechanism holds activity related to slow phase eye velocity during vestibular and optokinetic stimulation (Cohen Matsuo and Raphan, 1977; Raphan, Matsuo and Cohen, 1979). The most overt representation of velocity storage is OKAN. Velocity storage is dependent on the integrity of some parts of the labyrinth since bilateral labyrinthine destruction abolishes OKAN (Uemura and Cohen, 1973). Destruction of the utricles and saccules has no effect on OKAN (Takahashi, Igarashi and Homick, 1977). Therefore canal nerve section should theoretically abolish the response to OVAR. The present experiments were undertaken to determine how selective lesions of the peripheral vestibular system, which included plugging the semicircular canals and cutting the horizontal canal nerves would affect the velocity storage mechanism, and the sustained nystagmus induced by OVAR, OKN and OKAN.

METHODS:

Selective labyrinthine lesions were made in 10 monkeys (1 rhesus, 8 cynomologous and 1 nemestrina monkey). Operations were performed under anesthesia using an operating microscope. The labyrinth was approached through the mastoid bone, and the individual canals were identified. Canal plugging was accomplished by grinding across the canal with a diamond burr until the membranous canal was interrupted, using the technique of Money and Scott (1962). The region was packed with bone and covered with a small piece of muscle. To cut the lateral canal nerves, the area over the lateral canal ampulla was opened by shaving away the bone with a sharp scalpel. The canal nerve was cut with a sharp pointed blade without opening the membranous canal. The success of either operation was judged by determining if the response to rotation in the plane of the various canals had disappeared.

Eye movements were recorded by electrooculography (EOG) using silver-silver chloride electrodes placed in the bone around the eyes (Bond and Ho, 1970). The EOG was recorded with D-C coupling. It was electronically differentiated to obtain slow phase eye velocity. Voltages representing eye position, eye velocity and stimulus parameters were recorded on FM magnetic tape for playback and analysis. Animals were tested for horizontal and vertical OKN and OKAN and for the response to steps of yaw rotation about vertical and off-vertical axes. Accelerations were in the range of 2500 deg/sec^2 and velocities ranged from 0-180 deg/sec. The 2 axis vestibular and optokinetic stimulator used in these experiments was constructed by Contraves Goertz. It has been described in detail elsewhere (Raphan, Cohen and Henn, 1981).

RESULTS:

Normal Response to Off-vertical Axis Rotation (OVAR):

In the normal monkey, velocity steps of yaw rotation about a vertical axis in darkness produce nystagmus whose velocity is initially close to the velocity of the stimulus (Raphan, Matsuo and Cohen, 1979). The nystagmus characteristically has a slight plateau for several seconds and then declines to zero over 30-60 seconds. For yaw rotation about axes tilted from the vertical, the gain of the initial step in velocity is similar to that for rotation about a vertical axis (Raphan, Cohen and Henn, 1981). However, for stimulus velocities up to 50-60 deg/sec, slow phase velocity does not decline during OVAR but is maintained for as long as the stimulus continues at close to unity gain (eye velocity/stimulus velocity) (Fig. 1A). At the end of stimulation after-nystagmus is much weaker than after rotation about a vertical axis in darkness (Fig. 1A). Superimposed on the steady state velocity are small variations whose phase is related to the animal's head position with regard to gravity. The amplitude of the oscillations increases at higher velocities and with increasing angles of tilt of the axis of rotation from the vertical (Young and Henn, 1975).

The following experiment demonstrates that the velocity storage mechanism is involved in the production of the response to OVAR (Raphan, Cohen and Henn, 1981): The animal was rotated about a vertical axis in darkness until the per-rotatory nystagmus had disappeared. As rotation continued, the axis was tilted 30 deg from the vertical (upward arrow, Fig. 1B). In response to this, per-rotatory nystagmus reappeared and slowly built to a steady state level. The steady state level was the same as if the animal had been given a step of velocity about the tilted axis (Compare Fig. 1A & 1B). If the axis of rotation was tilted back to the vertical (downward arrow, Fig. 1B), the nystagmus again decayed to zero. The time course of the decay in slow phase velocity was approximately the same as the time course of the decay during OKAN or after rotation about a vertical axis (Raphan, Cohen and Henn, 1981). It was also about the same as the time course of the rise in nystagmus after the axis had been tilted (Fig. 1B, left). This experiment shows that activity stored during rotation about off-vertical axes is discharged when the axis of rotation is tilted back to the vertical. This activity can be used to cancel the post-rotatory response coming from the semicircular canals (Fig. 1A). Quantitative data are consistent with this hypothesis. The maximum velocity of the post-rotatory response after OVAR was reduced by the amount of steady state velocity (Raphan, Cohen and Henn, 1981).

Inactivation of the Semicircular Canals:

After all six semicircular canals had been plugged, nystagmus could no longer be induced by steps of velocity about a vertical axis in darkness (Fig. 2A). OKN and OKAN were present if the surround was rotated in the animal's yaw axis (Fig.

Fig. 1

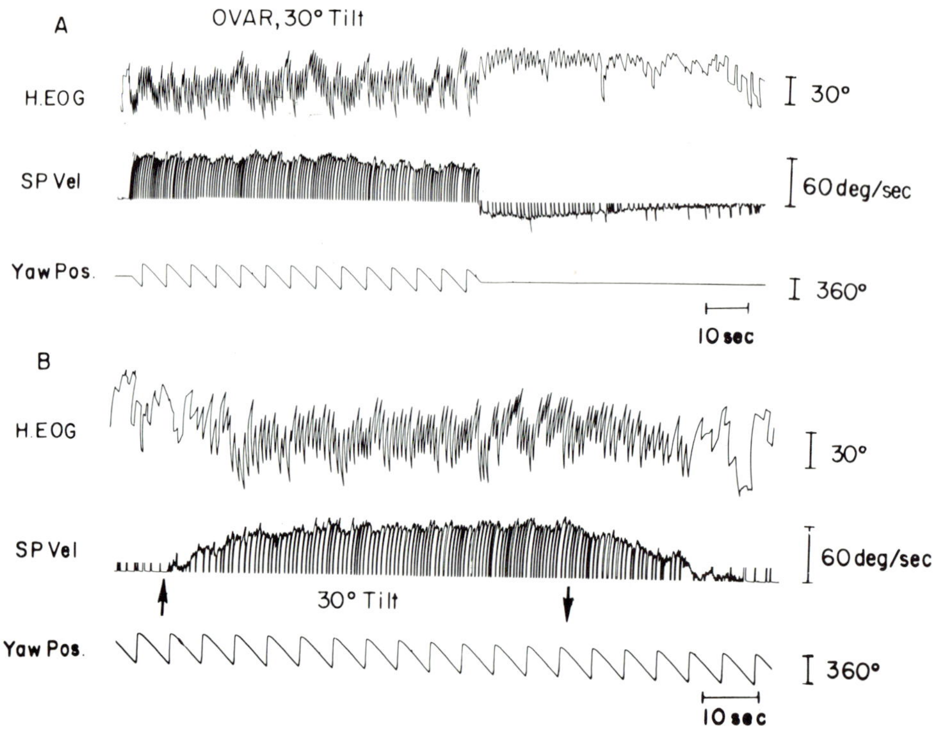

Fig. 1: A, Nystagmus induced by a step of head velocity of 60 deg/sec in darkness about an axis tilted 30 deg from the vertical. The top trace is the horizontal EOG, the second trace is horizontal slow phase eye velocity and the third trace shows position about the yaw axis. B, Nystagmus induced by tilting the yaw axis 30 deg during rotation in dark after the per-rotatory slow phase velocity had declined to zero. The moment of tilt is given by the upward arrow. After reaching a steady state eye velocity the subject was tilted back to the upright at the downward arrow and eye velocity again declined to zero. The steady state eye velocities were comparable in A and B.

2B). Brisk compensatory nystagmus was present during rotation in light, but it was OKN, as shown by the prominent OKAN that occurred at the end of stimulation when the animal was stopped and the lights were extinguished (Fig. 2C). The continuation of OKAN when the animal was stopped in darkness is consistent with the inactivation of the canals (Fig. 2A). That is, the stored activity was not cancelled by the counter-response of the semicircular canals (Raphan, Matsuo and Cohen, 1979). The gain of the OKAN was somewhat reduced after operation, with saturation velocities falling in this animal from 70 deg/sec to about 50 deg/sec.

Despite inactivation of the semicircular canals, there was a prominent response to OVAR. This agrees with the results of Correia and Money (1970). Fig. 2D shows an experiment similar to that in Fig. 1B. The animal was initially rotated about a vertical axis in darkness. There was no per-rotatory nystagmus (Fig. 2D, left). The axis of rotation was then tilted as rotation continued. Nystagmus velocity gradually built up to a steady state level (Fig. 2D, center).

Fig. 2

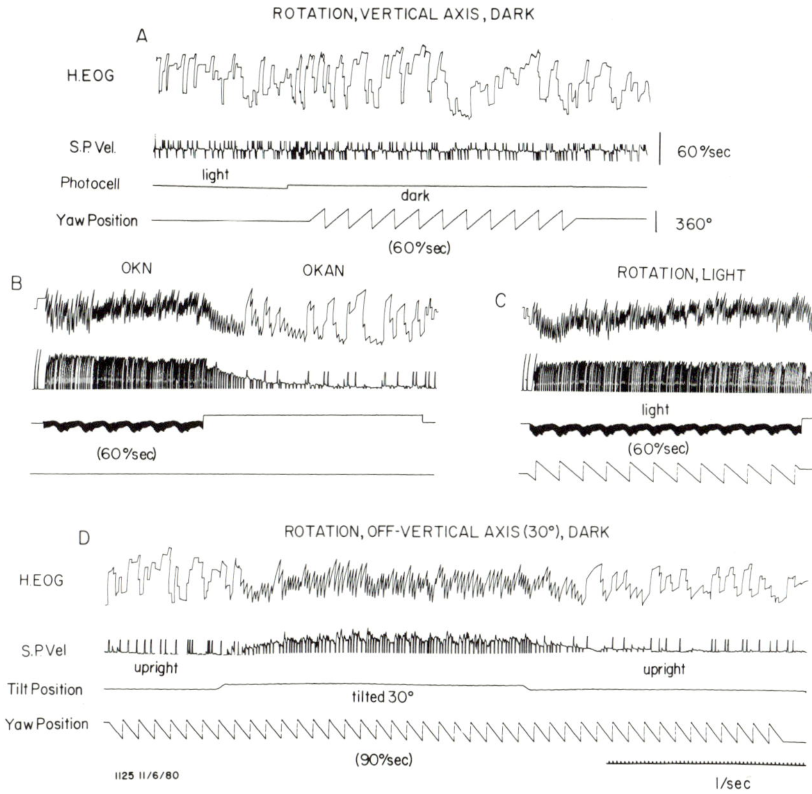

Fig. 2: Responses to rotation after all the semicircular canals had been inactivated by plugging. A, Rotation about a vertical axis in darkness. No nystagmus was induced. B, OKN and OKAN induced by surround rotation at 60 deg/sec. Both OKN and OKAN were preserved. C, Rotation in light in a stationary surround induced nystagmus that was similar to that seen during OKN and OKAN in B. The response was due to activation of the visual system, not the vestibular system. D, Rotation in dark about a vertical axis (at the left of the trace) produced no response. When the axis of rotation was tilted 30 deg, nystagmus developed along a slow time course to reach a steady state level. There were periodic modulations of eye velocity superimposed on the steady state velocity that were phase-locked to head position. When the axis of rotation was tilted back to the vertical, the nystagmus disappeared over the same time course as the decline of OKAN. There was no post-rotatory response at the end of rotation (extreme right side of trace). The time base is 1 mark/sec.

Superimposed on the steady state were oscillations that were phase-locked to the animal's position. When the axis of rotation was tilted back to the vertical, nystagmus velocity declined over the time course of OKAN (Fig. 2B), as in the normal animal.

The alteration in nystagmus during a step in yaw velocity about a tilted axis after canal inactivation is shown in Fig. 3. The response to rotation in light

Fig. 3

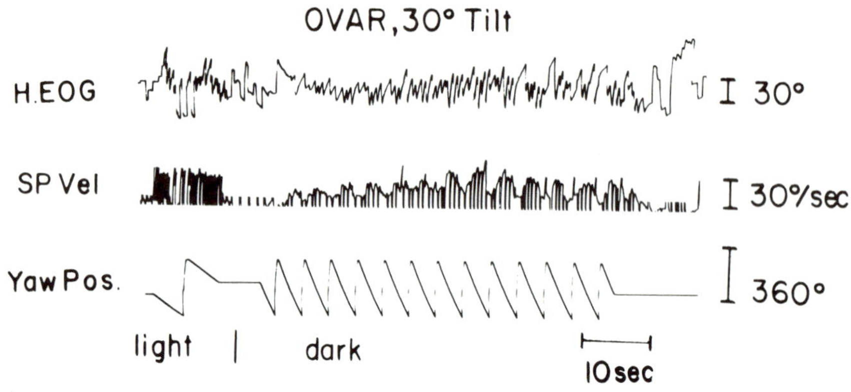

Fig. 3: Response to step in velocity of 90 deg/sec about a yaw axis tilted 30 deg from the vertical. On the left is a calibration response combining OVAR and optokinetic stimulation at 30 deg/sec. When the animal received the velocity step in darkness, the response built slowly to a peak velocity of about 30 deg/sec. It was similar to the response induced by tilting the axis during rotation (Fig. 2D). Note the reduced gain, the prominent peak to peak modulation of the steady state velocity, and the slow decline in slow phase velocity that outlasted the end of stimulation.

is shown on the left. During similar rotation in darkness there was a slow buildup in nystagmus velocity. The nystagmus outlasted the end of stimulation by some seconds. This can be compared to the response to the same stimulus shown in Fig. 1A. After canal plugging the rapid components produced by the semicircular canals were lost, but the slow response produced by the otolith organs was maintained. There were several differences in the response to OVAR before and after canal inactivation. Modulations in slow phase velocity that were phase-locked to position were more prominent after canal plugging, and the gain of the steady state response was reduced. Steady state velocities during OVAR did not exceed 30 deg/sec, which was about half the value in the normal animal (Raphan, Henn and Cohen, 1981). Despite these differences, characteristics of the nystagmus induced by OVAR before and after the canals had been inactivated were similar.

These data demonstrate that activity responsible for the continuous nystagmus during OVAR must arise mainly in the otolith organs. This is in accordance with findings of Correia and Money (1970). In addition, the slow time course of the buildup and decline of nystagmus indicate that the major coupling of otolithic information to the oculomotor system takes place through the velocity storage mechanism that is also activated by the semicircular canals and by the visual system (Raphan, Cohen and Henn, 1981).

Section of the Lateral Semicircular Canal Nerves:

The lateral semicicular canal nerves were sectioned in two animals. After nerve section, there was no response to rotation in the plane of the lateral semicircular canals. Optokinetic nystagmus after lateral canal nerve section is shown in Fig. 4A. There was an immediate jump in eye velocity to its steady state value at the onset of stimulation, and a prompt fall in eye velocity to zero at the end of stimulation. Primary OKAN, i.e. OKAN in the same direction

Fig. 4

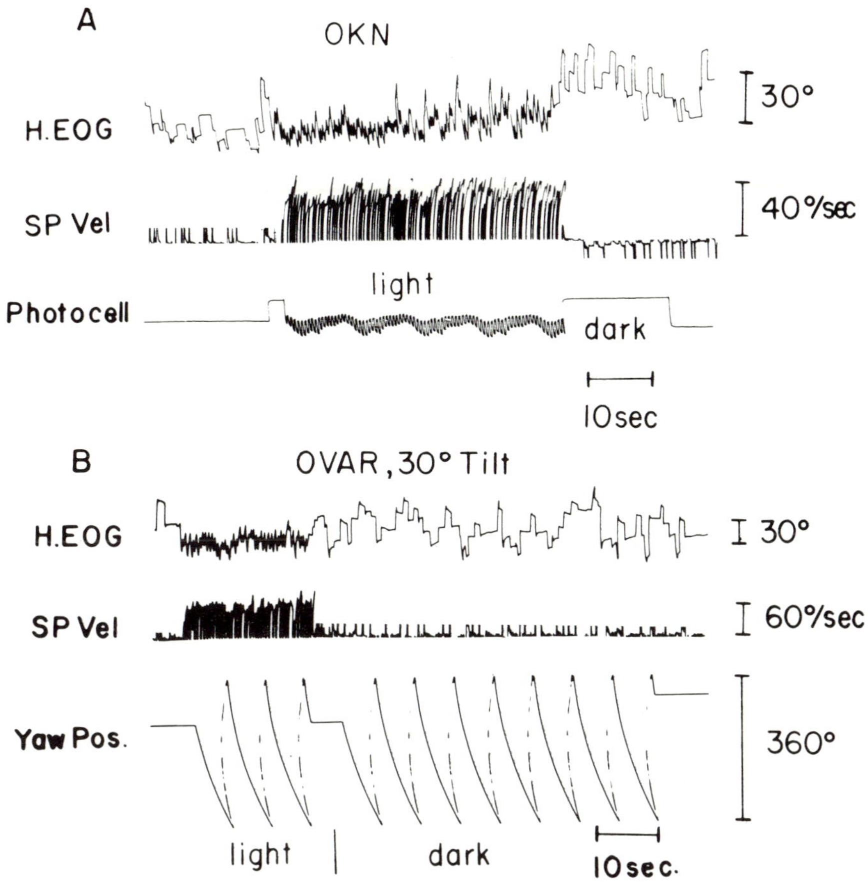

Fig. 4: Response to horizontal optokinetic stimulation (A) and OVAR (B) after the lateral canal nerves had been sectioned. A, OKN was characterized by a sudden rise in slow phase velocity to a peak level, by irregular maintenance of this steady state level for the duration of stimulation, and by a sudden fall in eye velocity at the end of stimulation. There was was no primary horizontal OKAN. B, Sustained nystagmus was not induced by rotation in darkness about a yaw axis tilted 30 deg from the vertical. The calibration response to optokinetic stimulation is shown on the left. Oscillations in horizontal eye position were induced by the OVAR.

as the preceding OKN, was absent. The altered characteristics of OKN and the loss of OKAN are consistent with the conclusion that the velocity storage mechanism was not activated during OKN after the canal nerve lesions. Taken together with the negative effects of utricular and saccular destruction on OKAN (Takahashi, Igarashi and Homick, 1977), the results indicate that the loss of horizontal OKAN after labyrinthectomy (Uemura and Cohen, 1973) was due to a loss of tonic activity arising in the lateral semicircular canals.

After the lateral canal nerves were cut and storage integrator function was lost, sustained nystagmus was no longer induced when the animals were rotated

Fig. 5

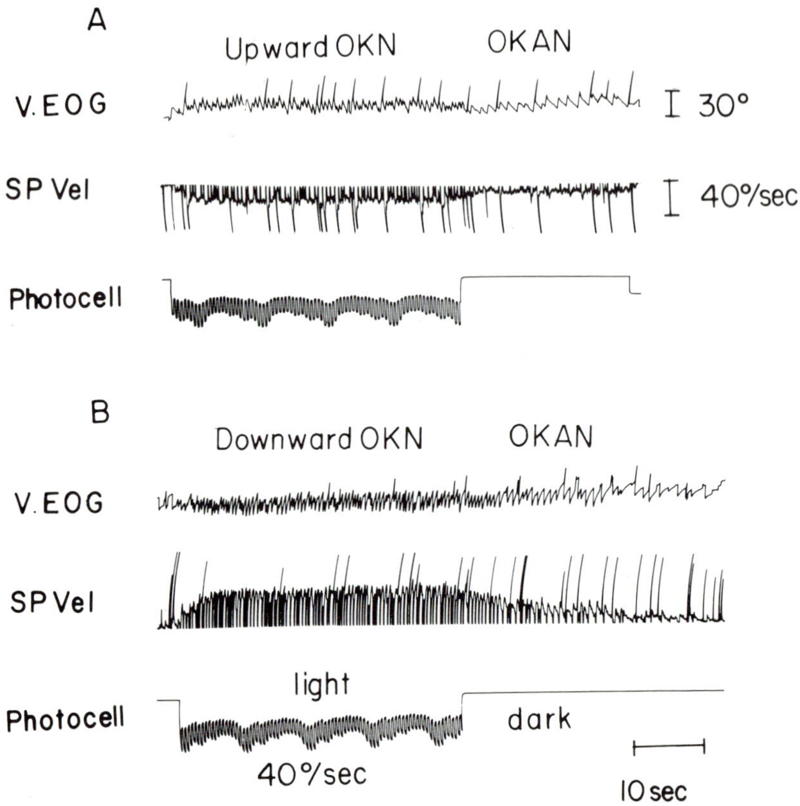

Fig. 5: Response to vertical optokinetic stimulation in the animal whose records are shown in Fig. 4. The animal was lying on its side during stimulation. These records were taken several months after the lateral semicircular canal nerves had been cut. At that time the characteristics of OKN and OKAN in the vertical plane were normal. As in the normal animal, there was stronger downward than upward OKN and OKAN. This reflected a difference in gain and in velocity storage for upward and downward nystagmus.

about axes tilted from the vertical (Fig. 4B). This supports the contention that the otoliths primarily couple to the oculomotor system through the velocity storage integrator. The lack of response in Fig. 4B is in contrast to the prominent nystagmus during OVAR when the canals were inactivated but storage integrator function was maintained (Figs. 2D & 3). There continued to be prominent oscillations in vertical eye position, and at higher velocities there were also oscillations in horizontal eye position when the animal was rotated about axes tilted more than 60 deg from the vertical or at higher velocities. This suggests that the otolith organs were functional in this animal.

Section of the Lateral Semicircular Canals and Vertical Nystagmus

There are a variety of data that suggest that the mechanisms that process velocity storage for vertical and horizontal nystagmus can be separated under certain circumstances. Characteristics of vertical and horizontal OKN and vestibular nystagmus are different, depending in large part on the amount of velocity storage that is available to add to the response. Velocity storage is more prominent for horizontal than vertical nystagmus and is generally left-right symmetrical (Matsuo, 1981; Matsuo and Cohen, 1981). In most animals velocity storage is weaker for upward than downward nystagmus (Matsuo and colleagues, 1979; Matsuo, 1981). Moreover, vertical OKAN is present only when animals are in the lateral position and disappears when they are upright (Matsuo, 1981; Matsuo and Cohen, 1981). This static effect of gravity on velocity storage is present only for vertical nystagmus, and is not manifested on horizontal nystagmus.

After selective destruction of the lateral semicircular canal nerves that caused a loss of horizontal OKAN (Fig. 4A), it was still possible to elicit upward and downward OKAN (Fig. 5A, B). As in the normal animal, there was a slow rise in OKN after the initial rapid rise. This was most prominent during downard OKN where stored velocity is greater (Fig. 5B). There was also a marked difference in upward and downward OKAN, with the latter lasting longer and having a higher saturation velocity (Fig. 5B). Vertical visual-vestibular interactions were intact, also demonstrating the presence of vertical storage, greater for downward than upward nystagmus. When the animal was upright, there was no OKAN, showing that the static gravity-dependence of storage for vertical OKAN was intact (Matsuo and Cohen, 1981). This indirectly indicates that the otolith organs were functional. This experiment demonstrates that the integrity of velocity storage for horizontal nystagmus depends on activity that arises in the lateral canals, and that this activity is not essential for production of storage for vertical nystagmus.

DISCUSSION:

When the otolith organs are dynamically activated under appropriate conditions, strong compensatory horizontal nystagmus and a sense of rotation can be induced. Nystagmus induced by OVAR in darkness in the normal animal (Fig. 1A) is similar to the nystagmus induced by a step of velocity in light. This indicates that the vestibular system is capable of maintaining compensatory eye velocities up to the saturation velocity of the storage integrator, without an additional contribution from the visual system.

The experiments on canal inactivation show that activity responsible for nystagmus during OVAR mainly arises in the otolith organs. This is in accord with the conclusions of Guedry (1965) and with our previous findings (Raphan, Cohen and Henn, 1981). Although it is clear that the otolith organs are excited by continuous changes in the orientation of the head with regard to gravity, until recently the nature of the central processing that produces the sustained nystagmus has been unclear. As shown by our recent studies (Raphan, Henn and Cohen, 1981) and the present experiments, this activity couples to the oculomotor system predominantly through the velocity storage mechanism that is responsible for prolongation of vestibular nystagmus and for the production of OKAN (Cohen, Matsuo and Raphan, 1977; Raphan and co-workers, 1977, 1979).

The persistence of the position-related oscillations in eye velocity during OVAR after the canals had been inactivated indicates that activity that produced these variations also arises in the otolith organs. There was also a prominent position-related oscillation in vertical eye position. It seems likely that these modulations were due to excitation of direct otolith-oculomotor pathways. Presumably, activation of these pathways is responsible for static counter-rolling during head tilt. It is unlikely that direct otolith-oculomotor pathways, being related to eye position, can produce eye velocity signals or sustained nystagmus. In support of this, nystagmus is not present in darkness in normal individuals when the head is tilted. Moreover, when the velocity storage integrator was inactivated, significant continuous nystagmus was no longer produced during OVAR (Fig. 4B).

If the otoliths couple to the oculomotor system primarily through the velocity storage integrator, it would explain why horizontal eye movements have not been elicited by electrical stimulation of the otolith organs. First, many stimulation studies have been done under anesthesia or in drowsy animals. The dynamic coupling that has been demonstrated must take place through polysynaptic pathways that would easily be depressed under these circumstances. More important, during dynamic otolith activation it appears that the nervous system is responding to a pattern of activation that sequentially excites elements across the utricular or saccular maculae. It is this pattern that we believe is used by the CNS to reconstruct the velocity of head movement (Raphan, Cohen and Henn, 1981). Electrical stimulation would produce synchronous activation of all elements in one macula. This would not be meaningful information to the CNS, and could not cause appropriate excitation of pattern recognition circuits which in turn would excite the velocity storage mechanism.

The finding that horizontal OKAN was selectively affected by cutting the lateral semicircular canal nerves is evidence that the velocity storage integrator for horizontal nystagmus is dependent on activity that arises in the lateral semicircular canals. By analogy, activity responsible for maintaining storage for vertical nystagmus probably comes from the semicircular canals that lie in or close to the plane of vertical nystagmus, i.e. the anterior and posterior canals. The otolith organs also play a role in conditioning this storage (Matsuo, 1981; Matsuo and Cohen, 1981). As yet it is not known how or where the storage mechanisms for vertical or horizontal nystgmus are realized in the nervous system. At the level of the vestibular nuclei vertical and horizontal storage mechanisms engage different sets of neurons that are related to specific canal planes. However, this is a summated signal from direct and indirect pathways and presumably activity related to storage arises elsewhere (Raphan and Cohen, 1981). Further experiments are necessary to provide a better understanding of the characteristics and site of origin of these mechanisms.

In summary, the velocity storage mechanism that we have previously characterized during optokinetic and vestibular nystagmus and visual-vestibular interactions appears to be the major mechanism by which the semicircular canal and otolith organs interact. When it is excited by the otoliths, it provides activity that could improve the low frequency characteristics of the VOR in the absence of vision. This activation would also help block vestibular after-responses and act to maintain a central signal that is proportional to head movement. We would emphasize that ocular compensation and the VOR are dependent not only on the semicircular canals and on vision, but on information that arises in the saccule and utricle. The key to demonstrating the powerful otolith-canal convergence and its role in producing compensatory eye movements and a sense of movement is dynamic activation of the otoliths and the velocity storage integrator in an alert subject.

ACKNOWLEDGEMENT

Supported by NIH Research Grant NS 00294, NEI Academic Investigator Award EY 00157 to Theodore Raphan, NEI Fellowship EY 07014 to Victor Matsuo and NEI Core Center Grant EY 01867.

VESTIBULAR DYSFUNCTION AND VISUAL ILLUSIONS IN WALLENBERG'S SYNDROME

G. HÖRNSTEN

Department of Neurology, Karolinska Institutet, Huddinge Hospital, S-141 86 Huddinge, Sweden

ABSTRACT

The ocular motor and visual disturbances of Wallenberg's syndrome are surveyed. In spite of the complex, clinical picture some consistent features are readily discerned. Absence of generalized posterior fossa pressure symptoms and the restricted area of the lesion offer an unusually advantageous opportunity for studies of ocular motor pathology at the level of the lateral medulla oblongata. Thoroughly analyzed clinical cases, however, still are few. Further studies are needed to correlate the clinical findings with current knowledge of central, ocular motor control.

KEYWORDS

Wallenberg's syndrome; vestibular dysfunction; Visual illusions

INTRODUCTION

At the last symposium held in Stockholm 1974 some of the clinical features of Wallenberg's syndrome were commented upon by Hoyt and Frisén (1975). They were at that time unable to precisely correlate the clinical disturbances with current knowledge of ocular motor control systems. Discordant retino-vestibular input by cerebellar deafferentiation was considered a major cause of the visuo-motor symptoms. I am afraid that the task of making clinico-pathological speculations in no way is easier today in spite of the overwhelmingly growing experimental literature. Efforts to offer possible explanations to the sum of the complex, clinical disturbances really make me feel walk on ice that is only one night old. So, I gratefully leave most of this mission to the basic scientists and neuro-ophthalmological authorities.

Disequilibrium, various oculomotor and visual disturbances are common features of Wallenberg's syndrome. Even though vestibular and ocular symptoms frequently were attended to in the earlier literature (e.g. Barré, 1927; Isch, 1957; Peterman and Siekert, 1960; Fisher and others, 1961) no typical or constant clinical pattern emerged. A variety of complex disorders related to the vestibular and vestibulo-ocular apparatus were found in the rather few cases reported by Silfverskiöld and co-workers (Bjerver and Silfverskiöld, 1968; Hagström and others, 1969; Moberg and others, 1962; Silfversköld, 1965). The vestibulo-ocular symptoms in these patients were intense and severely disabling. In some cases they dominated the persisting clinical course. Certain constant patterns were distinguished and confirmed in a greater series of patients (Hörnsten, 1974a). Even though our recording procedures did not satisfy today's demands upon exactness the application of cinematography and infrared video-tape recordings (Hörnsten, 1974b) made possible an evaluation of the totality of the ocular motor disturbances. In summary, our papers in broad and qualitatively outlined the various vestibulo-ocular features of Wallenberg's syndrome.

Lateropulsion of gaze and saccades

The ipsilateral falling tendency which accompanies the lateral medullary infarction was termed lateropulsion by Bjerver and Silfverskiöld (1968) and they clearly distinguished lateropulsion from body and limb ataxia. A lateropulsion comparable to that of the body may also affect the resting position of gaze. This sign originally was described in a case reported by Hagström and others (1969). In this patient the eyes slightly deviated to the side of infarction with open eyes. A very strong conjugate eye deviation appeared when fixation was interrupted or visual impulses were excluded. Turning of head and gaze vertically - causing transient loss of fixation - was accompanied by a deflection of the eyes towards the side of infarction. The range of ocular movements was normal and there were no signs of paresis of gaze. Saccades away from the side of infarction were slow and executed in steps. On combined turning of head and refixation of a target away from the side of infarction the eyes lagged behind the head with a latency of almost one second before they reached the target. A patient with features indicating the same ocular disability was analyzed in depth by Kommerell and Hoyt (1973). In this patient with a left lateral medullary infarction a strong leftward bias deeply influenced saccadic eye movements. In absence of visual contours the eyes deviated to the left. Spontaneous saccades to the right were small and made in steps, refixation saccades undershooted targets to the right, overshooted targets to the left. Undershooting rightward saccades were accomplished by a series of staircase-patterned small saccades, overshoot to the left was corrected by small, rightward saccades. Saccades between two vertically aligned visual targets were deflected towards the left producing an oblique trajectory. The authors chosed the designation "lateropulsion of saccadic eye movements" to characterize this ocular motor disability. Lateropulsion of gaze, notably in the dark, and typical saccadic disturbances appeared to be a frequent sign in our patients and has subsequently been reported in the literature (Frisén, 1978; Hamann, 1979).

Smooth pursuit movements

Smooth pursuit movements were in our patients only roughly evaluated and OKN reactions were not systematically studied. However, saccadic pursuit, in particular with objects moving away from the side of infarction was a common finding. In the case reported by Kommerell and Hoyt (1973) horizontal pursuit was slow and jerky, interrupted by saccadic steps, slightly more with pursuit to the right (away from the side of infarction). Optokinetic stimulation produced low frequency-high amplitude nystagmus with right-going stimuli, high frequency-low amplitude nystagmus with left-going stimuli. A principally identical defect of OKN appeared in the patient of Hamann (1979) and in the two cases reported by Frisén (1979) OKN "was poorly sustained" with stimulation away from the side of infarction.

Spontaneous nystagmus

In spite of great individual variations of intensity of the spontaneous nystagmus it shows a quite remarkable consistency. With open eyes in light and gaze in the approximate primary position nystagmus almost invariably beats away from the side of infarction. In addition to the horizontal vector of nystagmus there are superimposed rotatory-vertical (upward) components. With gaze towards the side of infarction the horizontal component is ipsilateral. With open eyes in darkness (or with closed eyes) nystagmus changes in mainly two respects: 1) the vertical-rotatory components increase, occasionally nystagmus is replaced by irregular and episodic vertical-rotatory oscillations; 2) the horizontal component is reduced and reversed. The changing nystagmic patterns evidently depend upon the ipsilateral gaze deviation in absence of vision. When gaze in darkness is directed away from the side of infarction the contralateral, horizontal vector reappears. When trying to keep contralateral gaze the eyes drift to the side of infarction; large corrective movements and superimposed nystagmus occurs in direction of attempted gaze. Some degree of dissociation of nystagmus is rather frequent; in our patients always an increase of the vertical-rotatory component of the eye ipsilateral to infarction. A very notable dissociation was noted in one patient (Hagström and others, 1969) with monocular down-beat nystagmus. Head position may occasionally reduce nystagmus when the patient is lying on the side of infarction; the reverse, however, was noted in the patient of Kommerell and Hoyt (1973). Gaze-evoked eye lid and ocular nystagmus inhibited by the near reflex is a unique manifestation reported by Daroff and others (1968).

Caloric reactions

The peripheral caloric reactivity essentially is normal. Typical caloric responses are reported by Kommerell and Hoyt (1973) and Hörnsten (1974b). Caloric nystagmus beating away from the side of infarction is low amplitude-high frequency, nystagmus beating towards the side of infarction is slow and of high amplitude. The latter reactions were in some cases of considerably shorter duration and in this respect there was a directional preponderance away from the side of infarction. Aberrant and paradoxical caloric reactions were described in three patients (Hamann, 1979; Kommerell and Hoyt, 1973; Moberg and others, 1962). A unifying feature in all of them was very brisk reactions behind closed lids when the ear on the "sound" side was irrigated by cold water. In one case (Moberg and others, 1962) there was a reversal of caloric nystagmus at eye opening.

Diplopia and skew deviation

Diplopia is a frequent early symptom. It may typically be episodic, change from one time to another and, like spontaneous nystagmus, exceptionally be reduced or disappear with change of head position (in our cases when the patient was placed on the side of infarction). Detailed analysis is difficult and bewildering because of superimposed spontaneous nystagmus, instability of ocular position and oscillopsia. Certain consistent features, however, are readily distinguished. Vertical diplopia dominates in combination with some degree of horizontal image separation. The image of the eye ipsilateral to the side of infarction is above that of the other eye and the images are tilted in relation to each other. Some degree of oscillation of the vertical double images is often present. A largely concomitant hypotropia of the eye ipsilateral to infarction in some cases may be easily observed. In other cases no significant disalignement of the eyes can be proved in spite of subjective complaints of diplopia. In none of our cases there was convincing evidence indicating paresis of individually acting vertical or horizontal eye muscles. One sole exception to the pattern described above was noted in a patient with monocular hypertropia and down-beat nystagmus of the eye on the side of infarction. The vertical double images incessantly jumped against each other and produced a very disabling oscillopsia (Hagström and others, 1969).

Tilt to 90° or even complete reversal of the visual surroundings is a most dramatic initial symptom which occurred in no less than one third of the patients in our whole series. The tilting sensations as a rule are momentary but may exceptionally persist for the first or second day. Similar tilting sensations have earlier been described in two patients (Fisher and others, 1961; Thompson, 1929).

Fixation instability and blurring of vision

Instability of fixation is common and results in blurring of vision. Severe fixation instability may bring about inability to fixate for more than a few seconds as reported in the case of Kommerell and Hoyt (1973). At interruption of fixation by a blink the eyes rapidly went to the side of infarction and back to the fixation target by several small saccades. Blurring may persist for a long time even when most of nystagmus, diplopia and oscillopsia have disappeared as in one of our patients. During the first month he was hardly able to recognize people entering the room because of blurred vision. Blurring was much more pronounced on the eye ipsilateral to infarction at monocular testing. Episodes of blurred vision persisted for years. Turning of head is particularly prone to blur the vision. It can persist for many seconds which was drastically exemplified at head turn away from the side of infarction in patients with simultaneous lagging of the eyes.

Reading difficulties

Difficulties in reading may be highly disabling. Scanning eye movements in reading are grossly disturbed. Some patients take up a compensatory position of head to reach the most stable position of gaze. Eye movements in following a text are partly supported by small head movements. For instance, in a case of left-sided infarction (Hagström and others, 1969) scanning eye movements in following the text to the right were extremely tedious and irregular. Reading was impossible for more than short whiles. On prolonged reading several of the ocular defects aggravated. Multidirectional eye movements appeared and the text became totally blurred. This patient, a manager, had to retire because of reading disability, which still is present fourteen years after infarction.

DISCUSSION

The lateral medullary infarction commonly involves the restiform body (Currier, 1969; Fisher and others, 1961; Grant, 1966) and a lesion at this level may disconnect important pathways subserving the coordination of head and eye movements. The various consequences, objective and subjective, of a unilateral disability of the side-lope control of the vestibulo-ocular open-loop reflex (VOR) and of the retinal velocity feed-back control during fixation and eye movements were excellently outlined by Hoyt and Frisén (1975). Discordant retino-vestibular input to the flocculus and resultant inadequate ocular motor output may account for most of the clinical symptoms; fixation instability, fleeting diplopia and visual disturbances during head and eye movements. The subjective symptoms may be compared to the perceptural delusions which normally may occur at conflicting or unphysiological visual and vestibular stimulation (Dichgans and Brandt, 1979).

The discussion to follow is an effort to elucidate one major quality of Wallenberg's syndrome, which presents itself to the clinician; the remarkable and constant lateralization of the ocular motor signs. I am quite aware of the hazards of making simple and unequivocal patho-physiological speculations and can just formulate some questions of where to search causative mechanisms and handle over possible interpretations to the basic scientists.

In the acute phase of the disease there is convincing, clinical evidence of a deep-going, unilateral vestibular imbalance; directionally appropriate spontaneous nystagmus and bodily lateropulsion. Lateropulsion of gaze, notably in the dark, certainly belongs to the same cathegory. However, the caloric reactions indicate no gross damage of primary vestibular connections or nuclear structures mediating impulses from the horizontal canals (Gacek, 1969; Shimazu and Precht, 1965; Stein and Carpenter, 1967). In addition, these structures are situated above the usual Wallenberg area and there were, in our patients, no clinical signs of extension of the infarction to the inferior pons. Thus, no evident mode of explanation is available for the acute vestibular signs.

The next mechanism to be considered concerns the floccular inhibition of the vestibular nuclei (Fukuda and others, 1972; Highstein, 1973; Ito and others, 1973) and its presumed role as a gain regulator of the VOR (Ito, 1972b). Visual suppression of vestibular nystagmus is lost after flocculectomy in the monkey (Takemori and Cohen, 1974). According to Lisberger and Fuchs (1977) VOR suppression is caused by a head and eye velocity signal (unrelated to vision) which both increase floccular inhibition of the VOR during ipsilateral rotation. During VOR in the dark the two signals cancel.

Some recent experimental evidence (Barmack and Hess, 1980 a, 1980 b; Barmack and Simpson, 1980) indicate that activation of the visuo-olivo-floccular projection produces a net decrease of the contralateral floccular inhibition of the vestibular nuclei. Cells of the dorsal cap of the inferior olive (rabbit) were sensitive exclusively to retinal slip velocity and not to eye movements or vestibular stimulation. Thus differential modulation of floccular activity on each side would work synergistically to minimize retinal slip during head-eye tracking movements. As for the clinical situation an interruption in the restiform body of head-velocity and retinal-velocity information would have opposing effects upon floccular P-cell activity. The normal increase and decrease respectively, of floccular inhibition would not be brought about at stimulation of either system. Normal pursuit, however, is essentially independent of head velocity (Miles and others, 1980) which would allow for the disruption of the olivo-floccular system to dominate. The complex, visual symptoms in Wallenberg's syndrome are indicative of a primarily disordered fixation-pursuit system, certainly caused by unilateral disruption of olivo-floccular projections. This projection constitutes the largest fiber group of the restiform body (Carpenter, 1976). Deficient pursuit movements away from the side of infarction manifest the lateralized dysfunction of the system.

However, other lateralized signs are much more prominent, in particular lateropulsion of saccades. This sign could be understandable in terms of a constant ocular motor bias towards the side of infarction. Clinical evidence favour a - yet not defined - vestibular origin. Ongoing saccades are normally modulated by vestibular activation during combined head-eye movements (Bizzi, 1975). An extraordinary example of deficient modulation is offered by the two patients with "lagging eyes" at simultaneous refixation and turning of head away from the side of infarction. A presumed mechanism is the added effects of disruption of fixation and an increase of a contralateral vestibular bias. Saccades become hypermetric during the adaptive phase after labyrinthectomy in the monkey (Dichgans and others, 1973). Clinically, a central, unilateral vestibular bias likewise could be responsible for saccadic hypermetria and deflection towards the side of infarction. This contrasts to saccadic dysmetria of "pure" cerebellar origin which is directionally appropriate (Ritchie, 1976; Selhorst and others, 1976a)and does not show the extreme degree of asymmetry which characterizes saccades in Wallenberg's syndrome. The dramatic dominance of the saccadic disorder may be related to the pulsative mode of release of saccadic eye movements (Robinson, 1975a). Lateropulsion of gaze was, for clinical reasons, presumed to be of a vestibular origin and this is supported by its notable appearance in the dark. It may represent the ultimate manifestation of a unilateral ocular motor bias which affects all classes of eye movements and saccadic movements in particular. In terms of current ocular motor, control models (Robinson, 1975a, it will be proposed, in accordance with Kommerell and Hoyt (1973), that the bias must be added before the common neural integrator. A constantly biased signal may be fed into the integrator and distort integration of velocity-to-position signals with the result of a highly lateralized "rest" position of gaze in the dark. The main function of the integrator is to hold gaze and a deficiency of the gaze holding function is particularly obvious in the dark. In particular the cerebellar flocculus is thought to improve the gaze holding function of the integrator which may become "leaky" in patients with cerebellar disease (Zee and others, 1980. Evidently, this mechanism can not adequately compensate for the lateral bias in Wallenberg's syndrome.

In conclusion it may be stated that Wallenberg's syndrome offers an unusually advantageous opportunity to study complex ocular motor problems. The syndrome is clinically well defined, the underlying lesion is restricted. With one exception (see below) all classes of eye movements have been studied only in the patient of Kommerell and Hoyt (1973) and much further investigation is needed.

An important contribution in this direction is offered in a very recent paper by Baloh and others (1981) who studied six patients with Wallenberg's syndrome. They postulated two types of ocular motor bias in their patients; a velocity bias and a position bias. The findings indicated an origin from different pathophysiological mechanisms. The velocity bias was responsible for spontaneous nystagmus and asymmetry of slow eye movements, the position bias was responsible for asymmetry of saccadic eye movements. Both contributed to the eye deviation towards the side of infarction. The velocity bias was thought to origin from central vestibular structures (preferentially lower parts of the ipsilateral vestibular nuclei). Disruption of the connections between cerebellar paravermal regions and PPRF prenuclear gaze centers was considered a critical element in the production of the position bias. As pointed out by the authors the pathophysiological speculations are limited by the lack of clinico-pathologically well correlated cases.

THE INFLUENCE OF CIRCULARVECTION (CV) ON OPTOKINETIC NYSTAGMUS (OKN) AND OPTOKINETIC AFTER-NYSTAGMUS (OKAN)

E. KOENIG, J. DICHGANS and D. SCHMUCKER

Neurologische Universitätsklinik Tübingen, Federal Republic of Germany

Summary:
With fast moving optokinetic stimuli eliciting circularvection humans reach higher slow phase velocities (SPV) of OKN than with optokinetic stimuli eliciting little or no CV. OKAN is stronger after optokinetic stimulation eliciting CV, but there was also rather strong OKAN when optokinetic stimulation did not elicit CV. The results partially support the hypothesis that visually induced vestibular activity is a source of OKAN, but suggest the contribution of an oculomotor after-effect that may independently cause OKAN.

Key Words:
Optokinetic nystagmus, optokinetic after-nystagmus, circularvection, circularvection-aftersensation, oculomotor after-nystagmus, vestibular system, pursuit.

Introduction:

In recent years the concept has been developed that OKAN may be a correlate of vestibular activity elicited by visual stimulation and that OKN is a result of stimulation of both, the pursuit system and the vestibular system (Cohen, Uemura and Takemori, 1973; Brandt, Dichgans and Buechele, 1974; Cohen, Matsuo and Raphan, 1977; Waespe and Henn, 1977 b). Projections from the vestibular nuclei to the vestibular cortex then carry vestibular activity not only during vestibular stimulation proper (i. e. body acceleration), but also during whole field visual stimulation without real body motion. Thereby a sensation of self-motion in the presence of visual stimuli without real body motion may be elicited, which may serve to monitor whether or not a visual stimulus excites the vestibular nuclei. In particular the sensation of turning about a vertical body axis (i. e. circularvection, CV) has been thouroughly studied (Brandt, Dichgans and Koenig, 1973). The summation of the two inputs supposedly contributing to OKN was studied using ample field visual stimuli, which elicit CV and others that do not elicit CV, but still evoke OKN. OKAN was also studied to determine whether it really was only elicited when the vestibular nuclei were driven.

Methods:

4 subjects aged between 24 and 32 years with normal vestibular function volunteered for our experiments. Subjects were seated on a chair, which was surrounded by a cylindrical drum serving as the visual surround. The drum was rotated about the vertical axis of the subject.

To present visual stimuli eliciting different amounts of CV the following stimuli were used:

Experiment I - full field stimulation: The unrestricted visual field was filled with a pattern of alternating black and white stripes, each subtending 7.5° of visual angle, covering the inner wall of the drum. A band at eye level covered with coloured comic strip figures served foveal pursuit.

Experiment II - ample field stimulation, restricted eye movement amplitude: To restrict the amplitude of eye movements to 60° the small band of comic strip figures, which the subject was asked to pursue, was masked peripherally from 30° off the midline to the right and left. The black and white stripe pattern above and below the band of comic strip figures, however, was visible.

Experiment III - low density stimulation along the horizontal meridian: To reduce CV, the number of contrasts in the visual field was decreased to 4 simultaneously visible faint light spots (LED's) moving around the subject at eye level, one every 45° of visual angle.

Experiment IV - low density stimulation - 60° range of eye movements: To exclude CV completely the arrangement of experiment III with one LED every 45° of visual angle was combined with the masks used in experiment II excluding the LED's in the periphery beyond 30° to left and right off the midline. Thus, within a central field of 60°, only 1 or 2 LED's were visible simultaneously. Subjects were asked to attentively pursue the comic strip pattern or LED's (look nystagmus) moving at angular velocities of 30, 60, 90, 120, and 180°/s for 1 minute. Subjects made estimates of CV magnitude. OKN was recorded by D-C-electrooculography. After 1 min. the light was switched off, OKAN was recorded and the subjects indicated the duration of CV after sensation.

Results:

Averages of the CV velocity estimates of the 4 subjects (Fig. 1 - open symbols) show that pure CV without surround motion is perceived with full field stimulation (exp. I) up to 120°/stimulus speed, above that additional surround motion is perceived. Estimates of CV are somewhat lower in experiment II with stimulus speeds exceeding 90°/s. The reduction of contrasts in exp. III results in a considerably lower estimated CV-velocity. With additional exclusion of contrasts in the peripheral retina in exp. IV none of our subjects perceived CV. With naive subjects also in exp. III CV is rarely elicited, by our experienced subjects, however, CV is perceived more readily.

At stimulus velocities of 30 and 60°/s slow phase velocity (SPV) of OKN is almost identical in all 4 subjects (Fig. 1 - dark symbols). With higher stimulus velocities, differences between OKN average SPV in the 4 experiments increase with increasing stimulus velocities. The effect of a reduction of the amplitude of eye movements and the concomitant slight reduction of CV (exp. II) on OKN-SPV is relatively small compared to a reduction of CV by the decreased number of contrasts (exp. III). OKN-SPV is lowest in exp. IV, where CV was not elicited and amplitude of eye movements was reduced to 60°. The sensation of CV outlasts optokinetic stimulation of 1 min. by several seconds (Fig. 2 - open symbols). It is longest with full field stimulation and somewhat shorter with the stimulus conditions of exp. II and III. Obviously there is no CV-aftersensation in exp. IV, as there was no CV during optokinetic stimulation. Cumulative amplitude of OKAN (Fig. 2 - dark symbols) is highest with full (exp. I) and ample field stimulation (exp. II) and with medium stimulus velocities. It tends to be lower with slow and fast stimulus velocities.

OKAN is considerably weaker after exp. III and IV, but still surprisingly strong in exp. IV, although CV was absent in this experiment.

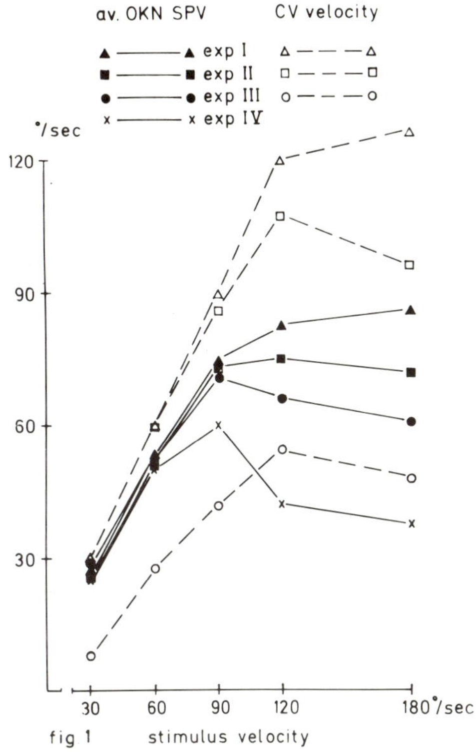

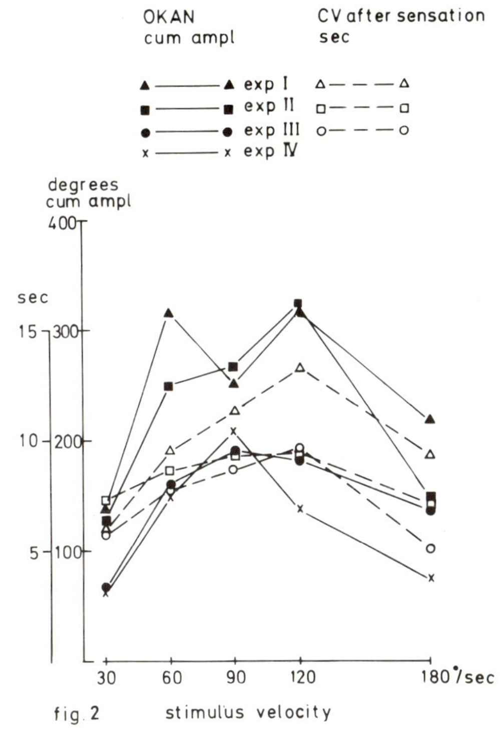

Fig. 1: Slow phase velocity (dark symbols) of OKN (averages of 4 subjects over 1 min) and estimates of CV velocity (open symbols) under conditions eliciting different amounts of CV (exp. I-IV). In exp. IV CV was not elicited.

Fig. 2: Cumulative amplitudes (dark symbols, degrees) of OKAN and duration (open symbols, sec) of CV aftersensation (averages of 4 subjects) after 1 min of stimulation. There was no CV aftersensation after exp. IV.

Discussion:

As expected from previous experiments (Brandt, Dichgans and Koenig, 1973) full field stimulation results in an increasing CV up to 120°/s stimulus speed. It leads to fast OKN and a strong OKAN and CV-aftersensation. Stimulation without CV reveals the rather low gain, especially at high stimulus velocities of the pursuit system alone. Target motion (retinal image motion + efference copy) drives both OKN and CV. The pursuit system is sufficient to drive OKN up to 30-60°/s stimulus velocities. Above this the large field dependent vestibular component becomes increasingly important. The fact that OKAN may be relatively strong without preceeding CV and without CV aftersensation suggests an additional mechanism (integrator) independent of the vestibular system. OKAN without CV or even with CV opposite to OKN (ambient stimulation, Brandt, Dichgans, and Buechele, 1973) may be an oculomotor aftereffect. Later Muratore and Zee (1979) described a similar phenomenon (pursuit afternystagmus).

EFFERENT MOTION PERCEPTION (σ–MOVEMENTS) AND σ–PURSUIT IN NEUROLOGICAL PATIENTS

U. W. BUETTNER, J. DICHGANS and O.-J. GRÜSSER

Neurologische Universitätsklinik Tübingen, Federal Republic of Germany

SUMMARY

Simultaneously flickering stationary periodic stimuli may induce an apparent σ-movement and σ-pursuit once initiated by pursuit of a real movement. σ-phenomena presumably are caused by the interaction of a premotor efference copy signal and afferent visual signals. Various central lesions cause smooth pursuit deficits. σ-pursuit has not yet been examined in patients. Therefore fifty patients with impaired smooth pursuit due to lesions of various origin were tested as to possibly localize the circuits involved. It could be shown that patients with brainstem lesions in contrast to patients with cerebellar lesions are able to perceive σ-movement and perform σ-pursuit, although target pursuit is cogwheeled.

KEY-WORDS: Smooth pursuit, σ-pursuit, apparent movement perception, efference copy, smooth pursuit deficits.

INTRODUCTION

An array of simultaneously flickering stationary periodic stimuli may elicit apparent motion perception and smooth pursuit eye movements or optokinetic nystagmus, once initiated by a brief real movement of the eye or the head. This in contrast to movement perception following successive illumination of discrete pattern elements (φ-movement and φ-pursuit) is called σ-motion perception and σ-pursuit (Stoper, 67; 73; Lamontagne, 73; Heywood, 73; Behrens & Grüsser, 79; Grüsser, Pause & Schreiter, 79). The conditions, which are necessary to elicit σ-movement perception and σ-pursuit have extensively been studied (Behrens & Grüsser, 79; Grüsser, Pause & Schreiter, 79). It has been argued that σ-phenomena are caused by the interaction of an efference copy signal of the smooth pursuit command and afferent visual signals (Behrens & Grüsser, 79). It is however open, where this interaction takes place and which nervous structures are responsible for the generation of σ-pursuit. It is generally accepted that brainstem, cerebellar, as well as cortical lesions may cause deficits of smooth pursuit. σ-pursuit has not yet been examined in patients. This was the aim of the present investigation. Patients with deficits of smooth pursuit caused by lesions of various sites and pathogenesis were examined with respect to their ability to perceive apparent motion and execute σ-pursuit.

METHODS

Fifty patients, who exhibited smooth pursuit deficits were tested with a machine, which consisted of 2 circles 10 mm apart (80 cm diameter) of 100 diodes each. The patient was seated in front of the device, so that the diameter of the circle corresponded to 40° of visual angle. The diodes could be illuminated at variable frequency and luminance. The diodes of the inner circle flickered simultaneously, thus producing a stationary pattern of discrete dots forming the circle, whereas the diodes of the outer circle were optionally illuminated successively clockwise or counterclockwise phase-locked to the diodes of the inner circle. The outer circle served to elicit φ-movement and to initiate σ-movement. φ-pursuit gain and its deficits are equivalent to real target pursuit. Horizontal and vertical eye movements were recorded by EOG on a strip chart. For data analysis a half-automatic programmed nystagmus analyzer was used, which calculated the smooth pursuit gain (deg/sec smooth pursuit/deg/sec stimulus velocity).

RESULTS

Based on clinical examination including computertomography it was tried to group patients according to the location of their lesion. Most (26) patients had lesions, which could not be well defined anatomically or were not restricted to one site, i. e. functional subunit. The remaining patients had unifocal lesions restricted to the lower brainstem (12), the cerebellum (7) or the supratentorial central nervous system (5). 1. The majority (70 %) of patients with target pursuit deficits were able to perceive the apparent motion of the stationary flickering circle at least for short times. Most of these patients performed smooth σ-pursuit only with the aid of φ-movement, but showed cogwheeled φ-pursuit without the flickering circle (Fig.1). Whenever apparent motion was perceived the smooth pursuit gain was approximately 1. 2. Only 12 % of the patients were able to perform pure σ-pursuit without the aid of the φ-stimulus (Fig. 2). 3. In many cases (50 %) the φ-pursuit gain was conspiciously low, whenever σ-pursuit was lost. The gain of φ then was much lower than prior to σ. This could be observed repeatedly in the same recordings. 4. σ-apparent motion perception and σ-pursuit may be unidirectionally disturbed. 5. Patients with lesions restricted to the cerebellum were not able to perceive σ-motion or to perform σ-pursuit, whereas all patients with isolated brainstem lesions, so far tested, could perform smooth σ-pursuit with the aid of φ despite their low pure φ-pursuit gain. Five out of the twelve patients could even perfectly follow the apparent target motion without support of φ. Among the five patients with supratentorial lesions, examined so far, two showed the σ-effects. 6. Changes of σ-pursuit and σ-perception over time could be detected in a patient with multiple sclerosis (Fig. 3). Smooth pursuit deficits at the time of the first recording were ascribed to a lesion in the left parietal white matter confirmed by CT-scan. At the time of the second recording symptoms pointed to a lower brainstem lesion. CT-scan showed marked improvement of the parietal lesion. Although smooth pursuit gain did not change considerably σ-pursuit was now easily performed.

DISCUSSION

σ-phenomena are thought to be generated by the interaction of an efference copy signal of the smooth pursuit command and the sensory afference (Behrens & Grüsser, 79). The present data suggest that σ-pursuit occasionally may be perfect, even if smooth pursuit is heavily

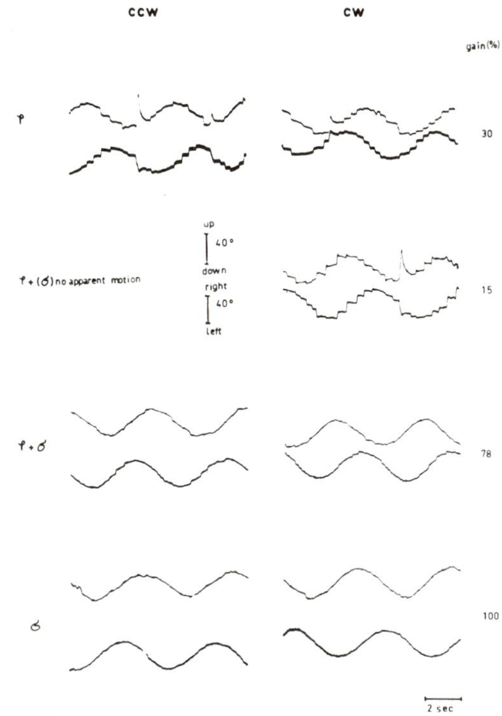

Fig. 1: Patient with suspected multiple sclerosis and isolated brainstem lesion. Severity of smooth pursuit disturbance depends on mode of pursuit. Perfect smooth pursuit is performed when σ-pursuit is possible without the aid of φ-motion.

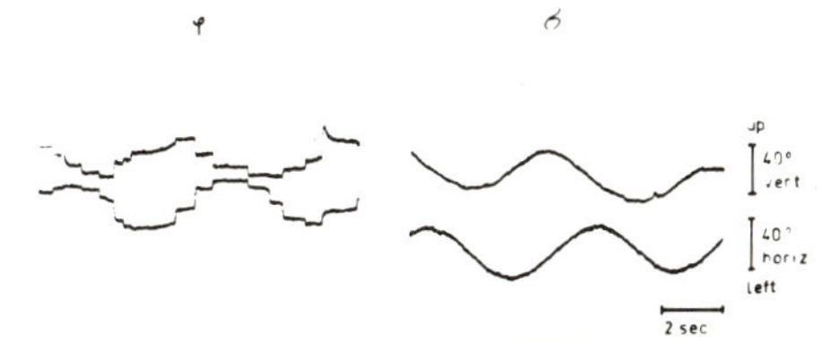

Fig. 2: Patient with isolated lesion of the lower brainstem. Although smooth pursuit was severely impaired, perfect σ-pursuit could be performed.

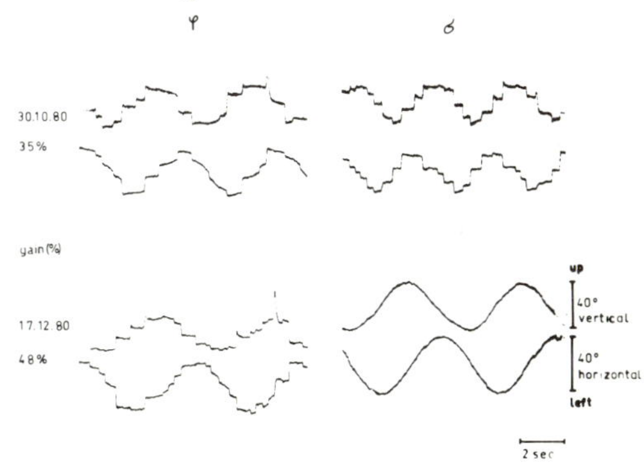

Fig. 3: Patient with different manifestations of multiple sclerosis. Perfect σ-pursuit after recovery from parietal lesion and newly acquired brainstem symptoms.

disturbed. It follows that in these cases the premotor and motor structures necessary for the performance of smooth pursuit are intact. Lower brainstem lesions, although causing deficits of φ-pursuit and real target pursuit, may allow for perfect σ. It may be concluded that the interaction between efference copy and afferent visual signals takes place outside the brainstem. This could be the case at various stations of the higher visual cortex. From our data it must be concluded that the cerebellum plays an important role also in σ-pursuit, since none of the patients with cerebellar degeneration could perceive σ. Generally the disturbances of smooth pursuit were severer in cerebellar patients than in others. So it cannot be excluded that the severity of the smooth pursuit defect by itself is important. It is likely that the cerebellum is involved in the generation of the efference copy signal. In conclusion preserved σ, but impaired real target pursuit is interpreted as the consequence of an impaired sensory afference with preserved efference copy and efferent motor capacity, as well as movement perception.

DISCUSSION

The discussion centered first on the NOT-Accessory Optic System and its pathways to the oculomotor system. Collewijn and coworkers studying the rabbit used autoradiography and found no direct projection to the nucleus reticularis tegmenti pontis (NRTP). This observation is in contrast to the findings of Maekawa and Kimura (1981), who describe this pathway in the rabbit. Collewijn found projections to the pontine nuclei which in turn project to the cerebellum. Heavy projections were seen to the nucleus praepositus hypoglossi. Projections to the abducens nucleus and to the dorsal rostral medullary reticular formation ventral to the nucleus praepositus hypoglossi were also found. Collewijn felt that these connections may be part of the Optokinetic-Vestibular-Integrator. Precht mentioned a very small zone of NRTP close to the midline in the rat and cat that clearly obtains direct input from NOT. From about this region projections to the cerebellar flocculus arise in these two animal species. In the monkey the pretectal-vestibular nuclei pathway carrying visual motion information is less well defined. Keller found very few cells in NRTP that responded to large visual field motion. The rare ones recorded showed velocity tuning curves that were different from the ones obtained when recording OKN-modulation in the vestibular nuclei. He concluded that in the monkey, NRTP is not a major relay station of the visual-vestibular pathway. Cells that looked more like the appropriate link between NOT and the vestibular nuclei were recorded within the medial pontine nuclei. In reference to the above mentioned findings of Collewijn and his own observations he commented about the fact that NRTP and pontine nuclei in more caudal sections are clearly separated by the medial lemniscus whereas more rostrally NRTP and what might be called medial pontine nuclei are not clearly separable. Considerations like these may partially explain the disagreements, but species differences are to be expected.

The question was then raised as to what extent man and monkey at all possess an NOT-Accessory Optic System. Precht conceeded that this system both anatomically and functionally is of much lesser importance in primates and man. He felt that the failure to find remarkable deficitis with pretectal lesions in the monkey may result from the complex organisation of the NOT-Accessory Optic System analogue with a rather widespread distribution within midbrain in this animal. Apparently, there is only one paper by Westheimer and Blair (1974) that reports on recordings of pretectal neurons that are modulated by optokinetic stimuli. These were situated in the nucleus of the transpeduncular tract, a possible homologue of the medial terminal nucleus (MTN) of the accessory optic system in the monkey. Both the nucleus of the transpeduncular tract and the MTN process vertical optokinetic information. Details about the anatomical organization of the accessory optic system in primates seem to be not known.

Strong interconnections between the different nuclei of the accessory optic system (MTN and LTN for vertical movements and NOT and DTN for horizontal) in the cat are considered to sharpen the directional selectivity (Hoffmann).

The question to which extent the NOT-Accessory Optic System is functional in primates and man could not sufficiently be answered. The earlier finding of the Pasik's who observed no OKN deficit after pretectal lesions in the monkey was mentioned by Cohen. Cohen himself obtained a clear deficit whenever the lesion extended laterally to the mesencephalic reticular formation. Midbrain lesions in man clearly affect OKN (Baloh), but are too large and nonselective so that they possibly damage efferent occipito-parietal-pontine pathways running through this region.

Without doubt the transcortical pathway in man and monkey is of exceeding importance. Hoffmann stated that his model could possibly still be applicable in man, if the cortico-pretectal input covers 80 - 90 %. In this case the pretectal relay would function only with cortex being functional. The phylogenetically old pathway via the pretectum to the brainstem could still be operative.

There is no evidence that a purely subcortical optokinetic system exists in man. The slow charge/discharge component of OKN is negligible in humans, as compared to the monkey. - "Whoever is blind cannot perform OKN and whoever performs OKN is not blind" was the firm statement of Dr. Daroff concerning this question. But recordings with prolonged very slowly moving optokinetic full field stimulation in cortically blind people are lacking. The other statement of Drs. Baloh and Daroff that patients presenting with a purely occipital cortical lesion and hemianopia show no OKN deficit ("Cogans rule", Daroff) does not hold for acute cases in whom a rapidly recovering asymmetry with slowed OKN particularly at high stimulus speeds is found when the stimulus moves to the ipsilateral side (Dichgans). Careful studies measuring OKN gain in chronic patients are lacking. Thus a symmetrical global gain reduction especially with high speed OKN stimuli (exceeding the 60 °/s used by Baloh) cannot be excluded.

Clinically the strongest OKN deficits of supratentorial origin are observed with parietal lobe lesions. Daroff stated that he is not aware of any convincing case in the literature who presented an OKN deficit due to an exclusively cortical parietal lesion. He felt that any parietal lesion causing an OKN deficit must involve the deep white matter and must cause hemianopia.

In this context Precht mentioned monkey data obtained by Kawano and Sasaki (1981) who in the parietal area 7 found neurons that possess all the features of OKN-pursuit. This area in the monkey projects to the pretectum. The possible function of area 7 in pursuit is further suggested by the data of Lynch (this volume) who with lesions limited to area 7 found pursuit deficits. OKN asymmetries were only observed when the lesion extended into prestriate cortex. Certainly it is not yet clear whether any deficit in pursuit exists that does not affect OKN at higher velocities or with small stimulus areas. In man, due to the high gain of pursuit as compared to the slow charge/discharge OKN component, any pursuit deficit should also affect OKN (Dichgans). OKN for an optimal gain clearly needs the contributions of both, foveally guided smooth pursuit and the retinal periphery dependent opto-vestibular system.

It was then discussed whether the OKN-vestibular integrator of Raphan and Cohen is charged via the cerebellum. Dr. Baloh's findings in cerebellar patients with almost complete absence of pursuit, but preserved slow charge OKN and OKAN may suggest that this is not the case. But the charge time constants are very much delayed both in the monkey and humans after lesions of the cerebellar flocculus (Cohen). Thus the flocculus cannot only be in the pursuit (direct) pathway, but must contribute to the brainstem optovestibular integrator.

The last subject addressed in the discussion was adaptation to visual rearrangement. The question of whether adaptation of VOR may be different for the two eyes was answered in reference to unpublished material of Collewijn and Steinmann who used +5 Dptr. lenses on one eye and -5 Dptr. lenses on the other. Adaptation of the VOR gain mostly did not occur or was extremely difficult and slow. In the latter case one eye took over and dominated vision and adaptation.

The general feeling after the talks presented in this session and the discussion was that neuroanatomical and neurophysiological studies of OKN and pursuit in animals now provide a great wealth of knowledge that may fruitfully be used by clinicians to better understand the specialities of the physiological organization of this system in humans and pathophysiology in patients.

SECTION VIII

Coordinator: A. Gresty

DISORDERS OF EYE-HEAD COORDINATION

EYE-HEAD COORDINATION IN MAN DURING THE PURSUIT OF MOVING TARGETS

H. COLLEWIJN, P. CONIJN and E. P. TAMMINGA

Department of Physiology I, Faculty of Medicine, Erasmus University, Rotterdam, P.O. Box 1738, 3000 DR Rotterdam, The Netherlands

ABSTRACT

Eye and head movements were measured during the pursuit of continuous, unpredictable movements of a target with a bandwidth of 1 Hz and a maximal excursion of 15-50°. Subjects were instructed to pursue without head movements, mainly with head movements or using their own strategy. Quality of pursuit, expressed in standard deviation (S.D.) of the error, was best with the free strategy and almost as good with the maximal use of head movements (S.D. about 1.5°). Pursuit by the eye alone was equally good for excursions up to 30°. Enlargement of target excursion (without increase in velocity) augmented pursuit errors. When subjects were forced - by feedback of eye position to target position - to pursue with the head only, errors increased threefold. Suppression of vestibulo-ocular reflexes was incomplete.

KEYWORDS

Eye movement; head movement; eye-head coordination; gaze control; pursuit.

INTRODUCTION

Whenever we want to observe a moving target in any detail, we have to pursue it to keep its image on the central part of the retina. The spatial orientation of the visual axis, the gaze, is most quickly changed by rotations of the eye in the head, the head on the body and the body in space. In addition, translations of head and body will occur. Voluntary gaze changes will interact and often apparently conflict with the compensatory systems of the vestibulo-ocular reflex (VOR) and optokinetic reflex (OKR) which tend to stabilize gaze. Obviously, the control of gaze in a completely "natural" situation - such as the walker observing a butterfly - is exceedingly complex to describe and moreover at present impossible to measure. As usually, in the laboratory we have to reduce the situation to a level of abstraction commensurate with our techniques of measurement and analysis. Recently (Collewijn, 1977), a system was developed which allows us to measure the angular direction of eye, head and gaze without narrow constraints on the mobility of the subject, which is an ideal situation for the investigation of coordinated eye- and head movements. First applications of this technique to human gaze control have been directed to the quality of fixation of stationary targets during voluntary and passive head movements (Steinman & Collewijn, 1980; Collewijn,

Martins and Steinman, 1981a). These studies revealed that the performance of our stabilizing systems is far from perfect, even though the systems are capable of rapid adaptive changes in overall gain.

We now address the pursuit of a continuously moving target by combined eye- and head movements. Most previous studies of eye-head coordination relate to the saccadic foveation of targets presented in the periphery, and only a few systematic studies of pursuit of continuous movement have been published (Fleming and co-workers, 1969; Gresty and Leech, 1977) for human subjects and for monkeys (Lanman, Bizzi and Allum, 1978). Those studies relate mainly to repetitive, highly predictable target movements. In our view this represents a special case of tracking. Also, the instructions to the subject may be important as the contribution of head movement to pursuit is to a large extent under voluntary control. Main features of our study are:

(1) Accurate measurement of angular eye- and head position;
(2) Pseudo-random (unpredictable), continuous target motion;
(3) Systematic variation of range of target motion;
(4) Systematic instruction of the subjects to use certain strategies;
(5) Optional feedback of eye- or head position to the target to make eye- or head movements ineffective in pursuit;
(6) Computer analysis of pursuit in the frequency domain (Bode plots) and time domain (distribution of pursuit error).

METHODS

Eye- and head orientation were measured with the rotating field technique (Collewijn, 1977). Briefly, a homogeneous a.c. magnetic field is generated which rotates in the horizontal plane with a frequency of 600 Hz. Induction coils are attached to the head and the eye (Collewijn, Van der Mark and Jansen, 1975). The phase of the induced potentials relative to that of the field is directly proportional to the eye and head position. The measurement is linear over 360° of rotation, has a bandwidth of about 100 Hz and is invariant for changes in the amplitude of the

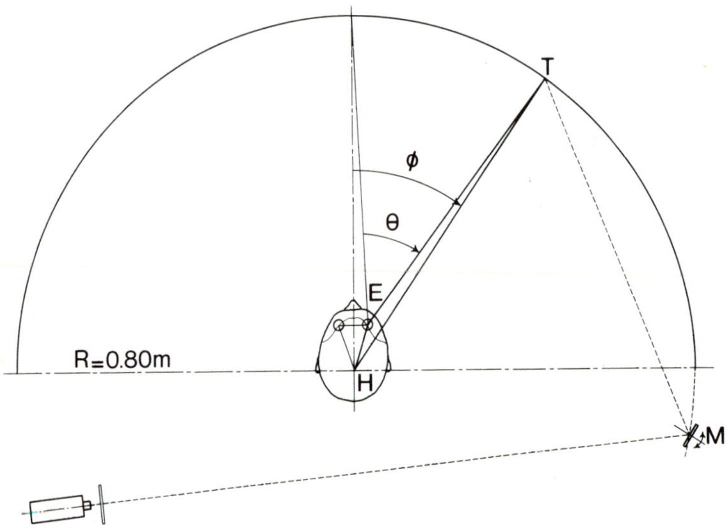

Fig. 1. Schematic diagram of the experimental arrangement. M: servocontrolled mirror; T: target; H: center of head rotation; E: center of eye rotation.

induced voltages as caused by the use of different coils etc. Calibration is therefore absolute and constant.

Inside the magnetic field coils a hemicylindrical, optically homogeneous screen with a radius (*R*) of 0.80 m was mounted. The target was a red spot created by a Helium-Neon laser beam, reflected on to the screen by a servo-controlled mirror (bandwidth about 200 Hz) and moved in a horizontal plane at eye level (Fig. 1). Target position was linearly controlled up to eccentricities of 60° and signalled by the internal position-transducer of the scanner.

All experiments were done monocularly, with the scleral annulus in the seeing eye. The system measures the eye and head angle in space, and the eye-in-head angle as a derived signal. However, as the rotation centers of eye and head do not coincide, the effective direction of gaze (intersection of the visual axis with the screen) is not equivalent to the sum of eye-in-head and head angle. This problem has been recognized and analyzed before by Blakemore and Donaghy (1980) and Brandt (personal communication).

The subject was placed, as precisely as possible, with the head rotation center (H) (assumed to be stationary in space) in the center of curvature of the screen. The eye rotation center (E) is located at a distance a in front of H. The relation between an eye rotation θ and an equivalent rotation ϕ (Fig. 2) around the axis of the screen is given by:

$$\sin\theta = \frac{\sin\phi}{\sqrt{\left(\frac{a}{R}\right)^2 - 2\frac{a}{R}\cos\phi + 1}} \qquad (1)$$

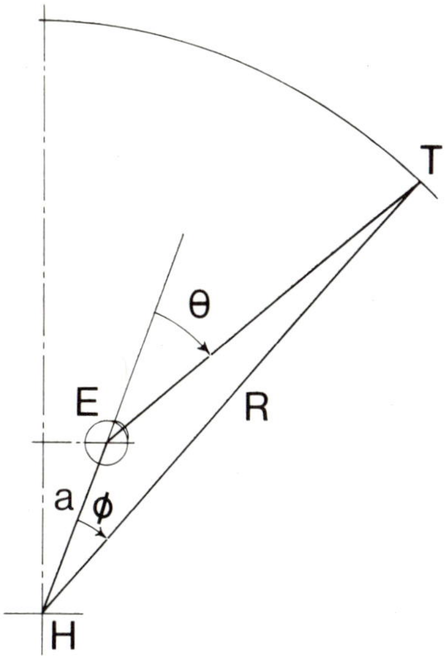

Fig. 2. The relation between the angle of eye rotation and an equivalent rotation around the center of the screen. See text.

The numerical solution of this equation is complex. For $a \ll R$ the following linear approximation can be used:

$$\phi = \frac{1}{1 + \frac{a}{R}}\theta \qquad (2)$$

For the case $a = 0.10$ m, $R = 0.80$ m this approximation is correct to within 0.3° for eye excursions up to 50°, and reduces to $\phi = 0.89\theta$. In practice the value of a is difficult to determine and probably varies between subjects.

Four target motion signals were generated by computer with different maximal excursions from the midposition ($15, 30, 40, 50^{\circ}$). Each signal consisted of a sum of six non-harmonic sinusoids. In addition to the overall amplitude ($15, 30, 40$ or 50°) the maximum velocity of the components was limited ($A\omega < 5^{\circ}/s$) to avoid target velocities out of the range of the smooth pursuit system.

Subjects were instructed to pursue the moving target as precisely as possible, using the following strategies:
(1) moving only the eye and keeping the head stationary (*Eye only*); (2) pursuing mainly with the head, moving the eye as little as possible (*Head only*); (3) using

a combination of eye and head movements of their own preference (*Free*). Two further conditions were added: (4) feedback of the head position to the target (*Feedback head*); (5) feedback of the eye-in-head position to the target (*Feedback eye*). Although in these latter conditions the subject was free to choose his own strategy, head movement and eye movement, respectively, had no effect on the retinal image position of the target, and effective pursuit was possible only with the eye (condition 4) or head (condition 5).

All conditions were used with maximal target excursions of 15,30 and 40°; at 50° the conditions requiring pursuit with the eye only were omitted in view of the mechanical limit of eye displacement to about 45°. Every measurement lasted about 60 s. Target, head equivalent eye and gaze positions as well as the error (target minus gaze) were registered on a penrecorder and sampled on line by a PDP 11/10 computer with a frequency of 150 Hz and stored on disk. The data on disk were corrected afterwards on the basis of two calibration measurements which were taken before every session. During one measurement, fixation on a stationary target at 15,30,40,50° eccentricity was achieved mainly by head movement. During the other, only eye movement was allowed.

RESULTS

General Pattern of Responses

Examples of recordings of one subject are shown in Fig. 3. When left free to use his own preferred combination of eye and head movements (*Free*) a subject usually used both. The degree to which the head was moved varied between subjects but could be modified very effectively by instruction. When the subject was instructed to move the *Eye only*, head movements were totally abolished. Under the instruction to pursue only with the head, head movements were greatly augmented and the amplitude of eye movements decreased. Most of smooth pursuit was done by the head and the eye executed mainly saccades. Both in the *Free* and *Head only* condition the smooth eye movements were often opposite in direction to the head movements, although smaller in amplitude. This indicates that the vestibulo-ocular reflex was only partly suppressed. A gross examination of the error signal shows no major differences in performance between these three normal pursuit strategies. Saccades tended to occur at similar moments in all three conditions and always decreased the error. In the feedback conditions, the error increased considerably. Surprisingly, the nature of the *Feedback head* condition was not perceived by naive subjects. Instead of avoiding all head movements, as was done by informed subjects to change the condition to an *Eye only* situation, they continued to generate large, erratic head movements. As these were added to the target motion, the pursuit task became much more difficult. The efficacy of the *Feedback eye* condition is shown by the absence of saccades in the error signal. The relative inefficiency of head pursuit is indicated by the large error signal.

Gain and Phase Relations

Gain and phase relations of the responses (eye, head and gaze) in relation to the target (position vs. position) are shown for one subject and for a maximal target excursion of 30° in the Bode plots of Fig. 4 and 5. They represent the over-all motions including smooth and saccadic components. Gaze corresponds to the *vectorial* sum of eye and head. The shape of these Bode plots may be partly determined by the specific composition of our stimulus.

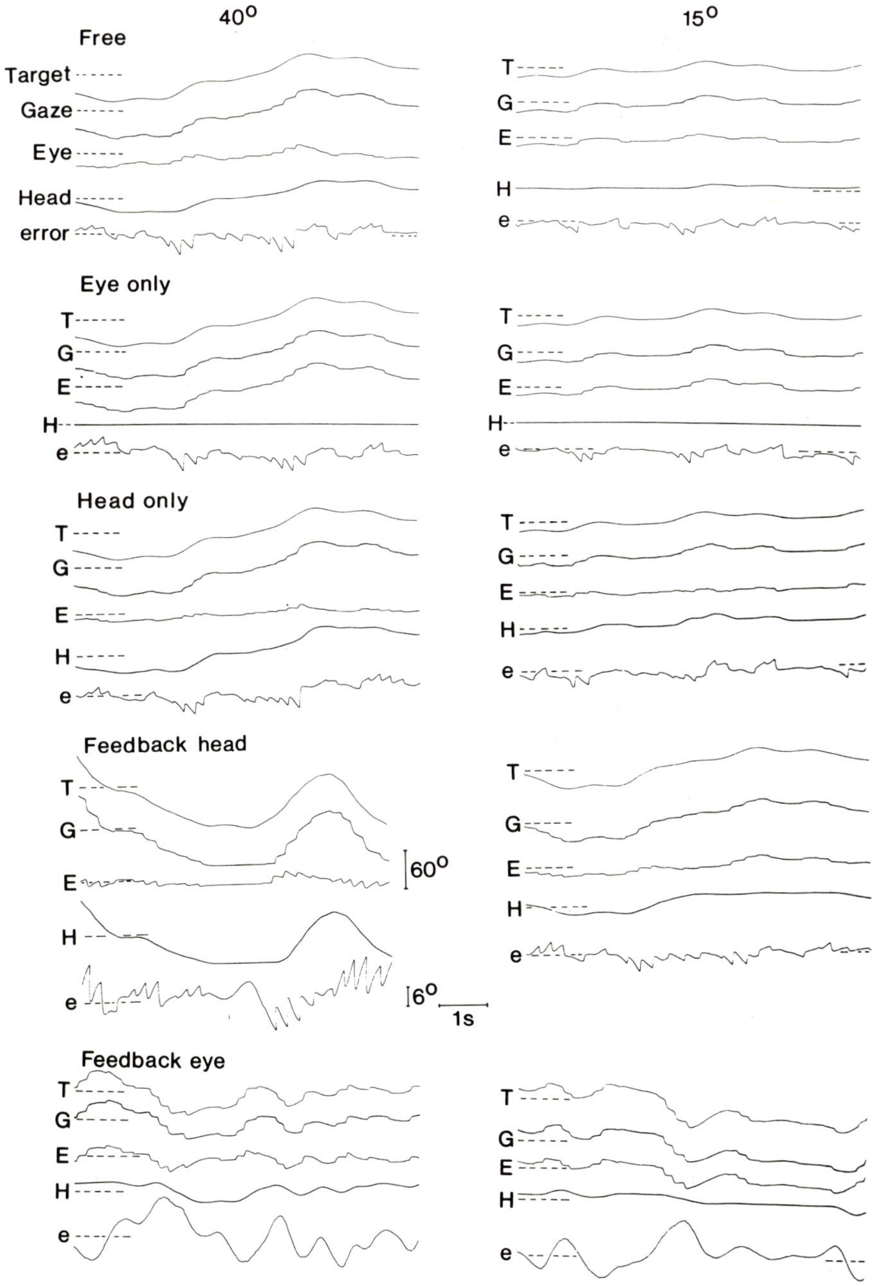

Fig. 3. Recordings of pursuit at two target ranges and under five instructions/conditions. Gaze = Head + Eye; Eye represents equivalent rotation around the center of the screen in all figures. Target, Gaze, Eye and Head have the same calibration (60° bar), upward is right. The error (Gaze - Target) is recorded at 5x higher sensitivity (6°). Interrupted lines indicate midposition or zero levels.

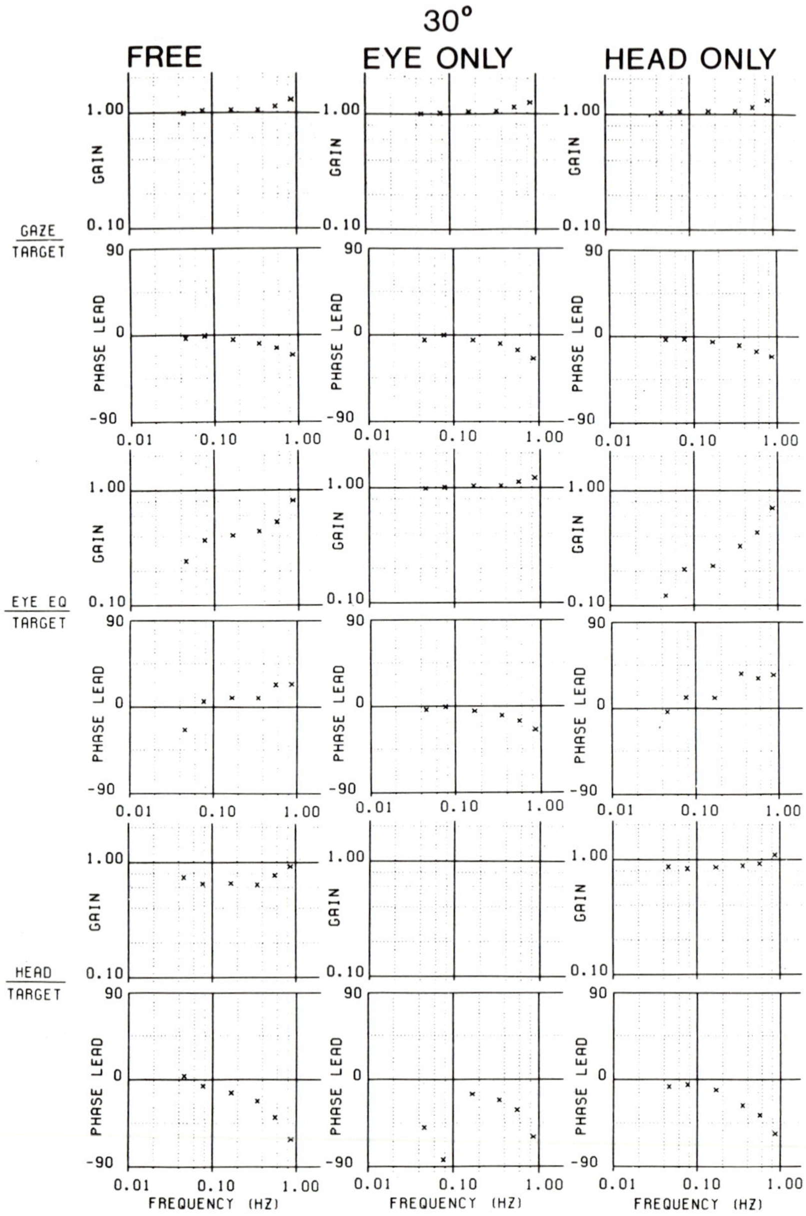

Fig. 4. Bode plots for one subject for different instructions and one target range.

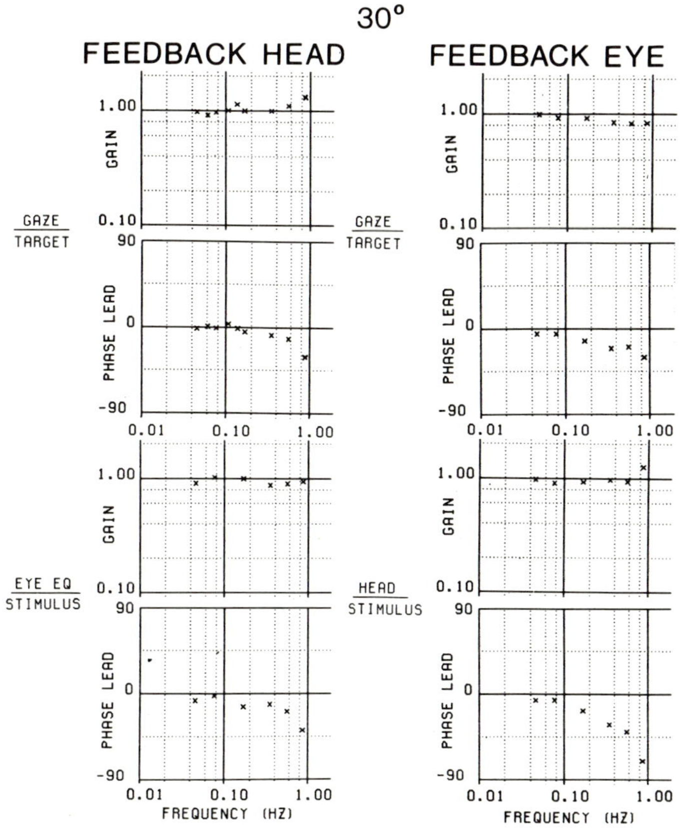

Fig. 5. Bode plots for pursuit in feedback situations.
Feedback head: stimulus = target - head
Feedback eye : stimulus = target - eye

The relation gaze/target. Gain and phase of gaze proved to be virtually independent of the instruction (*Free*, *Eye only* or *Head only*; Fig. 4) and also of the maximal excursion of the target (15,30,40 or 50°). Above 0.2 Hz an increasing phase lag was seen, accompanied by an increase in gain above unity. The reason is that subjects tended to overshoot the target and to be too late in changing the direction of pursuit of these higher frequencies. Accordingly, the overall error increased. Among subjects, the amount of increase in phase lag correlated strongly with the deterioration of pursuit accuracy.

Relative contribution of eye and head to gaze. This was strongly influenced by the instructions. Under the instruction *Eye only* the gain of head was essentially zero. Under the instruction *Head only* eye movements were decreased, but not completely suppressed. At low frequencies gain of the eye sometimes became lower than 0.1. Under the instructions *Head only* and *Free* gain increased markedly with the frequency for the eye, and slightly for the head. The phase relation for the head movement remained practically constant throughout all conditions and stimulus ranges, although it varied between subjects. Also in this case larger phase lag was correlated with poorer pursuit. The phase of the eye movement showed no consistent relation to instruction or target range, even within one subject.

Conditions with feedback. Bode plots for these conditions, in which head or (equivalent) eye-in-head position was added to target position, are shown in Fig. 5 (same naive subject as in Fig. 4). For the *Feedback head* condition the gaze/target relation resembles that in the normal conditions shown in Fig. 4. The eye/stimulus relation (stimulus = target - head) resembles that of the eye/target relation in the *Eye only* condition, although the gain is lower. However, the complex effects of feedback of head position to the target call for a cautious interpretation (see Discussion). For the *Feedback eye* condition the gaze/target relation shows the lowest gain of all conditions, in accordance with the poor pursuit. The head/stimulus relation (stimulus = target - eye) closely resembles the head/target relation in the *Head only* condition. Also in this situation the interpretation is complex.

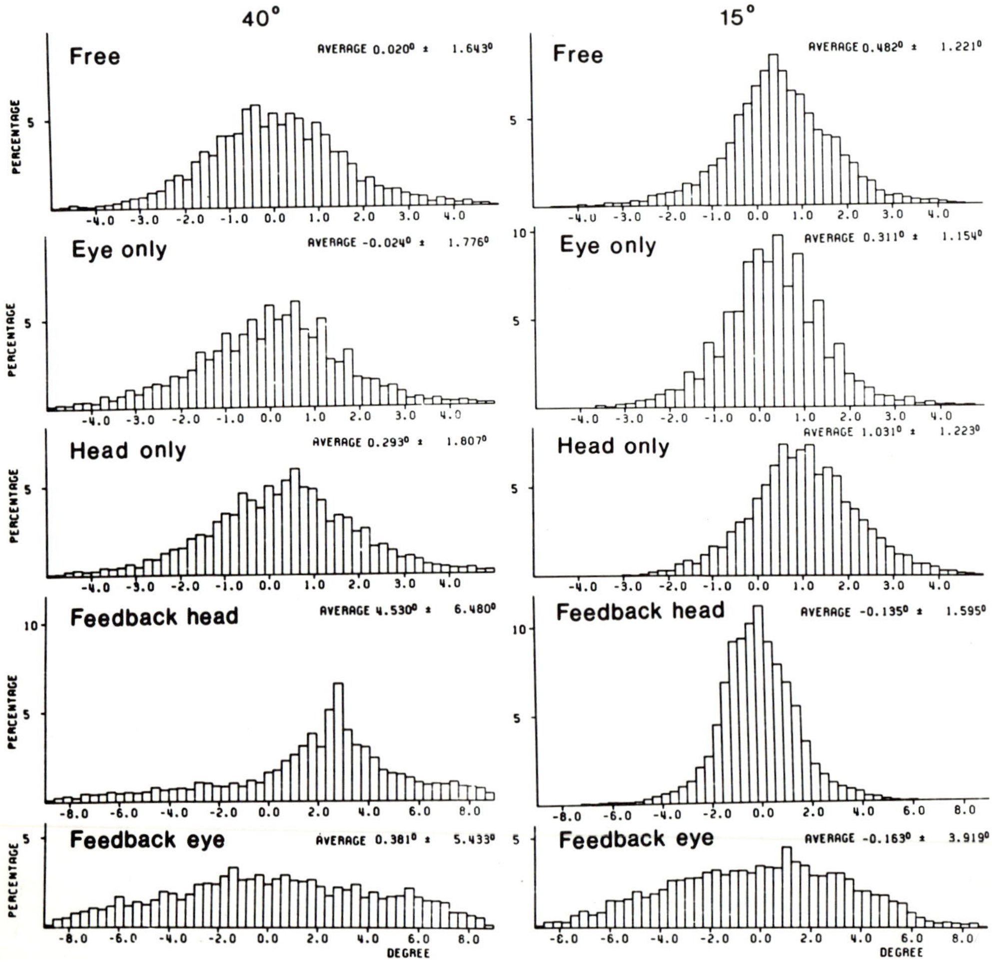

Fig. 6. Histograms of the distribution of error (Target-Gaze) for five conditions and two target ranges. Abscissa: pursuit error in degrees; ordinate: percentage of samples.

Distribution of the Error

The distribution of the error signal is shown for one (naive) subject in Fig. 6. The width of this distribution, expressed as standard deviation (S.D.) is a measure of the quality of the pursuit. A non-zero mean of the distribution could indicate a systematic deviation of pursuit in one direction, but is to be interpreted very cautiously as similar deviations may be caused by errors in the measurement. Essential, uncorrectible errors are caused by non-stationarity of the rotation axis of the head, although technical errors introduced by non-optimal settings of the controls of the equipment were largely corrected off-line on basis of the calibration trials.

While the general trends can be seen in Fig. 6, more precise results are given in Table 1, which shows the average S.D. (and their S.D.) for eight subjects, after optimal correction for technical errors.

TABLE 1 Standard Deviations of Pursuit Error Averaged over Eight Subjects

Target range	*Free*	*Eye only*	*Head only*	*Feedback eye*
15°	1.21 ± 0.29	1.18 ± 0.14	1.20 ± 0.16	3.38 ± 0.47
30°	1.46 ± 0.23	1.57 ± 0.25	1.55 ± 0.31	4.66 ± 0.34
40°	1.53 ± 0.20	2.65 ± 1.12	1.61 ± 0.24	5.19 ± 0.47
50°	1.64 ± 0.29		1.79 ± 0.29	6.12 ± 0.91

The S.D. of pursuit increased when the maximal deviation of the target increased, under all conditions. Pursuit was most accurate in the condition *Free*, except at a target range of 15° for which no difference between *Free*, *Head only* and *Eye only* was found. With a maximal excursion of 30°, pursuit under *Head only* and *Eye only* conditions was equal in quality. With target excursions of 40° (seen by the eye under an angle of about 45°) pursuit with *Eye only* was remarkably poor, while with *Head only* it was almost as good as under the *Free* instruction. In the *Feedback eye* condition all pursuit had to be done with the head. Not surprisingly, the errors were much higher (by about a factor 3) than in the normal conditions; the variability between subjects was relatively small and independent of their insight in the situation. On the other hand in the *Feedback head* condition the subjects split into an informed group, which stopped to move the head, and a naive group (Fig. 6). The informed subjects performed essentially *Eye only* pursuit, while the naive subjects created difficulties for themselves by increasing the target velocities and pursued with large errors. In view of this heterogeneity no averages of this condition are shown in Table 1.

DISCUSSION

A main purpose of this investigation was to see whether the precision of the gaze directed to a target in smooth, pseudo-random motion was strongly affected by the proportion of eye and head movements used in the pursuit. It appears that the quality of pursuit was practically equal under all strategies (Fig. 3,4,6 and Table 1) except that pursuit with the eye alone became poor for target excursions larger than 30-40°, which is not surprising in view of the mechanical limits of eye movements. Also for combined eye and head movements there was a tendency for pursuit errors to increase when the range of target motion was enlarged, independent of the strategy, even though target velocities were kept about constant. Lanman, Bizzi and Allum (1978) found in the monkey as well about equal precision of pursuit during head fixed and head free tracking of periodical target motion up to amplitudes of 30°. The gain and phase relations of gaze vs. target we found are different from those reported by Fleming and coworkers (1969) who found at 1 Hz a zero phase lag and a gain of about 0.75. This might be due to differences in spectral composition and predictability of the target motion. Gresty and Leech (1977) reported for tracking of predictable sinusoidal motion a phase lead of the head and a lag of the eye, both of about 20°, for frequencies between 0.2 and 1.0 Hz. With our unpredictable target movements, the head movements showed a definite phase lag in this frequency range (Fig. 4). Gresty and Leech (1977) reported a general tendency for the use of head movements to be detrimental, especially in the pursuit of random motion. This was attributed to incomplete suppression or even overcompensation of the VOR. Our findings do not substantiate any major adverse effect of the use of head movements. With all strategies the standard deviations of pursuit error were about 1.5°. We do agree, however, that suppression of the VOR is often very incomplete.

We introduced the *Feedback head* condition to force the subjects to pursue only with the eye, without restraining the head. For this purpose the conditions proved to be superfluous, as the simple instruction *Eye only* was completely effective in all subjects. Although the target followed all head movements in *Feedback head*, all naive subjects continued to make large head movements. In this condition it would be highly advantageous to completely suppress the VOR but, as shown in Fig. 3, this was not achieved. Although smooth gaze movements were in the direction of the target, the smooth eye-in-head movements were opposite to the head movements and thus compensatory. As a result, motion relative to the eye was augmented and pursuit error increased. This complex interaction makes interpretation of this condition difficult. The *Feedback eye* condition is more straightforward, as it simply cancels the effect of any eye-in-head movements on retinal image position. In this condition a VOR functioning at unity gain would prevent any effective smooth tracking, and the error would be equal to the stimulus signal. Actually, gaze pursuit was strongly saccadic and the eye moves mostly opposite to the head (Fig. 3). Once again, VOR suppression was very incomplete.

In the present paper, only a general description of coordinated eye and head pursuit is given. A more detailed analysis of the control system is still under development.

THE RELATIONSHIP BETWEEN RETINAL IMAGE SLIP, OSCILLOPSIA AND POSTURAL IMBALANCE

TH. BRANDT

Neurological Clinic with Clinical Neurophysiology, Alfried Krupp Hospital, Essen, Federal Republic of Germany

ABSTRACT

Oscillopsia as well as postural imbalance may be induced by head movements in patients with peripheral eye movement disorders or with acquired ocular oscillations. The amplitude of subjective oscillopsia is significantly smaller than the measurable net retinal slip of the visual scene. Suppression of oscillopsia may be due, in part, to an inhibitory interaction between self and object motion perception.

KEYWORDS

Retinal slip; oscillopsia; postural sway; motion detection threshold.

OSCILLOPSIA AND POSTURAL IMBALANCE INDUCED BY HEAD MOVEMENTS IN PERIPHERAL DISORDERS OF EYE MOVEMENTS

The sudden onset of an extraocular muscle paresis, such as in patients with ocular myasthenia, may induce "ocular vertigo" during voluntary head movements. The symptoms include perceptual illusions (oscillopsia) but also affect locomotion and cause postural imbalance (visual ataxia).

Oscillopsia, the illusory motion of the visual scene, results from an inappropriate gain of the vestibulo-ocular reflex. The latter stabilizes the direction of gaze in space (eye position in head summated with head position in space) by moving the eyes in the direction opposite to head movement. If the amplitude and/or the velocity of the eyes do not compensate for the head motion, the resulting shift in gaze causes displacement (slip) of the retinal image which may be perceived as apparent motion. The resulting symptoms reflect failure of compensation from either efference copy or afferent sensory signals which could detect the head and eye motion dissociation.

The postural imbalance can be attributed to an acute sensory deficiency of visual localization of objects in egocentric coordinates; this is calculated from both the position of targets on the retina and the awareness of the eye position in the head. Visually guided motor performance requires accurate information about gaze direction

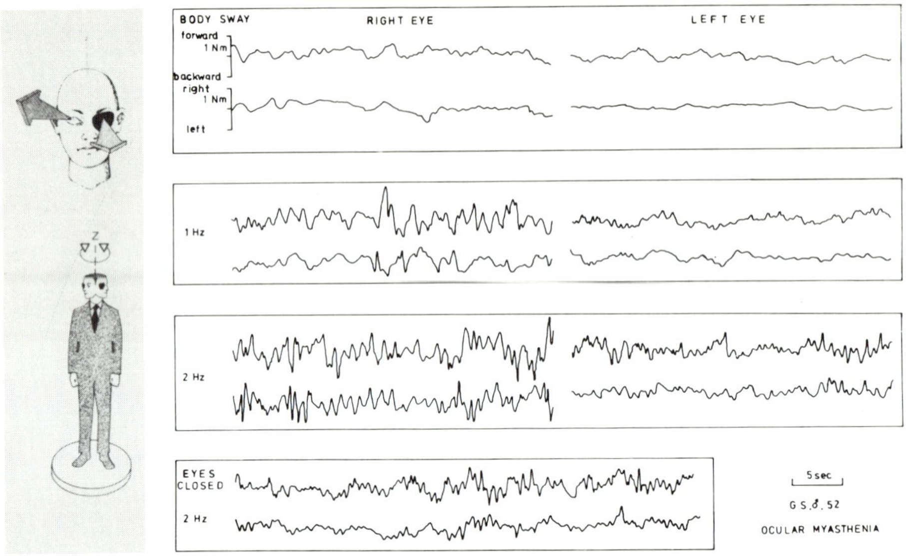

Fig. 1. Postural imbalance with acute extraocular muscle paresis of the right eye in a 52 year old man suffering from ocular myasthenia (upper left). The lateral deviation of the paretic right eye caused a dissociation of the subjective visual and somatosensory straight-ahead. Recordings of fore-aft and lateral body sway during free standing without voluntary movements (top) or with head oscillations in yaw ($\pm$ 20°; 1 or 2 Hz) revealed increased sway amplitudes with monocular vision of the affected right eye as compared to the normal left eye. With both eyes closed, the postural destabilization was less than with right eye fixation (Nm = Newton meters)

and body position relative to the surround. An extraocular muscle paresis causes a dissociation of subjective visual and somatosensory straight-ahead (Brandt and Büchele, 1979, Fig. 1) because the deviation from the "expected" eye position is not compensated by adequate afferent extraretinal information. The mismatch between expected and actual eye position is responsible for the direction-specific distorsion of locomotion and reaching movements. It can be interpreted as a visuo-spinal imbalance consequent to the disparate retinal slip as compared to the expected pattern calibrated prior to the disease onset. The disturbance of spatial localization, as well as the oscillopsia, are not restricted to the fovea but involve the entire visual field and therefore affect the two modes of visual processing, "focal" and "ambient", respectively. The ambient mode relies on afferent information from the peripheral field and subserves spatial orientation and postural balance (Dichgans and Brandt, 1978). Retinal image motion is a major cue for posture stabilization. Posturographic measurements of lateral and fore-aft body sway reveal increased sway amplitudes with monocular vision of the affected paretic eye as compared to the normal eye (Fig. 1). Postural imbalance is particularly

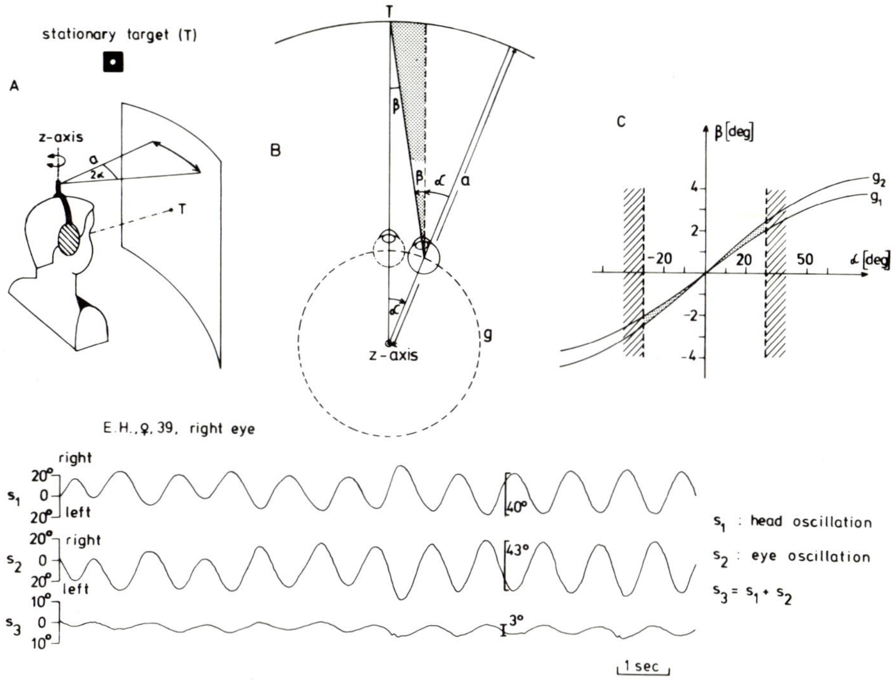

Fig. 2. Geometrical representation of the different angles of rotation (because of the two different axis) of eye and head required to maintain fixation on the target during head oscillation in yaw (top). For an accurate determination of eye-head coordination, it is necessary to calculate the additional rotation of the eye (ß), required by virtue of its displacement off the axis of rotation of the head. ß is a function of head oscillation amplitude and head circumference for a constant target distance. Original recordings of eye-head coordination during head oscillation obtained from a normal subject (bottom) exhibit this additional rotation ß (amplitude: 3°) in the bottom-line (adopted from Krafczyk in Wist, Brandt and Krafczyk, 1981).

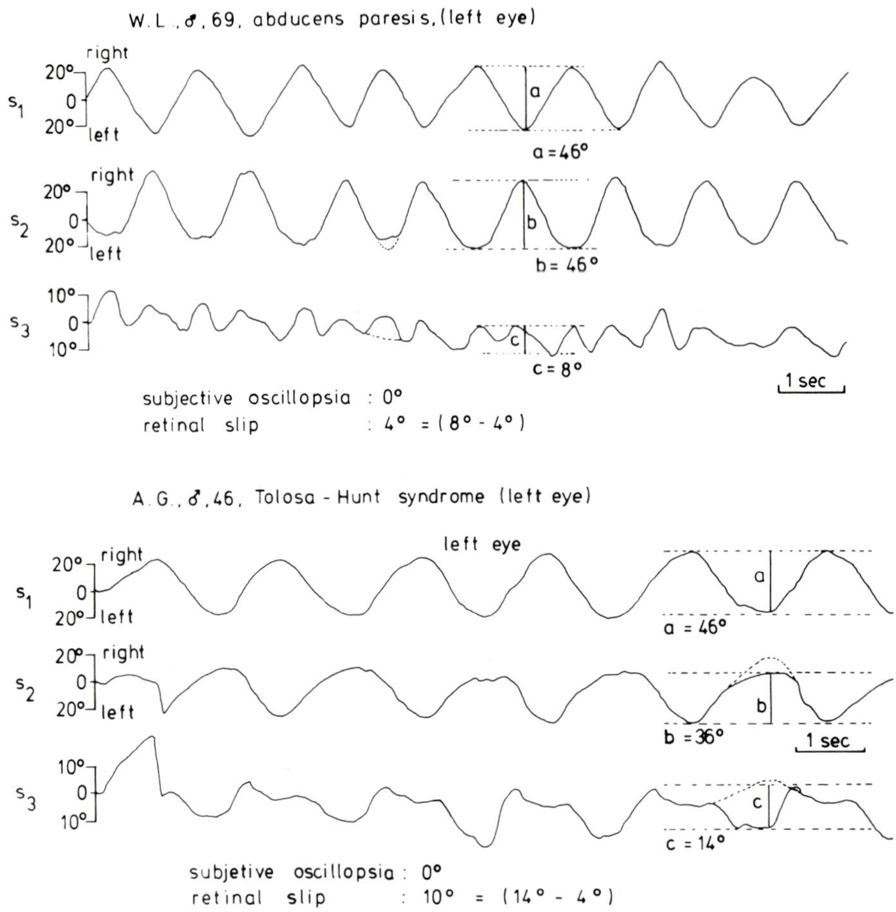

Fig. 3. Original recordings of eye-head coordination during head oscillation in yaw from a patient with a subacute abducens palsy (top) and from a patient with a subacute oculomotor palsy due to a Tolosa Hunt syndrome (bottom). The combined signals (S3) of the rotation of head (S1) and eye (S2) show oscillations with a net retinal slip of the target of four and ten degrees, respectively, but without the experience of concurrent subjective oscillopsia.

apparent when voluntary sinusoidal head movements are performed about the vertical Z-axis during free upright stance.

OSCILLOPSIA RELATED TO RETINAL SLIP DURING HEAD OSCILLATIONS

In patients with peripheral ocular motility disturbances, head exercises promote sensory rearrangement with subsequent diminution or disappearance of the previously described perceptual and postural symptoms and signs. This occurs despite persistance of the ocular paresis and reflects central nervous system plasticity which is consistant with the sensory and motor adaptation to prolonged optical reversal of vision by prisms (Kohler, 1956; Melvill Jones, 1977). Thus, the apparent motion of the visual field (oscillopsia) is not simply a direct result of the retinal image slip but must be related to an admixture of different mechanisms.

To compare quantitatively the relationship between oscillopsia and retinal slip, we recorded head and eye movements simultaneously during sinusoidal oscillations about the vertical Z-axis ($\pm$ 20°; 1 Hz) with subjects fixating on a stationary target (Fig. 2). In order for the VOR to be completely compensatory (maintaining a constant gaze direction in space), the eye must rotate with an angle exceeding that of the head since the eye and head have different axis (Fig. 2). The additional angle of eye motion (ß) depends on the circumference of the head (g) as well as the distance between the head and the fixated target (a). $\beta = \arccos \dfrac{2\pi a - g\cos\alpha}{\sqrt{(2\pi a)^2 + g^2 - 4\pi ag \times \cos\alpha}}$.

In patients with subacute peripheral extraocular muscle paresis, the psychophysically determined angle of subjective oscillopsia was considerably smaller or even absent (Fig. 3) when compared to the calculated net retinal slip (Wist, Brandt and Krafczyk, 1981). The patients were not able to detect the amount of actual displacement of the visual scene on the retina. Furthermore when tested with the head fixed, they exhibit an elevated threshold for detection of object motion with the paretic eye as compared to the normal eye.

OSCILLOPSIA AND POSTURAL IMBALANCE IN ACQUIRED OCULAR OSCILLATIONS

Involuntary ocular oscillations are not associated with an appropriate efference copy. In such situations there is oscillopsia and visually induced ataxia even without precipitating head movements which, as mentioned previously, is required to produce occillopsia in patients with paretic eye movement disturbances. The ocular oscillations associated with oscillopsia include acquired pendular nystagmus in demyelinating disease (Aschoff, Conrad and Kornhuber, 1974), intermittent monocular vertical or torsional eye movements in superior oblique myokymia (Hoyt and Keane, 197o) and downbeat nystagmus (Cogan, 1968; Zee, Friendlich and Robinson, 1974; Baloh and Spooner, 1981). Indeed, all acquired ocular oscillations in the primary position of gaze are associated with oscillopsia, at least in the acute phase prior to possible central compensation.

The illusory movement (oscillopsia) of a viewed stationary scene during ocular oscillations is perceptually different than that experience when the eyes are stable and the environment moves in a to-

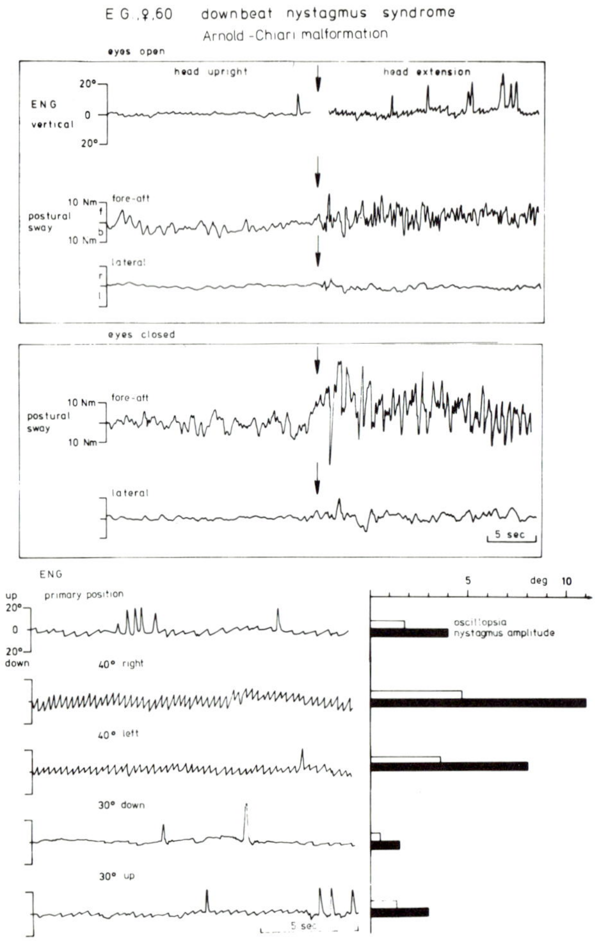

Fig. 4.

Simultaneous recordings in a patient with downbeat nystagmus of vertical ENG, and forward-backward and lateral body sway during standing with the head straight or maximally extended (top). The vestibulo-cerebellar lesion responsible for the nystagmus caused a pathological postural sway during head extension with the eyes closed; with the eyes open, visual control of balance was discernable but somewhat diminished by the concurrent activation of the downbeat nystagmus consequent to the head extension. Nystagmus amplitude was dependent on the direction of gaze as was the oscillopsia (bottom). The ratio, between the amplitude of subjective oscillopsia and net retinal slip in this patient was about 1:2.

and-fro direction since, with ocular oscillations, there is a visuo-proprioceptive mismatch. In downbeat nystagmus, oscillopsia usually is a permanent symptom but the amount of illusory motion is smaller than that which would be expected from the amplitude of the nystagmus (Fig. 4). The concurrent postural imbalance increases with the gaze dependent increased nystagmus amplitude. The postural imbalance in patients with downbeat nystagmus is secondary to both cerebellar and visual ataxia (Fig. 4)

RELATIONSHIP BETWEEN THE THRESHOLDS FOR OBJECT MOTION PERCEPTION AND CONCURRENT HEAD MOVEMENTS OR CIRCULARVECTION

The suppression of the detection of retinal image motion can, in part, be attributed to an inhibitory interaction between self- and object motion perception. We have shown that the thresholds for egocentric perception of object motion were significantly raised during concurrent head movements (sinusoidal head oscillations) about vertical Z-axis ($\pm 20^{\circ}$) by a factor of 2.9 at 1 Hz and 6.4 at 2 Hz oscillations

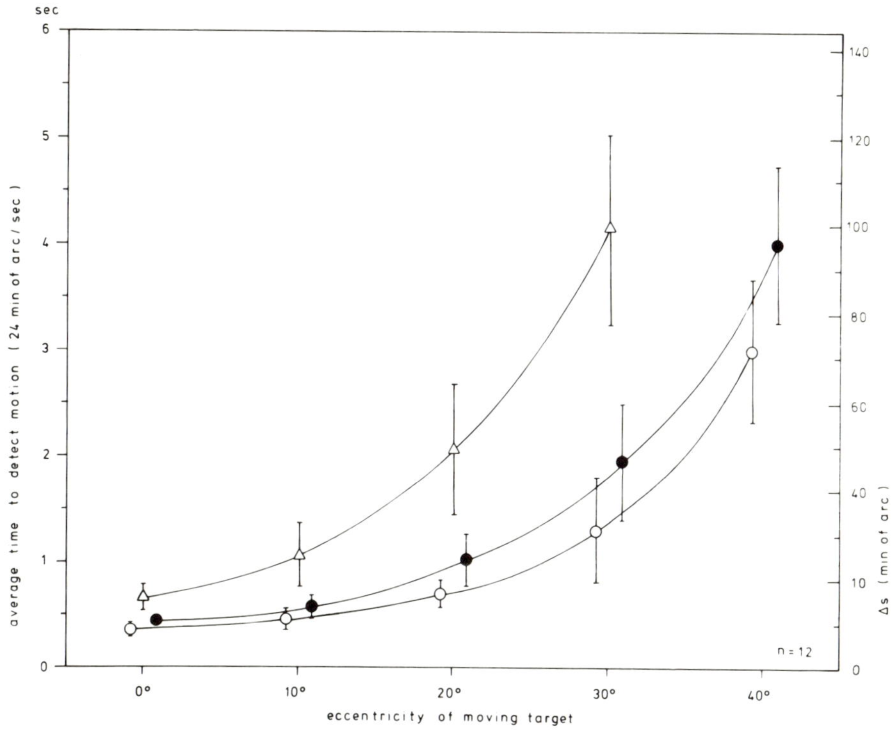

Fig. 5. Average time to detect motion, as a function of the eccentricity of the target on the retina, of a moving target (24 min of arc/sec) projected onto a screen with either the head fixed (lights on: O; darkness: ●) or with head oscillations in yaw (± 20°; 1 Hz) with lights on (Δ). Thresholds for egocentric detection of object motion are significantly raised by concurrent head motion.

(Büchele, Degner and Brandt, 198o; Degner and Brandt, 1981). This effect increases disproportionally with increasing eccentricity of the image of the moving stimulus on the retina (Fig. 5). With the head fixed, and the subjects experiencing horizontal optokinetically induced circularvection, the thresholds for perceiving vertical target motion were raised by a factor of 5.5; here the target motion was perpendicular to the direction of the horizontal pattern stimulus. However, with concurrent horizontal target motion during horizontal pattern motion , the thresholds were raised by a factor of 17.8. The increased thresholds during active head movements and during circularvection may reflect an inhibition of image motion perception related to the corollary discharge signal subserving the space constancy mechanism. This mechanism provides us with a stable world during self induced movements and locomotion. but has varying effects in vehicular transportation. For instance, during automobil driving, the latency required for active braking would be increased and thus the mechanism could be regarded as maladaptive. However, to the extend that this same mechanism alleviates the distressing oscillopsia and postural imbalance in ocular motor disorders is clearly beneficial to the organism.

VISUAL FACTORS AFFECTING SUPPRESSION OF THE VESTIBULO-OCULAR REFLEX

G. R. BARNES

RAF Institute of Aviation Medicine, Farnborough, Hampshire, UK

ABSTRACT

Experiments on human subjects exposed to angular oscillation whilst viewing a head-fixed display have indicated that the suppression of the vestibulo-ocular reflex is greatest when fixating a central target and decreases in a graded manner for targets placed more peripherally on the retina. During central fixation a low-velocity nystagmus is still evident and there is no indication of any complete cancellation of the vestibulo-ocular reflex.

KEYWORDS

Vestibulo-ocular reflex; visual suppression; fovea; peripheral retina.

INTRODUCTION

There has been considerable interest in recent years in the degree to which man is able to suppress reflex eye movements of vestibular origin. The mechanisms by which this suppression is carried out appear similar to those normally used during the visual control of eye movement (Barnes et al, 1978; Lau et al, 1978) and lesions which affect the pursuit reflex also generally affect both optokinetic nystagmus and suppression of the vestibulo-ocular reflex (Dichgans, 1979). However, one of the most important factors in achieving optimum suppression appears to be the acuity with which the display can be seen. This effect is typified in the clinical use of the de-focusing Frenzel glasses which have been shown by Baloh et al (1977) to allow a partial suppression of the response to caloric irrigation to be achieved. The relative effects of peripheral and foveal vision on eye movement control have been investigated for both the pursuit (Michalski et al, 1977), and optokinetic reflexes (Hood, 1967; Dichgans, 1977; Dubois & Collewijn, 1979), with the general conclusion that reduction of the peripheral field can lead to a substantial lowering of the peak velocity attainable. In the following experiment an attempt has been made to assess the relative contribution of foveal and peripheral mechanisms on suppression of the vestibulo-ocular reflex.

METHOD

The subject was seated on a turntable to which he was firmly harnessed with head clamped. He viewed a display, which was also rigidly coupled to the turntable, consisting of 9 red light-emitting diode (LED) target lights, placed on a periphery at 0°, $\pm2.5^o$, $\pm5^o$, $\pm10^o$ and $\pm20^o$ from the centre line in the horizontal plane. The diameter of each target light subtended an angle of 12 min arc at the eye and each had a luminance of 8 cd/m^2. The experiment was carried out in a completely darkened room so that the target lights appeared against a featureless black background. The subject was exposed to an oscillatory motion (peak velocity 60°/s) about the yaw axis of the body, stimulating the lateral semicircular canals. The stimulus was a sinusoidal waveform at six discrete frequencies: 0.25, 0.5, 0.75, 1.0, 1.5, and 2.0 Hz. Eye movements were recorded using an infra-red recording system which has been ruggedized for vibration environments.

Six subjects were each exposed to six experimental conditions at each of the stimulating frequencies in a balanced randomised order. In one condition the subject was presented with a single central target light and was instructed to maintain constant fixation on the target. In a second condition, eye movements were recorded whilst the subject was in complete darkness. In the remaining four conditions the subject was presented with a pair of target lights at one of four peripheral locations ($\pm2.5^o$, $\pm5^o$, $\pm10^o$, or $\pm20^o$) and was instructed to look fixedly at the black featureless space midway between the two peripheral target lights.

RESULTS

The recorded eye movements were analysed by computer (Barnes, 1981) and the ratio of slow-phase eye velocity to turntable velocity (gain) and the associated phase

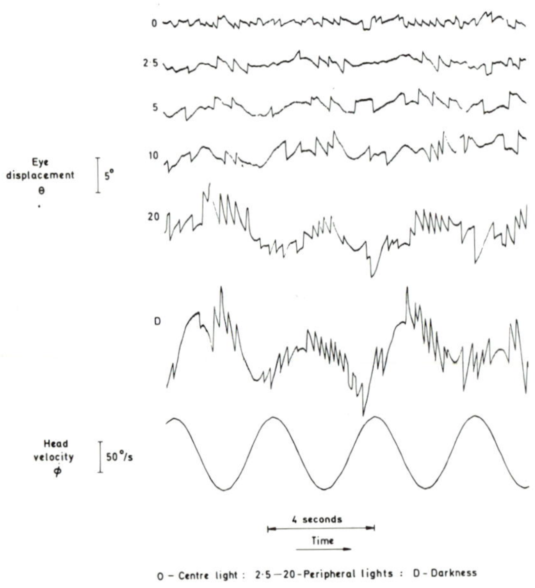

Fig 1. Eye movements evoked by sinusoidal head movements at 0.25 Hz when viewing a head-fixed display and in darkness.

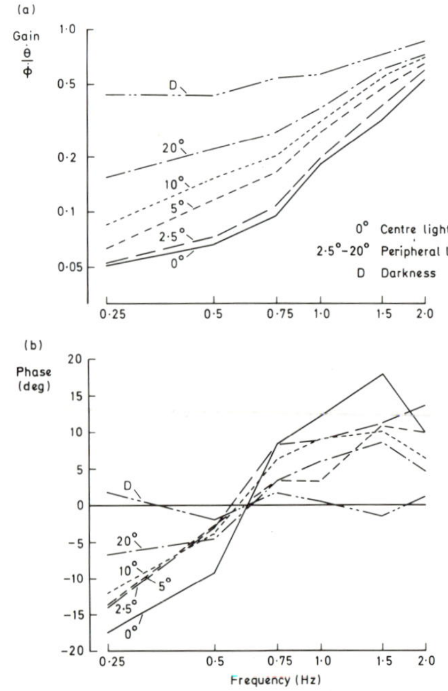

Fig 2. Gain (a) and phase (b) of the suppressed vestibulo-ocular reflex.

relationships were extracted using a least squares procedure. In Fig 1 sample raw eye displacement waveforms are shown for each of the visual target conditions from a typical subject at a frequency of 0.25 Hz. It is apparent from these records that the peripheral target lights did produce a marked suppression of the vestibularly induced eye movements observed in darkness, but that the suppression was not nearly as complete as that produced by fixation of the centre light. However, the feature of particular interest is that, even when the subject was fixating upon the central light, suppression was not complete; there was still a low-velocity nystagmus present. The overall eye movement, though, was small and was confined to the area of the fovea. There is thus no evidence of any cancellation of the vestibular response under these visual conditions. Rather, it seems that the presence of a fixation point leads to a restriction of the overall amplitude of nystagmus by reduction of saccade size and increase of saccadic frequency.

Analysis of the gain of the suppressed eye movements (Fig 2a) indicates that the degree of suppression which was achieved decreased as the target sources extended further into the periphery. However, the effect of peripheral location changed with the frequency of stimulation. At the lowest frequency, even the target sources at $\pm 20^{o}$ were able to exert a considerable degree of suppression (65% on average), whereas at the higher frequencies only the centrally located targets (0° and $\pm 2.5^{o}$) had any significant effect. In other words, the frequency response of the peripheral mechanisms exhibits a breakdown at a lower frequency than that of the parafoveal mechanisms. The responses to the central target and the $\pm 2.5^{o}$ targets were not significantly different, whereas the other visual conditions evoked responses which were highly significantly different ($P<0.001$) from each other. The changes in gain of the response were accompanied by changes of phase as indicated in Fig 2(b). At low frequencies, increasing levels of suppression were accompanied by increasing phase lag in the response, whereas at the higher frequencies a progressive phase lead was introduced.

DISCUSSION

The conditions of peripheral stimulation used in this experiment simulate the effects of a central scotoma, which Honrubia (1979) has shown leads to a deficit in pursuit and an impairment of optokinetic nystagmus. A particular feature of the impaired optokinetic response is that it exhibits a much slower build up (20-30 s) to terminal velocity compared with the normal, almost instantaneous, response. In the frequency domain this effect would be represented by a shift in the breakdown frequency of the response from a normally high frequency to a lower frequency for the scotomatous response. This is exactly the effect exhibited in Fig 2(a) by the breakdown of vestibular suppression as the peripheral location of the target is increased. It is evident that graded suppression can be achieved, but the exact manner by which this comes about is unclear at present. It is possible that the retinal location of the visual stimulus itself determines the gain of the feedback loop and thus the frequency response of visual-vestibular interaction. The relative movement of such a small, but high contrast edge across the retina clearly forms a sufficiently effective stimulus, whereas previous experiments have emphasised the effects of the area of the peripheral field upon the optokinetic response (Dichgans, 1977; Dubois & Collewijn, 1979). It remains to be seen how suppression is modified by the area of the peripheral field and what relation this bears to the effects of the peripheral location of the stimuli. The results have revealed no evidence of cancellation of the vestibular response during central fixation. Rather, it seems to be sufficient to keep the overall displacement within the fovea. At low frequencies the slow-phase velocity is sufficiently low (approximately 2-3 $^{o}/s$) that there is little blurring of the image (Barnes & Smith, 1981), so that there is no incentive to achieve complete suppression of the vestibulo-ocular response.

NORMAL MODES OF HEAD AND EYE CO-ORDINATION AND THE SYMPTOMATOLOGY OF THEIR DISORDERS

M. A. GRESTY and J. J. ELL

Medical Research Council Neuro-Otology Unit (formerly—MRC Hearing and Balance Unit), Institute of Neurology, National Hospital, Queen Square, London WC1N 3BG, UK

ABSTRACT

Normal patterns of head and eye co-ordination require complex inter-reactions between saccadic, pursuit and optokinetic systems and the vestibulo-ocular and otolith reflexes. Derangement of any one of these will lead to visual symptoms such as oscillopsia, transient blurring of vision on attempted refixation or whole body motion and diplopia, or to movement dependent symptoms ranging from vague sensations of imbalance and illusions of motion (subjective or objective) to motion sickness. In addition, certain head postures and movements may compensate for abnormalities of eye movement or macular fixation. These should be differentiated from involuntary head shaking or tremor occurring in conjunction with various disorders e.g. congenital nystagmus. The normal patterns of head and eye co-ordination during refixation, passive vibratory movements of the head and in moving vehicles are outlined. Clinically observed disorders of head/eye co-ordination are listed and discussed with respect to their symptomatology, aetiological mechanisms, investigation and analysis.

KEYWORDS

Vestibulo-ocular Reflex (VOR); Saccades; Smooth pursuit; Optokinetic Response (OKN); Oscillopsia; Head/Eye Synergy; Preservation of Visual Acuity; VOR Gain and Phase; Compensatory and Involuntary head movements; Visual/Vestibular mismatch

INTRODUCTION

The co-ordination of the position and movement of the head and eyes is one of the control mechanisms that maintain stability and orientation of the body in the physical environment. Head and eye co-ordination is of particular importance because in man the visual sense is predominant. Consequently, disordered co-ordination can cause disabling symptoms. Firstly, there may be a fall in visual acuity. Secondly, due to mismatch between visual and vestibular motion cues, a range of symptoms from vague unsteadiness to disorientation and frank motion sickness may ensue. These latter symptoms often result in secondary anxiety reactions. Co-ordinated movements of the head and eyes may be initiated under voluntary control (as in target refixation) or reflex (initiated in response to whole body activities such as running or riding in a vehicle). The primary functions of co-ordination are to transfer gaze to and maintain gaze upon visual targets and thereby to maintain visual acuity.

Head and Eye Posture

Head posture is determined by whole body attitude, the visual and acoustic environment and reactions to the vector sum of all forces (including gravity) which are acting on the vestibular apparatus. The primary posture of the head is in the upright position with respect to gravity and is determined largely by the otolith apparatus (Magnus 1924; Roberts 1967). In this position the eyes are orthophoric (or in vergence) with their principal axes intersecting at infinity or on a near target.

Voluntary Head and Eye Movements made for the purpose of refixation

The normal pattern of head and eye co-ordination during target acquisition in man has been described by Mowrer (1932), Bartz (1966), Crawford (1960), Gresty (1974), Barnes (1979), Uemura et al (1980) and Zangenmeister and Stark (1980). The essential components of the co-ordination sequence are as follows and in Fig. 1.

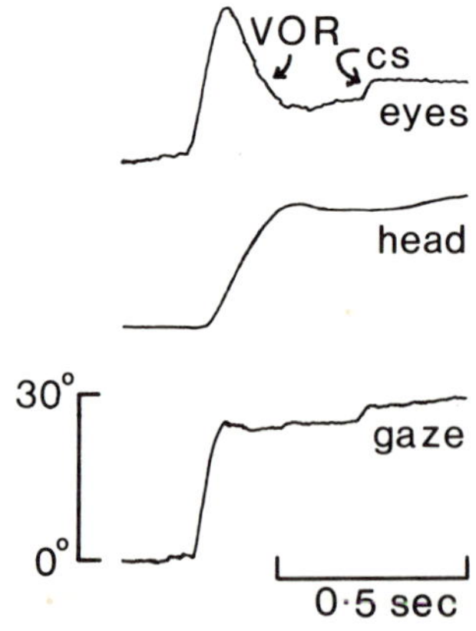

Fig. 1: Normal sequence of head and eye co-ordination during target acquisition.
EOG: Upper trace. CS = corrective saccade
Head position: Middle trace
Gaze (head and eye position): lower trace

Initially the eyes make a saccadic movement towards the target which, if made in isolation would bring the eyes to within about 10% of the target displacement. The head begins to rotate towards the target at about the same time as the initiation of the saccade but is much slower than the eyes. At the termination of the saccade the head is still turning. During this phase, due to the vestibulo-ocular reflex, the eyes move in an opposite direction to the head so compensating for its continued movement. Thus gaze is stabilized with respect to the visual environment and adequate visual acuity is preserved. In this phase corrective small saccadic movements achieve final, precise target localisation. In the case of an eccentric target, at the end of the acquisition sequence the head is turned towards the target by about 50 to 70% of the target displacement and the eyes move by the remaining amount. Disorders of this sequence which cause difficulties for patients arise either from an inability to generate voluntary saccades (as in oculomotor apraxia) or from a reduction in saccadic velocity or magnitude (as in progressive supranuclear palsy). Such patients find it difficult (and often frustrating) to attempt refixation. Minor derangement of this sequence is seen in disorders of the vestibulo-ocular reflex causing impairment of generation of adequate compensatory eye movements. In this instance patients experience transient oscillopsia during refixation because gaze is not stabilised.

Passive, vibratory movements of the head

Passive vibratory movements of the head caused by whole body activities such as running, jumping or riding in a vehicle are compensated for by the vestibulo-ocular reflex which produces eye movements which are equal in velocity to the head movements but opposite in direction so that the net result is that gaze is more or less held stable. The dynamics of the reflex have been described in man by Hixson (1974), Barnes (1980), Benson (1970), Barr et al,(1976), Wall et al,(1978), Takahashi et al,(1979). At low frequencies of movement the eyes lag with respect to the head and the gain is low. With increasing frequency the gain increases with concomitant phase advance until in the frequency band of natural head movements which is from about 0.2 Hz to 6 Hz (Benson and Gresty in Melville Jones, 1980) gain approaches unity with near perfect phase compensation.

Compensation for head movements with low frequency content is achieved by summation of vestibular with smooth pursuit and optokinetic mechanisms (Dichgans et al, 1973).

Disorders of the vestibulo-ocular reflex produce inappropriate gain and/or phase relationships between head and eye movements. These result in gaze instabilities which induce oscillopsia. Oscillopsia is only experienced with high frequency movements (Bender, 1965; Bender and Feldman, 1967; Atkin and Bender, 1968; Gresty et al, 1977). Compensation for inappropriate retinal slip at low frequencies is achieved by corrective saccades, smooth pursuit and optokinetic responses.

Head and Eye Co-ordination in moving vehicles

There are two situations in which pursuit and optokinetic mechanisms are in conflict with the vestibulo-ocular reflex. Firstly, in the pursuit of a moving target with active head turning and secondly when riding in a moving vehicle with visual fixation on a target within the vehicle, i.e. a target which is moving with the head. In these situations the vestibulo-ocular reflex tends to move the eyes away from the object of regard and thus has to be suppressed or cancelled to preserve visual fixation. It is commonly held that smooth pursuit has an important role in suppression of the vestibulo-ocular reflex. The dynamics of these situations have been described by Fleming et al, (1969), Barnes et al, (1978),

Sugie et al, (1970), Takahashi et al, (1981), Geudry, (1979), Gresty and Leech, (1977), Benson and Barnes, (1978).

Patients who have failure of vestibulo-ocular reflex suppression also have pursuit deficits (Halmagyi and Gresty, 1979; Dichgans et al, 1978). During target tracking they are unaware of a deficit presumably because the eye position with respect to the target is continually revised with corrective saccades. However, when riding in a moving vehicle which is vibrating they may experience a fall in visual acuity and oscillopsia when fixating objects such as a map or speedometer within the vehicle. These conditions can rapidly induce motion sickness (Reason and Brand, 1975).

DISEASES AFFECTING HEAD AND EYE CO-ORDINATION

Disordered Visual Input

Disorders of visual input predominately affect voluntary refixation movements and postural attitudes adopted during target fixation.

a) Impairment of vision produced by visual field defects:

The search strategies adopted by patients with acquired or congenital visual field defects, generally in the form of hemianopia, have been described by Meienberg et al, (1980) and Zangenmeister et al, in these proceedings. However, there are certain features of the movements which are worthy of further comment. We have examined head and eye movements during refixation in several patients with recently acquired hemianopia. Their strategies are all similar as exemplified in Fig. 2. When looking for a target whose approximate position in the blind field is known, these patients make a series of hypometric saccadic approximations to the target position. This strategy is not, however, the most efficient. If a single hypermetric saccade were generated then the target would be placed in the intact visual field and would be attained by one further saccade made under visual guidance.

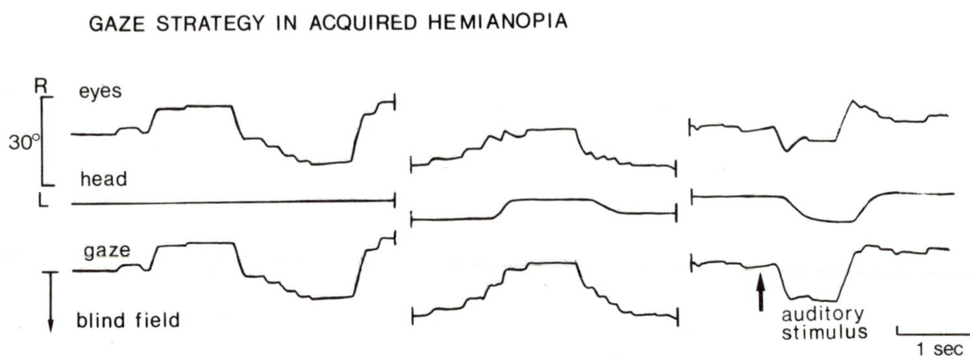

Fig. 2: Gaze strategies during target refixation in acquired hemianopia. The targets were presented in the blind field. Centering movements are random. Saccadic eye movements with and without accompanying head movements are similar. Head and eye co-ordination to a target presented with an acoustic position cue are indistinguishable from normal (EOG recording technique).

In everyday life, patients with acquired hemianopia behave similarly to normals insofar as they are able to extract reliable positional information from acoustic cues which can be used for the scaling of saccadic eye movements. In their absence, and once aware of field defects, some patients learn to execute hypermetric saccades into the hemianopic field.

b) Head and eye posture during target fixation in aphakism:

We have examined two brothers with the oculo-renal syndrome of Lowe. One of the characteristics of this syndrome is the early appearance of dense lenticular opacities which preclude the development of central fixation. Another feature is a nystagmus of early onset which is congenital in form being of the "jerk" variety in lateral gaze and pendular when the eyes are more central in the orbit. It is of note that central nervous white matter degeneration also occurs in this syndrome which may be relevant to the aetiology of the nystagmus.

Both brothers underwent early cataract extraction. The older brother has sufficient preservation of visual acuity to be able to read normal print at a normal distance without the aid of spectacles. When asked to look straight ahead at a target he adopts a characteristic posture. The head is turned to the right with the eyes in levoversion. Examination of what would be the visual axes in a normal person reveals that the image is not falling on the fovea. The patient appears to look down from and to the left of the target. In this position his nystagmus is of smallest amplitude.

This unusual strategy is likely to be the result of a combination of afoveate vision and use of the eye position with the smallest amplitude of nystagmus. To put things simply, when the patient seems to be looking away from you he is actually looking at you.

Disorders of Saccadic Eye Movements

Normal patterns of head and eye co-ordination may be altered when saccadic eye movements are absent or delayed in initiation, excessively slow or dysmetric. Dysmetria of saccadic eye movements, occurring typically in cerebellar disease, has been described by Zee et al, (1976) and Shimizu et al, (1981). Although dysmetria of saccades results in a gaze pattern (sum of head in space and eye in head) which is itself dysmetric, the disorder is not really one of co-ordination because the gaze movement is similar whether the head moves or not. Disorders of saccadic movements in which the mechanism of the co-ordination of head and eyes is intimately affected are typically the apraxias and progressive supranuclear palsy.

a) Acquired and congenital oculomotor apraxia:

The pattern of head and eye movements in congenital oculomotor apraxia has been described by Zee et al, (1976b). Of most interest to the present discussion is their observation that some children who were only capable of generating small saccades with the head fixed, could make much larger saccades when the head was free to move. This phenomenon we term a synergistic relationship between head and eye movement. It is not confined to congenital oculomotor apraxia. A similar phenomenon may be observed in progressive supranuclear palsy.

In an examination of six patients with the Steele-Richardson-Olszewski syndrome, three showed occasional synergy and one had a consistent augmentation of saccades with head movement. Her recordings are presented in Fig. 3. When the head was fixed she produced a series of five or six hypometric saccades in order to fixate eccentric targets. This is the familiar "staircase" type of eye movement which is so characteristic of the disease (David et al, 1968). In contrast, when her head was free to move, even though the movement could be small, her saccadic amplitudes increased to near normal. Finger pointing at the target did not augment saccadic amplitudes which is a demonstration that the effect is specific to head movement.

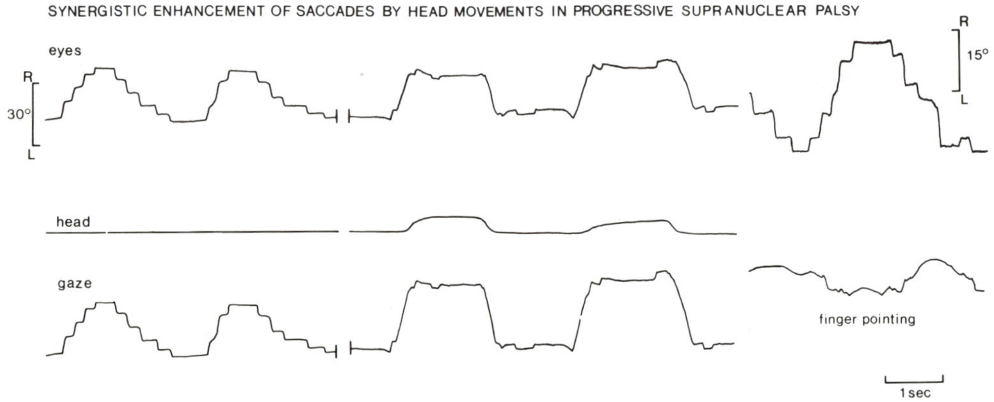

Fig. 3: Patterns of head and eye co-ordination in a patient with progressive supranuclear palsy.
Head fixed - left hand traces
Head free to move - centre traces
Finger pointing at the same targets - right hand traces
(nb change of scaling)

In several patients with cerebro-vascular disease we have observed a "saccadic release phenomenon". Recordings from a patient demonstrating this are presented in Fig. 4. Typically the patient is incapable of producing saccadic fixation movements to verbal command in the normal clinical testing situation in which the head is restrained. By contrast when the head is free to move a normal pattern of saccadic refixation movements is "released". This phenomenon is obviously complex, for patients with cerebro-vascular disease may suffer from many forms of sensory, ideational, motor and attentional deficits and it is not clear which of these faculties may be affected by the head turning.

An interesting variation upon this form of acquired oculo-motor apraxia is exhibited by patients who cannot turn head or eyes to refixate under voluntary command. Some of these patients can be instructed to point their head at a target upon which they execute a normal sequence of co-ordination.

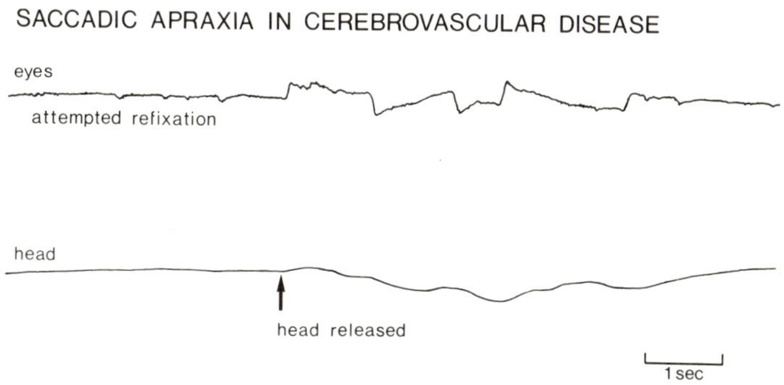

Fig. 4: Recordings of head and eye movements in a patient with cerebro-vascular disease. When asked to refixate with head fixed he was incapable of making saccades. With head released he made normal patterns of co-ordination with normal saccadic movements.
EOG: Upper traces
Head position: Lower traces
Head fixed to left of trace then free

b) Slow saccades:

Some patients with multiple sclerosis or system degenerations such as the Steele-Richardson-Olszewski syndrome have saccadic eye movements which are of very low velocity and also sometimes of small amplitude. When this is the case voluntary head and eye refixation movements give an appearance of the eyes remaining motionless in the orbit as the head turns. The patient also seems to have difficulty in making the refixation. He may turn his head around completely to look at the target whereas normally he would make up the displacement by proportional movements of the head and eyes. Recordings of these types of movement reveal that the patient is generating a saccadic movement which is of longer duration than a normal saccade. The saccade overlaps in time with the compensatory eye movements which are provoked by the head turning. Since the saccade and the compensatory movements are in opposite directions and because the velocity of the slowed saccade is comparable to that of the compensatory movement, the two tend to cancel each other out so that the eyes remain relatively motionless in the orbit. This sequence can give rise to a false impression that there is total absence of saccadic and slow phase eye movement.

Disorders of Vestibulo-ocular Reflex Eye Movements

Abnormalities of the vestibulo-ocular reflex may arise from peripheral or central lesions. Generally speaking, disordered vestibular function may be hypo or hyper-active. In both cases the result is that gaze is not stabilised with respect to the visual environment during active or passive head movements. This produces unacceptably high retinal slip velocities with a consequent blurring of vision or oscillopsia. The disorders may be symmetrical or lateralised to one labyrinth. An imbalance of vestibular function which remains uncompensated produces a vestibular nystagmus which can blurr vision if it is of the second or third degree.

The appropriate way to characterise vestibulo-ocular reflexes is by measurement of the gain and phase relationships between the head and eye movements at a range of frequencies of oscillation of the skull. This procedure enables one to plot the "transfer function" of the reflex. The transfer function following bilateral loss of labyrinthine function in patients with peripheral lesions has been described by Atkin and Bender (1968), Zee and Gresty (1977). There is typically a loss of gain and phase of the reflex with increasing velocities and frequencies of head movement. Abnormalities of the transfer function in central disorders have been described by Baloh et al, (1975), Zee et al, (1977) and Gresty et al, (1977) for "cerebellar disease" and by Gresty et al, (1977) for ponto-medullary lesions. In cerebellar disease there is typically an increase in gain of the reflex at high frequencies of oscillation which may be accompanied by phase lag. The elevated gain of the reflex corresponds to the exaggerated caloric responses seen in cerebellar disease. Disorders of the vestibulo-ocular reflex in lesions which are predominately ponto-medullary generally result in loss of gain and/or phase of the reflex. Certainly, in the case of ponto-medullary lesions the disorders may be asymmetrical. The characteristic features of disorders of vestibulo-ocular reflex function may readily be detected on clinical testing or eye movement recording (Fig. 5). Changes in gain may be detected in the light, with the dolls' head manoeuvre. Saccadic corrections (sometimes with the appearance of nystagmus) made in the opposite direction to the slow phase eye movement indicate elevated gain and saccades in the same direction indicate a reduction in gain. The detection of (left hand traces) phase changes is more difficult and requires recording of head and eye movements during sinusoidal oscillation of the skull.

Whilst disorders of the vestibulo-ocular reflex produce visual symptoms during high frequency head movements, it is possible that derangements of the low frequency performance of the reflex may cause sensations of "unsteadiness", "dizziness", disorientation and motion sickness. With the exception of simple right versus left imbalance of vestibular function these possibilities have not been explored.

a) Computerised measurement of the vestibulo-ocular reflex transfer function:

Observation of voluntary or manual oscillations of the head at various frequencies at the bedside can reveal much about vestibular function (Gresty et al, 1977). In addition, computerised measurement and analysis of the vestibulo-ocular reflex can be used to characterise symmetrical disorders of vestibular dysfunction. The method in our laboratory uses a 100 ft/lb torque motor to drive a Barany chair in yaw. The head is restrained with a chin rest and modified ear guards which clamp the skull. The stimulus profile consists of random amplitude velocity steps with a peak velocity limit of 30°/sec and a duty cycle of 2 Hz with a flat response to 1.5 Hz (Fig. 6, Auto-spec H). Eye movements are recorded in the dark using EOG. Saccades are detected using an on-line (dT = throughput delay) digital program similar to that described by Wall et al, (1978). The

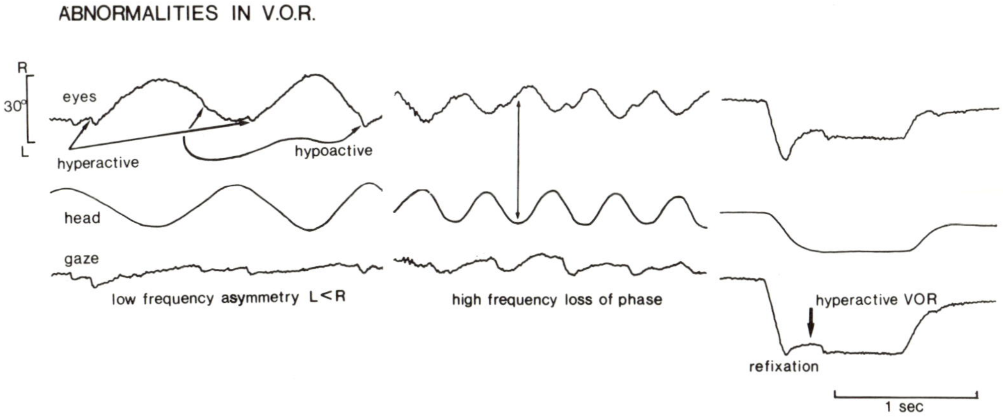

Fig. 5: Recordings of head and eye movements during active and passive head turning in a patient with multiple sclerosis.
With head movements to the left there is a hyperactivity of vestibulo-ocular reflexes and with movement to the right a hypoactivity (left hand traces). At high frequencies of oscillation there is a phase lag of about 60° (centre traces). Voluntary head turning in the direction which stimulates the hyperactive reflex produces a gaze displacement trajectory in which the eyes slip backwards off the target which is attained by the initial saccade; in the opposite direction the hypoactive reflex results in a hypometria of gaze (right hand traces).

saccades are detected using a velocity criterion and removed from the slow phase velocity to interpolate during the saccade to the next slow phase. The parameters are optimised for each subject, eye movement signal is then digitally filtered to exclude frequencies above 6 Hz (166 msec filter window). The transfer function of eye displacement/head velocity (E/H) is computed using a Hewlett Packard 5420A. The program employs a 1024 point transform on 42 second samples of data with averaging on successive overlapping samples. Typically between 1.5 and 3 minutes of recording are processed depending upon the patients' comfort and maintenance of arousal. Throughout the analysis the monitors the coherence function between E and H. With normal subjects data at frequencies associated with a coherence of less than 0.9 are rejected. The transfer function of eye velocity/head velocity (E/H) is computed using the jw operator.

The results for the mean of 11 normal subjects are presented in Fig. 6 (continuous lines). Gain and phase estimates above a frequency of 1.5 Hz are unreliable probably because of a tendency for the head to slip in the restraint above this frequency (see fall in coherence). The E/H gain plot is close to 0.6 for frequencies up to 0.6 Hz and thereafter climbs towards unity. Corresponding phase estimates are close to 0° (eye and head movement taken in the same direction). This data is similar to and in agreement with other reports on the use of passive stimuli. Although omitted in Fig. 6, the variance associated with the data is considerable, however, it is comparable with the estimates of other authors (particularly Wall et al, 1978). It is likely that the

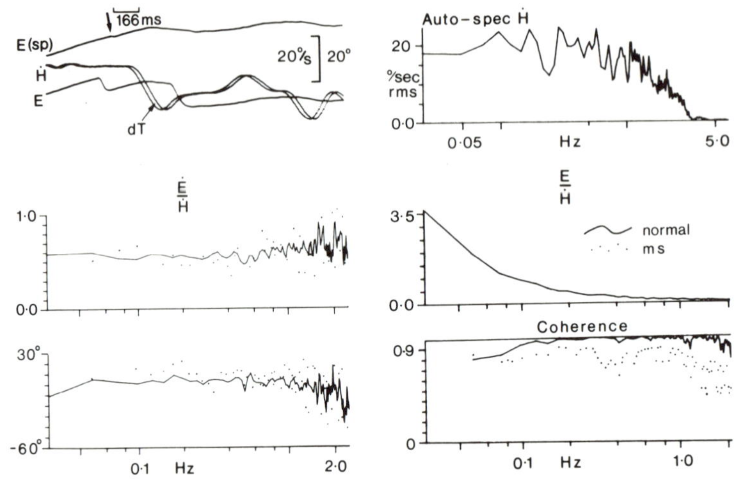

Fig. 6: Automated transfer function analysis of the vestibulo-ocular reflex (11 normal subjects).
Top left - raw data records showing stimulus velocity wave form (H) and eye displacement traces with (Esp) and without (E) the slow phase removed. Arrow indicates artefact remaining from detection of small saccades. This artefact would be lost in the digital filter window (166 msec). Auto-spectrum H shows the typical r.m.s. magnitude content of 1 minute of stimulus. E/H, displacement/velocity gain. E/H, velocity/velocity gain and phase. Coherence, typical for a single normal subject, averaged over 50, 41 sec overlapping samples. Dotted data points obtained from a 34 year old female patient with multiple sclerosis, averaged over 50 samples.

wide variability of normal subjects prevents the use of gain/phase comparisons to reveal subtle disorders of the vestibulo-ocular reflex. This point is of importance because, of course, much more simple (and inexpensive) tests can be used to reveal gross dysfunction. In this respect it is noteworthy that clinical applications of measurement of the vestibulo-ocular reflex transfer function are notably absent from the recent literature.

Our particular interest is in disorders of the central nervous system (particularly degenerative) which are associated with vertigo, unsteadiness and oscillopsia and the effect of drugs thereon. In this context there is promise for the use of the coherence function as an index of abnormality. This point may be illustrated in the case of a 34 year old female patient with multiple sclerosis whose main complaints were (vestibular) oscillopsia when walking or riding in a vehicle, a constant feeling of unsteadiness and gait ataxia. The gain and phase data for this patient are presented in Fig. 6 as dotted data points. Although gain and phase estimates fluctuate perhaps more widely than those of the average normal subject, the whole profile of her transfer function does lie within normal limits. By contrast the coherence associated with her data is consistently at or below a level of 0.8 up to a frequency of about 0.8 Hz and at higher frequencies (at which she experienced oscillopsia) drops to 0.4. The continuous line coherence function is typical for a normal subject. It is evident that there is complete separation between this and the coherence for the patient with multiple sclerosis at all frequency estimates. The coherence function is a measure of signal to noise ratio and so, in the context of multiple sclerosis, can be taken to indicate the reliability of signal processing through the vestibulo-ocular reflex at various frequencies of stimulation. This kind of abnormality is compatible with the disturbances of nerve conduction known to occur in primary demyelination.

Obviously this type of vestibular test requires rigorous standardisation and here we have only indicated possibilities for its application. Perhaps in the near future we can look forward to some agreement between groups on testing criteria and data processing.

b) Loss of vestibulo-ocular reflex suppression:

The clinical implications of loss of vestibulo-ocular reflex suppression during head turning have been described by Dichgans et al, (1978) and Halmagyi and Gresty (1979). This sign is always indicative of a central lesion and is part of the triad of broken pursuit plus failure of suppression with or without spontaneous nystagmus. Failure of suppression may only cause symptoms when the patient is riding in a vehicle and has to fixate on, say, the instrument panel or a map. Under these circumstances he may suffer a considerable loss of visual acuity and also motion sickness. There is probably no need for a specific test of suppression as all patients with failure of suppression also have broken pursuit which is much easier to examine. We have found the test to be of most value when presented with a nystagmus which is suspected to be of congenital origin. Patients with congenital nystagmus cannot suppress their vestibulo-ocular reflex and during attempted suppression the optokinetic stimulus of the background movement "releases" the nystagmus which the patient has in lateral gaze (Halmagyi and Gresty, 1981). As a consequence, during attempted suppression, a marked nystagmus appears which is disproportionate to the nystagmus or derangement of pursuit movements which the patient has in the region of primary gaze. The phenomenon of reversed optokinetic nystagmus also explains why patients with congenital nystagmus have blurred vision, sometimes with motion sickness when riding in and looking sideways out of a car.

c) Failure of adaptation to imbalance of vestibular tone:

There are two forms of vestibular adaptation. The first is the familiar adaptation to asymmetrical derangement of peripheral vestibular function which takes several days to accomplish. In addition, very recently, Steinman and Collewijn (1980) and Collewijn et al, (1980) have demonstrated that there is a very rapid adaptive process, taking only seconds to accomplish, which corrects for perspective distortions caused by corrective lenses. Failure of adaptation occurs characteristically in brain stem vascular disease (e.g. vertebro-basilar insufficiency and migraine). It is manifest symptomatically as motion sickness, feelings of unsteadiness or inability to adapt to the geometric distortions of the visual environment caused by wearing high dioptre spectacle lenses. Such perspective distortions are particularly evident during head movement. When failure of adaptation occurs there has usually been a disruption of vestibulo-cerebellar pathways (Rudge, 1981, personal communication). In the case of brain stem vascular disease, after the initial ictus the patient will complain (often for many months) of a continual sensation of "vertigo" which seems very difficult to categorise and is often interpreted as being functional in origin. A typical example of intolerance of high dioptre corrective lenses is that of the elderly patient with coexistant vertebro-basilar ischaemia who paradoxically seems unable to adjust to wearing spectacles following an apparently successful bilateral cataract extraction (Strachan, 1981).

d) Head and eye posture - otolith reflexes:

Disorders which affect the co-ordinated posture of the head and eyes arise through damage to the peripheral (Horsley, 1909; Halmagyi et al, 1978) or central (Brain, 1926) otolith pathways and result in head tilt with skew deviation and torsional rotation of the eyes; this is a pathological manifestation of the "ocular tilt reaction". In the case of peripheral lesions the tilt and rotation are towards the affected side whereas in central lesions the effects may be mixed. The ocular displacements prevent intersection of the visual axes and consequently the patient experiences diplopia with tilting and version of the images.

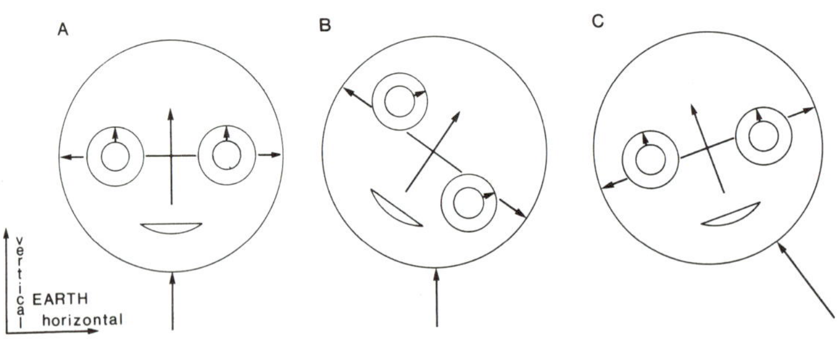

Fig. 7: The "ocular tilt reaction".
A - normal orientation with respect to gravity.
B - rotation of the head and eyes and skew deviation of the eyes resulting from a left sided otolith lesion.
C - normal tilt reaction to displacement of the vertical axis from upright.

Involuntary and Compensatory Movements of the Head and Eyes

a) Head nodding associated with nystagmus of early onset - "Congenital Nystagmus"

We recognise three distinct patterns of head and eye co-ordination in patients with congenital nystagmus. These have recently been reviewed by Gresty and Halmagyi (1981). The most common head movement encountered is a tremor. This is associated with the typical forms of congenital nystagmus which tend to be pendular in primary gaze and "jerk" on lateral gaze. The head movement is involuntary, at a similar frequency to the pendular nystagmus, in no way alters visual acuity when it occurs and can persist throughout adult life. A second form of "congenital nystagmus" (with the unfortunate name "Spasmus Nutans") manifests as a high frequency (10 - 12 Hz) oscillatory movement of the eyes. This nystagmus ceases, as if switched off, when the head is shaken from side to side. In its place can be seen normal compensatory eye movements. According to the early descriptions of Spasmus Nutans, the condition should remit. In the three patients we have examined who were exemplary of the disorder, two were undergoing considerable improvement. However, we have never observed full remission. A final form of nodding associated with congenital nystagmus is "compensatory head shaking". An example of a child showing this phenomenon is given in Fig. 8. His nystagmus is typically of jerk form with some pendular components and is of an unusually large amplitude. When his head is passively turned from side to side the nystagmus diminishes in amplitude and eye movements which are compensatory to the head movement appear. When visually fixating on objects of particular interest, as during reading, the child shakes his head from side to side. As he does so the nystagmus again diminishes and poorly formed compensatory movements appear. During the head shaking the child's visual acuity improved markedly. He was himself aware that he made the head movements deliberately in order to see better.

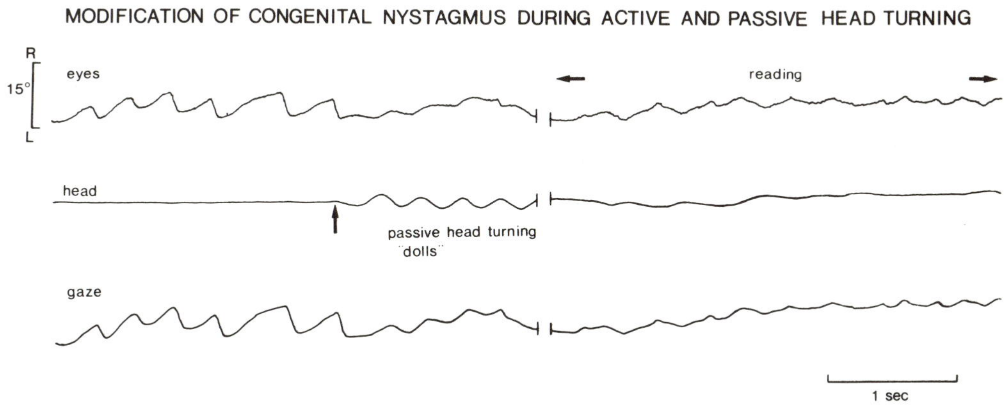

Fig. 8: Compensatory head shaking in a ten year old boy with congenital nystagmus.
Left hand trace: head still
Centre trace: passive head turning
Right hand trace: reading

There are obvious similarities between the compensatory head shakers and the children with Spasmus Nutans in that both produce head manoeuvres which reduce the nystagmus amplitude. An additional feature of the compensatory shaking is that during the movement the vestibulo-ocular reflex is also reduced in amplitude. If this were not so then the VOR would cancel the effect of head movement, leaving the nystagmus to determine the direction of gaze. Common to compensatory shaking and Spasmus Nutans is that both involve suppression of involuntary eye movements, a pathological nystagmus and the vestibulo-ocular reflex, accordingly they may both demonstrate examples of a similar physiological principle.

b) Pendular nystagmus and head tremor - "Oculo-palatal myoclonus":

We have recently reviewed 16 of our own patients and 32 more reported in the literature, with acquired pendular nystagmus, several of whom had associated somatic tremor including tremor of the head (Gresty et al, 1981). The nystagmus is typically a pendular oscillation of the eyes at a frequency of 3 to 4 Hz and may be monocular. Somatic tremor was at similar frequencies, within about 0.2 Hz. Although lesions of the cerebellar and inferior olivary nuclei are implicated in oculo-palatal myoclonus (Van Bogaert and Bertrand, 1928; Guillain et al, 1933) this cannot be the case for the eye movements. The existence of a monocular pendular nystagmus suggests that the mechanism responsible must lie close to the oculomotor nuclei. However, the similarity in frequency between the ocular and somatic tremors does suggest that the type of mechanism involved, whether this be a particular type of instability of the neuronal membrane or whatever, could be similar.

Miscellaneous disorders affecting Head and Eye Co-ordination:

a) Moebius' Syndrome:

We have examined head movements in a 23 year old male - a keen football player and boxer! with Moebius' Syndrome who had total absence of ocular movement accompanied by complete facial immobility. He experienced no oscillopsia during active and passive head movements in everyday life and had normal visual acuity. Recordings of his head movements made during target refixation revealed that they were much faster than normal, attaining peak velocities in the region of 400°/sec and hence comparable with saccadic velocities. During the head movements he denied oscillopsia. When moving his head slowly from side to side he admitted that the world looked blurred. The patient's hearing was normal and his rapid responses to alterations of posture indicated probable retention of vestibular function which is arguably why he was able to adapt to ocular immobility so well. By contrast we found that a 5 year old boy who had a more extensive form of the syndrome which included total deafness, absence of external auditory meati and pinnae, and absence of vestibular startle reflexes, was very "clumsy".

It is interesting that head movements in the older patient had become very much like eye movements: it is as if the head were being used like one cyclopean eye.

b) Dystonic postures:

Abnormal neck positions such as those occurring in torsion dystonia and spasmodic torticollis are accompanied by compensatory eye movement. As a corollary, eccentric eye positions encountered in Duane's and certain pontine syndromes are accompanied by compensatory head turning. Under both these circumstances the patients experience awkwardness in refixation manoeuvres and have a restricted range of peripheral vision.

In an ongoing survey of patients with spasmodic torticollis, the purpose of which is to screen for neuro-otological and neuro-ophthalmological abnormalities, we have found that whereas there is no evidence of abnormality in cases of isolated torticollis, patients with torticollis occurring as part of a more generalised neurological illness have deranged vestibular function. Specifically their responses to rotational stopping stimuli are reduced significantly in both amplitude and duration (to within one third of normal as measured by duration of nystagmus) and in addition are sometimes asymmetrical. These patients do not experience oscillopsia with normal head movements and so the derangement is confined to the low frequency performance of the vestibulo-ocular reflex. The asymmetries are not related to the direction of head turn and thus are unlikely to be in any sense "compensatory", whatever this term might mean in this disease.

Although one could argue that these observed abnormalities of vestibular function may be adaptive in nature we suspect that they are an intrinsic part of the illness.

CONCLUSIONS

From the point of view of the clinician a realisation that subtle derangement of head and eye co-ordination can give rise to symptoms is important because these are often obscure in nature and difficult for the patients to explain. The conventional methods of neurological examination are unlikely to reveal these disorders and one must employ specific co-ordination tests to demonstrate abnormalities.

NORMAL AND ABNORMAL GAZE TYPES AND ACTIVE HEAD MOVEMENTS

W. H. ZANGEMEISTER* and L. STARK**

*Department of Neurology, University of Hamburg, Federal Republic of Germany
**Department of Physiological Optics, University of California, Berkeley, USA

ABSTRACT

Eye-head coordinated gaze types that occur with active head movements in response to variable experimental conditions are described and analyzed in normals and neurological patients. Parameterization of dynamics (main sequence) and latencies (gaze plane) demonstrates differences of eye and head movements that are confirmed by modeling studies.

KEYWORDS

Active head movement dynamics; optimal control; main sequence; eye-head coordination; vestibulo-ocular reflex; neck muscle electromyography; eye-head latency; head movement model; neurological disorders; gaze plane analysis.

INTRODUCTION

Coordinated gaze movement normally has an initial eye-in-orbit saccade onto the target followed by a synkinetic much slower head movement. The vestibular ocular reflex (VOR) generated by head acceleration drives the compensatory eye movement (CEM), eye-in-orbit, in the opposite direction so that gaze, eye-in-space, remains on target. The CEM and its VOR component is influenced by visual input and other factors that modify gain (Sugie and Wakakuwa, 1970; Meienberg and others, 1981; Ito and others, 1974b; Zangemeister and Stark, 1980); resultant overshoots or undershoots are corrected by later saccades. These features have been defined in monkeys (Bizzi and others, 1971; Dichgans and others, 1974; Henn and Cohen, 1973; Morasso and others, 1973) and man (Atkin and Bender, 1968; Barnes, 1979; Bartz, 1965; Fleming and others, 1969; Gresty, 1974; Stark and others, 1962; Sugie and Wakakuwa, 1970; Zangemeister and others, 1981a; Zangemeister and others, 1981c), and some clinical studies have begun exploration of pathological changes (Kasai and Zee, 1978; Meienberg and others, 1981). Beside this classical coordinated gaze movement (type I) other gaze patterns exist, generally determined by asynchronicity of the neural controller signals as reflected in the experimentally recorded EMGs.

LATENCY OF EYE AND HEAD MOVEMENT IN COORDINATED GAZE

The classical coordinated gaze movement may be described as a saccadic eye movement followed by a head movement. Synchronously with the head movement the compensatory eye movement returns the eye to its primary position in the orbit as an exchange of head movement for eye movement. In this way coordinated gaze obtains a first advantage of the fast eye saccade to rapidly place gaze onto a target in space. It obtains a second advantage of having the eye in primary position at end of the movement for equal ease of next moving in either direction. Although this classical description of a coordinated gaze movement has head movement occuring with a longer latency than eye movement, it must be realized, that the head being a larger mechanical object than the eyeball requires an increased dynamical lag period in order to move.

Thus we could expect that the neck EMG might begin synchronously with eye movement EMG. Indeed neck EMG occured synchronously with eye movement (Fig. 1), since the eye movement is almost synchronous with its own EMG (about 8 to 12 msec) (Bizzi and others, 1971; Henn and Cohen, 1973; Zangemeister and others, 1981b); this synchronicity suggests the clarification obtained by measuring latency with respect to the control signal and not to the behavioral movement which has its own dynamical lags.

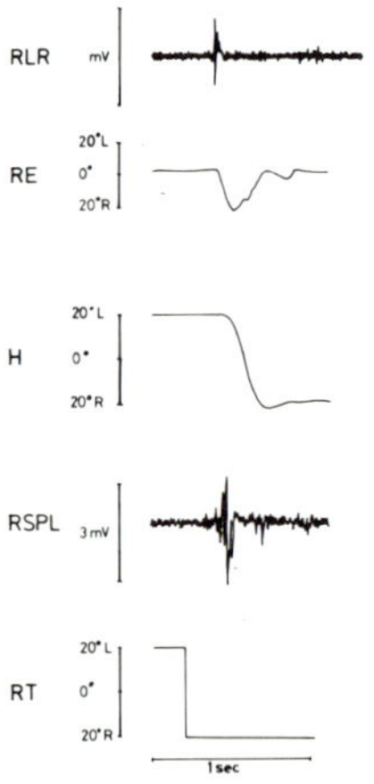

Fig. 1. Response to a 40 degree target shift from left (L) to right (R). Random (RT) target shift. Eye movement precedes head (45 msec), whereas right splenius EMG (R SPL) starts about 10 msec before initial eye position changes; (RE) right eye, (RLR) right lateral rectus (calibration: 1 mV).

The movement of Fig. 1 shows a large amplitude head movement with the agonistic neck muscle EMG trace turning on approximately 45 msec before the head movement occurs. Latency studies demonstrate the causal chain from target input to agonistic electromyogram (EMG) (200 msec), to head acceleration (20 msec) and initial change in head position (45 msec), to final head position (240 msec) for 20 degree head rotations. Antagonistic EMG, obeying reciprocal innervation, begins about 70 msec after agonistic EMG begins.

Comparison of mean latencies of eye movements with fixed head, with head and arm movements demonstrates the better prediction in head movements, such that the increased dynamical lag of the head movement can be overcome by the better prediction operator of the head (Zangemeister and Stark, 1980). This is of importance when understanding the different gaze types.

DYNAMICS AND CONTROL OF HEAD MOVEMENTS

The parameterization of the dynamics of head trajectories (Main Sequence (Bahill and others, 1975b;Zangemeister and others, 1981a) Fig. 2) shows lawful relationships over a wide range of amplitudes that are comparable to eye and arm movements, even though they have different mechanics.

This is also true for a comparison with human and animal data from the literature. The main sequence demonstrates on a log-log scale the different dynamical properties of head and eye movements: the head being a visco-inertial load as compared to the eye being a visco-elastic load (Zangemeister and others, 1981d). Examples of the main sequence of neurological patients demonstrate the slow velocity and increased duration of head movements of a parkinson patient, whereas in a cerebellar patient head movements can be performed optimally but with much greater variance (see Zangemeister and Stark, this volume).

INFLUENCE OF EXPERIMENTAL CONDITIONS ON GAZE TYPES AND GAZE ERROR

Errors, or differences between gaze angle and target angle are important to study, because both eye and head movement are visual feedback error actuated movement patterns. This error function monitored continually by the subject is the important variable to be minimized as the off-fovea eccentricity of the target.

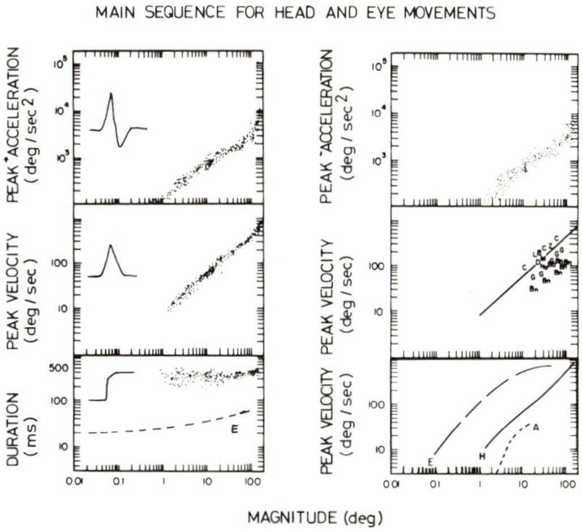

Fig. 2. Head main sequence. Over 100 fast intended head movements of a normal subject. Continuous line is a head movement model line. Middle right shows comparative data from the literature. Eye (E) and arm (A) movement main sequence data on the lower right show similar slopes but differing intercepts. Note the comparatively small increase of duration with large head movements.

An additional aid in understanding the gaze error that occurs with respect to certain gaze types is the "gaze plane". In the gaze plane plot time is only an implicit function of eye and head position (Fig. 3) that are displayed as functions of one another; arrows show movement of only the eye (vertical arrow) or the coordinated eye-head movement (diagonal arrow, CEM).

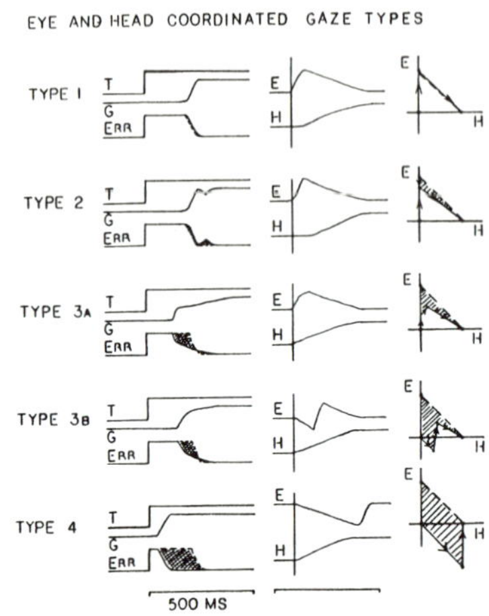

Fig. 3. Left: error displays, cross hatched lines excess error (Err) with respect to gaze (G) and target (T) position. Middle: Eye (E) and head (H) position, vertical line indicating the relative eye and head latency. Right: Gaze plane display with time as an implicit function showing excess error (dashed lines) and eye head interaction for the gaze types in normal subjects.

Error is minimized in the type I gaze movement (Fig. 3), where it persists only for the short eye latency and during the very rapid eye saccade, which is time optimal (Lehman and Stark, 1981). An excess error does not occur. Since head acceleration can vary greatly in this type, additional errors due to non-unity CEM gain and quick-phase-like saccades occasionally take place. It is not favoured by a particular experimental condition (Fig. 4).

Gaze type II shows the delayed head movement condition with an early gaze acquisition of the target. Typically, an anticipatory compensatory eye movement (ACEM) occurs, that does not depend on the VOR. The ACEM moves gaze off target until the head movement again brings it back onto target. This type is highly favoured by two conditions: forced intent and small amplitude; the latter relates it to slow fragmented head accelerations. The excess error shows up after the first target acquisition has occured. Although ACEM velocity often merges indistinguishably with the subsequent CEM, its beginning (vertical line, Fig. 3) demonstrates its important distinction from the VOR. Low gain CEMs frequently occur that relate closely to particularly slow head velocities (Zangemeister and Stark, 1980).

The early head movement in type III is not due to delay in the occurence of the eye saccade but rather to the early appearance of the head movement with its greater flexibility in predicting the target.

GAZE TYPE / CONDITION	I SYNCHRONOUS EYE NECK EMG (34%)	II LATE HEAD MOVEMENT (4%)	III EARLY HEAD MOVEMENT (43%)	IV LATE EYE SACCADE AND EARLY HEAD MOVEMENT (19%)
AMPLITUDE: 60°/15°	↓ 0,90	↓ 0,09	↑ 3,05	↑ 2,10
INTENT: forced/natural	↓ 0,73	↑ 3,80	↑ 2,20	↑ 3,50
PREDICTABILITY: high/low	↓ 0,71	↓ 0,85	↑ 1,60	↑ 2,90
ACCELERATION TYPE				

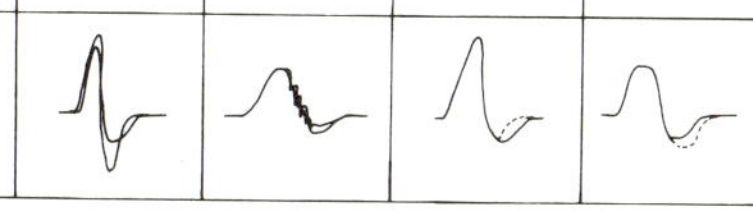

Fig. 4. Influences on frequency of gaze types. The four coordinated gaze types (columns) and the three most influencing experimental protocol conditions (rows). For each condition a ratio is formed (length of arrows) to indicate the influence of that condition on the probability of different gaze types. Mean percentage of frequency of occurence in parentheses. Lowermost row: head acceleration types that match with certain gaze types.

Thus the excess error with respect to type I frequently is not nearly as great as it might be seen with random targets. With enough prediction it may even be a negative quantity. This type is favoured by large amplitudes and, to a lower extent, by forced intent and increased predictability. Being fast, head accelerations in type III become high peaked in the positive part, long and rounded in the negative part. Head movement often occurs early with respect to the occurence of the eye movement, and the dynamical interactions are therefore a significant and major consideration. Two varieties are shown in the abstracted diagrams. Type IIIa shows a saccade occuring early during the head trajectory, but late enough to interact with the VOR which slows the saccade down.

When the eye saccade occurs later in the trajectory, as in type IIIb, it may be truncated due to its synchrony with a maximally active VOR occuring at peak positive head acceleration. Often this truncation is compensated for by a lowered CEM gain, which in fact may be the result of the influence of a saccade on the ongoing VOR. Thus truncation of the saccade could be due to neuromuscular and peripheral biomechanical interactions depending upon the different initial conditions of an oppositely going VOR and influencing the forces of the muscles attempting to generate the saccade (Lehman and Stark, 1981; Stark, 1968). Another explanation for this interaction type could be given by an interaction of the control signals on a higher central nervous system level (Morasso and others, 1973).

In the type IV gaze response there is a much longer period, before the fovea acquires the target, since the head movement finishes its trajectory following the head movement latency, before the eye even begins its saccadic trajectory.

Thus the error function has a large value for the long time period of approximately 600 msec, that includes the latency of 250 msec of the head movement, a long head trajectory of 300 msec, and a subsequent fast eye saccadic trajectory of approximately 50 msec. This additional "excess error", present in type IV compares with the minimal error present in type I. The extreme lateness of the eye saccade in type IV provides for a great deal of excess error, when the very early head movement did not anticipate target movement. However, the importance of the prediction operator is demonstrated in Fig. 3 (lower left) showing negative excess error. This means that with high prediction the very late eye saccade actually occurs earlier than the early eye saccade of type I with its minimal standard latency error. Forced intent, high predictability, and large amplitude favour this gaze type. Its head acceleration traces are high and rounded, i.e. saturating, sometimes with a higher negative than positive acceleration (Fig. 4).

When the head movement is large and also predicted, a highly efficient and time optimal neural controller signal can be generated, also described in EMG studies (Zangemeister and others, 1981). With the "classical" gaze type I both fast and slow head accelerations can be seen. The possible variability of the head trajectory is particularly noted in this type. It contrasts with the rather stereotyped eye movement trajectory. In concluding our observations in normal subjects we see, how the more intentionally governed head movement influences the eye and gaze patterns on different levels of the central nervous system in the sense of Hughling Jackson. It changes on a higher level with various experimental conditions (e.g. prediction), and it acts on a lower level through its variant dynamical trajectories on the VOR and therefore the eye movement.

MAIN SEQUENCE ANALYSIS IN NEUROLOGICAL PATIENTS

Parkinson patients show slow saccades, especially for large amplitudes (Chan and others, 1979; Traub and others, 1980). Our results (Fig. 5) demonstrate that for saccades of low amplitude their main sequence values are close to normal. Their head movements, however, demonstrate obvious slowness, so that normal main sequence values are significantly faster for these time optimally intended head movements.

Saturation of peak velocity and peak acceleration can be noted, particularly in movements of medium and large amplitudes. As earlier described in hand and arm rotations (Stark, 1968), a relative increase of the visco-elastic muscle forces could cause this slowness. Consequently, duration of head movements becomes increasingly longer with large amplitudes. This increase with magnitude of the movement is much more pronounced than in normal subjects, where it is considerably low.

Cerebellar patients can adjust their head movements to the task "to be time optimal"; therefore some of their main sequence data appear to be normal. However, a highly increased variability can be noted. This could be caused by an adaptation to dysmetric movements; it would be a compromise between time optimal and highly dysmetric, and slow but more accurate head movements. The dynamic behaviour of eye movements of cerebellar patients does not differ significantly from normal values.

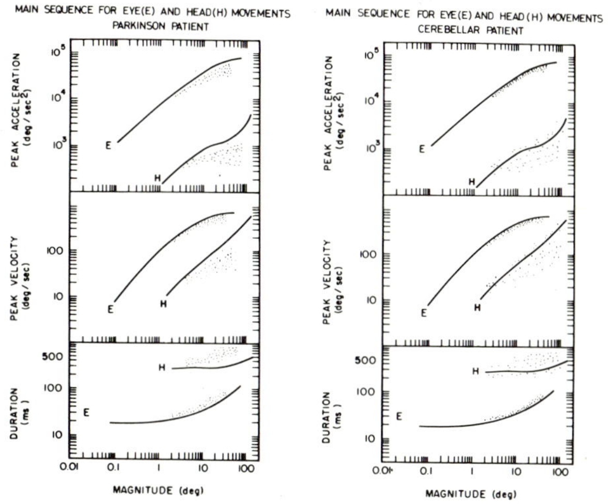

Fig. 5. Main sequence of a Parkinson and a cerebellar patient. Continous lines represent normal data for eye (E) and head (H) movements.

ABNORMAL COORDINATED GAZE TYPES

The earlier described experimental time functions of coordinated eye and head gaze movements give an idea of the variability found and suggest a classification for better understanding. To understand these gaze types and their relation to active head trajectories it is most helpful to discuss them in terms of a model. This model, the "gaze plane", has the advantage that eye and head movement are displayed as functions of one another with time as only an implicit function of eye and head position (Fig. 6, right part). In the gaze plane plot we see the fast eye saccade occuring first (Fig. 6, vertical arrow starting from the origin). The diagonally downwards pointing line exemplifies the CEM and the head movement occuring at the same time. Eye position is exchanged for head position, and gaze that is eye in space remains on target (dashed line) throughout for a typical (type I, Zangemeister and Stark, 1980) gaze movement.

This is only achieved when the CEM gain equals unity; higher or lower gains would slightly move gaze off the target during the head trajectory. Normally this would not be a severe disturbance of the target acquisition, since the "post-saccadic snapshot" already had occured. Therefore, the target did not need to remain exactly on the fovea; after an intersaccadic interval occured, corrective saccades could return target onto the fovea. However, in neurological patients particularly the unpredictability of a visual target leads to increased frequency of gaze errors, so that variants of the "normal" gaze types most often occur.

Depending upon the gaze type or a certain pathological condition deviations from the optimal target line (dashed line in gaze plane display, Fig. 6) can be noted. It can be seen that parkinson patients showing hypometria keep the target on fovea once they have it slowly acquired. Additionally, parkinson patients tend to move their head much later than healthy subjects in response to visual targets. Gaze type 2 with its anticipatory compensatory eye movement (ACEM) is therefore favoured by them (see also C. Kennard and others, this volume).

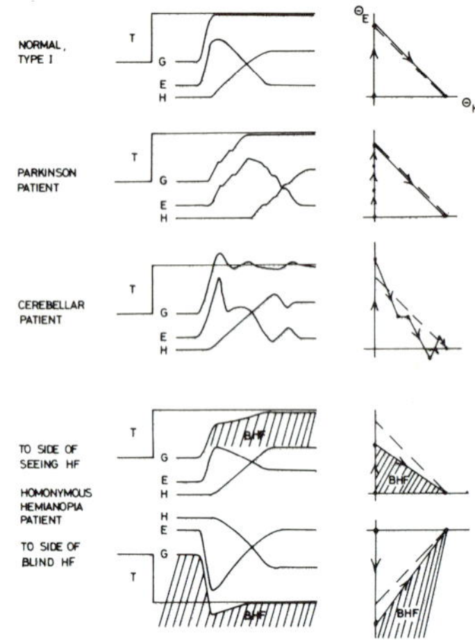

Fig. 6. Time functions (left) and gaze planes (right) of a normal gaze type I and neurological patients. Target (T; up = left), gaze (G), eye (E), head (H) position. Θ_E, Θ_H: eye and head position. BHF: blind hemifield (HF).

Cerebellar patients with hypermetria, however, demonstrate a comparably longer lasting difficulty in catching a random target and getting their gaze finally adjusted to it. When prediction is permitted, cerebellar patients show significantly less dysmetria, that is less overshooting gaze movements. Obviously some of the dysmetria can be overcome by the better head movement predictor. The main sequence of eye movements of cerebellar patients does not show a significant difference to normal values. However, the more intentionally governed head movements show a high variability of their dynamical behaviour. Therefore, as soon as the movement is unpredicted and intended to be fast this increased dynamical variability leads to more variable eye movement patterns: Compensatory eye movements (CEM) of relatively too high gain, because of a diminished cerebellar suppression of the VOR, and dysmetric corrective saccades.

Cerebellar patients show more frequently gaze type I and IIIa (44 %; 39 %). The frequency of occurence of gaze types II, IIIb and IV is greatly diminished. The fact that movements that show a high amount of prediction as the eye in type II (anticipatory compensatory eye movement, ACEM) or the head in types IIIb and IV only seldom occur could indicate either a decreased ability to predict visual targets in general or to adapt rapidly to a given predictive situation.

Of special interest is the behaviour of coordinated gaze in patients that suffer from an isolated sensory defect with homonymous hemianopia.
If they try to acquire a predictable target they tend to overshoot the target when viewing to the side of the blind hemifield, and they tend to undershoot the target when viewing to the side of the seeing hemifield such that target always stays on the safe side. A high gain CEM when viewing to the side of the blind hemifield and vice versa brings target accurately onto the fovea. However, when confronted with random targets these patients tend to eliminate this complicated strategy by keeping their head still. In case they move, a great variety of gaze errors is likely to occur (Meienberg and others, 1981; Zangemeister and Stark, 1980), that are analyzed in detail in the following part.

CLINICAL EXAMPLES OF A GAZE PLANE ANALYSIS

Clinical examples (Fig. 7) demonstrate the variety of interactions of eye and head coordinated gaze movements in patients with homonymous hemianopia. Upper left shows a gaze movement towards the seeing hemifield (SHF), placed in upper right direction in this figure, (directions are plotted positively in graphs, ΘE ordinate, ΘH abscissa), with eye movement undershooting target, so that the right hemianopic field (represented by diagonal slashes) does not obscure view of target: neither after the first eye saccade nor during head movement and compensatory eye movement (CEM), nor with the second eye saccade compensating or correcting for initial undershoot (small upward vertical arrow).

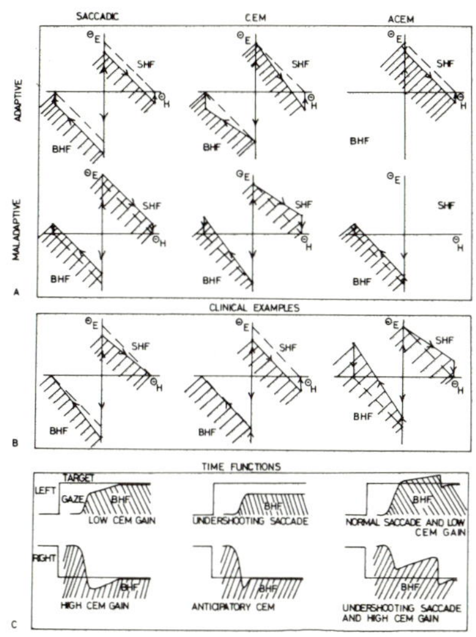

Fig. 7. Gaze plane display for patients with homonymous hemianopia. Columns show saccadic, CEM and ACEM mechanisms compensating for the field defect, while acquiring targets. Rows show adaptive, maladaptive and clinically more frequent examples.

Upper left also shows a gaze movement toward the blind homonymous hemifield (BHF) which overshoots target on initial eye movement saccade (vertical arrow downward from the origin) so that the right hemianopic field does not obscure view of target. This upper left part of Fig. 7 shows saccadic eye movements adaptive for safe acquisition of target. Contrariwise, maladaptive saccadic eye movements (lower left) overshoot a target in the SHF or undershoot a target in the BHF, so that its view is obscured by the hemianopic field.

Similarily, a change in CEM gain can be adaptive (upper middle) or maladaptive (lower middle). Unity gain has a minus 45 degree slope in contrast to CEM gains greater, with greater slope, or lower, with less slope. Corrective saccades (small vertical arrow) are required to compensate for non-unity CEM gains. The effect of the ACEM, occuring before actual head movement, is shown on upper and lower right (Fig. 7). On gaze to target in the SHF with accurate eye saccade, the occurence of an adaptive ACEM places the hemianopic field away from target and permits safe viewing of target during head movement and CEM. A corrective saccade is necessary (small vertical upward arrow) at the end of gaze movement. A maladaptive ACEM (lower right) moves gaze off the target so that the BHF obscures its view.

More frequently occuring clinical examples (Fig. 7b, c) are easily interpreted in the light of these less often occuring examples. For comparison the typical time functions are also given (Fig. 7c). Compensating discrepancies (left) permit safe viewing. With gaze to the SHF an undershooting saccade (upward vertical arrow) prevents low CEM gain (downward oblique arrow) from obscuring view of target in many instances (about 60 %). Similarily, an overshooting saccade (downward vertical arrow) with gaze to the BHF prevents high CEM gain (upward oblique arrow) from obscuring target in many instances (about 60 %).

An especially interesting compensatory discrepancy sometimes occurs (about 25 %; Fig. 7b, c, middle), when saccadic overshoot (large downward vertical arrow) with gaze to the BHF is corrected by an ACEM (small upward vertical arrow), so that fovea is on target, but without a safety margin. A pure saccadic undershoot discrepancy also sometimes occurs (about 25 %; upward vertical arrow) which permits safe target acquisition.
Maladaptive discrepancies may occur (right) with low CEM gain (downward oblique arrow) on gaze to the SHF and ACEM (small upward vertical arrow), or high CEM gain (upward oblique arrow). Both place target into the hemianopic field during CEM and require corrective saccades into the BHF.

In conclusion our observations and analyses demonstrate the clinical application of the main sequence and gaze plane analysis as an aid in understanding pathological conditions of gaze movements. Further clinical and modeling studies should analyze the underlying physiological conditions and also validate particular clinical tests of gaze shifts in neurological patients.

DISCUSSION:

Dr. Ian Strachan was invited to present his findings relating to adaptation to aphakic spectacles in patients with cataract extraction. Approximately one third of the patients reviewed by Dr. Strachan did not adapt to aphakic spectacles which introduce a telescopic magnification of 1.25 to 1.3. Such patients were generally elderly and predominately female and their degree of handicap could render them housebound. All of the non-adapting patients were found to have broken pursuit on an oscilloscope tracking test and failure to suppress their vestibulo-ocular reflex. Some had hypometric saccades during refixation movements. Dr. Strachan was reluctant to conclude that the non-adapting patients had neurological disease because of the preponderance of women in the group. Furthermore the form in which suppression was broken frequently consisted of saccadic intrusions rather than nystagmus, which suggests that the subjects were anxious and the anxiety state was inhibiting the adaptive process.

Dr. M. Gresty commented that some people, particularly the elderly, regardless of whether they were aphakic, had difficulty in adapting to the perspective and magnification distortions introduced by spectacles and asked Dr. Strachan whether he had any views on possibile underlying disorders of eye movement which might explain this. Dr. Strachan replied that he felt such people did have oculomotor disorders but that he had not characterised them and was not convinced that there was a one to one relationship between the presence of oculomotor disorders and inability to adapt to spectacles.

Dr. L. Stark offered an explanation of the surprising finding of Steinman and Collewijn that during active head rotations made during target fixation, retinal image speed could be of the order of 4°/sec and disparity between the two eyes could be of the order of 3°/sec. Dr. Stark asserted that his calculations showed that misalignment of the coil eye movement recording device with respect to the visual axes and failure to take into account the fact that horizontal rotations of the head induce pitching and rolling movements due to kinematic cross coupling could account for these high retinal slip velocities. Dr. H. Collewijn agreed that cross coupling effects may well account for the high retinal slip velocities and disparities he found, however, experiments performed by both Dr. Collewijn and Dr. G. Barnes involving head shaking during the fixation of strobed targets and multiple after images had demonstrated that there was some retinal image motion during compensatory eye movements. According to Dr. Collewijn's investigations the retinal slip as judged by after images was about half that as measured by coil recording techniques.

Dr. Barnes described feelings of motion sickness and disorientation experienced by normal subjects in the experiments he had conducted on head and eye co-ordination. Subjects asked to try to suppress their compensatory eye movements with targets placed in the peripheral visual field became disoriented and lost sense of the "straight ahead" direction. In addition they felt as if the small targets were dragging them sideways. In another situation in which targets were pursued with a collimated sight attached rigidly to the head, subjects moving rapidly became motion sick particularly during pursuit of targets moving rapidly with trajectories of high frequency content. This situation is comparable with the pursuit with head only condition in the experiments of Dr. Collewijn who asserted that this had occasionally induced motion sickness in his subjects. Describing his own experience,

Dr. Zangenmeister related the onset of motion sickness to the speed and frequency of target motion during fixation on a pointer attached to the moving head. Dr. T. Brandt reported that in his experiments normal subjects began to feel nauseous when making head movements at frequencies and velocities which produced oscillopsia. Dr. Barnes pointed out that motion sickness is more commonly related to low frequency, whole body movements such as "wallowing" in a ship, and yet the situations reported in the present discussion were concerned with high frequency movement. Dr. Brandt offered an explanation of this apparent incongruity in that the oscillopsia which was associated with high frequency and high velocity head movements produced a visual/vestibular mismatch as did low frequency movements. According to the theory of Reason and Brand this mismatch was the factor inducing motion sickness.

Dr. Gresty raised the question of why patients with multiple sclerosis who had vestibular pathway lesions complained frequently of oscillopsia whereas those with inter- and supra-nuclear ophthalmoplegia, both producing considerable degrees of retinal slip during head movements, did not report oscillopsia. Dr. G. Kommerell stated that whether or not oscillopsia was experienced depended upon how peripheral the lesion was in the oculomotor machinery. Patients with extra-ocular muscle palsy with an immobile eye could adapt through central mechanisms to retinal image slip. Similarly, since internuclear ophthalmoplegia involved lesions at a more peripheral level than lesions of the vestibular projection pathways, more central mechanisms capable of adaptation were left intact. Dr. Gresty commented that supra-nuclear ophthalmoplegia could hardly be considered as a peripheral phenomenon and that there was doubt as to whether patients with multiple sclerosis would necessarily have mechanisms of adaptation left intact. Dr. R. Daroff extended the problem by pointing out that not only were patients with internuclear ophthalmoplegia oblivious to retinal image slip but in addition they denied diplopia, despite the fact that they could have considerable misalignment of the visual axes. In general the discussion was divided as to whether or not there was a reasonable explanation for these observations.

Dr. Barnes was asked whether size of target and velocity of rotation had any effects on the ability to suppress the vestibulo-ocular reflex in the presence of peripherally placed targets which were stabilised with respect to the head. In reply he stated he had found that stability to suppress improved with target size which was in agreement with earlier findings of Dr. J. Dichgans and Dr. Collewijn. In respect of the velocity of oscillation, he had found a non-linear relationship between suppression ability and velocity that the faster the subject went the less well able he was to suppress. There was also a "spatio-temporal integration" effect on suppression in that if targets in the periphery were strobed suppression deteriorated with a proportional relationship between rate of strobing and suppressive ability.

Dr. Gresty put the general question to the audience of whether vestibulo-ocular reflex suppression was always related to the quality of pursuit eye movements in patients with nervous diseases. Dr. J. Dichgans expressed the opinion that there was a one to one relationship and that failure of VOR suppression could be more easily tested at the bedside than pursuit and could be taken to indicate the quality of pursuit. Dr. Gresty stated that he had examined suppression and pursuit in many patients and had always found that their respective performances went hand in hand. This view was challenged by Dr. Daroff who asserted that he had encountered both patients with abnormal pursuit who could suppress their VOR and patients with normal pursuit who could not suppress their VOR. Dr. Gresty raised the problem that one must be sure that the patient undergoing testing is not making vergence eye movements which would override VOR movements. Dr. J. Sharpe suggested that there may be several ways in which the VOR may be suppressed, one simply being through will so that intact pursuit is not singly necessary for suppression. Dr. Barnes pointed out that if large targets are used then the optokinetic reflex may be responsible for VOR suppression.

Finally, Dr. Buettner highlighted the fact that in the sort of patients being discussed the VOR gain itself might be low and be the major factor responsible for apparent suppression. In general the clinical opinion was divided as to whether or not the quality of VOR suppression and of pursuit went hand in hand.

SECTION IX

Coordinator: D. S. Zee

DISORDERS OF THE CEREBELLUM

OCULAR MOTOR ABNORMALITIES RELATED TO LESIONS IN THE VESTIBULOCEREBELLUM IN PRIMATE

D. S. ZEE

Johns Hopkins University, School of Medicine, Baltimore, Maryland, USA

ABSTRACT

Removal of the flocculus and paraflocculus in monkeys causes a number of ocular motor abnormalities including variable changes in VOR gain, impaired smooth tracking with the head still (pursuit) or moving (VOR cancellation), gaze-paretic, rebound and downbeat nystagmus, post-saccadic drift (glissades), and loss of ability to adaptively modify VOR gain or the saccadic pulse-step match. All these abnormalities reflect disorders of mechanisms that insure best visual acuity by preventing retinal slip. The ocular motor cerebellar syndrome of human patients is, in large part, reproduced by flocculectomy in monkeys with the important exception of disorders of saccadic amplitude (saccadic dysmetria). The latter probably reflects dysfunction in the dorsal cerebellar vermis and underlying deep cerebellar nuclei.

KEYWORDS

Cerebellum; vestibulocerebellum; flocculus; eye movements; vestibulo-ocular reflex; smooth pursuit; saccades; nystagmus.

INTRODUCTION

A major advance in ocular motor neuro-ophthalmology has been the recognition of a specific, cerebellar, ocular motor syndrome. A group of ocular motor signs (Table 1) have been described in patients with lesions restricted to the cerebellum (Daroff, this symposium; Leigh and Zee, 1982; Zee and others, 1976b). Recent experimental studies have suggested an anatomical basis for many of them. (Interestingly most of these ocular motor signs had long ago been attributed to cerebellar dysfunction by Holmes (1922) and Cogan (1948)). Control of saccadic amplitude and its pathological expression -- saccadic dysmetria -- appear to reflect ocular motor functions of the dorsal vermis and underlying fastigial nuclei (see E. Keller and L. Optican, this symposium). On the other hand, stabilization of images upon the retina during smooth tracking and fixation, with or without accompanying head rotation, are a function of the vestibulocerebellum and the flocculus (and possibly paraflocculus) in particular. Thus pursuit deficits (head still or moving), gaze-paretic, downbeat and rebound nystagmus, and post-saccadic drift (glissades) may reflect dysfunction in the flocculus.

TABLE 1 Ocular Motor Abnormalities in "Pure" Cerebellar Degenerations

1. Inaccurate (dysmetric) saccades; normal velocities and latencies
2. Fixation abnormalities: square wave jerks (saccadic intrusions) and increased slow drift
3. Impaired smooth pursuit (head still or moving (VOR cancellation)); impaired OKN; impaired fixation suppression of caloric-induced nystagmus
4. Post-saccadic drift (glissades)
5. Gaze-paretic nystagmus (occasionally centripetal nystagmus)
6. Rebound nystagmus
7. Downbeat nystagmus
8. Positional nystagmus
9. Increased VOR gain
10. Skew deviation
11. Impaired head pursuit

Floccular Ablations

The flocculus and paraflocculus contain a number of neurons that discharge in relation to eye movements of all types (both versions and vergence) (see Buttner, Waespe and Henn, this symposium). Not all cells discharge for each type of movement but a variety of combinations have been observed. Important for the interpretation of lesion studies is that, in a given flocculus, Purkinje cells related to smooth tracking of small targets tend to increase their discharge rate for ipsilateral (horizontal gaze velocity Purkinje cells) or downward (vertical gaze velocity Purkinje cells) movements.

We recently investigated the ocular motor defects in monkeys with bilateral ablations of the flocculus and portions of the paraflocculus ("flocculectomy") (Zee and others, 1981). The vestibulo-ocular reflex (VOR) gain (eye velocity/head velocity) in darkness was variably affected by flocculectomy. In some monkeys, it went up, in others down and sometimes it did not change. In human patients with cerebellar (Baloh and others, 1981; Estanol, Romero and Corvera, 1979; Zee and others, 1976) or vestibulocerebellar (Baloh and others, 1981; Zee, Friendlich and Robinson, 1974) lesions, the VOR gain is often increased. In flocculectomized monkeys, the ability to smoothly track targets moving in space was decreased (gain (eye velocity/target velocity) about 0.65 in the horizontal plane) but not abolished. Vertical pursuit was also impaired after flocculectomy. Smooth tracking deficits were comparable whether the head was still (pursuit) or moving (VOR cancellation). Since pursuit is nearly completely abolished after total cerebellectomy (gain $<$ 0.2) (Optican and Robinson, 1980), but not after flocculectomy alone, other cerebellar structures -- possibly residual paraflocculus, nodulus or even the cerebellar hemispheres -- may also participate in pursuit. (Igarashi and others (1975) have shown a high velocity OKN deficit after uvulonodulectomy in monkey. This may reflect a pursuit deficit.) The ability to generate high velocity OKN was also impaired after flocculectomy and, in response to a constant velocity stimulus, the rise to a steady state was prolonged. An identical pattern of optokinetic response has been reported in patients with the Arnold-Chiari malformation or selective posterior vermian atrophy (Baloh and others, 1981; Yee and others, 1979; Zee and others, 1976b). However, one must be cautious when comparing optokinetic responses of monkeys and human beings. The latter show a much weaker and less consistent OKAN which saturates at about 30 deg/sec (Cohen and others, 1982) and OKN (as opposed to pursuit) appears to have a longer rise time (as shown by the rate of charging of OKAN) in human beings (3-4x that of monkey). Furthermore, in human beings, the initial nystagmus response in a revolving optokinetic drum appears to be almost exclusively generated by the pursuit system.

Flocculectomized monkeys also showed horizontally, gaze-paretic and rebound nystagmus and vertically, downbeating nystagmus -- all cardinal features of the human ocular motor cerebellar syndrome. Gaze-paretic nystagmus, with its exponentially decaying slow phases, implies that an important function of the flocculus is to improve the fidelity of the brain stem neural integrator that normally functions to hold positions of gaze. Holmes (1922) had already recognized this specific cerebellar function: "The essential component of (cerebellar) nystagmus is consequently the slow phase of the jerk and this is obviously due to a failure of the eyes to maintain postures. Consequently nystagmus can be attributed to a disturbance of the tonic contractions of the ocular muscles by which postures are maintained".

Rebound nystagmus has recently been reported in a patient with a tumor involving the flocculus (Yamazaki and Zee, 1979). While the mechanism of rebound nystagmus is not completely understood it has been suggested that it represents a bias (position? velocity?), possibly developed in the vestibular system, to help hold eccentric positions of gaze (Hood, in press; Yamazaki and Zee, 1979). Recent clinical studies continue to support the localizing value of rebound nystagmus as a cerebellar sign (Morales-Garcia and others, 1978) although exceptions may occur. In fact, any condition that impairs smooth pursuit may theoretically lead to rebound nystagmus since if the lights are turned out (eliminating pursuit) when a normal subject returns the eyes to the primary position after prolonged eccentric gaze, rebound nystagmus occurs (Zee and others, 1976b).

Downbeat nystagmus has long been recognized as a sign of lesions in the posterior fossa and its occurrence in the flocculectomized monkey suggests a possible anatomical locus. However, downbeat nystagmus can also be produced experimentally by midsaggital section in the rostral medulla (de Jong and others, 1980), or by nodulus lesions (Takemori and Suzuki, 1977). Downbeat nystagmus may relate to a loss of inhibition of the anterior (superior) semicircular canal VOR (which mediates upward slow phases). This could occur after lesions of either the flocculus or midsaggital portion of the medulla since both may interrupt pathways that inhibit anterior canal reflexes. Downbeat nystagmus might also be caused by a pursuit imbalance. Most vertical gaze velocity Purkinje cells in the flocculus increase their discharge rate during downward pursuit eye movements; hence their loss could create an upward bias with consequent downbeat nystagmus. Finally downbeat nystagmus might also occur if the vertical neural integrators (for up and down) become unbalanced. Thus one can envision a number of mechanisms by which posterior fossa lesions might produce "downbeat nystagmus". All probably occur.

Experimental flocculectomy produces downbeat nystagmus with slow phases that have exponentially decaying waveforms in some animals and exponentially increasing waveforms in others. In the former, downbeat nystagmus is worse on down gaze; in the latter, worse on upward gaze. A similar, exponentially increasing waveform has been reported in a human patient with downbeat nystagmus (Zee, Leigh and Mathieu-Millaire, 1980) associated with a presumed paraneoplastic cerebellar degeneration and in a patient with the Arnold-Chiari malformation (Pedersen and others, 1980). We have presented an analysis of the variable waveforms and position dependency of downbeat nystagmus using a positive feedback loop hypothesis for the cerebellar control of the brain-stem neural integrators (Fig. 1). In this hypothesis, the cerebellum and especially flocculus is thought to improve the performance of the brain stem neural integrator by positively feeding the integrator's output back into its input. If the feedback loop gain is too low, exponentially decaying slow phases occur; if too high, exponentially increasing slow phases occur. A theoretical consequence of nystagmus produced by imbalance in a pair of push-pull integrators (working reciprocally in a given plane of rotation) is that if the slow phase is exponentially increasing, nystagmus becomes more prominent when the eyes are moved in the direction of the slow phase; if the slow phase is exponentially decaying, nystagmus becomes more prominent when the eyes are moved in the direction of the quick phase.

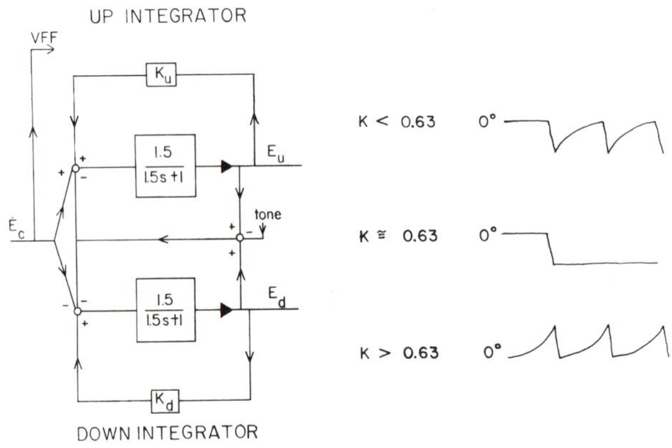

Fig. 1. Positive feedback scheme to boost the time constant of the brain stem neural integrator. Two integrators, one producing upward (E_u), the other, downward (E_d), position commands, work in push-pull. Solid arrows indicate that the output of an integrator can never be negative. The integrators are connected together to keep the sum of their outputs constant and provide a source of tone. In this way the integrators work reciprocally around a steady, primary-position level. A positive feedback loop, with gain k, was placed around each "leaky" brain stem integrator. (k) was assumed to be under the control of the flocculus and/or paraflocculus. Based on the results in flocculectomized monkeys we have assumed that the time constant of the brain stem "leaky" integrator is 1.5 sec. Thus the transfer function of the brain stem integrator becomes 1.5/(1.5s + 1). With positive feedback the transfer function of the integrator becomes 1.5/(1.5s + (1 - 1.5k)) and its time constant 1.5/(1 - 1.5k). If the time constant of the integrator in the intact monkey is about

25 sec then k = 0.63. If k > 0.63 the integrator becomes unstable, if k < 0.63 the integrator becomes leaky, and if k = 0.63 the integrator functions properly. The corresponding waveforms of nystagmus are depicted. s = Laplace complex frequency. k_u = feedback gain of up integrator, k_d = feedback gain of down integrator, $\dot{E}$ = eye velocity command, and VFF = velocity feed forward pathway by which eye velocity commands are passed directly to the ocular motor neurons. From Zee and others, Effects of ablation of flocculus and paraflocculus on eye movement in primate, J. Neurophysiol., 1981, in press.

Flocculectomized monkeys show saccades of normal velocity and accuracy but with brief (50-200 msec) post-saccadic drift. This is thought to reflect a mismatch between the phasic and tonic innervation (pulse-step) that creates saccades. In the horizontal plane the eyes usually drifted onward but the patterns in the vertical plane were variable from monkey to monkey. We recently have recorded eye movements (magnetic field search coil technique) of three patients with familial cerebellar degeneration and they showed a similar pattern of post-saccadic drift to flocculectomized monkeys (Kennard, Zee, Leigh and Newman, unpublished observations) (Fig. 2 and Table 2). Our age-matched control was Dr. D. G. Cogan.

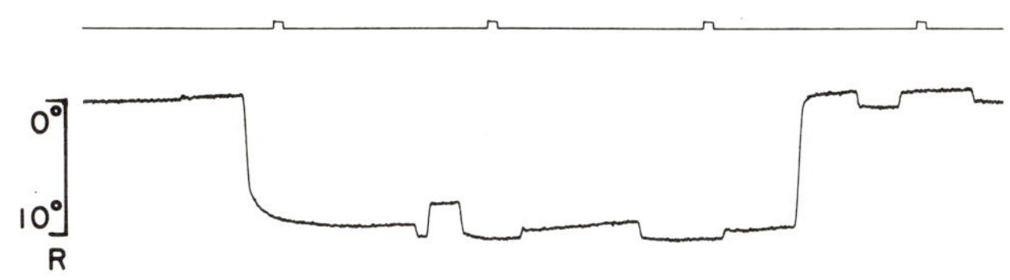

Fig. 2. Post-saccadic drift in a patient with familial cerebellar degeneration. Note the prominent mismatch between the pulse and step components of his rightward saccades (pulse < step). Time marks indicate 1 second.

TABLE 2 Post-Saccadic Drift

Pulse-Step Ratio[1]: 10 Degree Saccades

Horizontal

	Rightward		Leftward	
	Centripetal	Centrifugal	Centripetal	Centrifugal
Patient No. 1	.83	.75	.97	.99
2	.94	.88	.88	.86
3	.99	.97	.87	.90
Normal	.96	.92	.97	.97

Vertical

	Upward		Downward	
	Centripetal	Centrifugal	Centripetal	Centrifugal
Patient No. 1	.84	1.05	.99	.92
2	.98	.97	.89	.77
3	.99	.84	.94	.98
Normal	1.00	.86	1.01	1.00

[1]Pulse = amplitude of high velocity portion of saccade; step = total amplitude of saccade taken from onset of the saccade to when the eye comes to rest.

In sum, flocculectomized monkeys show a number of ocular motor abnormalities and each reflects an inability to hold images stable on the retina. Thus impaired pursuit and VOR cancellation, gaze-paretic, rebound and downbeat nystagmus and post-saccadic drift all emerge after removal of the flocculus and portions of the paraflocculus. Similar findings have been reported in human patients with presumed floccular lesions (Baloh and others, 1981; von Reutern and Dichgans, 1977; Yamazaki and Zee, 1979).

Flocculus and Adaptation

The flocculus has also been implicated in long term, plastic, adaptive changes that insure that retinal image-stabilizing reflexes such as the VOR remain appropriate to the visual stimulus (see Miles, this symposium). Experimentally, the VOR can be made to seem inappropriate using optical devices such as reversing prisms (which cause the seen world to appear to move in the same direction as the head) or magnifying (or minifying) spectacles (which change the velocity of image motion on the retina during head rotation). In response to such optically-imposed retinal image motion; the amplitude, direction and phase of the VOR can be adjusted appropriately so that eye movements compensate for any type of image motion that occurs during movements of the head. These changes persist even in the absence of continuous stimulation and are present when the VOR is measured in darkness.

Experimentally, flocculectomy in monkeys (Optican and others, 1980) and vestibulo-cerebellectomy in cats (Robinson, 1976) interferes with these VOR adaptive capabilities. However, removal of the flocculus does not appear to interfere with adaptation (by rebalancing the vestibular nuclei) to a unilateral peripheral vestibular lesion (Haddad, Friendlich and Robinson, 1977; Takemori and Cohen, 1974). Recently the adaptive capabilities of the VOR have been tested in human patients with various brain stem and cerebellar lesions using reversing prisms (Yagi and others, in press). As in experimental animals, human beings with cerebellar lesions show a decreased ability to adaptively modify the gain of the VOR. Finally another form of vestibular learning, habituation to a repetitive vestibular stimulus is impaired after midline cerebellar lesions that include the nodulus and uvula (Blair and Gavin, 1979).

Experimental studies have also suggested that monkeys with floccular lesions are unable to adjust the match between the saccadic pulse and step so as to eliminate post-saccadic drift (Optican and others, 1980; Optican, this symposium). In the face of a brief period (several hundred milliseconds) of optically-imposed, post-saccadic retinal slip, normal monkeys readily learn to program a nearly matching post-saccadic drift of the eyes which in turn compensates for the artificially-induced image movement upon the retina. Presumably this is accomplished by adjusting the match between the saccadic step and pulse. However, flocculectomized monkeys show a strikingly reduced ability to carry out such adaptation.

By considering the long-term adaptive functions of the cerebellum one might explain the unpredictable effects of flocculectomy on VOR gain, vertical nystagmus waveforms and patterns of post-saccadic drift. Since the flocculus normally optimizes ocular motor performance, its removal may expose inherent imperfections in brain stem and peripheral ocular motor mechanisms. Naturally, these are idiosyncratic from monkey to monkey (or patient to patient) so that flocculectomy need not cause the exact same ocular motor abnormality to emerge in each animal. As another example, patients with longstanding blindness show ocular motor abnormalities similar to those of patients with cerebellar lesions (Leigh and Zee, 1980). These may also reflect cerebellar dysfunction but in this case blindness deprives the flocculus of the necessary visual feedback to appropriately modify ocular motor performance.

How the flocculus participates in ocular motor adaptation is unknown. It may be that the visual information used by the flocculus for long-term adaptation arrives on climbing fibers via the inferior olive while visual information for immediate use -- required for smooth pursuit or VOR cancellation -- arrives on mossy fibers via pontine relay nuclei (Miyashita, 1980). However, Miles and others have suggested that the adaptive changes do not take place on floccular Purkinje cells but rather the flocculus provides an error signal to other neurons -- probably in the brain stem -- where the adaptive changes actually occur (Miles, this symposium).

Floccular Connections

An important and as yet unanswered question is by what anatomical pathways does the cerebellum influence brain stem ocular motor mechanisms. The flocculus projects strongly to the vestibular nuclei but vestibular neurons that discharge in relation to gaze velocity have not yet been reported. Chubb and Fuchs (in press) have recorded from the dentate nucleus and adjacent Y-group of the vestibular complex and found cells that discharge in relationship to upward smooth tracking during both pursuit and VOR cancellation. Stimulation here also elicits upward smooth movements. Since 1) floccular Purkinje cells that relate to vertical tracking discharge primarily for downward pursuit, 2) the flocculus is known to project to the dentate and Y-group, and 3) Purkinje cells are inhibitory; one can hypothesize that the flocculus facilitates downward tracking by inhibiting upward tracking cells in the Y-group. The Y-group has a number of brain stem projections, some traverse the MLF (Stanton, 1980). The flocculus also has important reciprocal connections to another important ocular motor structure, the nucleus prepositus, lying just behind the abducens nucleus as part of the perihypoglossal complex, in the rostral medulla (McCrea, Baker and Delgado-Garcia, 1979). This may be an important relay by which the flocculus influences brain-stem ocular motor mechanisms.

Conclusions

We can now, at least tentatively, relegate specific ocular motor functions to the vestibulocerebellum and flocculus and paraflocculus in particular (Table 3). These structures function in the control of a number of retinal image stabilizing reflexes including smooth pursuit, visual modulation of the vestibulo-ocular reflex, holding positions of gaze and suppression of post-saccadic drift. Furthermore, the elaboration of long term, adaptive changes in ocular motor performance depends on these same structures.

TABLE 3 Summary of Vestibulocerebellar Function and Pathology

Function	Disorder
Retinal-image stabilization (smooth tracking, suppression of inappropriate vestibular nystagmus, holding positions of gaze, long-term adjustments in VOR gain and the saccadic pulse-step match), habituation of the VOR to repetitive stimuli.	Impaired smooth pursuit, VOR cancellation and fixation suppression of caloric nystagmus; gaze-evoked, rebound and downbeat nystagmus; post-saccadic drift; inappropriate VOR.

Even so, a number of questions remain about floccular, parafloccular and nodular function. What do the floccular vergence units do? Do they modulate VOR gain as a function of vergence angle (a necessity for stabilization of images of close objects during head rotation)? Or are they responsible for some aspect of vergence tone that accounts for the divergence nystagmus and occasional convergence spasm observed in patients with the Arnold-Chiari malformation? What is the cause of the transient convergence paralysis after acute cerebellar lesions in both monkeys and human beings. Still unclear is the pathophysiology of the complete pursuit and optokinetic deficit after total cerebellectomy versus the partial deficits after flocculectomy. Does the nodulus participate in pursuit? Furthermore, cerebellectomy in cats only minimally affects OKN while a devastating OKN deficit is produced in the monkey. Why the species difference? What cerebellar lesions cause upbeating nystagmus or alternating skew deviations on lateral gaze? Do flocculus lesions cause a deficit of pursuit movements of the head as has been observed in patients with cerebellar degeneration? By what routes does the flocculus influence brain stem vestibular, pursuit and gaze-holding mechanisms? How does the flocculus participate in VOR adaptation and control of the match between the saccadic pulse and step?

THE ROLE OF THE CEREBELLUM IN THE CONTROL OF SLOW CONJUGATE EYE MOVEMENTS

U. BÜTTNER*, W. WAESPE** and V. HENN

Department of Neurology, University of Zürich, 8091 Zürich, Switzerland

ABSTRACT

Single units have been recorded in the vestibulo-cerebellum and the cerebellar nuclei, and their contribution to the generation of smooth pursuit eye movements and nystagmus has been analyzed in alert animals. In most of these studies the flocculus of the monkey was investigated. For natural stimulation animals were exposed to angular accelerations in the horizontal plane (vestibular) or large moving visual fields (optokinetic). They were also trained to fixate on small moving light spots (smooth pursuit) or to suppress their vestibulo-ocular reflex (VOR). The results demonstrate that in the vestibulo-cerebellum vestibular, oculomotor and visual input activity can be distinguished. Furthermore output activity from Purkinje cells (PC) and in the deep cerebellar nuclei can be related to various oculomotor tasks, for example smooth pursuit eye movements, high velocity optokinetic nystagmus (OKN), and VOR-suppression. On the other hand little or no activity change is observed in these elements during vestibular stimulation in the dark, low velocity OKN and optokinetic after-nystagmus (OKAN). Finally by comparing unit activity in the vestibular nuclei with that in the vestibulo-cerebellum it is shown that the vestibulo-cerebellum becomes active when the visual environment requires an oculomotor performance which cannot be provided by the vestibular nuclei.

KEY WORDS

Vestibulo-cerebellum; cerebellar nuclei; flocculus; alert monkey; smooth pursuit; VOR-suppression; optokinetic nystagmus.

INTRODUCTION

For a long time cerebellar involvement in eye movement control has been known (Hitzig, 1874; Ferrier, 1876). Clinical and lesion studies over the last years

---

Present address:
* Dept. of Neurology, University of Düsseldorf, D-4 Düsseldorf (Germany)
**Dept. of Neurology, Mount Sinai School of Medicine, New York, N.Y. 10029 (U.S.A)

permitted certain oculomotor deficits to be related to pathology of specific cerebellar structures. From these studies it was concluded that the vestibulo-cerebellum (flocculus, paraflocculus, nodulus, uvula) is important for the correct performance of slow conjugate eye movements (smooth pursuit, slow phases of optokinetic and vestibular nystagmus). Other cerebellar structures have been related to different eye movement functions, e.g. saccadic dysmetria to dysfunction of the dorsal vermis (Ritchie, 1976; see Keller and Optican, this volume).

The neuronal mechanisms underlying these various oculomotor deficits are still only partly understood. Over the last few years single unit studies in alert behaving animals allowed neuronal activity to be related directly to oculomotor behavior. Some of the results of these studies will be summarized below. It will be shown how these single unit studies can contribute to understanding the functions of the cerebellum and provide a basis for the interpretation of some clinical findings. This report will concentrate on the role of the cerebellum in immediate changes of oculomotor behavior and not on long term plasticity changes (Miles and Lisberger, 1981a).

SINGLE UNIT STUDIES IN ALERT ANIMALS

The vestibulo-cerebellum (flocculus, paraflocculus, nodulus, uvula) receives, as well as the rest of the cerebellum, input activity via mossy (MF) and climbing (CF) fibers - the latter arising from the inferior olive. The output activity is carried via Purkinje cells (PC) to deep cerebellar nuclei or directly to brain stem structures.

Most single unit studies in alert animals have been performed on the flocculus of the monkey. Animals were exposed to natural vestibular and optokinetic stimulation and trained to fixate small stationary or moving light spots. This allowed the distinction to be made between vestibular, oculomotor and visual mossy fiber (MF) input activity to the vestibulo-cerebellum and to relate PC activity to specific oculomotor paradigms.

FLOCCULUS

Mossy Fiber (MF) Activity

Vestibular input. Responses of central vestibular neurons to horizontal rotation have been classified as type I (activation during rotation to the ipsilateral side) or type II (rotation to the contralateral side) (Duensing and Schaefer, 1958). MF units having responses correlated with vestibular stimulation originate mainly from type I vestibular nuclei neurons on both sides (Waespe and others, 1981): They have a long dominant time constant of 15-20 s (Fig. 1A); and the majority of neurons shows an additional modulation with either fast eye movements or eye position, or both. They also modulate their firing frequency during optokinetic nystagmus. An activation occurs when the optokinetic stimulus moves in the direction opposite to that which elicits a vestibular activation. Under this condition optokinetic and vestibular nystagmus beat in the same direction. During OKN the activity increases up to stimulus velocities of 60 deg/s, on average, and saturates at higher velocities, as it is found for neurons in the vestibular nuclei (Fig. 4, Waespe and Henn, 1977a). When the optokinetic stimulus moves in the opposite direction activity of vestibular input neurons is suppressed (Fig. 1b).

Thus there is a close correlation between the activity of vestibular MF input neurons and vestibular nystagmus and optokinetic nystagmus velocity up to about 60 deg/s. However in many instances these two parameters, neuronal activity and

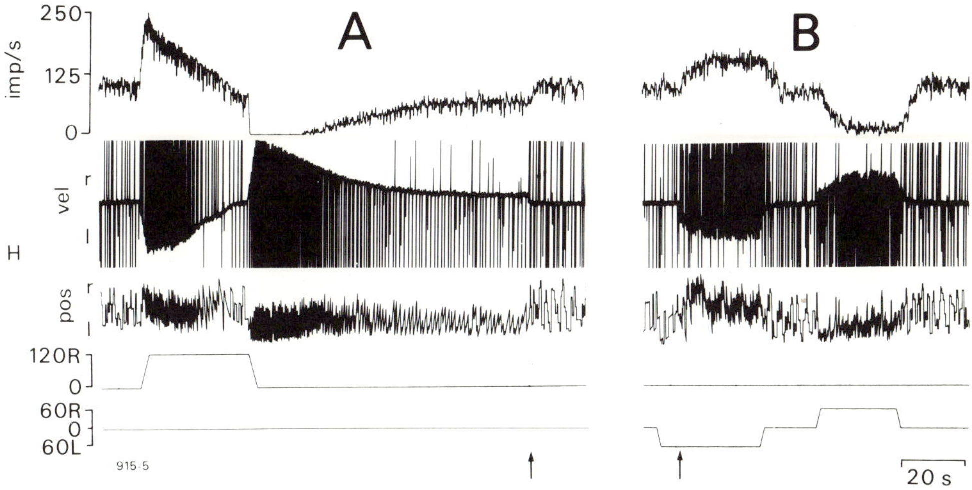

Fig. 1. Type II unit in flocculus driven by vestibular MF input during vestibular (A) and optokinetic stimulation (B). From above: neuronal activity (running average over 250 msec); horizontal eye velocity (first derivative of eye position, velocity of fast phases of nystagmus clipped at an arbitrary level), horizontal eye position, turntable (vestibular) and cylinder (optokinetic) velocity. In (A) the monkey was rotated in clomplete darkness with a velocity trapezoid (acceleration and deceleration 40 deg/s^2, constant velocity 120 deg/s) about a vertical axis. After acceleration and deceleration neuronal activity and nystagmus velocity return to the baseline level with the same time course. Time constant of decay after acceleration is 15-20 s for both neuronal activity and nystagmus velocity. In (B) the rotation of a striped cylinder (constant velocity 60 deg/s) around the stationary monkey leads to an increase or decrease (depending on stimulus direction) in neuronal activity and to optokinetic nystagmus. The arrow in (A) and (B) indicates light on.

nystagmus velocity, dissociate. This can be seen during high velocity OKN or during suppression of vestibular nystagmus either by fixation of a small light spot or in a visual-vestibular conflict situation. In the latter instance input neurons are still modulated (Waespe and others, 1981). A further example of such a dissociation is shown in Fig. 2. The optokinetic drum was stopped in the light and nystagmus ceased, however MF input activity continued at an increased level for another 2-4 s before returning to baseline.

Type I input activity from ipsilateral primary vestibular afferents has not been encountered in the flocculus (Waespe and others, 1981) despite the well known anatomical evidence for such a projection (Carpenter and others, 1972). Physiologically it should be characterized by a short (5-6 s) time constant, no OKN response and no eye movement modulation (Büttner and Waespe, 1981).

Oculomotor input. The majority of MF recorded in the flocculus responds only in relation to eye movements (Miles and others, 1980). Their discharge pattern allows one to distinguish two main classes (Noda and Suzuki, 1979c):

1. Burst neurons are active only prior to and during saccades. They may have a preferred direction or fire with saccades in all directions. Between saccades they are silent. Units can be classified according to their onset of activity as long lead burst neurons (activity starts 50-150 msec before the saccade) or burst neurons (0-20 msec before the saccade).

2. The activity of tonic neurons is related, often linearly, to eye position, increasing as the eye moves in the preferred direction. During sacccades most of these neurons burst in the on-direction and pause in the off-direction in a manner similar to motoneurons. During smooth pursuit and vestibular stimulation tonic neurons show some additional modulation related to eye velocity.

Visual input. A small percentage of neurons (less than 5%) responds exclusively to visual stimulation and not during vestibular stimulation in the dark (Miles and others, 1980; Waespe and others, 1981). Neurons do not respond to light on or off. Response latencies after sudden displacement of a visual scene range from 70-125 msec, suggesting polysynaptic pathways. When eye movements are suppressed during optokinetic stimulation by fixating a small target light, neurons are activated up to velocities of 30 deg/s and saturate at higher velocities. During OKN neuronal responses reflect retinal slip velocity. At higher stimulus velocities the response is related to the difference between nystagmus and stimulus velocity. If the optokinetic stimulus is presented suddenly, there is an initial large response which decreases as nystagmus velocity builds up.

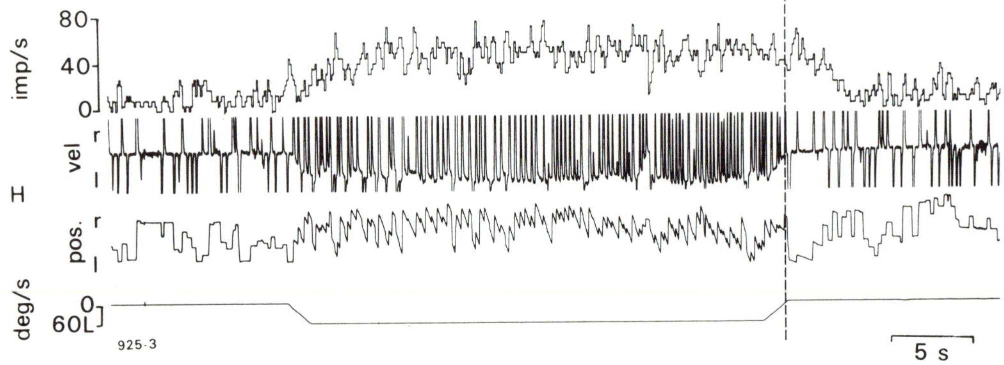

Fig. 2. Typ II unit in flocculus driven by vestibular MF input during and after optokinetic stimulation. From above: neuronal activity (running average), horizontal eye velocity and position, stimulus profile of optokinetic cylinder. Optokinetic stimulation (constant velocity 60 deg/s) leads to an increase in neuronal activity and OKN. OKN stops with end of stimulation (broken line). However, neuronal activity is increased for another 3 sec.

Purkinje Cell (PC) Activity

Spontaneous eye movements. The vast majority of PC in the flocculus of the monkey alter their activity with spontaneous eye movements (Lisberger and Fuchs, 1978; Miles and others, 1980; Waespe and Henn, 1981). In general, PC activity is more irregular and variable than the MF input neurons. During saccades neurons usually pause either in all or only in particular directions. Other neurons show a burst, or a burst and pause, pattern of activity. Activity changes start immediately before saccade onset, too late to allow these neurons to play a role in saccade initiation (Noda and Suzuki, 1979a). While some PC only alter their activity with saccades most of them show an additional modulation with eye position, although their eye position sensitivity is low in comparison to motoneurons (Miles and others, 1980).

Smooth pursuit. 60% of the PC respond specifically during smooth pursuit eye movements (Miles and others, 1980). During sinusoidal tracking the activity is in phase with eye velocity. For these neurons the activity changes during spontaneous eye movements are small compared to those during smooth pursuit. For most neurons the preferred direction is ipsilateral or downward, although contralateral and upward preferred directions are also represented (Miles and others, 1980).

Vestibulo-ocular reflex (VOR) and its suppression. PC show little or no modulation during vestibular stimulation in the dark (Fig. 3A; Lisberger and Fuchs, 1978 ; Miles and others, 1980). If a monkey suppresses his VOR by fixating a small target light, some PC increase their firing rate. Activation occurs for most neurons during VOR suppression to the ipsilateral side. These are the same neurons which increase their firing rate during ipsilateral smooth pursuit. During VOR-suppression neural activity is in phase with head velocity (Fig. 3A). During vestibular stimulation with a fixed visual field (visual-vestibular conflict: optokinetic cylinder mechanically coupled to the turntable; Waespe and Henn, 1981) PC respond weakly at low vestibular accelerations (10 deg/s^2), despite full nystagmus suppression. Only at higher accelerations (40 deg/s^2) do PC show a vigorous response.

The activity pattern of PC during VOR-suppression, either by light-spot fixation or with a fixed visual field, has to be compared with the activity pattern found in the vestibular nuclei. Here the response amplitude is smaller in a fixed visual field (visual-vestibular conflict) situation at low accelerations (10 deg/s^2), but with little or no attenuation at higher accelerations (40 deg/s^2) (Waespe and Henn, 1978). During light-spot fixation the response amplitude is not decreased (Keller and Daniels, 1975; Buettner and Büttner, 1979). Thus vestibular nuclei activity is suppressed during fixed field visual stimulation at low accelerations, a condition under which PC are not active. However PC are active, when vestibular nuclei neurons show a response and nystagmus is suppressed. As will be discussed below, this demonstrates two points. First, under alert conditions modulation of PC activity does not affect vestibular nuclei activity. Second, the suppression of vestibular nuclei activity during fixed field stimulation must originate from structures outside the flocculus which are not yet identified.

Optokinetic nystagmus (OKN) and optokinetic after-nystagmus (OKAN). About 50% of PC which are active during VOR suppression by fixed field stimulation can also be activated by constant velocity optokinetic stimulation (Waespe and Henn, 1981). For type I PC (activation during ipsilateral VOR suppression) the optokinetic stimulus has to move to the ipsilateral side to produce an activation. This is different from the activity pattern in the vestibular nuclei, where the optokinetic and vestibular stimuli have to move in opposite directions to elicit an activation (Waespe and Henn, 1977a). PC only respond at OKN velocities above

30 deg/s. At higher velocities activity increases in parallel with nystagmus velocity (Fig. 4).

PC also show transient responses to optokinetic stimuli. This is particularly evident for type I PC when an optokinetic stimulus is suddenly stopped in the light (Fig. 3B). Then activity shows a transient increase for 2-4 s.

These activity changes have to be compared to those found in the vestibular nuclei. Vestibular nuclei neurons respond already at low nystagmus velocities and saturate at nystagmus velocities above 60 deg/s. During high velocity optokinetic stimulation to the ipsilateral side vestibular nuclei and PC activity act synergistically

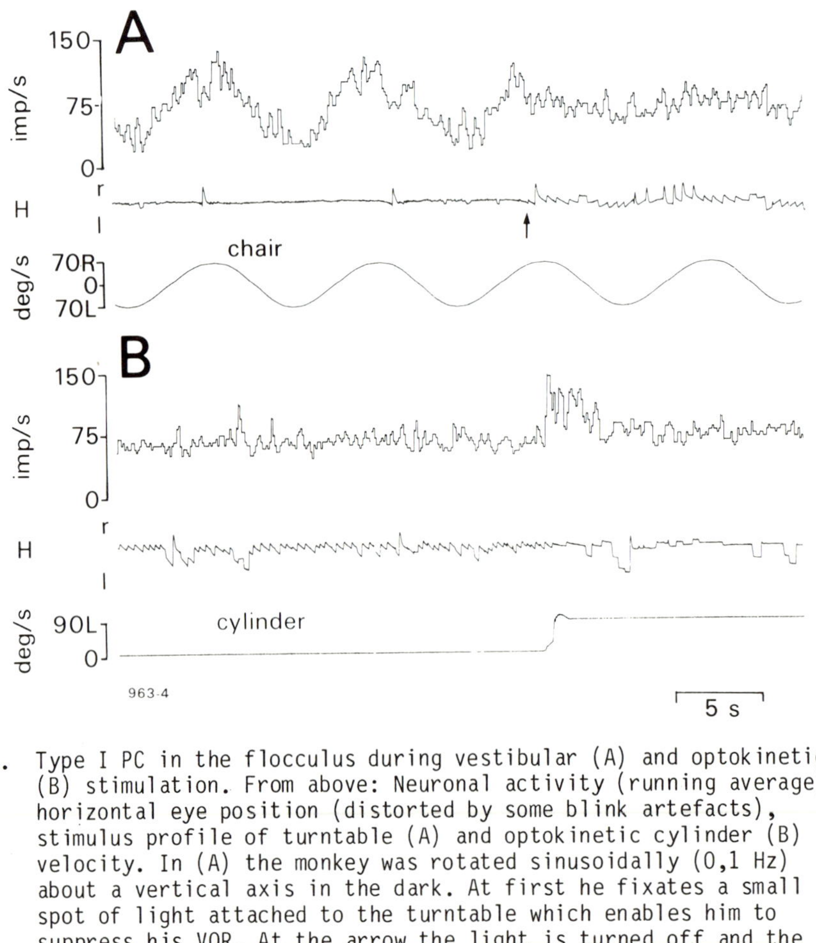

Fig. 3. Type I PC in the flocculus during vestibular (A) and optokinetic (B) stimulation. From above: Neuronal activity (running average), horizontal eye position (distorted by some blink artefacts), stimulus profile of turntable (A) and optokinetic cylinder (B) velocity. In (A) the monkey was rotated sinusoidally (0,1 Hz) about a vertical axis in the dark. At first he fixates a small spot of light attached to the turntable which enables him to suppress his VOR. At the arrow the light is turned off and the monkey has compensatory eye movements. PC activity is deeply modulated during VOR suppression but virtually not during VOR. Activity increases during rotation to the ipsilateral side and is in phase with head velocity. In (B) the monkey was stationary while an optokinetic cylinder rotated with constant velocity to the contralateral side. A transient (ca. 3 s) activity increase occurs when the cylinder is suddenly stopped.

(Fig. 4; Waespe and Henn, 1981; Büttner and Waespe, 1981). The transient PC activity increase after optokinetic stimulation to the contralateral side should have an antagonistic effect and might be used to cancel the vestibular nuclei activity outlasting the optokinetic stimulation (Fig. 2).

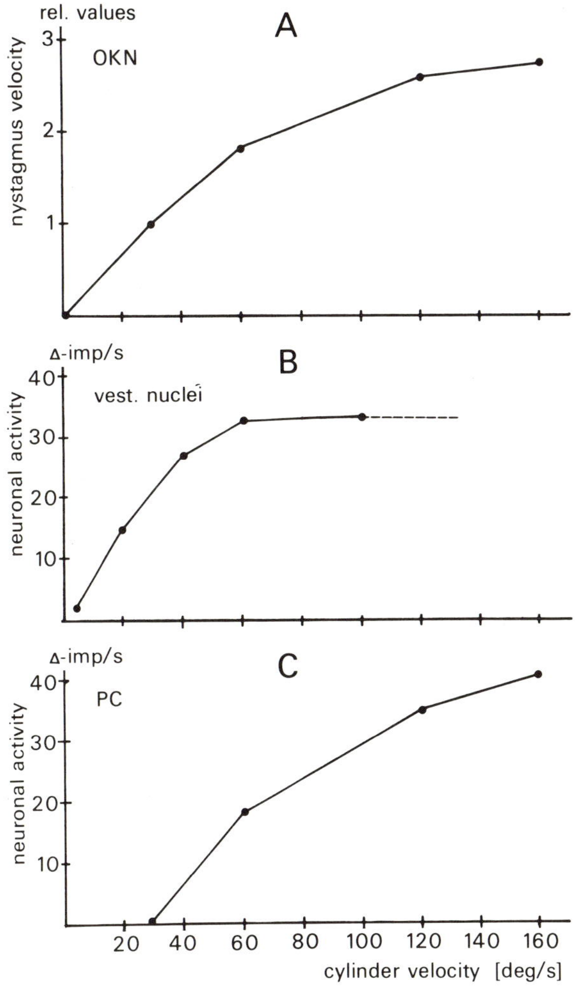

Fig. 4. The activity changes of vestibular nuclei neurons (B) and floccular Purkinje cells (C) in the alert monkey during different velocities of optokinetic stimulation. Optokinetic nystagmus velocity (A) was normalized in relation to values recorded at a stimulus velocity of 30 deg/s. (B) and (C) show the activity increase above resting discharge. Vestibular nuclei activity increases already at low nystagmus velocities, but tends to saturate at stimulus velocities above 60 deg/s. In contrast PC activity only starts to increase at nystagmus velocities above 30 deg/s. At higher nystagmus velocities neuronal activity increases in parallel. Thus the combination of vestibular nuclei and PC activity could provide a signal to drive the eyes over the whole range of optokinetic nystagmus velocities.

If lights are switched off during optokinetic stimulation, nystagmus continues as OKAN, but PC activity immediately returns to baseline levels (Waespe and Henn, 1981). This activity pattern is different from that found in the vestibular nuclei during OKAN (Waespe and Henn, 1977b). During OKAN vestibular nuclei activity decreases in parallel with nystagmus velocity.

PARAFLOCCULUS

A recent single unit study in the paraflocculus of the alert monkey showed that activity during eye movements does not differ significantly from that found in the flocculus (Mikami and others, 1981). In the white matter of the paraflocculus, burst and burst tonic MF eye movement neurons were encountered. PC altered their activity during saccades. Some also showed position related tonic activity. Unit studies to investigate specifically the role of the paraflocculus in slow, conjugate eye movements have not been performed so far.

NODULUS, UVULA

Nodulus and uvula activity has not yet been studied in trained, alert animals. In the anaesthetized rabbit Precht and others (1976) found type I and II vestibular MF responding to angular acceleration with low thresholds and high sensitivity, whereas PC showed high thresholds and low sensitivity.

DEEP CEREBELLAR NUCLEI

Chubb and Fuchs (1981) investigated neurons in the dentate nucleus and the adjacent Y-group of the vestibular nuclei during vertical smooth pursuit. For most neurons an activity increase could be related to eye velocity during upward smooth pursuit and upward head velocity during VOR-suppression. Thus an activity pattern was found similar to that for PC in the flocculus, except that the preferred vertical direction for most floccular PC is downward.

Neurons in the fastigial nucleus were found to respond during vestibular stimulation. They did not show an additional eye movement modulation (Gardner and Fuchs, 1975).

Eye movement related neurons were recently found in all deep cerebellar nuclei of the monkey. The relation of these neurons to slow, conjugate eye movements has yet to be investigated (Hepp and others, 1981).

COMMENT

In the flocculus PC activity has been investigated under a variety of rather specialized paradigms, which makes it difficult to compare results from different laboratories. However there seems to be agreement in some common features.

PC activity is modulated with smooth pursuit, high velocity OKN and VOR suppression either with small target lights, or fixed field stimulation. These oculomotor functions are impaired after floccular lesions in man (Dichgans and others, 1978) and monkey (Takemori and Cohen, 1974; Zee and others, 1981). In contrast, PC show little or no modulation with vestibular nystagmus in the dark, low velocity OKN and OKAN. For the latter conditions the range of activity in the vestibular nuclei is sufficient to drive the oculomotor system. Activity in the vestibular nuclei is proportional to slow phase eye velocity during vestibular nystagmus (Buettner and others, 1978), low velocity OKN and OKAN (Waespe and Henn, 1977a,b). This close correlation between unit activity and eye velocity makes it likely that vestibular nuclei neurons are the principle input for eye velocity under these conditions. However, during high velocity OKN or during VOR suppression vestibular nuclei activity dissociates from eye velocity. Also during smooth pursuit there is no vestibular nuclei activity modulation (Keller and Daniels, 1975). Under these conditions, when oculomotor performance requires an additional signal besides that provided by the vestibular nuclei, the flocculus PC become active.

Therefore we view the flocculus as an important input structure for the oculomotor system which works in synergy with the vestibular nuclei to either modulate eye velocity up or down.

So far it is not clear where this interaction between the flocculus and the vestibular nuclei takes place. Anatomical and electrophysiological evidence suggests an interaction at the vestibular nuclei level (Angaut and Brodal, 1967), which however is not confirmed by single unit recordings in alert animals. Alternatively floccular-brainstem interaction could occur in the perihypoglossal complex, since anatomical connections exist in both directions and neuronal activity can be related to oculomotor, vestibular and visual parameters (Lopez-Barneo and others, 1979).

Since extensive unit studies have been performed only in the flocculus, very little is known about the specific role of the paraflocculus, nodulus, uvula and the deep cerebellar nuclei in the control of slow conjugate eye movements.

As for the motor system in general the cerebellum has a modulating effect on fast eye movements. They are not lost after cerebellectomy (Westheimer and Blair, 1974). For smooth pursuit eye movements however, the cerebellum might play a more basic role. After complete cerebellectomy smooth pursuit is greatly impaired (Westheimer and Blair, 1974). This suggests that the cerebellum does not only improve or correct smooth pursuit, but it plays a role in generating eye movements. After flocculectomy smooth pursuit is partly preserved (Zee and others, 1981), which suggests the participation of other cerebellar structures as well. With this in mind it is interesting to know that in the monkey vermis PC activity similar to the flocculus was recorded during smooth pursuit (Kase and others, 1979).

ACKNOWLEDGEMENTS

Supported by Swiss National Foundation 3.343-78. The authors wish to thank B. Gähler for typing the manuscript, V. Isoviita for assistance during the experiments and J. Müller for photographic work.

SACCADIC DYSMETRIA

L. M. OPTICAN

Laboratory of Sensorimotor Research, National Eye Institute, Bethesda, Maryland, USA

ABSTRACT

Cerebellar ablations in monkeys cause deficiencies in the control of saccadic eye movements. Amplitude dysmetria follows lesions of the dorsal vermis and the fastigial nuclei. Post-saccadic ocular drift appears after lesions of the flocculus. Complete removal of the cerebellum results in both extreme hypermetria and post-saccadic drift. Lesions of the superior colliculus, posterior-medial thalamus and pretectum cause hypometria without corrective saccades. These lesions do not directly alter the saccade generating mechanisms, but rather reveal the cerebellum's involvement with the adaptive mechanisms that maintain orthometria and suppress post-saccadic drift.

A model of the saccadic system with four adaptive gain elements can be used to explain and group the oculomotor signs seen in cerebellar disease, and also provide a hypothetical role for corrective saccades. This scheme suggests that hypermetria, macrosaccadic oscillations, and post-saccadic drift indicate cerebellar dysfunction, while increased saccadic latency, slow saccades, square wave jerks, macro square wave jerks, and hypometria without corrective saccades may indicate involvement of areas outside the cerebellum. The proposed function of the corrective system is to provide an amplitude error signal for adaptive control of dysmetria.

KEYWORDS

Cerebellum; pretectum; posterior-medial thalamus; saccades; dysmetria; corrective saccades; adaptive gain control; vermis; flocculus; vestibulocerebellum.

INTRODUCTION

Saccades are the rapid eye movements used to voluntarily change fixation. In normal, alert subjects saccades are stereotyped. They occur shortly after an unpredictable target jump, are very fast, stop abruptly when the movement is over and are fairly accurate (Fuchs, 1971). The saccades of human beings and monkeys are similar. Over the last few decades studies in both species have helped to elucidate the mechanisms responsible for producing normal saccades. By understanding how normal saccades are generated, it is possible to explain many clinical signs observed in abnormal states.

The saccadic system can be divided into four functional parts: the visual target selection mechanism, the oculomotor periphery (often called the plant), the innervation generator, and the adaptive controllers (sometimes called calibrators). The selection of a target requires consideration of more than just visual information. Saccades can be made to imaginary, auditory or tactile stimuli. Once the target has been selected a command is sent to tell the brainstem saccade generators where to go. It appears that the target selection command does not simply echo the target position, but rather stages a sequence of movements. This part of the system is called the corrective saccade system. It makes a primary saccade short of the target (especially for large movements (Erlandson and Fleming, 1974)), then a corrective saccade to get on target. Retinal error is not required for this corrective saccade. The peripheral oculomotor apparatus is divided functionally into the active force generating elements in the muscle, and all the other elements, which possess both elasticity and viscosity. To make a saccade the innervation generator must produce a high-frequency burst (a pulse of innervation) followed by a sustained, lower, frequency (a step of innervation). The pulse creates a phasic increase in muscle tension that moves the eye rapidly despite the viscous drag of the orbital tissues. The step causes a tonic change in muscle force that holds the eye in its new position against the elastic restoring forces of the orbital tissues (Collins, 1975; Robinson, 1964). The adaptive controllers keep the amplitude of the pulse, and the ratio of the step to the pulse, appropriate (Kommerell, Olivier, and Theopold, 1976; Optican and Robinson, 1980). These adaptive controllers enable the brain to compensate for peripheral or central disorders, making them important in interpreting clinical findings. Studying the effects of ablating different parts of the brain on saccadic control gives insights into the functioning and distribution of the saccadic mechanisms.

EFFECTS OF ABLATIONS ON PRIMATE SACCADES

Cerebellar Lesions

Aschoff and Cohen (1971) reported that saccades in monkeys with cerebellar ablations appeared normal, except for an increase in the number of saccades toward the side of unilateral cerebellar cortical lesions. Westheimer and Blair (1973) reported that saccadic eye movements appeared qualitatively normal after cerebellectomy in monkeys. Blair and Gavin (1979) reported that saccades in vermisectomized monkeys had a higher spontaneous frequency, occurred in short trains of repetitive alternating saccades, and appeared dysmetric. Blair and Gavin also reported an increase in the frequency of vestibular nystagmus in the dark, which might indicate a deficit in the quick-phase mechanism. These three studies used untrained animals, and saccadic accuracy was not assessed.

The first study of the quantitative effects of cerebellar lesions in trained monkeys was carried out by Ritchie (1976). Following lesions of the cerebellar vermis Ritchie noted that saccades made toward the primary position (centripetal movements) were markedly hypermetric, while those made away from the primary position (centrifugal movements) were hypometric. Ritchie also reported that the duration of these dysmetric saccades was constant, i.e., for a 30° target displacement the duration of a hypermetric, centripetal saccade of 40° amplitude was the same as the duration of a hypometric, centrifugal saccade of 24° amplitude. Since these saccades have the same duration but different amplitudes, they cannot lie on the so-called main-sequence of normal saccades (Bahill, Clark, and Stark, 1975 a).

Vilis and Hore (1980) reversibly cooled the fastigial and interposed nuclei in trained monkeys. They found a transient saccadic dysmetria. Centripetal saccades were hypermetric, while centrifugal saccades were either hypermetric or hypometric. These dysmetric saccades, however, had normal main-sequence relationships, with large amplitude saccades having longer durations than small amplitude saccades.

In another study Optican and Robinson (1980) ablated the midline vermis and fastigial nuclei in two monkeys (see Fig. 1A). One monkey (LZ) had a large lesion of the vermian cortex and an 80% complete ablation of the fastigial nuclei. The centripetal saccades in this monkey were hypermetric in both directions (to the left and right). The gain (expressed as the ratio of the amplitude of the initial saccade to the amplitude of the target jump) for 20° centripetal target movements was 1.6. The centrifugal saccades in this animal were only slightly hypermetric, having a gain for 20° target movements of 1.1. In all the monkeys studied, the gain was always higher for centripetal than for centrifugal saccades (see below).

A second monkey's (ML) lesion was more extensive in the midline and more restricted laterally. All of the vermian cortex from Larsell's lobe IVb to lobe IX was removed, as well as all of the fastigial nuclei bilaterally. In this animal saccades in both directions were markedly hypermetric. The gain for centripetal saccades to 20° target displacements in this monkey was 2.1, while the gain for centrifugal movements to the same size target displacement was 1.5. The time course of each individual saccade appeared normal, but comparisons were difficult because of variability in the amplitude-duration relationship.

The difference between Ritchie's findings and those of Vilis and Hore and Optican and Robinson on the constancy of saccadic duration have not been resolved. The differences in the findings about the amplitude dysmetria can be understood if the hypothesis is made that the larger the lesion, the more hypermetric saccades are in all directions. The ablations of Optican and Robinson and the effects of cooling the deep cerebellar nuclei, as done by Vilis and Hore, appear to involve a larger area of the dorsal vermis than that lesioned by Ritchie. Centrifugal saccades are usually a little hypometric even in normal animals (Optican and Robinson, 1980; Ritchie, 1976). Thus a pattern of hypermetric centripetal and hypometric centrifugal saccades would appear after small lesions. (It must be emphasized that large cerebellar lesions result in large gains in animals for all directions. The large gains might be offset by movement strategies that call for many small saccades to acquire the target. This would make subjects with high gains appear hypometric unless accuracy were quantified in a special paradigm that defeated the strategy of making small steps. It is also possible to transiently decrease saccadic gain after the primary saccade (see below). Therefore, one must always specify how saccadic gain was measured.)

Glissades (saccades with post-saccadic, exponentially slowing, ocular drift) have been observed in totally cerebellectomized monkeys (Optican and Robinson, 1980) and in monkeys with floccular lobe ablations (Optican and colleagues, 1980; Zee, this symposium). In animals with bilateral floccular lesions, the saccades appeared to have normal amplitude, but were followed by post-saccadic drift. This drift was presumed due to a step of innervation that was inappropriate for the pulse of the antecedent saccade.

Saccades in the totally cerebellectomized monkeys were also hypermetric (Fig. 1B). The gains in one monkey for a 10° target jump were 2.4 for centripetal and 2.1 for centrifugal saccades. The post-saccadic drift carried the eyes onward after the saccade, and the gains of the final, or step-determined positions relative to the target amplitudes were 2.7 for centripetal and 3.0 for centrifugal movements. Expressing the amount of drift as a percentage of the pulse-driven saccadic amplitude, a simple measure results: the pulse-step mismatch, which was -15% for

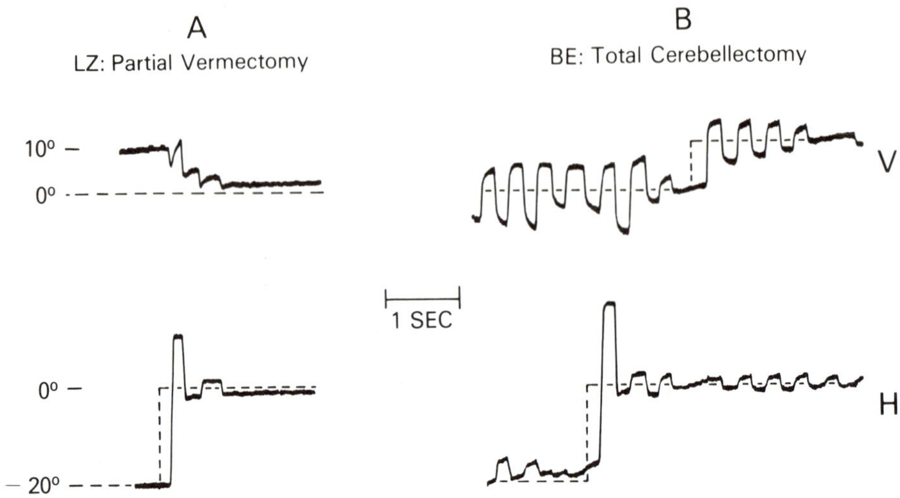

Fig. 1. Refixation saccades in monkeys with cerebellar ablations. A. Monkey with partial ablations of the dorsal vermis and fastigial nuclei. The target jumps from 20° left to zero. Monkey LZ responds with a series of hypermetric saccades. Note that there is no post-saccadic drift in the horizontal direction. B. Monkey with complete ablation of cerebellum. The target jumps from 20° left to zero, then to 10° up. Monkey BE responds with a series of hypermetric saccades. Note the presence of post-saccadic drift and macrosaccadic oscillations. H is horizontal, V is vertical component of eye movement. Dashed lines indicate target position.

centripetal and -47% for centrifugal saccades.

In intact animals saccadic dysmetrias of this magnitude created by peripheral disorders (Optican and Robinson, 1980) or optically-induced retinal slips (Optican and Miles, 1979) can be compensated within a few days. Yet the ocular dysmetria following cerebellar lesions is enduring. Attempts to elicit adaptation in cerebellectomized animals have revealed that the area of the posterior vermis and the fastigial nuclei is essential for the adaptive control of the pulse of innervation, which determines the rapid part of the saccade, and the area of the cerebellar flocculus is essential for the adaptive control of the step of innervation, which determines the final eye position (Optican and colleagues, 1980; Optican and Robinson, 1980).

Lesions of the Posterior-medial Thalamus and Pretectum

Recent studies by Albano and Wurtz (1981) have discovered a new type of saccadic dysmetria. In attempts to make a complete lesion of the superior colliculus, they found that in some monkeys areas farther anterior were also damaged. In the one animal whose lesion was restricted to the superior colliculus alone, saccades were essentially normal. Three animals with unilateral lesions of the superior colliculus, the mesodiencephalic junction, and the posterior-medial region of the dorsal thalamus could not acquire targets on the contralateral side. A target jump was followed by a single, hypometric saccade. No contralateral corrective saccades were seen at any time. Even though the target remained lit for several seconds, these monkeys never made another saccade to acquire the target. Except for the zero target position, all saccades ended with a steady-state position error. These steady-state position errors were larger for more eccentric positions of the target. The hypometria and loss of corrective saccades endured for as long as four months (when the monkey was sacrificed).

AN ADAPTIVE-CONTROL MODEL OF SACCADE GENERATION

Hypermetria and post-saccadic drift onward after cerebellar lesions are consistent with the hypothesis that the pulse gain and the step gain of the brainstem saccade generating system are normally greater than one (Optican, 1978). The function of the cerebellum would then be to exert an inhibitory controlling influence over the brainstem to lower the gains to unity. Since the amplitude-peak-velocity and amplitude-duration characteristics of saccades do not change during adaptation (Optican, 1978), the control of the pulse gain must be accomplished indirectly. A model incorporating these results can explain how the adaptive influences of the cerebellum are exerted on the brainstem saccadic system.

A model that simplifies the relationship between the brain and the sensorimotor periphery is shown in Fig. 2. (All the dynamic components and time delays have been removed.) The viscosity of the orbital tissues is the dominant factor in the mechanics of the orbit (Robinson, 1964). Hence some mechanism for generating both a pulse and a step of force is needed to make a saccade (Collins, 1975; Robinson, 1973). It has been proposed that the pulse of innervation needed to move the eye is generated, and then (mathematically) integrated to derive the step of innervation needed to hold the eye in the new position. This mechanism is plausible, since the presence of a neural integrator has been established in the vestibular system (Fernandez and Goldberg, 1971; Skavenski and Robinson, 1973). The model in Fig. 2 is based on a continuous saccadic pulse generator that works in spatial coordinates (Robinson, 1975a). Variable gain elements have been added to allow adaptive control of saccades (Optican, 1978). The gains of the pulse and step are independent, which fixes the placement of G_s, and the saccade dynamics do not change during adaptation, which restricts the location of $G_{\hat{T}}$ and $G_{\hat{E}}$ to be before the pulse generator.

Consider how the model makes a saccade to a visual target. After the target (T) moves, the eye position (E) is no longer appropriate, creating a retinal error (e_r). This error is added to a neural estimate ($\hat{E}$) of the eye position to convert the retinocentric error into a target position in spatial coordinates. This reconstruction of the target in space is scaled by the gain $G_{\hat{T}}$ to obtain a neural estimate ($\hat{T}$) of the point in space where the fovea will align with the target. This desired point in space is fed into the corrective subsystem. This subsystem generates the neural command for desired eye position (E_d). E_d immediately assumes the value G_{ps} times $\hat{T}$ (giving rise to the primary saccade), and after a delay (normally) jumps to the value $\hat{T}$ (making a corrective saccade). The pulse generator (PG) makes a burst of innervation appropriate for the value of E_d. This pulse is turned into the step of innervation by the neural integrator (NI). The output of the neural integrator is used in two ways. After being weighted by G_s, it becomes the step of innervation sent to the oculomotor plant. After being scaled by $G_{\hat{E}}$ it becomes $\hat{E}$, the neural estimate of eye position which is used to transform from retinal to spatial coordinates. The combined pulse and step of innervation drive the plant, which has gain G_p, making an eye movement.

Considerable evidence now exists to support the continuous generation of the pulse of innervation by local feedback (Jürgens, Becker, and Kornhuber, 1981; Mays and Sparks, 1980), but the lack of direct evidence in the past has caused many to question the concept of spatial coordinates in saccadic control. However, an exciting inference can be drawn from the recent results of Albano and Wurtz (1981). Their monkeys with extensive lesions made hypometric saccades which were

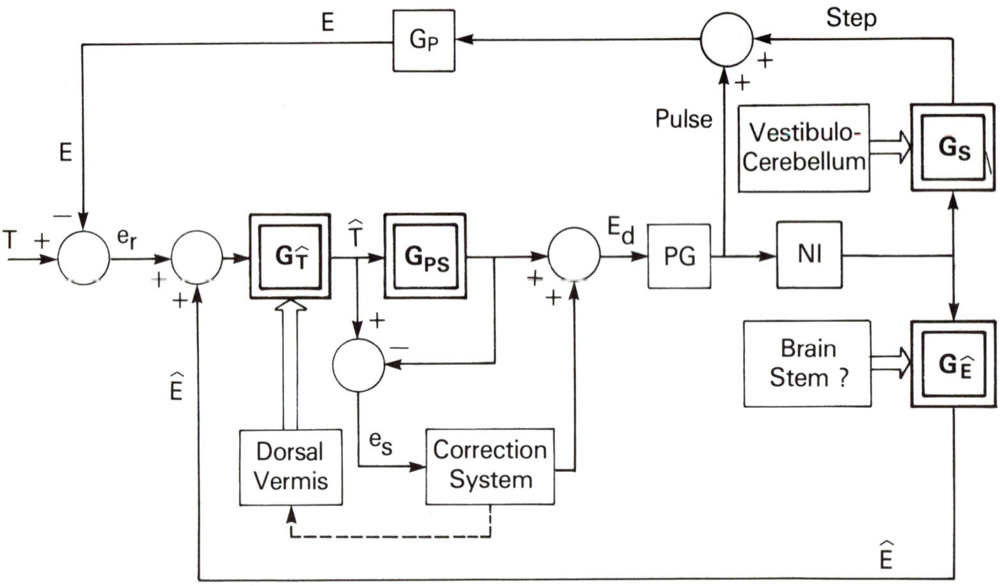

Fig. 2. Adaptive control of the saccadic system. The task of the saccadic system is to provide the proper input for the plant, which has a gain of G_P. Four variable gains (double boxes) are needed. $G_{\hat{T}}$ is adjusted to be approximately $1/G_P$, so that saccades are essentially orthometric. $G_{\hat{E}}$ is adjusted to be equal to $1/G_{\hat{T}}$, so that steady-state eye position matches target position. G_{PS} is the gain of the primary saccade in the corrective saccade system. It is adjusted to be less than one, so that the adaptive controller of $G_{\hat{T}}$ can obtain an error signal from the corrective system (dashed line). G_S is the gain of the step of innervation. It is adjusted to make the pulse-step ratio match the viscoelastic ratio of the plant, to suppress post-saccadic ocular drift.

not corrected, even after several seconds. That means that their animal's saccadic systems were tolerating a non-zero retinal error. A retinocentric saccadic system, by definition, attempts to reduce retinal errors. The retinal error after a saccade is not qualitatively different from the retinal error before a saccade. Hence a sustained, or steady-state, retinal error indicates that the saccadic system is not using retinal error directly. This finding provides strong support for working in spatial coordinates.

The spatial coordinate model of Robinson (1975a) can be modified to allow an elegant interpretation of the lesion results from both the cerebellum and the pretectum and posterior-medial thalamus. The new model provides hypotheses for why normal primary saccades usually fall short, why a corrective system exists at all, and why the hypometric saccades in the pretectum and posterior-medial thalamus lesioned monkeys were not compensated by the adaptive gain controller. The modification is to add a subsystem that allows the model to make corrective saccades. The new hypothesis of this model is that the corrective system exists to provide the error signal for the adaptive control of saccadic amplitude. (The subsystem shown in Fig. 2 is an oversimplification of corrective saccadic properties, but serves for this purpose.) Since the saccadic system is working in spatial coordinates and is inside the efference copy feedback loop (which cancels the physical feedback of eye position), it is difficult for it to obtain an error signal indicating the presence of dysmetria. The corrective system, however, is ideal for this, since it can determine the retinal error remaining between the fovea and the selected target and compare that with the expected retinal error obtained by commanding a short primary saccade. The simple corrective subsystem used here consists of two parts. The first is a direct pathway that establishes a gain for the primary saccade (G_{ps}). This gain must be less than one (see below), and there appears to be an adaptive control system that adjusts this gain to be less than one after only a few saccades (Henson, 1978). The second is an indirect pathway that looks at the expected retinal error after the primary saccade, e_s, and compares it with the real retinal error. If nothing is amiss, the correction is issued. If the errors do not match closely enough, the corrective saccade is not issued, and a new, visually guided saccade is generated. In addition, the corrective system sends an error signal (dashed line in Fig. 2) to the adaptive controller responsible for dysmetria compensation. If the purpose of the corrective system is to provide an amplitude error signal to an adaptive controller, it explains why the primary saccade falls short. It takes much longer to make a corrective saccade in the direction opposite to that of the primary saccade, presumably because the correction command must be generated on the other side of the brain. In order to reduce the probability that an unexpected retinal error is due to the motion of the target, it makes sense to keep the correction computations as short as possible. That means making G_{ps} less than one, so that the expected correction will usually be in the same direction as the primary saccade.

The purpose of the adaptive control systems is to keep the performance of the saccadic system appropriate despite degradation of individual components of the oculomotor system. For example, while G_p is normally one, disease, trauma or ageing can make it decline in value. Also, due to changes in the orbital tissues, the viscoelastic ratio of the plant might change. If the viscoelastic ratio changes, the ratio of the pulse to the step of innervation would be inappropriate, and there would be post-saccadic drift. This ocular drift would give rise to a retinal image slip that would be correlated with the direction of the antecedent saccade. An adaptive control system depending on the vestibulocerebellum would adjust the gain of the step, G_s, so that the post-saccadic slip would be suppressed. If the static gain of the plant were decreased, saccades would fall short (hypometria). The estimated saccadic error, e_s, would no longer match the true retinal error, e_r, after each primary saccade. This mismatch would give rise to an amplitude error signal (dashed line in Fig. 2) that would be sent to an adaptive control system depending on the dorsal vermis. The gain of the desired target position in space, $G_{\hat{T}}$, would be changed until it would be approximately the reciprocal of G_p. While $G_{\hat{T}}$ was changing, another adaptive control system (at this time its location is unknown, except that cerebellectomy does not seem to affect it) would be keeping $G_{\hat{E}}$ equal to the reciprocal of $G_{\hat{T}}$. (This is essential in order for the saccadic system to acquire the target in the steady-state.)

With this model all the results of cerebellar and brainstem lesions in monkeys can be understood. Cerebellar lesions leave the brainstem saccadic pulse generator intact. Since it is the pulse-generator that determines the saccadic waveform, qualitative assessments of saccade performance will appear normal (see Keller, this symposium). Lesions of the dorsal vermis release the adaptive control mechanism's inhibition of the brainstem gain $G_{\hat{T}}$, resulting in hypermetria. The more extensive the damage to the vermian cortex and fastigial nuclei, the greater the saccadic hypermetria. Since normal centrifugal saccades are a little hypometric, this means that incomplete lesions will result in a pattern of centripetal hypermetria and centrifugal hypometria. Lesions of the vestibulocerebellum release the brainstem gain G_s from inhibition, causing the step to be too large for the pulse. This results in a post-saccadic drift onward. In general, enduring saccadic dysmetrias imply a lesion of the the midline vermis and fastigial nuclei, while enduring post-saccadic drifts, or glissades, imply a lesion of the vestibulocerebellum.

Lesions of the other two gains would give rise to very interesting behavior. If G_{ps} were lesioned, saccades would become hypometric. If the corrective pathway were intact, the eye would get to the target by making many small steps. This would cause the adaptive controller to increase $G_{\hat{T}}$ to compensate for the hypometria. If the corrective saccade subsystem were lesioned, say by removing the pathway which delays the expected error and compares it with the actual post-saccadic error, then no corrective saccades could occur. Because G_{ps} is less than one, all saccades would now be hypometric. Furthermore, since there would be no error signal for the amplitude adaptive controller, no compensation for these hypometric saccades could occur. Hence lesions of the corrective system result in an enduring hypometria without corrective saccades. Since $G_{\hat{T}}$ and $G_{\hat{E}}$ are assumed to be appropriate in this case, the neural feedback of $\hat{E}$ would cancel the physical feedback of E. Thus the saccadic system would be operating essentially open-loop, with a gain less than one. The steady-state error would simply be proportional to the eccentricity of the target. Because this is a true position dependent error, and not a retinocentric error, the saccade system can acquire the zero position accurately from any orbital position. This behavior of hypometria without corrective saccades, and steady-state error proportional to target eccentricity, is exactly what has been seen by Albano and Wurtz (1981).

If $G_{\hat{E}}$ were not equal to $1/G_{\hat{T}}$, the neural estimate of the target's position in space ($\hat{T}$) would be inappropriate. After every saccade, the target would appear to move, and corrective saccades would occur until the eye finally stopped away from the true target. Hence a lesion of $G_{\hat{E}}$ would cause the eye to exhibit dysmetria with corrective saccades that acquire an incorrect final position. There has not yet been a report of this type of behavior in animals or patients.

SACCADIC DYSMETRIA IN HUMAN CEREBELLAR DISEASE

The model in Fig. 2 has been based largely on data from monkey experiments. However, the adaptive behavior of human patients is very similar to that of monkeys (Abel and colleagues, 1978; Kommerell, Olivier, and Theopold, 1976; Zee, this symposium), so it seems reasonable to use this model to examine oculomotor dysfunction seen in human patients. A patient with a central neurological disorder can present with three basic types of saccadic abnormality: errors in timing, errors in waveform, or errors in saccadic accuracy. According to the model, the cerebellum influences only saccadic accuracy and post-saccadic drift, all other deficits originating elsewhere.

Errors In Saccade Timing

On examination a patient may make saccades with inappropriate timing. These might be either saccades with a latency beyond 250 msec, or unexpected saccades. Saccadic latency in monkeys with cerebellar lesions appears normal (Vilis and Hore, 1980). In cerebellar diseases where increased saccadic latency has been reported, there is also an involvement of brainstem structures (Baloh, Yee and Boder, 1978). Increased latency is also found in brainstem diseases, such as Parkinson's, that do not involve the cerebellum (DeJong and Melvill Jones, 1971). Hence it is inferred that increased latency is a sign of brainstem, and not cerebellar, dysfunction.

A frequently observed sign in cerebellar patients is an inappropriate saccade away from the fixation point followed immediately by a return saccade (see Daroff, this symposium). These are of two types: square wave jerks and macro square wave jerks. Square wave jerks (SWJ) are small (less than 3°) and include a normal intersaccadic interval of about 200 msec before the return to fixation. Macro square wave jerks (MSWJ) are large (4° to 50°) but have reduced intersaccadic latency, from 50 to 150 msec, before the return saccade. Neither SWJ nor MSWJ have been reported in cerebellectomized monkeys. Since the eye returns accurately to the fixation point after the SWJ or MSWJ, it seems unlikely that these reflect cerebellar dysfunction. It might be supposed that SWJ or MSWJ occur when spurious initiation commands are generated. Because of the diffuse nature of the diseases associated with SWJ and MSWJ (multiple sclerosis (Dell'Osso, Troost, and Daroff, 1975), presenile dementia of the Alzheimer type (Feldon and Langston, 1977), acute encephalopathy (Dell'Osso, Abel, and Daroff, 1977), and Friedreich's ataxia (Dale, Kirby, and Jampel, 1978)), it is possible that they are caused by cerebral or brainstem dysfunction, and not directly by cerebellar dysfunction.

Errors In Waveform

Patients may present with various forms of abnormal saccadic waveform; the two most common being slow saccades and glissades. Slow saccades are not seen in monkeys with cerebellar lesions. In patients with slow saccades, there is often also an involvement of the brainstem. The speed of a saccade appears to be determined by the short-lead burst cells in the pontine reticular formation (horizontal saccades) and in the mesencephalic reticular formation (vertical saccades) (Keller, 1974; King and Fuchs, 1979). Hence, slow saccades are nosologic for lesions of the brainstem and not the cerebellum (Avanzini and colleagues, 1979; Larmande and Autret, 1980; Zee and colleagues, 1976a).

When a patient presents with glissadic eye movements it indicates a mismatch between the pulse and step of innervation. If this problem is chronic, and not due to a peripheral motor deficit, the adaptive control system responsible for controlling the step gain must itself be deficient. Otherwise, irrespective of the pulse gain, the step gain would always be adjusted to minimize retinal slip (Optican and Robinson, 1980). Hence enduring post-saccadic drift indicates a vestibulocerebellar lesion.

If the condition is acute (less than a day or two), however, it could be that the pulse gain is inappropriate, and the adaptive controller for the step gain has not yet had time to adjust for the orbital-position dependent viscoelasticity. The difference can be revealed by examining the patient's ability to refixate between two targets held about 20° apart, with one directly in front of the patient. On refixation from the peripheral to the central target, a marked undershoot or overshoot of the rapid part of the movement would indicate midline cerebellar involvement (see below) while a floating or drifting movement as the eye approaches the central target would indicate a vestibulocerebellar lesion. (Note that even normal subjects occasionally exhibit glissades, especially when fatigued (Bahill and Stark, 1975).) An enduring combination of dysmetria and drift would indicate lesions in both areas.

Errors In Saccade Metrics

The most common finding in cerebellar disorders in both patients and monkeys is saccadic amplitude dysmetria. This disorder is usually a hypermetria (Cogan, 1956), although depending on amplitude, direction, and whether it is centrifugal or centripetal it can also manifest as a hypometria.

Hypermetric saccades, often associated with hypometric saccades, are seen in cerebellar lesions (Avanzini and colleagues, 1979; Larmande and Autret, 1980; Selhorst and colleagues, 1976a; Zee and colleagues, 1976b). Hypometria and hypermetria do not seem to be of any use in localizing the site of the lesion, except that

Larmande and Autret (1980) have noted that in some patients with asymmetrical dysmetrias to the right and left, the centrifugal saccades toward the lesion were regularly hypometric.

In some patients, the saccadic hypermetria is so great that saccadic oscillations occur. These saccadic oscillations are centered about the fixation point, and saccades are separated by normal intersaccadic intervals. Selhorst and colleagues (1976b) have explained these oscillations as being due to a saccade gain greater than two. Such oscillations then result because the attempt to fixate carries the eye beyond the target, requiring a series of refixation saccades. In principal, each saccade should be a little larger than the previous one, but some system acts to reduce the gain of subsequent saccades, so that their envelope is shaped like a spindle: growing in size and then shrinking (see Stark, this symposium).

Perhaps the reason that hypometria and hypermetria are of such little use clinically lies in the existence of other adaptive mechanisms which function at other levels when the cerebellum is affected. For example, Estanol, Romero and Corvera (1979) have reported a patient with an almost total functional cerebellectomy: one half of the cerebellum was removed surgically, and seven years later a tumor developed in the remaining hemisphere. Surprisingly, this patient showed no saccadic dysmetria (although other oculomotor signs, such as inability to maintain eccentric gaze, failure of smooth pursuit, etc. were noted). Perhaps when the loss of the cerebellum occurs gradually, or in stages, the brainstem gains (which are intrinsically greater than one) can be lowered. Alternatively, the visual system processing might be altered, so that sequences of short eye movement commands are sent to the brainstem generator.

Although dysmetric saccades in human patients seem to be of limited diagnostic use, the results of animal studies suggest that careful, quantitative clinical testing can improve their usefulness in localizing the site and extent of cerebellar and brainstem lesions. Testing of saccadic performance must allow accurate recording of absolute eye and target position (i.e., DC-coupled). The test must require the patient to follow a small target light that can jump unexpectedly to unpredictable locations. the patient should be instructed to follow the light as quickly and accurately as possible. The test should include target amplitudes up to 30°, and both left and right directions. The target should be made to jump both away from the center (centrifugal) and toward the center (centripetal). The records should have a temporal resolution of at least 25 mm/sec.

The evaluation of saccadic performance should be based only on those saccades that follow target jumps with the shortest latency. The gain of these primary saccades can be calculated (as the ratio of the saccadic amplitude to the antecedent retinal error) to give a measure of performance. From the monkey studies it can be inferred that the more pronounced the hypermetria the more extensive is the lesion of the posterior vermis, paravermis and fastigial nuclei. If centripetal saccades are hypermetric while centrifugal saccades are hypometric, small lesions of the dorsal vermis or fastigial nuclei should be suspected. Also, the presence of steady-state errors or lack of corrective saccades must be looked for. If saccadic hypometria is associated with a loss of corrective saccades and a steady-state non-zero retinal error proportional to target eccentricity, one might suspect damage to the mesodiencephalic junction and posterior-medial region of the dorsal thalamus (Albano and Wurtz, 1981), rather than a cerebellar disorder.

CONCLUSION

Basic scientific investigations into the effects of cerebellar lesions on saccadic eye movements have provided new insights into the mechanisms underlying saccadic oculomotor signs in patients with cerebellar disease. Some signs, such as transient loss of fixation due to back-to-back saccades or increased latency are not seen in monkeys, which suggests that they might be due to lesions outside the cerebellum. Enduring hypermetria of saccadic eye movements appears nosologic for lesions of posterior, midline cerebellar structures (particularly the vermis and paravermis, Larsell's lobes IV to VII, and the fastigial nuclei), while enduring post-saccadic drifts, or glissades, indicate lesions of the vestibulocerebellum.

An enduring hypometria without corrective saccades, where the steady-state error is proportional to eccentricity, has been seen in monkeys with lesions of the superior colliculus, pretectum and posterior-medial thalamus. Similar deficits can be looked for in patients. A new deficit, dysmetria with corrective saccades converging to the wrong point, has been predicted by an adaptive-control model. This predicted deficit awaits clinical or experimental confirmation. The simple model described above summarizes the relationship between different parts of the brain and different functions of the saccadic system. Analysis of the model shows that clinical testing of saccades must be conducted with careful attention to whether or not the saccades actually acquire the correct target position. Observing that the eye jumps in the direction of the target, and perhaps even makes a few corrective saccades in the vicinity of the target, is no longer sufficient. Failure to acquire the target must now be recognized as a sign of possible brainstem lesions, rather than merely a failure of vision or motivation.

Further studies joining clinical examples with laboratory experiments can provide a better understanding of the eye movements seen in health and disease, and help to define more specific clinical tests. Quantitative models of normal and abnormal behavior are essential to our understanding of neurology and neurophysiology. Even very simple models, such as the functional block diagram in Fig. 2, can help organize data from diverse sources, and establish test procedures capable of distinguishing deficits of different origins. Such models can act as mnemonic aids to clinicians and investigators, delineating areas of ignorance as well as knowledge.

NEURONAL DISCHARGE IN THE POSTERIOR CEREBELLUM: ITS RELATIONSHIP TO SACCADIC EYE MOVEMENT GENERATION

J. G. MCELLIGOTT* and E. L. KELLER**

**Department of Pharmacology, Temple University School of Medicine, 3420 N. Broad Street, Philadelphia, PA 19140, USA*
***Smith-Kettlewell Institute of Visual Sciences, 2232 Webster Street, San Francisco, CA 94115 and Department of Electrical Engineering and Computer Science, University of California, Berkeley, California, USA*

ABSTRACT

Experiments were conducted in trained monkeys to clarify the role played by neurons in the posterior vermis of the cerebellum in regulating voluntary saccadic eye movements. Major findings include the following: (1) Purkinje cells of the vermal region in the primate are involved in the preprogamming of saccadic eye movements; (2) there is almost a direct relationship between saccadic amplitude and magnitude of cell firing; (3) a majority of Purkinje cells show dramatic differences in saccade-related discharge modulation related to initial eye position. Since input fibers do not show this dependence, the cerebellar cortex is implicated in its development; (4) stimulation studies support the idea of major cerebellar involvement in the compensation for initial eye position so that saccades directed into the primary position have the same velocity profiles as outward directed movements.

KEYWORDS

Cerebellar vermis; saccadic control; eye movements; oculomotor system; saccadic dysmetria.

INTRODUCTION

Certain pathological disturbances within the saccadic system have long been associated with cerebellar dysfunction and in particular with lesions of the posterior vermal region (Cogan, 1956; Daroff and Hoyt, 1971). Recent clinical studies have more precisely defined these deficits to include saccadic dysmetria, macrosaccadic oscillations and square-wave jerks (Zee and others, 1976b, Selhorst and others, 1976b). Confirmation of these findings have been produced in monkeys with experimentally induced lesions of the posterior vermis (see Optican, this volume).

Such studies, including extensive vermal ablations, indicate that dysmetric saccades are made following the lesions (Ritchie, 1976), but that these animals produce saccades with normal amplitude-velocity relationships (Aschoff and Cohen, 1971; Westheimer and Blair, 1974). In addition, Ritchie (1976) showed that the degree and sign of the dysmetria was dependent on initial eye position in the orbit. Finally, lesion studies in the vermis of monkeys suggest that this structure plays a role in the compensatory correction of saccadic dysmetria induced by other neural or ocular muscle injuries (Optican and Robinson, 1980).

Recently, rather spectacular advances have been made in understanding the neural organization of the oculomotor system in other regions of the brain. These advances have been generated by the knowledge gained from lesion studies followed by single-unit recording studies of the same region in intact, waking monkeys. The best example of this approach has been concerned with the organization of the medial pontine reticular formation. Lesion studies first circumscribed a small region of the brain stem core (Bender and Shanzer, 1964), which is essential for the production of horizontal gaze shifts. Subsequent detailed single-unit studies of this region (Luschei and Fuchs, 1972; Keller, 1974; Henn and Cohen, 1976) provided considerable data on the types of local neurons involved in saccadic eye movements and led to a model (Robinson, 1975a)which is now widely accepted as a working hypothesis of how the immediate supranuclear saccadic system is organized.

With respect to the vermis, only a limited number of single-unit recording studies have been carried out to aid in the interpretation of the cerebellar lesion studies. Llinas and Wolfe (1977) reported that vermal Purkinje cells could be found whose discharge occurred in bursts which preceded certain saccadic eye movements. Furthermore, the intensity of these bursts was inversely related to the size of the saccade. In more quantitative studies in the cat (McElligott, 1979; Waterhouse and McElligott, 1980) and in the monkey (Kase and others, 1980) several interesting but complex temporal relationships between vermal unit discharge and various parameters of saccadic eye movements have been reported. Studies of this type have the added advantage that the same microelectrode recording penetrations can be used to record from identified Purkinje cells (cerebellar output) and from directly underlying mossy fibers (cerebellar input). Therefore, it should be possible to deduce how the cerebellar cortex has processed and elaborated saccadic control signals. One overriding characteristic of cerebellar unit discharge severely limits this optimistic assessment. This characteristic is the irregular, high-frequency spontaneous discharge of Purkinje cells and their apparent high degree of response variability. Taken together these factors require that discharge responses of each cell be averaged for a number of similar saccades in order to uncover possible systematic movement related unit modulations. We have undertaken such an approach in well trained monkeys using a computer program previously developed for this purpose in the cat (Mays and McElligott, 1976).

RESULTS

The discharge patterns of Purkinje cells and mossy fiber axons were recorded in those specific vermal regions (lobules V, VI and VII) implicated in the control of the saccadic system by previous lesion and stimulation studies. All units isolated in each microelectrode penetration in this region were recorded with the monkey training on a standard oculomotor paradigm to be described below. Possible unit relationship to various saccadic metrics were subsequently examined off-line by computer analysis.

Purkinje cells (P-cells) were identified by the presence of a climbing fiber response. We also recorded from a number of other cells with similar simple spike discharge patterns in which we did not positively see a complex spike discharge. These cells have been included within the P-cell category because there were no obvious differences in their quantitative discharge relations to saccades.

In these same monkeys we were able to record from fibers projecting into the vermal cortex. These units were identified as fibers by the standard extracellular criterion (King and others, 1976) and also by their patterns of activity. The discharge of these units occurred in short, transient bursts of activity without the high-frequency irregular background always seen in identified P-cells. However, since we cannot positively identify the origin of these units, we will call them vermal input elements following the similar terminology of Miles and others (1980) in the flocculus.

In the standard paradigm the monkey sat facing a screen in a dimly lighted room. The target image was backprojected on the screen and consisted of a single spot subtending about one-half degree of visual angle on an otherwise featureless background. An auditory cue (buzzer) sounded at a fixed interval before light presentation to alert the animal to an upcoming trial. The target spot then appeared at an eccentric position (up, down, left, or right with equal probability). The monkey was required to foveate the target and hold fixation for a one-second period. If this condition were met, the target jumped to the primary position, a condition which required an inward directed saccade and a new period of fixation. The target then jumped in the same direction to the opposite eccentric position. When the monkey had again fixated on the final target position, a small liquid reward was automatically delivered. Thus a successful trial consisted of two saccades, separated by a period of steady gaze. Both saccades were in the same direction and of the same size, but one was directed toward the primary position, while the other went from primary out to an eccentric position. The direction varied at random from trial to trial, but the amplitude remained fixed at 10 or 20 deg for a block of trials.

The evoked saccades in a given direction induced by the automated target movements were almost identical in terms of latency, amplitude, and peak velocities. The trials in a given direction, although interspersed with trials in other directions during the actual neural recordings, were later separated by computer analysis. The unit discharge associated with a block of trials (usually 15) could be aligned with a number of behavioral or stimulus related events present in each trial. In this paper we emphasize the results produced by aligning the discharge rasters and cumulative histograms on saccade onset. Figure 1 shows several of the characteristic features of the discharge patterns seen in individual Purkinje cells during these highly stereotyped movements. The eye movement synchronized histograms and the individual trial rasters show the irregular ongoing discharge during the presaccadic interval that was associated with every P-cell we studied. When the cumulative discharge remained above or below two standard deviations from the mean ongoing discharge rate for several consecutive bins (10 ms/bin), a significant response was defined to have occurred. Time measurements were made from the initial point of such crossings.

For the cell shown in Fig. 1B, a clearly evident, transient modulation of this background, which in this cell was excitatory, occurred in association with the saccadic eye movement. The onset of the modulation in this cell preceded the beginning of the eye movement by about 50 msec. This temporal relationship varied widely over the population of cells studied, from 60 msec before saccade onset to synchrony with or just following saccade termination. Among those cells (n = 38) which showed a modulation epoch which began at least by saccade onset, the average lead was 22 msec ($\pm$ 20 SD). In addition the sign of the modulation could be a suppression of discharge (11 out of 38 cells) or excitation (27 out of 38 cells). A consistent feature of the modulation in all P-cells was the transient nature of the response (e.g., there were no steady state responses correlated with fixation eye position). Another characteristic well illustrated by Fig. 1 is the extreme variability of the modulation found from trial to trial even though the eye movements were identical.

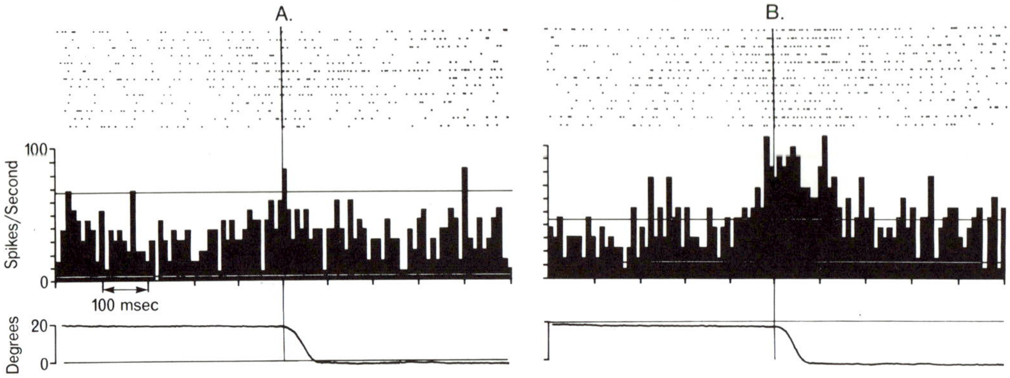

Fig. 1. Example of a vermal Purkinje cell which showed an excitatory modulation for outward (B) directed left saccades but not inward saccades (A) in the same direction. In each plate discharge rasters for individual trials, cumulative histograms, and averaged horizontal eye movements are displayed from top to bottom. In each histogram the individual discharges are summed in 10 ms bins and then are divided by the number of trials to yield average frequency. Neuronal activity was aligned in time with saccade onset (vertical line). Horizontal lines represent discharge rates which are plus or minus two standard deviations from the mean ongoing discharge rate. On eye movement traces the rightward direction of movement is shown as up and horizontal lines show the primary position.

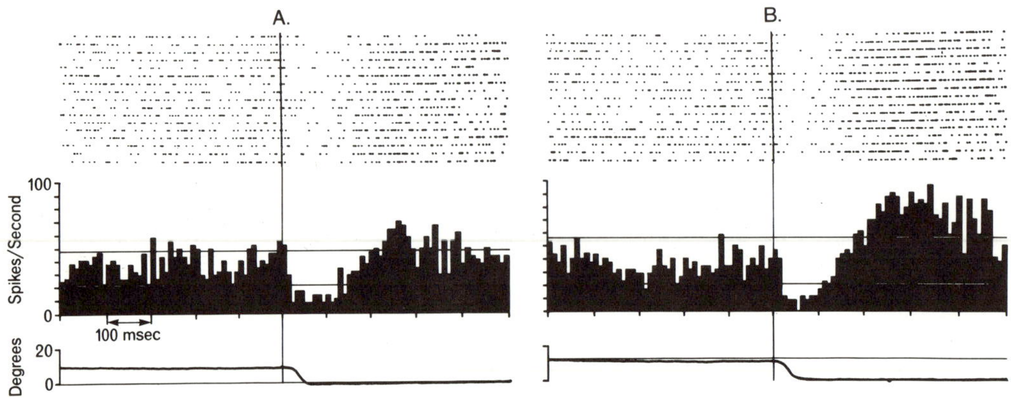

Fig. 2. Purkinje cell which shows suppressed discharge during left saccades and a late excitatory modulation well after saccade termination. This late component is smaller for inward (A) as compared to outward saccades (B) of the same size. All other conventions the same as Fig. 1.

Figure 2B illustrates another unusual feature of saccade-related P-cell discharge - the appearance of multicomponent modulations which, although they were transient in nature and time-locked to the saccade, could extend well beyond the termination of the movement. The second (late) component in Fig. 2A was a transient excitation beginning at about 200 msec following the saccade and extended out to about 450 msec after the movement.

The activity then returned to background levels of discharge. Significant modulations extending well after the termination of the saccade was a common feature of P-cell activity (15 out of 38 cells) and could be either a transient increase or decrease of activity extending out as long as 500 msec following the saccade.

Since the modulations of P-cell discharge were so complex, it was obviously very difficult to relate the patterns to specific saccadic metrics. Nevertheless there were a number of properties that showed consistent correlations with saccadic parameters. The one most easily related to saccadic production was a clear initial-position dependency that was noted in the discharge pattern for families of saccades with the same amplitude and direction but oriented centrifugally or centripetally with respect to primary position. Figure 1 illustrates a P-cell which showed a burst of activity before and during leftward outgoing saccades (Fig. 1B) but no modulation at all for saccades in the same direction when directed toward the primary position (Fig. 1A). Figure 2 illustrates the same principle, but in this case the early transient component (a suppression of discharge) occurring at saccade termination remained about the same, but the late component (an excitation) showed a clear accentuation for outward (Fig. 2B) as compared to inward saccades (Fig. 2A) of the same size and direction. Figure 3 shows another variation of the same theme.

In this case the early modulation remains the same for rightward saccades from all initial positions, but for outward saccades a late inhibitory component appeared (Fig. 3B) that was not present for inward saccades in the same direction (Fig. 3A).

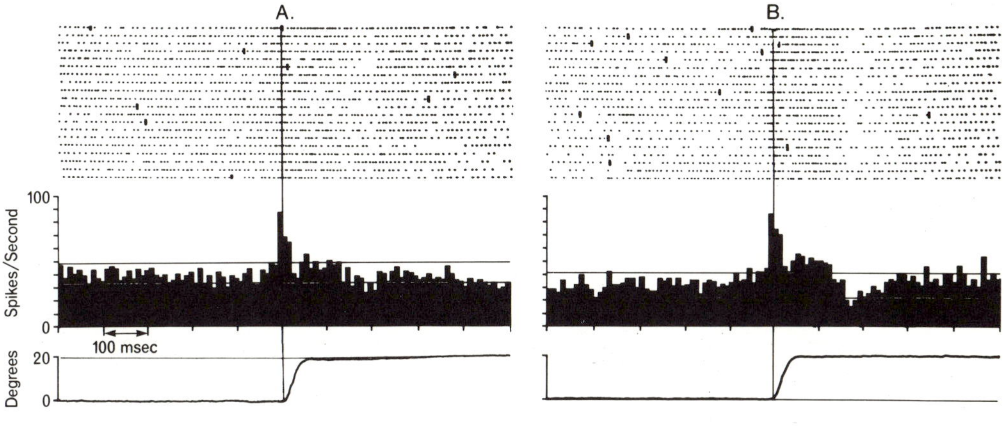

Fig. 3. Purkinje cell which shows an initial excitatory component and a position dependent late inhibitory modulation for right going saccades. Inward directed movement (A) and outward directed movement (B). All other conventions the same as Fig. 1, except horizontal eye movements show one representative saccade from the block of trials. Solid bars in the discharge raster indicate the times of occurrence of complex spikes.

A typical vermal input element is shown in Fig. 4. Several features of these input elements' discharge are particularly noteworthy. Those units (18 out of 25) which were eye movement related showed a burst of activity in association with saccades. Most units burst for saccades in all directions but showed a clear directional preference. The directional preferences were not sharply tuned and usually included two or more of the cardinal directions (e.g., down and right). The onset of these bursts led saccade onset in 16 of the 18 saccade related units (average lead = 30 ms ± 9.6 SD). In clear contrast to the marked initial position dependency noted in P-cell modulations, no differences were noted in burst parameters (duration and peak frequency) for any of the vermal input elements for inward or outward saccades. The unit shown in Fig. 4 discharged best for right saccades and had indistinguishable burst profiles for inward (Fig. 4A) or outward (Fig. 4B) movements. Also in clear contrast to P-cell modulations, the bursts observed in input elements were over close to saccade termination in all but two units.

The appearance of late components in the saccade-related modulation in the time period 100 to 500 ms after the saccade, which was a common feature in P-cells was not seen in the vermal input elements.

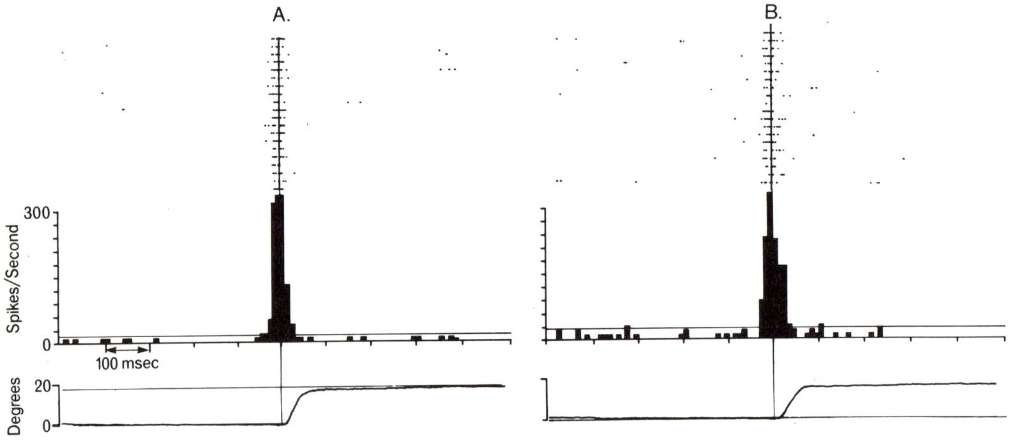

Fig. 4. Vermal input element discharge during inward (A) and outward (B) directed right saccades. All conventions the same as Fig. 1.

In these same monkeys we made a systematic attempt to map the effect of focal electrical microstimulation of the same vermal regions in which we recorded unit responses. Our results generally agreed with the detailed cerebellar stimulation study in the monkey by Ron and Robinson (1973). Two features of our results seem worthy of note here because they are closely related to our neural recording results. First, focal electrical stimulations produced ipsilaterally directed saccades (usually with a vertical component), but as noted by Ron and Robinson (1973) the amplitude of the evoked saccades were initial position dependent.

Figure 5 shows the results for one stimulation site where a 21-deg rightward (inward) saccade was induced when the gaze was initially directed at the 20-deg leftward target (Fig. 5A), but a 15-deg movement (outward) was evoked when gaze was initially at the primary position (Fig. 5B). When gaze was directed out 20 deg, the evoked saccade was only 8 deg in amplitude (Fig. 5C). The evoked vertical component (upper traces) in these stimulations remained the same, but it also varied in amplitude when the initial vertical position was varied. The second unique feature noted during these stimulations was the frequent appearance of postsaccadic drift (glissades) associated with the evoked saccades. In the stimulated saccades shown in Fig. 5, a horizontal backward drift was present whenever the initial position was 20 deg in the direction of the evoked movement (Fig. 5C). A smaller onward directed drift can also be seen following the vertical component of each evoked saccade.

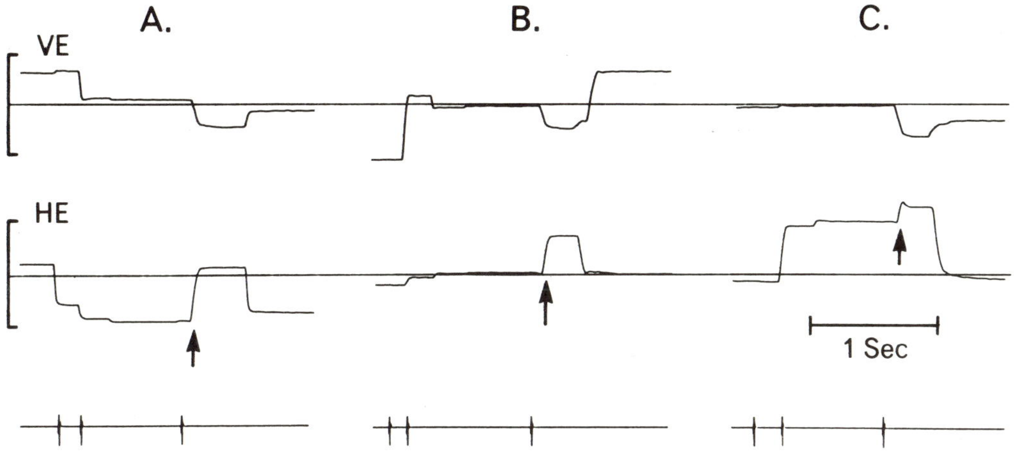

Fig. 5. Electrical microstimulation (50 ms pulse train, 200 Hz, 20 μA) of saccades from the vermis. Each plate shows one evoked saccade (arrow) with the monkey fixating the target at different horizontal positions. In each case an oblique movement with a rightward horizontal component resulted, but this component became smaller as the initial position was moved from 20 deg left (A), to the primary position (B), and to 20 deg right (C). VE = vertical eye position. HE = horizontal eye position (rightward movements shown as up). The light horizontal lines indicate the primary position. Eye position calibrations are $\pm$ 20 deg. The lower traces show the computer generated event marks. In each trace the first mark indicates target light on, the second trace indicates the monkey's eye position has become close to target position (after voluntary foveating saccade is made), and the third mark shows the time of electrical stimulation onset.

DISCUSSION

Primates with permanent (Ritchie, 1976; Optican and Robinson, 1980) or reversible (Villis and Hore, in press) vermal lesions produce highly dysmetric saccades. However, since these saccades have normal velocity profiles and durations for their size, the saccadic pulse generators appear to be left intact in the lesioned animals. These observations suggest that the cerebellar input to these generators occurs at the level of spatial-to-temporal translation in the saccadic system. For example, in the case of hypermetric saccades, a spatially coded visual signal indicating a 20-deg target eccentricity results in pulse generator, temporal (frequency and duration) activity appropriate for perhaps a 30-deg saccade. The mechanism for this conversion during normal saccades is not made specific in the Robinson (1975a pulse-generator model, but amplifications of this model (Keller, 1981; Wurtz and Albano, 1980) suggest that different spatial target locations are coded in separate input fiber projections to the pulse generator. These inputs each produce different intensity graded activations of the generator through differential synaptic weighting (fibers coding small target eccentricities would produce smaller post-synaptic effects in burst generator neurons than equivalently discharging fibers coding larger eccentricities). Cerebellar input at the level of this weighting mechanism, either pre- or postsynaptic, could insure a proper correspondence between target location as coded by the input fibers and their level of pulse-generator activation. Several features of P-cell activity recorded in the present study are consistent with this role for the cerebellum. First, many of these cells are directionally selective indicating they could project to different pulse generators which exist for the cardinal directions of eye movement (Robinson and Fuchs, 1969). Units with different directional preferences were found intermixed throughout the posterior vermis. Therefore, lesions of this cerebellar cortex would be expected to lead to saccadic dysmetria in all directions, an effect reported by Vilis and Hore (in press).

One way of viewing the extreme variability in an individual P-cell's discharge pattern for similar saccades would be to assume that the hypothesized synaptic weighting controlled by the cerebellum is made manifest by averaging the activities of many loosely correlated P-cells at the site within the pulse generator where they make their effect. This view is implicitly assumed in our method of averaging the discharge patterns of a single unit for successive saccades and the further assumption of ergodicity, i.e. that the averaged output of the vermis from many P-cells involved in a saccade can be approximated by the average over many trials of a single representative cell. If this view is correct, then the effect of vermal lesions would be expected to be cumulative. The larger the area destroyed, the larger would be the expected dysmetria. In this regard, it is interesting to note that we recorded many of our saccade related P-cells with similar properties out to 6 mm from the midline of the vermis.

The results of reversible lesions of cerebellar nuclei (Vilis and Hore, in press) suggest that the cerebellar influence on the saccadic pulse generator is continuously mediated, that is, an output signal from the cerebellum to the pulse generators is required for every orthometric saccade. Our unit results are consistent with this view. In addition, the timing of the early response components was consistent with the idea that it could play a role in pulse generator function. Previous recordings of primate vermal P-cells indicated that the transient change in their activity preceded saccadic onset by only a millisecond or so (Kase and others, 1980). Our average lead time of 22 ms corresponds very closely in time to that when the brain stem saccadic pulse generators are activated by higher visual centers like the superior colliculus (Raybourn and Keller, 1977; Sparks and others, 1976). Thus these P-cells could effect the earliest programming of the burst generators. It should be noted that brain stem neurons called long-lead bursters show discharge that can be related to the metrics of saccades as early as 100 to 150 ms preceding the saccade (Henn and Cohen, 1976), but that the relationships are crude and such cells seem not to be included in the actual burst generator which is believed to consist of short-lead burst neurons and pause cells.

Since our monkeys were making normometric saccades during the trials in which the related activity shown here was recorded, it is difficult to relate their discharge specifically to dysmetric saccades. Our P-cell recordings should be viewed as baseline data giving the time frame and modulation amplitudes of cerebellar units during normal saccades. Similar recordings in monkeys made dysmetric by peripheral lesions (Optican and Robinson, 1980) can now be carried out with the purpose of comparing cerebellar activity in these animals with our normal data.

The dramatic differences in many P-cells' saccade related modulation for inward vs. outward movements is a feature not previously found in brain stem saccadic units (Luschei and Fuchs, 1972; Keller, 1974; Henn and Cohen, 1976). Furthermore, since we could find no evidence of such dependencies present on the cerebellar input elements, we suggest that its development is a cerebellar cortical property. This property seems to be a general characteristic of the cerebellum since it is found both in the monkey and the cat (McElligott, 1979). Initial position dependency as a characteristic of cerebellar P-cell discharge is also consistent with the vermal electrical stimulation results which showed that the size of the evoked saccades were highly eye position dependent. This again contrasts with the eye movements evoked by the stimulation of other saccadic control areas (superior colliculus and frontal eye fields) where a given size saccade is normally elicited at each stimulation site.

The question remains as to the role played by P-cell initial position dependent discharge. The inward and outward directed saccades generated by the monkeys in our study had almost identical velocity profiles, which would be expected if the burst-generating mechanism and oculomotor plant were strictly linear systems. The linearity of the peripheral oculomotor mechanics with respect to position in the orbit has been emphasized, but mainly with respect to steady-state elastic forces (Robinson, 1973). There is some suggestive evidence from studies in the human orbit during saccades (Collins, 1975) that position dependent non-linearities may exist and the discharge of at least some oculomotor neurons is different during inward and outward directed saccades (Robinson, 1970). Nevertheless, it should be emphasized that position dependent effects at the level of the burst generators, motoneurons, or orbital mechanics have not been carefully investigated, and our present results provide an impetus for such studies in the future.

The late components (from the end of saccades out to several hundred milliseconds beyond), which we observed in many P-cells' discharge patterns, have also not been previously reported in brain stem saccadic units. Since the discharge rates of oculomotor neurons have settled to their steady rates well within 100 msec following saccade termination (Robinson, 1970; Fuchs and Luschei, 1970; Schiller, 1970), it seems unlikely that this late discharge could be related to controlling the saccade. The hypothesis of Optican and Robinson (1980) that the vermis plays a role in detecting the presence of saccadic dysmetria and provides compensation for this effect over the long term, requires that some cerebellar units reflect the accuracy of completed saccades. The time frame of the late responses seen in this study is consistent with the idea that a comparison of movement accuracy could be made in individual P-cells immediately following each saccade. Thus we suggest that these late responses could represent visual or orbital proprioceptive input on units which were often active earlier during the saccade. Since our monkeys' saccades were usually normometric, our data would again represent baseline data which should be compared to any late responses seen in animals making dysmetric saccades.

ACKNOWLEDGEMENTS

The authors would like to express their gratitude to William Crandall for technical assistance and to Jona Countie for typing and preparing the camera ready manuscript. The research was supported by grants BNS 79-14107 from the NSF EY03280 and EY01186 from the NIH, and Smith-Kettlewell Eye Research Foundation.

EYE SIGNS IN HUMANS WITH CEREBELLAR DYSFUNCTION

R. B. DAROFF

Department of Neurology, Case Western Reserve University, School of Medicine, Cleveland, Ohio and Neurology Service, Cleveland Veterans Administration Medical Center, Cleveland, Ohio, USA

ABSTRACT

A brief review of putative mechanisms of the various eye signs encountered in patients with cerebellar disease is presented.

KEYWORDS

Eye movements; cerebellum; cerebellar disease; nystagmus.

What have we (more precisely, I) learned about the disturbances of eye movements in patients with cerebellar lesions since the last Stockholm Symposium in 1974? In my published chapter (Daroff, 1975), 12 such eye signs with 4 different types of nystagmus were listed. In the interval, more precise oculographic studies justify increasing the list to 21 signs with 12 different types of nystagmus (Table 1) but with the same reservations expressed previously (Daroff, 1975) concerning the clinical difficulty in distinguishing the manifestations of pure cerebellar dysfunction from those secondary to coexisting, or even isolated, brain stem involvement. Undoubtedly, many of the signs in Table 1, such as skew deviation and periodic alternating nystagmus, can be removed safely from future tables. However, in this short discussion, probably it is best to list even dubious signs rather than defending exclusions of some clinical favorites. Shortening the list with any certainty would be quite difficult. We can establish that a sign is "cerebellar" if it occurs following discrete cerebellar lesions in primates. Isolated cerebellar lesions in humans are rare and the fact that certain signs are never produced with animal lesions cannot be used to negate the causal relationship in human disease states which, unlike experimental conditions, may evolve slowly and/or diffusely throughout the cerebellum. Moreover, keeping with the concept of the cerebellum as the "repair shop" (Hoyt and Frisen, 1975; Robinson, 1975b, a silent brain stem lesion may be unmasked by later cerebellar dysfunction and produce an eye sign that would not have been present with either lesion alone. A more complicated situation is with pendular vertical nystagmus (ocular myoclonus) which is associated with hypertrophy of the inferior olivary nuclei in the medulla, a morphological change occurring after a latency of months to years after a lesion of the dentate nucleus of the cerebellum (Matsuo and Ajax, 1979).

TABLE 1 Cerebellar Eye Signs

Gaze Palsy (Daroff, 1970) (Daroff & Hoyt, 1971)
Pseudo Abducens Palsy (Fisher et al, 1965)
Skew Deviation (Keane, 1975)
Saccadic Pursuit (Zee et al, 1976)
Slow-to-No Saccades (Osorio & Daroff, 1980)
Hypometric Saccades (Zee et al, 1976)
Post Saccadic Drift (Zee, in press)
Slow Drifts in Darkness (Leach et al, 1977)
Overshoot Dysmetria (Selhorst et al, 1976a)
Flutter (Zee & Robinson, 1979)
Flutter Dysmetria (Daroff & Dell'Osso, 1979; Zee & Robinson, 1979)
Opsoclonus (Zee & Robinson, 1979)
Square Wave Jerks (Dell'Osso, et al, 1977)
Macro Square Wave Jerks (Dell'Osso et al, 1975)
Macro Saccadic Oscillations (Selhorst et al, 1976b)
Increased VOR Gain (Zee et al, 1976)
Inability to Suppress VOR (Zee et al, 1976; Dell'Osso et al, 1981)
Loss of VOR Plasticity (Yagi et al, in press)
Impaired OKN Gain (Yee et al, 1979)
Prolonged Rise to Steady State OKN (Yee et al, 1979)
Nystagmus
- Gaze Paretic (Zee et al, 1976)
- Vestib.-like (Duncan et al, 1975)
- Period. Altern. (Baloh et al, 1976)
- Centripetal (Leach et al, 1976)
- Upbeat (Mehdorn et al, 1979)
- Downbeat
  - Linear (Zee et al, 1976)
  - Decreasing Velocity Exponential (Abel et al, in Preparation)
  - Increasing Velocity Exponential (Zee et al, 1980)
- Pendular Vert. (Ocular Myoclonus) (Daroff et al, 1978)
- Circular-Elliptical Pendular (Aschoff et al, 1974)
- Rebound (Zee et al, 1976)
- Positional (Harrison & Ozahinoglu, 1975)

Inferring functional properties to a structure by analysis of the manifestations of dysfunction is indirect, yet the best approach presently available. Based upon animal experimentation, Zee (in this volume) has attributed the control of saccadic amplitude to the dorsal vermis and underlying fastigial nuclei, and the stabilization of images upon the retina to the vestibulo-cerebellum. The pathological eye sign related to the dorsal vermis is overshoot dysmetria whereas signs of vestibulo-cerebellar disease include: saccadic pursuit; inability to suppress the vestibulo-ocular reflex (VOR); post saccadic drift; and gaze paretic, downbeat, and rebound nystagmus.

A tentative classification of cerebellar eye signs related to the presumed pathophysiological or control system mechanism appears in Table 2. Some of the mechanisms undoubtedly will be proven to be incorrect. Others are admittedly simplistic. The classification was formulated without anatomical consideration. To provoke correlation, the signs which have been produced by experimental lesions of the vestibulo-cerebellum (VC) or dorsal vermis and underlying nuclei (DV) are followed by the appropriate abbreviation in Table 2.

It is possible that the prolonged buildup of slow phase OKN velocity, secondary to VC lesions, is related to decreased slow eye movement gain. If so, there would appear to be a mechanistic consistency in the manifestations of VC dysfunction which is quite consistent with Zee's proposed role of this structure in the stabilization of retinal images. The notion is particularly compelling if one accepts Yarbus' (1967) conceptualization of fixation as merely pursuit at zero velocity.

Patients, unlike animals with discrete lesions, often have eye signs reflecting different mechanistic derangements such as a combination of macro square wave jerks and macro saccadic oscillations (Dell'Osso et al, 1977). We have recently recorded a patient with cerebellar disease who manifested overshoot dysmetria, flutter, flutter dysmetria, and macro saccadic oscillations (Doslak et al., in preparation). This probably reflects the diffuseness of cerebellar lesions in clinical disease states in humans.

TABLE 2 Mechanisms of Cerebellar Eye Signs

- I. Main System Loop Gains
  - A. Saccadic [Position Sensitive]
    - 1. Decreased Gain
      - a. Hypometric Saccades
    - 2. Increased Gain
      - a. Overshoot Dysmetria (DV)
      - b. Macro Saccadic Oscillations
  - B. Slow Eye Movement (Pursuit and Other) [Velocity Sensitive]
    - 1. Decreased Gain
      - a. Saccadic Pursuit (VC)
      - b. Decreased OKN Slow Phase Gain (VC)
    - 2. Increased Gain (Dell'Osso and Daroff, in press)
      - a. Pendular Vertical Nystagmus (Ocular myoclonus)
      - b. Circular-elliptical Nystagmus (Horizontal and vertical pendular nystagmus 90° out of phase)
- II. Cerebellar - PPRF Loop
  - A. Tonic Cell (Leaky Integrator) Positive Feedback Loop
    - 1. Decreased Gain
      - a. Gaze Paretic Horizontal Nystagmus (VC)
      - b. Decreasing Velocity Exponential Downbeat Nystagmus (VC)
    - 2. Increased Gain
      - a. Increasing Velocity Exponential Downbeat Nystagmus (VC)
  - B. Burst Cell Dysfunction
    - 1. Slow-to-No Saccades
  - C. Pause Cell Dysfunction
    - 1. Flutter
    - 2. Opsoclonus
    - 3. Flutter Dysmetria
    - 4. Square Wave Jerks
    - 5. Macro Square Wave Jerks
  - D. PPRF Dysfunction
    - 1. Ipsilateral Gaze (Saccades and Pursuit) Palsy
- III. Position Bias Control
  - A. Periodic Alternating Nystagmus
  - B. Rebound Nystagmus (VC)
  - C. Centripetal Nystagmus
  - D. Slow Drifts in Darkness
- IV. Defective Vestibular Inhibition or Control
  - A. Increased VOR Gain (VC)
  - B. Inability to Suppress VOR (VC)
  - C. Vestibular-like Nystagmus
  - D. Loss of VOR Plasticity (VC)
  - E. Periodic Alternating Nystagmus (?)
  - F. Positional Nystagmus
- V. Tonic Vertical Imbalance
  - A. Upbeat Nystagmus with Linear Slow Phase
  - B. Downbeat Nystagmus with Linear Slow Phase
- VI. Pulse-step Mismatch
  - A. Post Saccadic Drifts (Glissades)
- VII. Defective Yoking
  - A. Skew Deviation
  - B. Pseudo-abducens Palsy
- VIII. Defective OKN Control
  - A. Prolonged Slow Phase Velocity Buildup (VC)

THE CEREBELLUM AS A CALIBRATOR ORGAN

L. STARK

Neurology Unit, University of California, Berkeley, USA

The cerebellum is a marvelous organ with beautiful structures at many levels of anatomical scale; not being accessible to input-output studies that might quickly disprove inadequate theories, it has remained the focus of neurophysiological concepts. A seminal idea was that of Braitenberg & Atwood (1958) that Purkinje cells act to cross-correlate the temporal-spatial information in parallel fibers; this now appears not to be feasible because of the shorter length of parallel fibers than previously estimated. On the occasion of the 'Salisan Conference on Cerebellum', I speculated on "Three Nonexclusive Hypotheses of the Physiology of the Cerebellum" (Stark, 1967). These were: "that the cerebellum regulates the interaction between the intermittent cortical-spinal voluntary input and the postural reflexes, that the cerebellum is the site of an output adaptation mechanism to compensate for changing plant dynamics, and that the cerebellum is the mechanism for motor learning, whereby the substitution of successive automatic postures is made for voluntary movements." For the present discussion, I wish to support the adaptive role of the cerebellum as a 'calibrator organ' with evidence from three of our recent studies.

i.- Cerebellar stimulation has a powerful effect in producing rapid conjugate eye movements (Gauthier, 1970; Gauthier & Stark, 1979; Ron & Robinson, 1973). From Bode diagram analysis of eye movements produced by cerebellar, ocular motor and combined stimulation, we inferred that reciprocal innervation was obeyed and pulse-step signals activated the ocular motor nuclei. The eye movements were somewhat below the main sequence data for humans, a common finding in spontaneous eye movement in the cat. The data were compatible with the cerebellum acting "as a 'calibrator organ' that continually adjusted the forward loop gain and thus eventually influenced the output of lower motor neurons to allow proper amplitude, velocity, and stability of eye movements."

ii.- Clinical Recordings of patients with saccadic overshoot dysmetria (Selhorst, Stark, Ochs, and Hoyt 1976a) using photocell glasses (Stark, Vossius, and Young, 1962) give an impression of a short series of sequentially diminishing square waves (Ashoff & Cohen, 1971; Optican & Robinson, 1980) (Fig. 1B). In control system terms, square or flat-topped oscillations signify a discrete position-correcting mechanism holding position during intersaccadic intervals; also, step discharge rate is precomputed along with saccade pulse duration and that this rate does not change until the next corrective saccade occurs. More specifically, the system follows a discrete sampled data control rule and thus is in the 'open loop' mode between saccades (Young & Stark 1963). These theoretical deductions are supported by EMG recordings in man and by microelectrode data in monkeys on the pulse-step envelope of discharges in ocular motor neurons during eye position changes.

Saccadic overshoot dysmetria in patients with cerebellar involvement may be related to the minor dysmetric errors recorded in normal subjects. Occurrence of these minor undershoots and overshoots suggests that feed-forward gain normally fluctuates within narrow limits. The control system abnormality in saccadic overshoot dysmetria is an abnormally high gain in the brain's feed-forward path. We suggest that it is the cerebellum that continuously modulates saccadic gain, although it may not lie directly in the visual ocular motor (feed-forward) path. Thus rapid correction by saccades of off-foveal target position is possible, while longer-term adaptive modulation by the cerebellum provides parametric control over saccadic precision without interposing an additional delay in the saccadic system. Cerebellar gain control of VOR is perhaps similar (Gonsher & Melvill Jones, 1976a;Ito, Shida, Yagi, and Yamamoto, 1974b, Miles & Fuller, 1974).

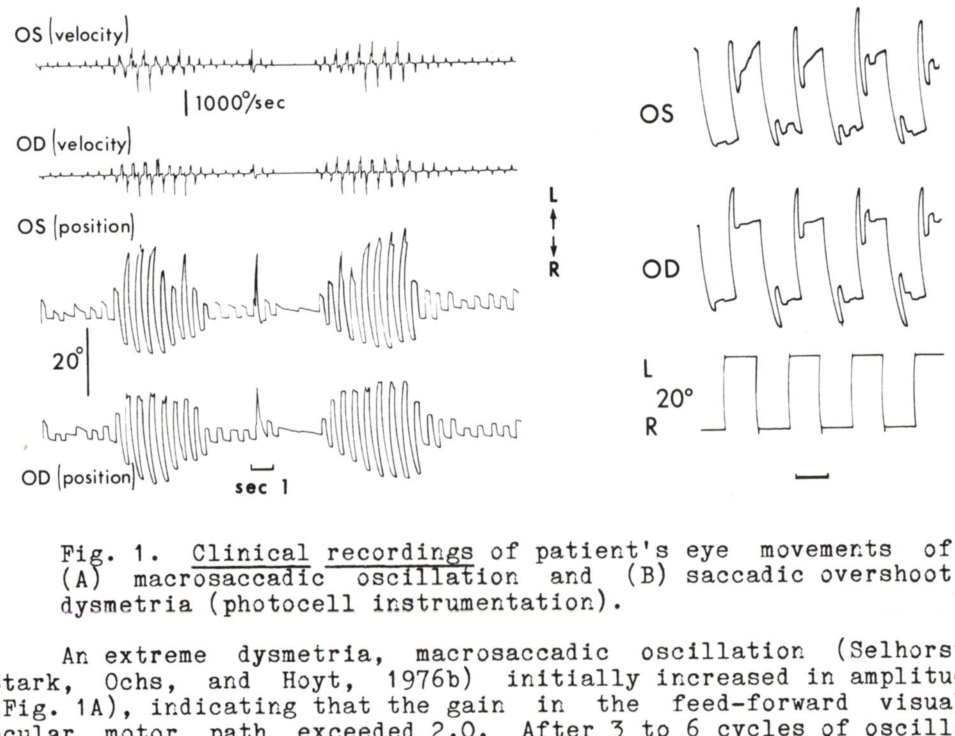

Fig. 1. Clinical recordings of patient's eye movements of (A) macrosaccadic oscillation and (B) saccadic overshoot dysmetria (photocell instrumentation).

An extreme dysmetria, macrosaccadic oscillation (Selhorst, Stark, Ochs, and Hoyt, 1976b) initially increased in amplitude (Fig. 1A), indicating that the gain in the feed-forward visual-ocular motor path exceeded 2.0. After 3 to 6 cycles of oscillation, amplitude remained constant for several additional cycles. Amplitude then diminished, but the eye continued to overshoot the target, indicating a gain between 2.0 and 1.0, as in saccadic overshoot dysmetria. Initial increase in gain occurred either suddenly after a large saccade or after a series of small oscillations of constant amplitude.

Computer simulation approximated saccadic overshoot dysmetria (Fig. 2B) and macrosaccadic oscillation (Fig. 2C) using the variable gain forward loop model (Fig. 2A) (Hsu, Krishnan, and Stark, 1976). Macrosaccadic oscillation requires an intact visual feed-back loop; clinical evidence for this is its exacerbation by visually guided attempts at fixation or smooth pursuit. An elegant observation is that in the dark, the oscillation stops abruptly and is not induced by saccades or vergence. [This finding was not confirmed by Ritchie (1976) in animal experiments.]

In the tradition of Hughlings Jackson we emphasize that there are separable lower and higher levels of supranuclear ocular motor control acting in cerebellar macrosaccadic oscillation. At the lower level of control, gain in the feed-forward loop drifts away from its normal value; at the higher level, the cerebellum's adaptive role as a gain calibrator is suspended by acute loss of function of the vermis. Macrosaccadic oscillation results from gain fluctuation about the uncompensated high gain value of 2.0. Similar control abnormality and the loss of vermis function also underlie the clinical phenomena of saccadic overshoot dysmetria.

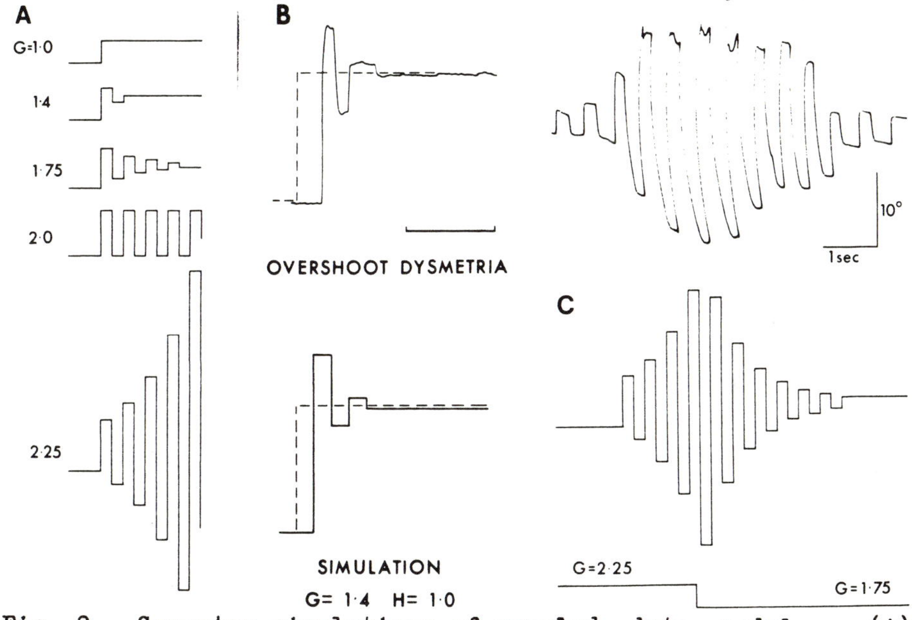

Fig. 2. Computer simulations of sampled data model. (A) variable feed-forward gains; (B) simulation (lower) of overshoot dysmetria recording (upper); (C) simulation (lower) of macrosaccadic oscillation (upper); note gain change switch below to account for spindle.

iii.- In an adaptation paradigm experiment dealing with hand-eye coordination only a patient with cerebellar and olivary disease showed inability to adapt (Gauthier, Hofferer, Hoyt, and Stark, 1979). The adaptation paradigm included change of viewing lenses and open loop and closed loop hand and eye movements (Buchtel, 1970; Harris, 1965). Inability to adapt was supported when the adapting lenses were removed (Fig. 3). We believe that the absence of visual motor adaptation displayed by our patient paralleled his persistent motor deficits. Inability to recalibrate would relate both the patient's saccadic overshoot dysmetria and the absence of visual motor adaptation.

The patient's initial course 17 years ago was complicated by a two-month episode of palatal, pharyngeal, paraspinal, and diaphragmatic myoclonus implicating the olivary system (Llinas, 1975). Normal 'main sequence' saccades and Hering's Law conjugacy of his eye movements suggest preservation of ocular motor brain stem mechanisms. The question of exact anatomical localization is always a difficult one with clinical lesions even though CT scan was available. However, the neurological deficits in this patient may shed some light on the role of climbing fibers for motor coordination in the still illusive cerebellar 'machinery'.

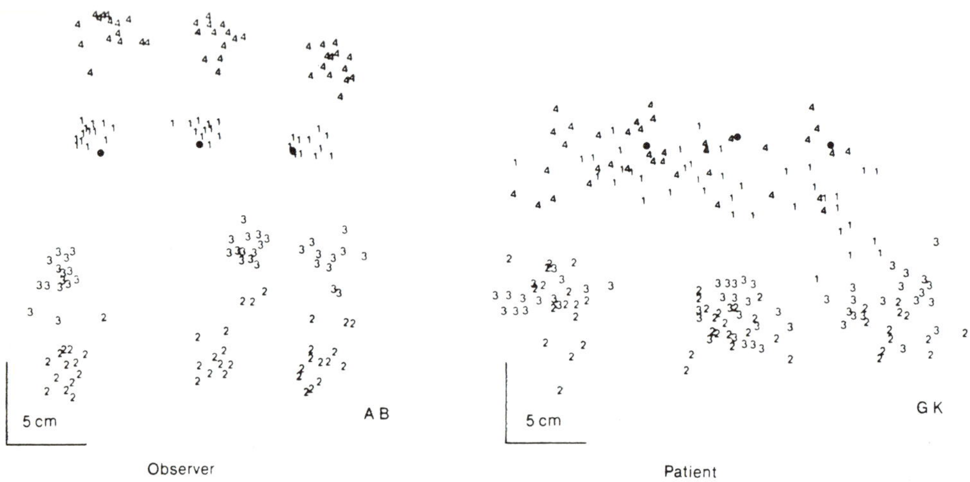

Fig. 3. Visual-motor adaptation experiment. Note patient showed no adaptation (points 2 & 3 are not separated) and no rebound after-effect (points 1 & 4 are not separated). Observer (and patient) showed optical effect of lens (points 2, after lenses, are displaced from points 1, initial viewing); observer demonstrated adaption after closed loop visual-motor trials (points 3 have moved halfway to actual light location from optical distortion of distance, points 2).

I would like to thank my colleagues Drs. Gabriel Gauthier, William Hoyt and Valentino Braitenberg for exciting discussions, and NASA-Ames Research Center for partial support (NCC 2-86).

VISUAL SUPPRESSION AND ACTIVATION OF FIXATION EYE MOVEMENTS IN CEREBELLAR DISORDERS

J. R. HOTSON

Department of Neurology, Stanford University School of Medicine, Stanford, California 94305 and Santa Clara Valley Medical Center, San Jose, California 95128, USA

During visual fixation spontaneous saccades, slow drifts, square waves, saccadic oscillations, flutter, and vertical nystagmus occur in both patients with degenerative cerebellar disorders and normal subjects (Hotson, 1979, 1981). In normal subjects these eye movements are so small that they are not detected by routine observation. However in patients these spontaneous eye movements become enlarged. Also horizontally coupled saccades (i.e., square waves and saccadic oscillations) become more frequent and clinically appear as saccadic fixation instability.

The enlargement of fixation eye movements may be due to an inability to visually suppress or reduce the gain of saccade and slow drift generators. This possibility was studied by recording the spontaneous eye movements of 9 control subjects and 4 patients with degenerative cerebellar disorders. The methods have been previously described, (Hotson, 1981) though in this study a chin and head support was used rather than a bite bar.

The subjects were studied during different test situations, namely, a. fixation on a target, b. fixation on a remembered target in darkness, and c. in darkness with no target and performing mental arithmetic. In all situations the amplitude of fixation saccades and velocity of slow drift was increased in patients compared to controls. Also the degree of visual suppression was reduced in the patients (Table 1; % visual supression = no target-target/no target x 100). These findings indicate that while the overall gain of saccade and slow drift generators was increased in all test situations a more selective defect in the active reduction of gain by vision was present in patients with cerebellar disorders.

The mean coefficient of variation for fixation saccades (standard deviation/saccade amplitude x 100) was 49 for controls and 47 for patients. This measurement may provide an estimate in the variation or fluctuations in the gain of fixation saccade generators. The similarity in the variation of saccade amplitudes does not provide support for the proposal that some forms of saccadic oscillations are due to increased fluctuations of gain (Selhorst, 1976b).

Cerebellar disorders also increased the frequency of horizontal saccade coupling in the form of square waves and saccadic oscillations (Fig. 1, Hotson, 1981). Disorders of supranuclear control other than cerebellar may also increase saccadic coupling (Ciuffreda, 1979a;Dell'Osso, 1975; Feldon, 1977; Herishanu, 1981; Troost, 1976). It is possible that diseases that impair either afferents to the cerebellum or its efferent control may predispose to saccadic coupling.

TABLE 1

	Target (SD)	Remembered Target (SD)	No Target (SD)	% Visual Suppression
Saccade Amplitude (min arc)				
Controls	9.7 (4.4)	24 (9)	54 (19)	82
Patients	68 (47)	70 (42)	93 (35)*	27
Drift Velocity (min arc/sec				
Controls	3.6 (1.2)	8.7 (3.7)	13.6 (8)	73
Patients	13.4 (5.2)	14.5 (2.5)	28 (14)*	52*
Coupled Saccades (#/min)				
Controls	8.4 (8.4)	9.1 (7.7)	2.8 (4.3)	
Patients	28 (14)	17.7 (12.8)*	8 (7.2)*	

*Significance of difference between controls and patients 0.1>p>0.05; otherwise p <0.5.

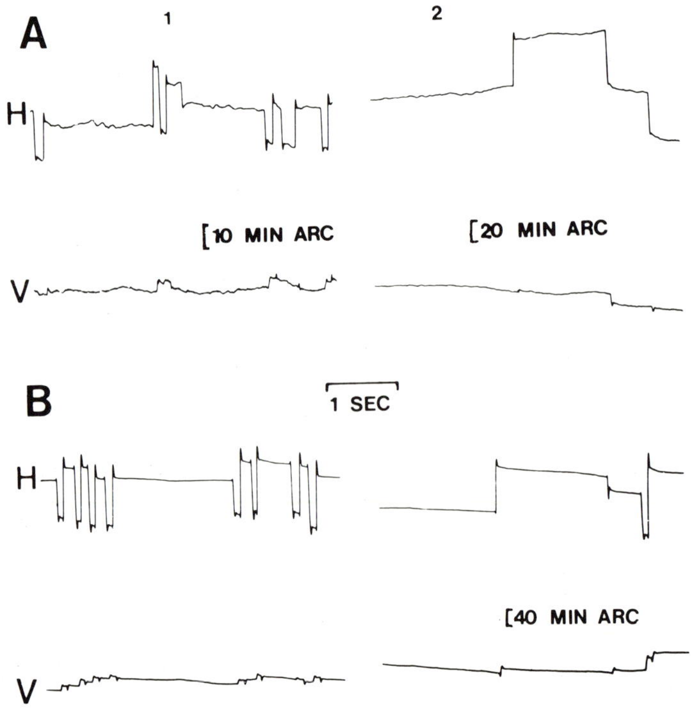

Fig. 1 A.1. Saccade coupling in control subject fixating on target. A.2. Coupling decreases with no target. B. 1,2. Similar reduction in saccade coupling in a patient.

To test the effect of altering the visual afferent input to the cerebellum the frequency of square waves and saccadic oscillations was determined in the three test situations outlined above for both control subjects and patients. In addition the acuity of 5 normal subjects was progressively decreased using +1 to +7 diopter lens and the frequency of saccade coupling determined.

Decreasing acuity to 0.05 (20/400) did not significantly alter the frequency of coupled saccades and changed other fixation movements little (Fig. 2). For clinical purposes decreasing acuity to 0.2 (20/100) has no effect on the stability of fixation. Fixation in darkness on a remembered target also did not consistently alter the frequency of saccadic coupling. In contrast coupling frequency decreased in darkness with no target (Table 1, Fig. 2; $p > 0.001$ for combined control and patient results).

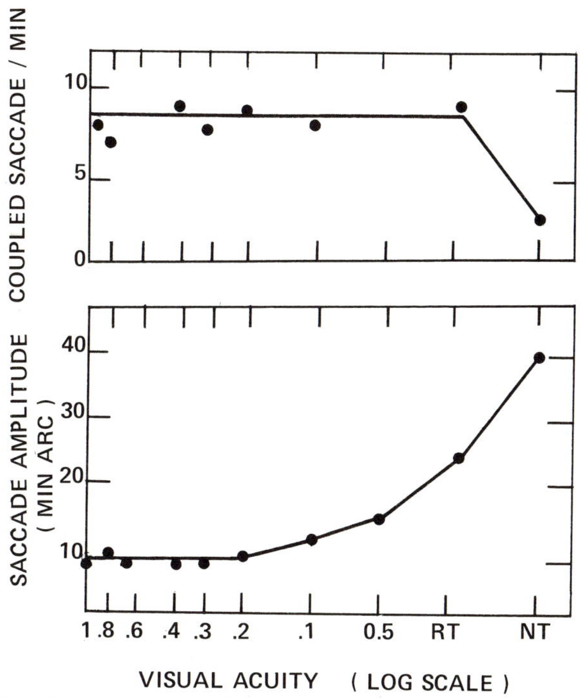

Fig. 2 Saccade amplitude, coupling versus acuity. RT = remembered target; NT = no target.

These and other observations (Dale, 1978; Herishanu, 1981) indicate that square waves and saccadic oscillations occur in normal subjects, persist and are increased with disorders of the cerebellum, and are visually activated horizontal events. Therefore it seems plausible to suggest that spontaneous coupling of fixation saccades is mediated by a visually activated pathway to the pontine saccade generators; while this pathway may be modulated by the cerebellum it persists in degenerative and destructive disorders of the cerebellum.

Supported by NEI Grant # 1 R01 EY03387-01 and the Institute for Medical Research, San Jose, California

DISCUSSION

J. Dichgans and R. Daroff clarified the distinction between opsoclonus (wild chaotic multivectorial saccadomania) and ocular myoclonus (pendular, usually vertical, oscillations of the eyes associated with rhythmic movements of the palate). R. Daroff queried the relationship between pause cell dysfunction, opsoclonus and macro square wave jerks. D. Zee answered that while part of the problem in opsoclonus may be that pause cells are not appropriately inhibiting burst cells between voluntary saccades, the pulse generator itself might be triggered inappropriately from any one of a number of places that are connected to burst cells (e.g. cerebellum, brain stem or even cerebral hemispheres). In this case opsoclonus may result when there is associated pause cell disease; macro square wave jerks, when there is not.

M. Goldberg asked about the lack of precision in the discharge rates of saccade-related units in the cerebellar vermis as reported by E. Keller and K. Hepp reported that saccade-related neurons in the fastigial nucleus behave in a similar way. L. Stark emphasized the possible role for cerebellar vermis Purkinje cells in the recalibrating process necessary for accurate eye-head coordination. D. Guitton pointed out that in Keller's experiments the animals were so well trained to make accurate saccades that no adaptation would be necessary. Hence the Purkinje cell discharge might not show a precise relation to any eye movement parameter. Keller agreed and pointed out the necessity of studying vermal Purkinje cells in animals making dysmetric saccades.

Keller also pointed out that there were Purkinje cells in the vermis that discharged in relationship to pursuit of a small target or just movement of a small spot in the background during fixation. He raised the question about a vermal function in pursuit. Zee suggested that even the saccadic system needs to know target velocity in order to accurately acquire a moving target.

Barmack queried Buttner about the source of vestibular information in the flocculus and Buttner replied that the head movement related activity fit the firing patterns of neurons in the vestibular nucleus much better than the eighth nerve.

Finally, the question about saccadic dysmetria and direction was discussed. Optican emphasized that since monkeys normally have a slight degree of centrifugal hypometria then the first hint of saccadic hypermetria would be centripetal hypermetria since centrifugal saccades now might only be orthometric. Daroff reported that he didn't find much difference between centripetal and centrifugal saccade accuracy in human beings and Stark commented that any difference was idiosyncratic from subject to subject and also related to saccade size.

SECTION X

Coordinator: L. Frisén

DISORDERS OF CEREBRAL CONTROL OF EYE MOVEMENTS

CEREBRAL OCULAR MOTOR DEFICITS

J. A. SHARPE

Division of Neurology, Playfair Neuroscience Unit, and the Neuro-ophthalmology Unit, Toronto Western Hospital, Departments of Medicine and Ophthalmology, University of Toronto, Toronto, Canada

ABSTRACT

Cerebral hemispheric disease causes distinct disorders of saccadic, smooth pursuit and vestibulo-ocular reflex (VOR) control. Paralysis of saccades after acute hemispheric lesions is attributed to combined cerebral damage and a remote effect of frontal eye field projections upon saccadic triggering by the superior colliculus. Recovery of saccades is near complete but mild slowing and delay in both horizontal directions are enduring defects after unilateral decortication. Low amplitude square wave jerks intrude upon fixation in patients with focal cerebral lesions.

Unidirectional smooth pursuit is evidenced by saccadic tracking toward the side of patietal lobe lesions. It signifies prestriate cerebral damage or intrahemispheric disconnection of prestriate cortex from visual information from the intact fellow hemisphere. Acute parietal lesions can also impair contralateral pursuit, although less severely than ipsilateral pursuit. During head motion toward the side of parietal lesions visual cancellation of the contralateral VOR is defective. Visual enhancement of the ipsilateral VOR is mildly impaired during head motion away from the side of the lesion. Voluntary (non-visual) VOR control shows parallel defects. One hemisphere regulates ipsilateral smooth eye movements that achieve voluntary and visual control of the VOR. Defective voluntary modulation in darkness indicates that cerebral hemispheric control of the VOR can be independent of the smooth pursuit system.

KEYWORDS

Cerebrum; saccades; smooth pursuit; vestibulo-ocular reflex; apraxia; nystagmus.

INTRODUCTION

The neurology of cerebral hemispheric ocular motor function has been advanced in the past decade by progressive understanding of brain stem and cerebellar ocular motor control. The apparently normal eye movements reported after focal cerebral lesions and fleeting deficits after occipital lobectomy or complete hemidecortication in the monkey suggested that different extrastriate cerebral areas might be equally potent (Pasik and Pasik, 1964a). Failure to demonstrate cortical neurons that discharge before eye movements (Bizzi and Schiller, 1970) led to the impression that the cerebrum might merely relay retinal spatial information to the brain stem. Nonetheless, neurologists are familiar with distinct disorders of saccadic and pursuit function after focal cerebral lesions in humans. This chapter describes clinical observations and quantitative studies of ocular motor dysfunction in cerebral hemispheric disease.

SACCADIC SYSTEM

Resolution of the conflict between observation of patients and animal studies is promised by recent reports of units in the frontal eye fields and posterior parietal cortex of the monkey that are active before visually guided saccades (Bushnell and Goldberg, 1979; Robinson, Goldberg and Stanton, 1978; Lynch and others, 1977b)and by recordings of thalamic neurons in the internal medullary lamina that discharge before saccades whether evoked by vision or volition (Schlag and Schlag-Rey, 1980; Schlag and others, 1980). Cerebral blood flow studies in man indicate that the frontal eye field, parieto-occipital cortex, and a zone presumed to be the supplementary motor area are metabolically active during saccades (Melamed and Larsen, 1979). Blood flow patterns do not reveal temporal sequences of cerebral activation to establish whether these regions are monitoring visual inflow or processing saccadic commands.

Computer averaged cortical potentials recorded from the frontal and parietal scalp yield bilateral premotion positive waves (PMP) preceding saccades in either horizontal direction by some 50-200 msec, and negative readiness potentials (RP) beginning about one second before saccades (Becker and co-workers, 1972; Kurtzberg and Vaughan, 1977). A unilateral negative motor potential (MP) immediately precedes movements of contralateral fingers but no such potential precedes saccades. If these potentials represent motor programs, the PMP being a motor command and the MP actual cortical motor activity (Deecke and others, 1976), then programs for limb and eye movements have disparate cerebral representation. This interpretation is consistent with enduring paresis of contralateral finger movements but fleeting paresis of contralateral saccades after unilateral cerebral lesions.

Saccadic Paralysis

Acute unilateral cerebral lesions cause ipsilateral deviation of the eyes and head. Contralateral saccades cannot be triggered by volitional or optical stimuli. Contralateral refixation to the mid-position, but not beyond, is soon possible. After variable intervals of hours to weeks, full bidirectional saccadic excursions are evident. This acute saccadic paralysis is often attributed to frontal lobe damage (Holmes, 1938; Daroff and Hoyt, 1971) but extensive deep hemispheric involvement is the rule. Frontal eye field ablation in the monkey causes transient ipsilateral head and eye rotation and neglect of the contralateral visual field but contralateral saccades can be elicited (Latto and Cowey, 1971). Paralysis of saccades has not been documented after lesions confined to any discrete region of the cerebral cortex in man.

Defective saccadic triggering appears to comprise the saccadic paralysis after extensive acute lesions. Saccades are initiated by supranuclear trigger signals that may disinhibit pontine burst units by inhibiting saccadic pause cells (Chun and Robinson, 1978). Schiller, True and Conway (1980) found that bilateral frontal eye field ablation in the monkey causes only temporary partial visual neglect and reduced saccadic frequency. Ablation of both frontal eye fields and the superior colliculi produces virtual paralysis of saccades, suggesting that redundant pathways from the frontal eye fields and colliculi mediate saccadic triggering. Acute saccadic palsy in humans might represent a remote effect of corticofugal projections upon activity of the superior colliculus, *collicular shock,* analogous to the diaschisis of spinal shock.

Acute hemidecortication in the monkey causes ipsilateral deviation but contralateral saccades are evoked by auditory stimuli and all ocular motor functions appear intact within months (Pasik, Pasik and Bender, 1960). After chronic hemidecortication in man, saccadic velocities are equal in both horizontal directions but peak velocities are significantly lower and durations significantly longer than normal (Sharpe, Lo and Rabinovitch, 1979). The mild saccadic slowing suggests cerebral modulation of brain stem burst unit frequency. Horizontal symmetry of saccadic velocity demonstrates intact reciprocal function of rightward and leftward pontine saccadic pulse generators long after unilateral cortical ablation. However, saccadic latencies to unpredictable target steps are prolonged in both horizontal directions, indicating delayed release of brain stem burst units. Rehabilitation of contralateral saccades after unilateral damage may be mediated by the other hemisphere. Unilateral cerebral stimulation elicits predominantly contralateral saccades but some are ipsilateral (Robinson and Fuchs, 1979; Penfield and Jasper, 1954) and bilateral frontal lobe lesions are reported to cause persistent bilateral saccadic palsy (Cogan, 1956; Daroff and Hoyt, 1971).

In a patient studied a decade after hemispherectomy, Troost and his associates (1972) documented inaccuracy of contralateral saccades, manifested by multiple hypometric steps. They argued that these inaccuracies were not explained entirely by the hemianopia since saccadic hypometria persisted in darkness. Meienberg and co-workers (1981) found hypometria of saccades to contralateral target presentations in three patients with recent occipital lobe lesions. Hypometric saccades into the blind hemifield are eventually replaced by hypermetric overshoots that place the target image on the seeing hemiretina. The blind hemifield is like a curtain that moves with the eyes. Hypometria of saccades to targets in the seeing hemifield is another adaptation which insures against loss of the target in the blind hemifield.

Correspondence between the position of refixational eye movements and the position of targets transiently presented in the blind hemifield of patients with cerebral lesions has been invoked as evidence of midbrain processing of retinal information (Pöppel, Held and Frost, 1973; Weiskrantz and colleagues, 1974; Perenin and Jeannerod, 1978). This accuracy of saccades to cerebrally blind retinal targets is not confirmed in patients with recent occipital lesions (Meienberg and others, 1981). Perenin and Jeannerod (1978) studied saccadic latencies in two hemidecorticate patients using a forced choice paradigm wherein patients had to seek a target as soon as it escaped fixation. They found no difference in saccadic latencies to target amplitudes over 15° in the blind and seeing hemifields. Sharpe, Lo and Rabinovitch (1979) found disparity in the latencies to 5° paracentral targets and 20° and 40° eccentric targets presented in the blind hemifields of hemidecorticate patients. Latencies to forced-choice target presentations were significantly longer to 5° steps in the blind field than in the intact field but latencies to peripheral targets were symmetrical in both horizontal directions. The results suggest retinotopic dissociation of saccadic processing. Symmetrical latencies of saccades to peripheral targets might be mediated by direct retinocollicular projections subserving the blind hemifield.

Presumed collicular triggering of saccades to blind retinal targets has not withstood the rigorous test of random on-off presentation in the blind field. Random on-off target presentations elicit genuine ocular motor responses to the target which are distinct from forced-choice reactions to target disappearance as it jumps from view into the blind field. In the random on-off paradigm, patients with recent occipital lobe lesions do not react to targets in the blind field (Meienberg and others, 1981). In man, midbrain processing of saccades to cerebrally blind retinal targets lacks such compelling evidence.

Ocular Motor Apraxia

A congenital disorder of triggering voluntary horizontal gaze with the head immobile is called apraxia (Cogan, 1966). Head thrusts are utilized to activate gaze shifts. Saccadic delay and hypometria are fundamental defects (Zee, Yee and Singer, 1977). Combined head and eye motor programs compensate for saccadic delay by dispatching saccades or nystagmus fast phases in the direction of head motion. Some cases studied radiologically show dysgenesis of the corpus callosum (Orrison and Robertson, 1979) suggesting that a cerebral hemispheric defect might be responsible. However, the callosal defect might be coincidental and is not universal in patients with congenital ocular motor apraxia. The rare occurrence of structural brain stem lesions in children with presumed apraxia (Zaret et al, 1980), who have impaired generation of both nystagmus fast phases and voluntary saccades, makes CT scanning a mandatory diagnostic precaution.

Acquired intrahemispheric lesions cause gaze defects that have also been considered apraxic (Cogan and Adams, 1953; Waltz, 1961). In one variant voluntary and optically elicited refixation is defective but fixation and pursuit are relatively preserved. Fixation, once attained, is not readily shifted. This spasmodic fixation (Holmes, 1938) is attributed to bilateral frontal lobe lesions but pathological confirmation of discrete damage is unavailable. A report of a unilateral dominant frontal lesion associated with bidirectional impairment of voluntary, visual, and auditory evoked saccades (Waltz, 1961) suggests that one hemisphere exceptionally exerts predominant control of bidirectional eye movements.

Absence or misdirection of optically elicited saccades, and intact saccades to command, are associated with impaired visual guidance of limb movements (optic ataxia) and visual inattention in Balint's syndrome. Pursuit is severely impaired. Although the extent of lesions and clinical findings are quite variable, bilateral parieto-occipital damage is the common structural correlate (Hausser, Robert and Giard, 1980). The refixational saccadic deficit might correspond to damage to simian parietal lobe neurons which discharge before optically elicited saccades in all directions but not before voluntary saccades (Lynch and others, 1977b) or to disconnection of those units from frontal eye field neurons whose presaccadic discharge requires visual guidance (Bushnell and Goldberg, 1979).

The semantic propriety of apraxia in these disorders of saccadic programing is moot. Quantitative analysis of saccadic and head movement responses to volition and visual, vestibular, auditory and proprioceptive stimuli should pre-empt prevailing concepts of ocular motor apraxia.

Fixation Instability

Impaired fixation is manifested by square wave jerks (SWJ) in patients with focal frontal, parieto-temporal, or occipito-parietal lesions. These saccadic intrusions consist of 0.5° to 3° horizontal excursions followed some 200 msec later by refixation. They occurred in 70% of patients with acute and chronic cerebral lesions studied in our laboratory (Sharpe, Herishanu and White, 1982). Cerebral SWJ, like the physiological SWJ that occur at low frequency in some normal subjects (Herishanu and Sharpe, 1981), may be sporadically enlarged microsaccades. Mean amplitudes of cerebral SWJ are lower than those in cerebellar system disease but their frequency and duration do not differ. The amplitude duration, and frequency of SWJ are uniform regardless of the site of focal hemispheric damage. Cerebral SWJ are directed in either horizontal direction regardless of the side or site of cerebral lesions. In patients with complete homonymous hemianopia, SWJ toward the blind hemifield place the target on the seeing hemiretina, but SWJ toward the intact hemifield occlude the target by moving the blind hemifield across it. SWJ are not an adaptive strategy of visual search, because frequent SWJ toward the seeing hemifield occlude the target. Patients with hemianopia also make intermittent large searching saccades toward the blind hemifield, despite instructions to maintain steady fixation. Moreover, refixation saccades in patients with hemianopia often show adaptive, not disruptive, trajectories. Refixation saccades toward the blind hemifield may overshoot, placing the target image on the seeing hemiretina. Overshoots are corrected by return drifts (glissades) or saccades that place the target image at the seeing hemifovea (Meienberg and others, 1981). Precise refixation saccades toward the seeing hemifield that attain hemifoveation are often followed immediately by searching saccades toward the blind hemifield that place the target off-fovea on the seeing side of the macula. Hemifoveation is then attained promptly, once again, by backward drifts or saccades.

Omnipause cells in the pontine tegmentum are thought to inhibit saccadic burst neurons. They are independently activated by stimulation of the visual cortex or superior colliculus (King, Precht and Dierenger, 1980a). The dorsal lateral nucleus of the monkey thalamus also contains omnipause neurons (Schlag-Rey and Schlag, 1980) that could comprise an interface between cortical visual information and brain stem pause cells. Focal hemispheric damage apparently causes SWJ by releasing trigger signals that dispatch intrusive saccades followed by refoveating saccades. In contrast to focal cerebral lesions, complete hemidecortication causes fixational nystagmus (vide infra), not SWJ.

SMOOTH PURSUIT AND OPTOKINETIC SYSTEMS

Unilateral parieto-occipital lesions commonly cause ipsilateral impairment of smooth pursuit, evidenced by saccadic tracking. In contrast to rehabilitation of saccadic paralysis, ipsilateral pursuit paresis endures after hemidecortication (Sharpe, Lo and Rabinovitch, 1979). Ipsilateral pursuit gain, the ratio of smooth eye movement velocity to target velocity is subnormal at all target frequencies but contralateral pursuit gain is somewhat above unity at predictable target frequencies under 1.0 hertz. This pursuit pattern maintains the target on the seeing hemiretina during tracking in both horizontal directions. Compensatory foveating saccades are directed one way, toward the decorticate hemisphere. Although ipsilateral pursuit paresis is usually associated with contralateral homonymous hemianopia, the disorder does not appear to be simply a strategic adaptation to the field defect since smooth eye movement asymmetry does not accompany hemianopia caused by pregeniculate lesions, or recent damage to the optic radiation or striate cortex (Sharpe and Deck, 1978; Pasik and Pasik, 1964a).

Conventional clinical testing of optokinetic nystagmus (OKN) with hand-held striped drums or tapes may fail to appreciably activate the optokinetic system. The resulting nystagmus pattern may consist of sequential smooth pursuit and corrective saccades, rather than genuine OKN slow and fast phases which are assured by the illusionary self rotation and OKN-after nystagmus achieved by full field stimulation (Zee and others, 1976c). This does not negate the value of hand-held OKN stimuli in a clinical setting since paretic pursuit typically accompanies impaired OKN. However, the smooth pursuit and optokinetic tracking modes can be dissociated; foveal pursuit may be impaired disproportionately to OKN.

Severe impairment of foveal pursuit, together with little impairment of full field OKN during tracking toward the side of parietal lesions has been reported in two patients (Baloh, Yee and Honrubia, 1980 a). Baloh and his associates invoked disparity between pursuit and OKN as evidence of subcortical OKN in humans, perhaps mediated by the accessory optic system. Although ipsilateral OKN slow phase velocities did not attain normal gain in their study, integrity of peripheral retinal tracking was evidenced by slow build-up of OKN over 20 to 30 seconds. ter Braak, Schenk and Van Vliet (1971) recorded similar build-up of OKN in a case of long-standing bilateral occipital lobe and geniculate infarction; the patient claimed total blindness. These provocative reports suggest that extrafoveal optokinetic tracking in man, as in the monkey (Pasik and Pasik, 1964a; ter Braak and Van Vliet, 1964), may be independent of occipital or parietal lobe function. Foveal pursuit, on the contrary, requires integrity of prestriate cerebral function.

If one hemisphere is deprived of visual input by interruption of the classic optic pathway (Pasik and Pasik, 1964b), transfer of visual information from the intact fellow hemisphere, across the corpus callosum, is necessary for symmetrical OKN in the monkey. Unidirectional impairment of OKN elicited by hand-held targets moving toward the side of parietal lobe lesions in humans is typically associated with impaired pursuit in the same direction. Subcortical prestriate lesions may cause asymmetrical pursuit by disrupting commissural connections that transmit retinal velocity information from the intact hemisphere to prestriate cortex of the blind hemisphere. Pursuit asymmetry without hemianopia might result from disconnection of one parietal lobe from retinal information from both hemifields (Sharpe, Lo and Rabinovitch, 1979).

Unilateral lesions of prestriate cortex and subjacent white matter also lower contralateral pursuit gain, although less severely than ipsilateral gain (Fig. 1). The effect of a pure prestriate cortical lesion in humans is unknown. Each hemisphere participates in pursuit in both directions, an observation consonant with activity of simian parietal cortex units that discharge before and during pursuit in either horizontal direction (Lynch and others, 1977b). This neuronal activity may be the correlate of visual attention rather than of pursuit commands (Robinson, Goldberg and Stanton, 1978), but vigilance is prerequisite for normal pursuit.

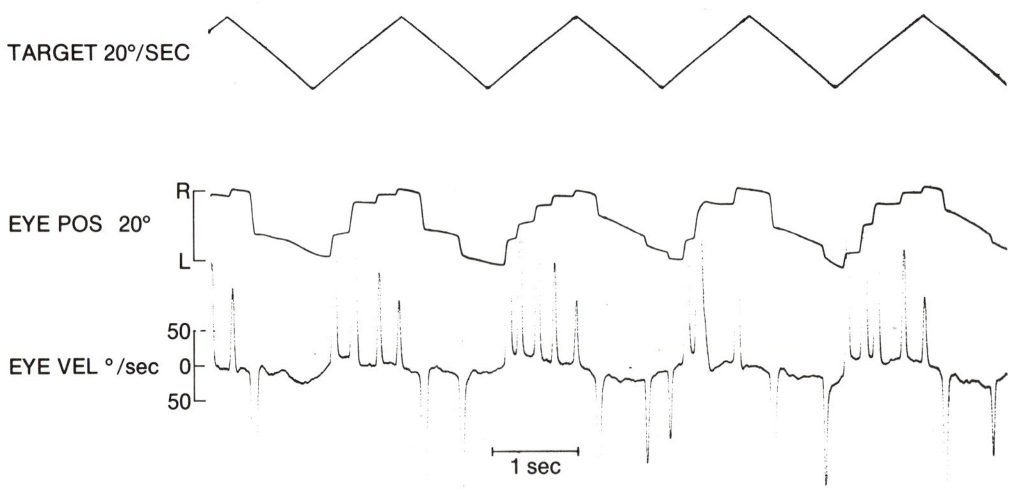

Fig. 1. Pursuit of triangular waveform target at 0.5 hertz in 46 year old male patient with right parietal tumor was asymmetrical, but subnormal in both horizontal directions. Mean rightward gain was 0.46 and leftward gain was 0.79.

VESTIBULO-OCULAR SYSTEM

The conjugate deviation that occurs after acute hemispheric damage may be overcome only by vigorous oculocephalic manoeuvres combined with caloric vestibular stimulation. Contralateral caloric nystagmus fast phases are lost transiently after extensive lesions in both man (Merwarth and Feiring, 1939; Daroff and Hoyt, 1971) and the monkey (Pasik, Pasik and Bender, 1960). The loss of contralateral nystagmus suggests that the primate cerebrum can participate in triggering fast phases, perhaps together with efferent motor programs which normally dispatch the voluntary saccades and head movements that achieve gaze shifts. Acute loss of vestibular slow phases in the direction of the saccadic palsy implicates a remote effect of cerebral projections upon brain stem vestibulo-ocular reflex (VOR) activity (Rosenberg, Sharpe and Hoyt, 1975). This transient vestibulo-ocular areflexia can be thought of as *vestibular shock*. With recovery, fast phases appear horizontally symmetrical (Sharpe and Lo, 1981), indicating intact reciprocal function of burst neurons for horizontal fast eye movements. Smooth eye movements, however, show enduring asymmetry.

The asymmetry is evident as directional preponderance of vestibular nystagmus induced toward the side of parieto-temporal lesions in man. The directional preponderance is abolished when fixation is eliminated (Carmichael and others, 1961). This indicates a cerebral effect on the VOR that is mediated by vision. In hemidecorticate humans contralateral VOR gain is slightly higher than ipsilateral gain when tested in darkness during sinusoidal whole body rotation at frequencies under one hertz (Sharpe and Lo, 1981). This smooth eye movement asymmetry in darkness is augmented by visual and voluntary (non-visual) modulation of the VOR.

Visual Control of the VOR

While following objects with the moving head, normal subjects cancel the VOR and the eyes remain relatively stationary in the orbit. Fixation of a stationary target during low frequency head motion normally enhances VOR gain to near unity so that the eyes remain stationary in space. In hemidecorticate patients, enhancement of the ipsilateral VOR is defective during low frequency head rotation away from the side of ablation (Sharpe and Lo, 1981). Cancellation of the contralateral VOR is defective during head rotation toward the side of posterior hemispheric lesions (Dichgans, Von Reutern and Rommelt, 1978; Sharpe and Lo, 1981). Although paresis of ipsilateral pursuit accompanies this unidirectional impairment of visual control of the VOR, voluntary modulation of the reflex in darkness is also asymmetrical. Asymmetrical voluntary control indicates that cerebral control of the VOR can be independent of the pursuit system.

Voluntary Control of the VOR

Normal subjects can voluntarily change the gain of the reflex by attempted fixation of imaginary targets during rotation in darkness. Fixation of imagined stationary targets elevates the gain while fixation of imagined targets moving with the head decreases it (Barr, Schultheis and Robinson, 1976; Sharpe and colleagues, 1981). Hemidecorticate patients exhibit impaired enhancement of the ipsilateral VOR and impaired cancellation of the contralateral VOR. Whether fixating an imaginary or a real target, patients have nystagmus toward the decorticate hemisphere during rotation (Fig. 2). Horizontal nystagmus also occurs toward the side of decortication in the absence of vestibular stimulation, with the head immobile.

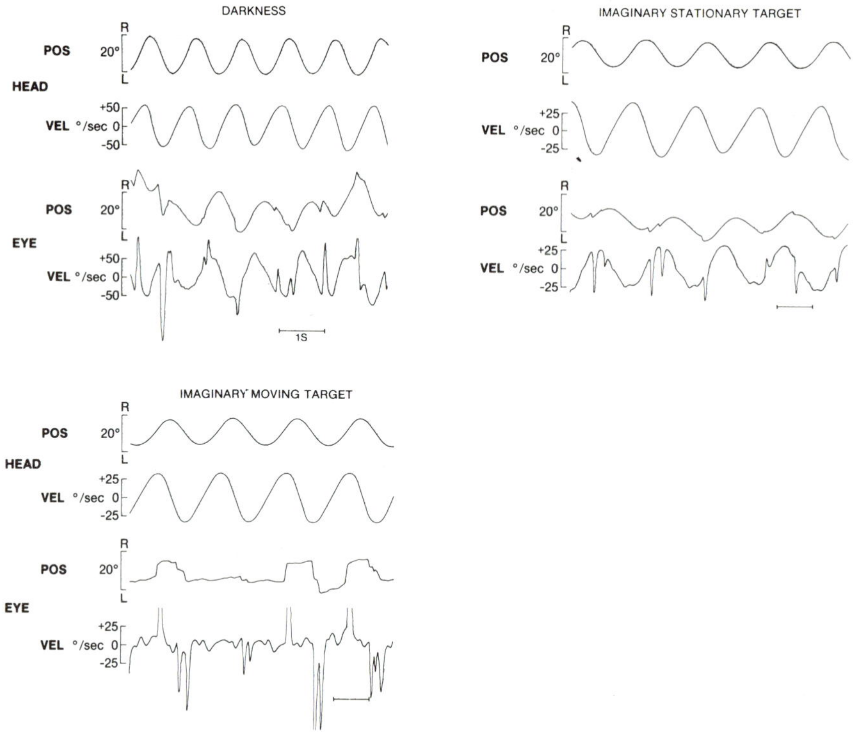

Fig. 2. Voluntary control of the VOR in patient with left hemidecortication. In darkness, nystagmus fast phases are bidirectional (upper left). Fixation of an imaginary target in darkness increases VOR asymmetry. Nystagmus is leftward, toward the decorticate hemisphere. Voluntary enhancement of the ipsilateral VOR (imaginary stationary target) and voluntary cancellation of the contralateral VOR (imaginary moving target) are defective.

The marked pursuit imbalance after hemidecortication is associated with static asymmetry of smooth eye movement control during fixation, evidenced by nystagmus toward the decorticate hemisphere, and it is associated with dynamic asymmetry of the VOR during rotation. The pursuit imbalance may cause both the static and the dynamic asymmetry. Zee and his associates (1974) proposed that impaired downward pursuit causes downbeat nystagmus by imbalancing vertical pursuit. Unlike nystagmus caused by primary vestibular imbalance, the nystagmus after hemidecortication does not increase in darkness, and it is not inhibited by fixation. Unlike vestibular nystagmus, it occurs during the effort to fixate an actual or an imagined target. Physiological nystagmus occurs after repetitive unidirectional pursuit stimulation. This pursuit after-nystagmus (Muratore and Zee, 1979) indicates that pursuit imbalance can cause nystagmus and supports the concept that nystagmus after hemidecortication is *pursuit paretic nystagmus* (Sharpe, Lo and Rabinovitch, 1979).

The distinction between nystagmus caused by vestibular imbalance and that caused by pursuit imbalance may be, in part, semantic, since the vestibulo-ocular and smooth pursuit systems may share neural circuits (see Fig. 3). Although this fixational nystagmus correlates with severe unidirectional paresis of pursuit, asymmetrical voluntary modulation of the VOR in darkness cannot be explained by imbalance in the pursuit system alone. Asymmetrical cerebral smooth eye movement velocity input to a brain stem site of vestibular interaction is a credible source of this horizontal imbalance.

When the retinal feedback loop of the pursuit system is opened by darkness, perceived location of an imaginary target can activate voluntary smooth eye movements to enhance or cancel the VOR. Non-visual regulation of the VOR requires spatial localization of the imagined target relative to the moving head and eyes (Barr, Schultheis and Robinson, 1976; Sharpe and Lo, 1981). Spatial localization of an imagined target in darkness utilizes information about gaze position, the sum of head position in space and eye position in the orbit. During whole body rotation vestibular signals of head velocity in either horizontal direction are relayed to parietal lobe neurons which receive visual input (Kawano, Sasaki and Yamashita, 1980). Eye position information utilized for spatial localization in darkness must be derived from feedback of either orbital proprioceptive inflow or eye position outflow—an efference copy that internally monitors smooth eye movement commands (Yasui and Young, 1975a; Barr, Schultheis and Robinson, 1976).

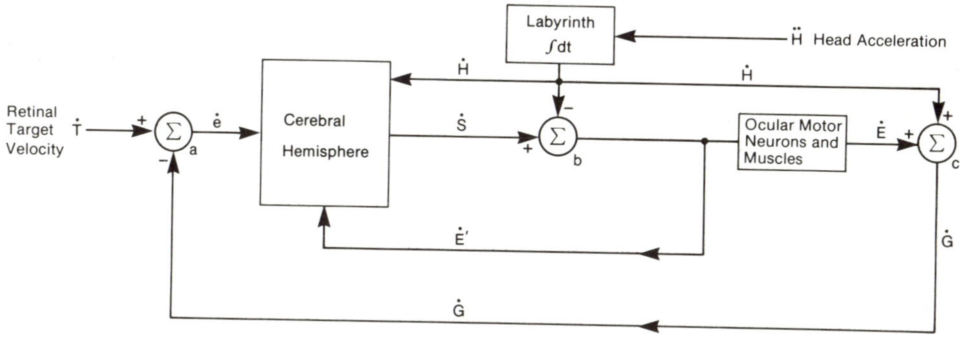

Fig. 3. Schematic cerebral control of the VOR by visual and voluntary smooth eye movement velocity commands ($\dot{S}$) at summing junction b. Gaze velocity ($\dot{G}$) is the sum of eye velocity in the orbit ($\dot{E}$) and head velocity in space ($\dot{H}$). When the pursuit feedback loop is opened by darkness at retinal summing junction a, an internal target percept activates an internal feedback loop. The cerebrum uses an internal estimate of eye velocity ($\dot{E}'$, efference copy) and a head velocity signal ($\dot{H}$) to direct voluntary smooth eye movements toward the perceived target location. One cerebral hemisphere processes the perpetual and retinal velocity error ($\dot{e}$) signals that generate ipsilateral smooth eye movements.

The cerebrum may use an efference copy of eye velocity and a head velocity signal to direct gaze toward the desired target position (Fig. 3). Pursuit feedback could then act in concert with internal efference feedback to achieve foveation by smooth eye movements during head or environmental motion. Since few normal subjects can generate any voluntary smooth eye movements with their heads immobile (Heywood, 1972), activation of non-retinal feedback utilizes a head motion signal. When parafoveal retinal image slip, the stimulus to smooth pursuit, is reduced to zero during effective tracking, this non-retinal positive feedback could sustain pursuit at unity gain.

One cerebral hemisphere regulates ipsilateral smooth eye movements that achieve both voluntary and visual control of the VOR. Cerebral hemispheric regulation of this visual-vestibular interaction probably depends on the same prestriate corticofugal pathways that mediate smooth pursuit. Proximate or identical cerebral, cerebellar and brain stem circuits may achieve voluntary and visual control of the VOR. Complete operation of the vestibulo-ocular system requires normal cerebral hemispheric function.

ACKNOWLEDGEMENTS

Supported by M.R.C. of Canada grants ME5509 and MT5404 and by the Physicians' Services Incorporated Foundation of Ontario. Mrs. Ruth Armstrong provided editorial assistance.

SUPRANUCLEAR CONTROL OF SACCADIC EYE MOVEMENTS

M. E. GOLDBERG

Laboratory of Sensorimotor Research, National Eye Institute, Bethesda, MD, and Department of Neurology, Georgetown University, Washington, DC, USA

ABSTRACT

Since the brainstem can program rapid eye movements without the intervention of supranuclear structures, the role of these structures is to trigger saccades at appropriate times. Three supranuclear structures have been shown to have activity preceding saccades: the superior colliculus, the posterior parietal cortex, and the frontal eye fields. Single cell recording in awake monkeys has shown that all three areas have visual activity, and that this visual activity is enhanced before purposive eye movements. In the parietal cortex this enhancement also occurs when the animal attends to the stimulus without making an eye movement. In frontal eye fields and superior colliculus the enhancement only occurs in association with eye movements. We postulate that this enhanced discharge is a trigger signal which tells the brainstem to make a saccade of certain amplitude and direction.

KEYWORDS

Saccades, monkey, frontal eye fields, posterior parietal cortex, superior colliculus, single cell recording, oculomotor control, visual responsiveness.

INTRODUCTION

The exact mechanism of the supranuclear control of eye movements is far from understood. No lesion above the reticular formation leaves man or monkey soundly ophthalmoplegic, and it is clear that no single structure is obligately required for the generation of saccades. However, since the 19th century (Adamuk, 1870; Ferrier, 1875) stimulation of cerebral cortex and superior colliculus has been known to elicit saccadic eye movements. Clinical evidence has also implicated these structures and it would be strange if the oculomotor system were in fact independent of these supranuclear structures (Sharpe, 1981).

It is clear that supranuclear structures do not participate in the motor programming of saccadic eye movements. The brainstem and cerebellar systems involved in the slow and quick phases of vestibular nystagmus can solve the motor problem of moving the eyeball quickly or slowly without help from the cerebral cortex or superior colliculus. The cortical centers have little or no direct projection to the oculomotor nuclear complexes (Kunzle and Akert, 1977; Kuypers and Lawrence, 1967; Leichnetz, 1980) This relative independence of the motor program from the cortex differs markedly from the skeletal motor system, especially that evolved to control the distal extremities, where single neurons in the cortex directly control a few muscle fibers (Asanuma, 1975), predict the force at a joint (Evarts, 1968), and project strongly monosynaptically to the motor neuron. Instead, it is more likely that the contributions to the guidance of eye movements is involved in functions germane to the selection and analysis of suitable targets for eye movements, and the transmission of that information to the brainstem.

EVIDENCE FROM STIMULATION EXPERIMENTS

The amplitude and direction of electrically evoked saccades is determined by the placement of the stimulating electrode. More intense stimulation does not result in larger saccades, and prolonged stimulation results in repetitive saccades of the same direction and amplitude, rather than prolonged or lengthened single saccades. (Robinson, 1972; Robinson and Fuchs, 1969). Stimulation of two points simultaneously results in the generation of saccades whose amplitude and direction is roughly the vector sum of the saccades evoked at either point. This vector addition phenomenon is true even when one stimulated point is in the frontal eye field and the other in the superior colliculus (True, Schiller, and Conway, 1979). The effects of stimulating cortex and colliculus differs sharply from stimulating the reticular formation, where the amplitude of the evoked eye movement depends on the length of the train of stimulating impulses. Thus, the activity in a certain collection of cortical neurons must imply a desired eye movement, and the brainstem saccade generating system must turn signals from differents parts of the supranuclear structure into the temporal code that actually drives the eye.

EVIDENCE FROM LESION EXPERIMENTS

No supranuclear structure alone is necessary for saccades. Lesions of the superior colliculus alone result in a transient loss of accuracy and reaction time, which recovers almost entirely. (Mohler and Wurtz, 1977; Wurtz and Goldberg, 1972b). Lesions of the frontal eye fields result in a slight diminution of saccade size and frequency. Recently, Albano and Wurtz (1981) have shown that a lesion which involves both superior colliculus and posterior and medial thalamus results in a monkey's inability to make accurate saccades to or from eccentric eye positions. Lynch (1980a) has shown that parietal-occipital lesions result only in increased latencies of eye movements. Schiller, True, and Conway (1980) have shown that superior colliculus lesions combined with frontal eye field lesions have a devastating effect on visually guided saccades in the monkey. These animals, trained to pick bits of food from a board in front of them tend to keep their eyes in the center of the orbit, and acquire targets with head saccades, if at all. This evidence provides the most compelling evidence that the cerebral cortex and the superior colliculus participate in some kinds of saccadic eye movements.

EVIDENCE FROM SINGLE NEURON EXPERIMENTS IN SUPERIOR COLLICULUS

Single neuron studies in these areas have indicated the mechanisms by which these centers might accomplish their contribution to the processes of oculomotor control. The superior colliculus provides a model for oculomotor processes. This six layered structure is divided into two physiologically distinct regions (Goldberg and Wurtz, 1972a, 1972b; Schiller and Koerner, 1971; Wurtz and Goldberg, 1972a, 1972b) the superficial layers (zonale, stratum griseum superficiale, and stratum opticum) and the deep layers (stratum grisum intermedium, stratum album intermedium, stratum griseum profundum, and stratum album profundum). In the monkey the great majority of cells in the superficial layers have visual receptive fields. (Goldberg and Wurtz, 1972a). In the deeper layers the majority of cells are not visually responsive, but have a discharge before eye movements of particular amplitudes and directions (Wurtz and Goldberg, 1972a). The superficial layer has a retinotopic map of the contralateral visual field, and the deep layers have a similar map of potential eye movement. The two maps are in register, so that neurons with receptive fields in a certain part of the visual field lie over neurons in the deep layers that discharge before eye movements to targets in that same area of the visual field.

The neurons in the deep layers discharge obligately before all rapid eye movements: even the quick phases of vestibular nystagmus. (Wurtz and Goldberg, 1971). Neurons in the superficial layers discharge in the response to the onset of spots of light in their receptive fields. These neurons do not discharge in association with spontaneous saccadic eye movements, and for some neurons their spontaneous discharge can be suppressed during saccades in any direction (Goldberg and Wurtz, 1972a). However, fifty percent of these neurons exhibit a phenomenon which is the model for eye movement related activity in higher centers: a neuron which has a visual response to a stimulus will have that response significantly enhanced when the animal makes a saccade to a stimulus in the receptive field. (Goldberg and Wurtz, 1972b). This enhancment is spatially specific: it only occurs when the animal is actually making a saccade to the area of the receptive, and does not occur when the animal makes a saccade elsewhere. Thus the cells in the superficial layers of the superior colliculus participate in the process of analyzing the visual environment and selecting targets for saccades. Although the visual stimulus is necessary for evoking cellular activity, only the combination of the visual stimulus and the selection of that stimulus results in the development by the cell of the maximum enhanced response.

EVIDENCE FROM SINGLE NEURON STUDIES IN CEREBRAL CORTEX

Much cortical activity that precedes saccadic eye movement can also be interpreted as an enhanced response resulting in the selection of a visual stimulus similar to that found in the superficial layers of the superior colliculus. The first efforts to show a presaccadic signal in cerebral cortex were significant in that they conclusively demonstrated that the cerebral cortex does not participate in the events preceding all saccades. Bizzi (1968) studied neurons in the monkey frontal eye fields while a monkey was making spontaneous eye movemetns in darkness. He found a population of neurons that discharged during and after saccades, and one that discharged in association with certain eye positions, but failed to show a neuronal class that discharged before spontaneous movements. The bulk of neurons in this study were undrivable by eye movements.

Mohler, Goldberg, and Wurtz (1973) subsequently showed that many of the cells in the monkey frontal eye fields that could not be driven with eye movements were responsive to visual stimuli. The cells had large receptive fields generally located in the contralateral visual field, and responded better to small spots than to larger stimuli. Like neurons in the superior colliculus, cells in the frontal eye fields yielded an enhanced response when the stimulus in the receptive field was a target for an eye movement. (Wurtz and Mohler, 1976b).

The second cortical association area with a discharge that precedes saccades in the posterior parietal cortex. Hyvarinen and Poranen (1974), and Mountcastle and his group, (Mountcastle, Lynch, Georgopoulis, Sakata and Acuna, 1975), showed that neurons in area 7 discharged before saccades, and Mountcastle observed that this was not an obligate discharge, but rather one that only preceded saccades relevant to the animal's behavior. They postulated that area 7 was important in direction visual attention, and that area 7 accomplished this direction by commanding saccades (Lynch, Mountcastle, Talbot, and Yin, 1977 a). These results were highly important and original, because although it had been known that electrical stimulation of the posterior parietal cortex could result in eye movements (Wagman, 1964), this area was in general thought of as a higher order somatosensory area (Jones and Powell, 1970). Hyvarinen's and Mountcastle's work showed that the regions were not so much a somatosensory area, but a region important in the analysis of extrapersonal space. Hyvarinen and Poranen (1974) interpreted this function as being accomplished by the association of somatosensory and visual inputs. Mountcastle interpreted this function as analysis of space through the command of movement (Mountcastle, 1976).

Our laboratory formulated a different interpretation (Bushnell, Goldberg and Robinson, 1981; Goldberg and Robinson, 1977; Robinson, Goldberg, and Stanton, 1978). It is apparent that many neurons in area 7 discharge before saccades. However, in our experience, such neurons could inevitably be driven by some visual stimulus in the absence of the eye movements. In many instances, this visual response, especially that to the small stimuli used to evoke eye movements, was very weak. These experiments showed that the discharge before saccadic eye movements could be interpreted as an enhancement of the visual response. Like neurons in the superior colliculus and the frontal eye fields, a main role of the posterior parietal cortex could be construed as the enhancement of visual responses so that a stimulus could have a greater effect on the oculomotor system.

RELATION OF EYE MOVEMENTS AND VISUAL ATTENTION

However, when a monkey makes a saccade to a visual target there are two ongoing neural processes. The first is the act of attending to the stimulus. The second is the act of actually performing the saccade to that stimulus. In primates with foveate retinas the processes of attention and eye movement are closely intertwined (Yarbus, 1967) but they are separable. Showing that a neuron discharges before a saccade is therefore not sufficient. One must also determine how that neuron responds when the animal attends to a stimulus without making an eye movement to it. By dissociating the act of a saccade from the fact of attention it is possible to determine how the enhanced discharges to visual stimuli relate to the process of eye movement.

Wurtz and Mohler (1976a) trained animals to attend to stimuli in the peripheral visual fields. The animals were trained to respond to the dimming of a light by releasing a lever. The animals were presented with two visual stimuli, one a small fixation point and the other a larger stimulus which could be placed in the receptive field of a neuron. Either the small fixation point or the peripheral visual field could provide the signal for the monkey's responses. The central fixation point was so small that the monkey had to fixate it in order to perform the task, but the animal could easily perceive the dimming of the larger stimulus with its peripheral vision. The animal's response to the dimming of the larger stimulus implied that the animal was in fact attending to it, but this attention occurred in the absence of an eye movement. When Wurtz and Mohler (1976a) studied neurons in the superior colliculus under this paradigm, they were unable to find neurons that gave an enhanced response to a stimulus that was not the target for an eye movement, and they concluded that enhancement in the superior colliculus was specific to eye movements.

We studied neurons in the posterior parietal cortex and the frontal eye fields in a similar task (Bushnell, Goldberg, and Robinson, 1981; Goldberg and Bushnell, 1981a, 1981b). In the posterior parietal cortex enhancement of the visual response occurred in roughly half of the neurons studied either before an eye movement to the stimulus in the receptive field or when the animal attended to the stimulus without making an eye movement. The quantitative intensity of the enhancement was equivalent in both tasks. Thirty-one neurons were studied in both tasks. Those neurons that gave an enhanced response in the peripheral attention task also yielded an enhanced response in the saccade task. Those that failed to yield an enhanced response in the peripheral attention task also failed to yield an enhanced response in the saccade task. These results imply that the attention is an important factor determining the response to which the attention may lead. Figure 1 shows the response of a neuron in the rhesus monkey posterior parietal cortex to the onset of a stimulus when that stimulus is irrelevant to behavior (A), when the stimulus is a target for an eye movement (B), or when the stimulus is used as a cue in a peripheral attention task (C). The response is enhanced in both cases where the animal must pay attention to the stimulus and not when the stimulus is irrelevant.

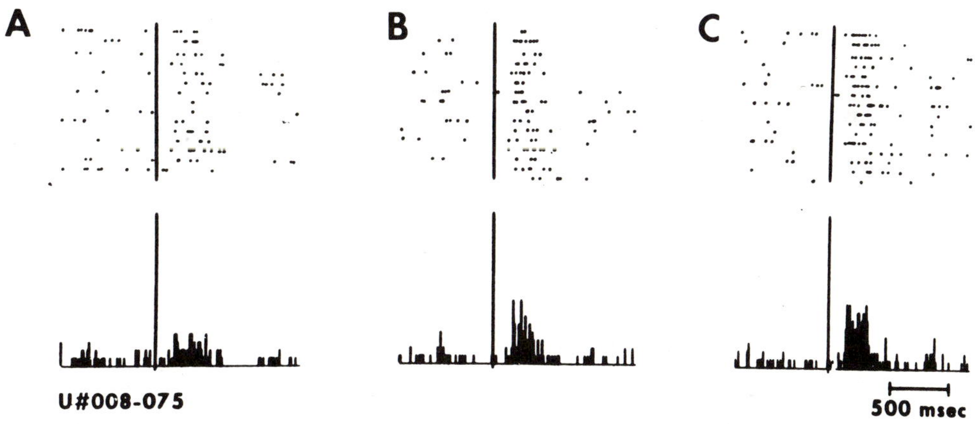

Figure 1. Dissociation of visual enhancement from eye movements in posterior parietal cortex. Each diagram consists of a raster (top) and related post stimulus histogram. Each dot in the raster signifies the occurrence of an action potential. Each line of a raster represents a two second epoch of cell activity. Successive trials are aligned on the stimulus onset, which occurs at the vertical line. Each histogram represents the sum of the activity in the raster above. The vertical line in the histogram corresponds to a discharge frequency of 114hz; bin width is 12 msec. A. Shows the response of a neuron when the stimulus is irrelevant. B. Shows the response of the same neuron when the stimulus is the target for an eye movement. C. Shows the response of the neuron when the animal attends to but does not make a saccade to the stimulus. Reproduced with permission from the Journal of Neurophysiology (Bushnell, Goldberg, and Robinson, 1981).

In a similar experiment we trained rhesus monkeys to reach out and touch stimuli without concurrently making an eye movement to fixate them (Bushnell, Goldberg, and Robinson, 1981). Parietal neurons which yielded an enhanced response in this hand reach task also yielded an enhanced response in the saccade task. The behavioral signal from the neurons in posterior parietal cortex shows that the stimulus in its receptive field is important, but the signal does not carry the information about the motor strategy that the animal will adopt in order to deal effectively with a stimulus.

The frontal eye fields present a very different picture. Although half of the neurons in the frontal eye fields of the monkey yield an ehanced response to stimuli that are the targets for eye movements, enhanced responses to stimuli in the peripheral attention task or hand reach tasks are found in fewer than five percent of cells (Goldberg and Bushnell, 1981a). Figure 2 shows the responses of a neuron in the frontal eye field of the monkey when the stimulus is irrelevant (A), used in the peripheral attention task (B), or used as the target for a saccade (C). Note that only in the saccade task does the stimulus evoke an enhanced response.

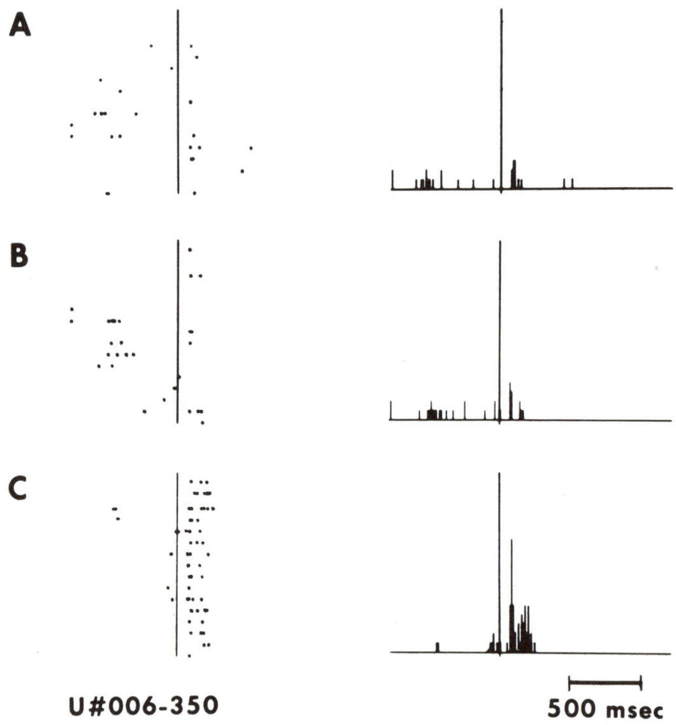

Figure 2. Saccade specific enhancement in frontal eye fields. A. Shows the response of a neuron in monkey frontal eye fields when the stimulus is irrelevant to the animal. B. Shows the response of the same neuron when the animal attends to the stimulus but does not make a saccade. C. Shows the response to the stimulus when the animal must make a saccade to it. Vertical lines signify stimulus onset. Reproduced with permission from the Journal of Neurophysiology (Goldberg and Bushnell, 1981b).

There is a direct relationship between the eye movements evoked by electrical stimulation from the frontal eye fields and the position of the receptive fields of presaccadic neurons. Eye movements evoked by electrical stimulation through the recording microelectrode are those which would be made to fixate stimuli in the receptive fields of neurons at the site of stimulation (Goldberg and Bushnell, 1981b).

These results imply that the frontal eye fields send a signal which is turned by the brainstem into a saccade. This signal must not be the only one which the brainstem can use to generate a saccade, since saccades can be made in the absence of the frontal eye fields, nor do the frontal eye fields participate in the neural events preceding all saccades: they participate only in the generation of purposeful, visually guided saccades.

The single neuron experiments above show that the frontal eye fields participate in certain visually guided saccades, but not in other saccades that are not involved in active visually guided behavior. Other experiments show that the brainstem saccadic system is more sensitive to frontal eye field stimulation when the animal is not performing a visual task than when it was. We (Goldberg and Bushnell, 1980) stimulated the frontal eye fields of rhesus monkeys when the monkey was at rest in a dimly lit environment, and when the monkey was actively looking at a small spot of light. Seventy msec trains of bipolar constant current pulses, 400 usec in duration, 350 hz in frequency were used throughout. Inevitably the current threshold, defined as that current which had a 0.5 probability of evoking a saccade, doubled when the monkey was actively fixating, as opposed to resting. In addition, the saccades evoked during fixation are slower and of shorter amplitude than those evoked at rest. These data imply that the brainstem can integrate a spurious saccade signal with the process of active fixation, and that visual fixation that is a part of purposive behavior is somehow less amenable to disruption from the frontal eye fields.

CONCLUSIONS

These three areas give us some insight into how higher centers control eye movements. Activity in these areas begins with some stimulus to make an eye movement, and continues until after the eye movement is accomplished. The activity can be triggered by the onset of some stimulus in the receptive field of the neuron, or it can be triggered by some other cue to the animal to make an eye movement (for example, the offset of the fixation point). Ongoing activity implies the impending occurrence of an eye movement of certain size and duration, and activity in a certain place in these supranuclear structures implies an eye movement of a certain direction. The length of the discharge is not related to any parameter of the eye movement except for its reaction time. Finally, the higher centers, because they provide this directional trigger signal rather than any code for the dynamic parameters of the movement, are not necessary for the eye movements nor do they control all saccade-like eye movements. However, as the brain evolved more complex structures to deal with the cognitive problems implied in higher functioning, cortical mechanisms evolved to control the already well functioning oculomotor system to participate in the process of visual analysis. When eye movements are an integral part of such purposive visual behavior the cerebral cortex is an active participant; when eye movements are not involved directly in some mode of higher behavioral processing, the cortex is not needed.

ACKNOWLEDGMENTS

Drs. David Lee Robinson and M. Catherine Bushnell participated in the experiments herein described. Jean Steinberg was invaluable in preparing the manuscript.

DISTURBANCES OF VOLUNTARY SACCADIC EYE MOVEMENT MECHANISMS FOLLOWING DISCRETE UNILATERAL FRONTAL LOBE REMOVALS

D. GUITTON, H. A. BUCHTEL and R. M. DOUGLAS

Montreal Neurological Institute, McGill University, 3801 University Street, Montreal, Quebec, Canada

ABSTRACT

Frontal patients made normal saccades to cue stimuli but were markedly abnormal in looking away. Their deficit was an inability to suppress a disallowed reflexive glance at the stimulus.

KEYWORDS

Frontal lobes, temporal lobes, frontal eye fields, eye movements, saccades, orienting response, foveation, visual grasp reflex.

INTRODUCTION

Each frontal lobe contains a region, called the frontal eye field (FEF), which has been implicated in the control of saccadic eye movements. Schiller, True and Conway (1980) have shown that ablation of both the FEF and superior colliculus (SC) together eliminates the primate's ability to make saccadic eye movements. However the synergistic role of these two structures remains unclear. Classically, the SC has been considered central to the programming of reflexive eye movements (the "visual grasp reflex"). The FEF, a cortical structure, could therefore be thought to impose some higher level control on this reflexive foveating mechanism (Holmes, 1938). We have examined the ability of human patients with frontal lobe lesions to perform a simple task requiring a presumably higher level control of foveation: the "anti-saccade" task first used by Hallett (1978), Hallett and Adams (1980).

METHODS

Nine patients having discrete unilateral removal of frontal lobe tissue for the relief of intractable epilepsy were studied during the second week that followed the operation. Three of these had probable FEF lesions. The control group consisted of 9 normal subjects and 5 patients having discrete temporal lobe removals performed 2 weeks earlier.

Each subject faced a large cathode ray oscilloscope screen onto which there first appeared a central fixation point (FP). After a short random time, the FP was extinguished and a stimulus cue appeared for 100 msec randomly 12° either to the left or right. In the standard foveation task (Hallett's N-task) the subject was told to look at the location of the cue. In the "anti-saccade" task (Hallett's A-task), run separately, the subject was told to look not at the location of the cue but in the opposite direction, an equal distance from FP. A symbol (a square with a gap on one side) eventually appeared briefly at the required goal and the correct identification of the gap location required the eyes to be already on target. In all patients the first anti-saccade test was an easy task with a time between cue and symbol of approximately 500 msec. Whenever possible this time was progressively shortened in subsequent runs. The response of a subject was non-verbal: the gap location was indicated by orienting the right thumb in the proper direction. No feedback on correctiveness of response was given during the tests. Eye movements were measured using EOG.

RESULTS

N-task

All patients with temporal or frontal lobe lesions (including those with probable lesions of the FEF) could perform, with normal latency and accuracy, the standard foveation task.

A-task

Both the normal subjects and the temporal lobe patients were able to make anti-saccades in almost 80% of the trials. In the remaining 20% there was typically a short latency saccade aimed at the cue similar to those seen in the N-task, followed by a large corrective saccade in the opposite direction to the location at which the target symbol was to appear. The frontal lobe patients exhibited deficits in direction, precision and timing. The most consistent and conspicuous feature of the deficits was in the direction of the initial saccade, and because of space limitations only this aspect of the results will be considered here.

All frontal patients experienced considerable difficulty in suppressing a reflex-like saccade to the cue stimulus in the A-task (Fig. 1). In 5 patients (Y.G., R.M., E.K., L.G., J.H.) the deficit was present in the first "easy" run and was generally worse when the cue stimulus was presented to the side contralateral to their lesion. In the remaining 4 patients (S.K., S.B., J.R., J.F.) the deficit appeared only when the task was made difficult by reducing the time between cue and symbol. In 3 of these patients the disturbance strongly depended on the direction of the required "anti-saccade". They had difficulty in suppressing a reflex-like saccade to the cue when it was located in the visual field contralateral to their lesion. When the cue was presented to their ipsilateral field, and therefore projected initially to their intact cerebral hemisphere they were normal in their ability to prevent the reflex-like saccade and thus to generate an "anti-saccade".

Deficits were also seen in the corrective saccade that followed the many incorrect reflexive responses. Four of the 5 patients (Y.G., E.K., L.G., J.H.) that exhibited directional deficits in the "easy" tests also had difficulty making corrective saccades (i.e. ones organized by their lesioned hemisphere) back to the contralateral anti-saccade goal. This abnormality was reflected in timing and accuracy and in 1 case (Y.G.) by the total incapacity to generate this movement. By contrast a corrective return movement organized by the good hemisphere was, in all patients, essentially normal.

DISCUSSION

Frontal lobe lesions, particularly in the dorsolateral region, have been associated with unilateral neglect in monkey (Kennard and Ectors 1938; Welch and Stuteville, 1958) and man (Heilman and Valenstein, 1972). The present results do not agree with these observations. None of our frontal lobe patients neglected visual targets in the N-task. Indeed, in the anti-saccade task they had difficulty in neglecting the cue stimulus and usually made a saccade to its location, even though they were asked not to look.

It is noteworthy that the temporal lobe patients showed absolutely no deficit on either the N or A tasks and that in those patients that had both frontal and temporal lesions (S.K. and J.F.) the deficits were indistinguishable from the frontal group. The site of the ablation as well as electrical stimulation during surgery suggest that patients Y.G., E.K., L.G. and J.H. probably had FEF lesions. It is of interest that these FEF patients essentially form the group that experienced the most difficulty in suppressing a reflexive glance at the cue even in the easy test runs. All of these patients, save J.H. showed strong bilateral effects. These patients were also unique in their difficulty in generating a corrective return saccade organized by the bad hemisphere.

In general the data is in agreement with the hypothesis that the frontal lobes - and possibly specifically the FEF - modulate a reflexive foveating mechanism: i.e. they play a role in inhibiting saccades to inappropriate but visually attractive stimuli.

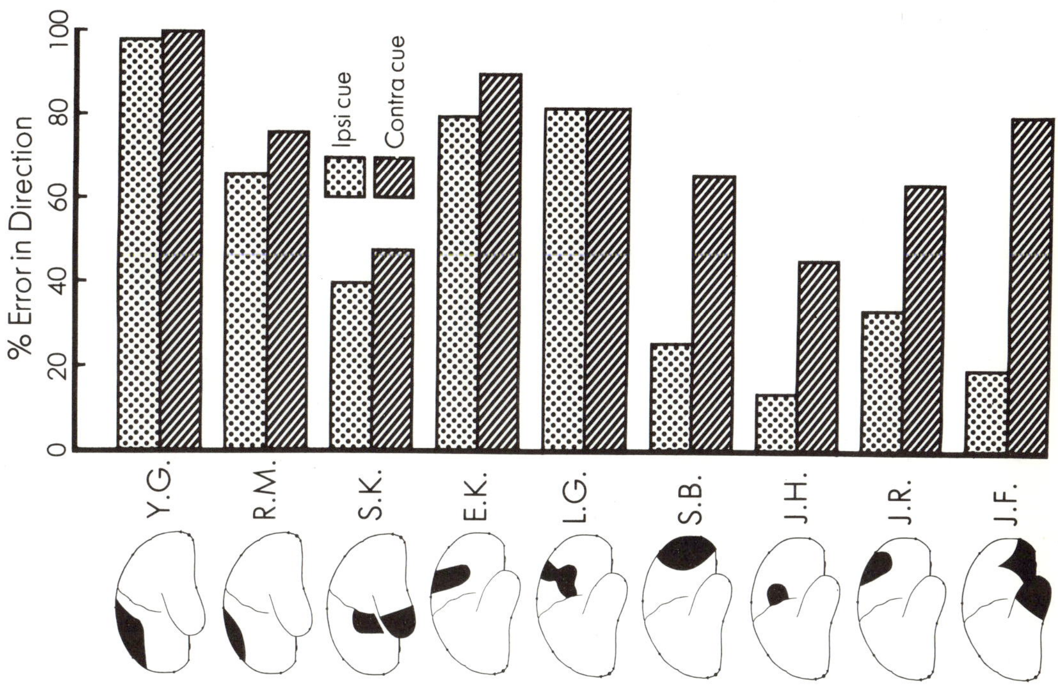

Fig. 1. Anti-saccade task. The number of incorrect "reflexive" glances relative to the total number of trials made by the frontal patients. The darkened areas on the brain maps indicate the lesioned areas. Normal and temporal lobe subjects were similar to each other and had, on the average, a 20% error in direction. Contra; Ipsi cue: cue flashed respectively contralateral and ipsilateral to the lesion.

Supported by The Medical Research Council of Canada.

THE CONTRIBUTION OF PARIETO-OCCIPITAL ASSOCIATION CORTEX TO THE CONTROL OF SLOW EYE MOVEMENTS

J. C. LYNCH[1] and J. W. MCLAREN[2]

Department of Physiology and Biophysics, Mayo Clinic and Foundation, Rochester, Minnesota, USA

ABSTRACT

Slow eye movements were studied in monkeys during optokinetic nystagmus (OKN) and visual tracking before and after surgical lesions of posterior association cortex. OKN was impaired, with reduced slow phase velocity toward the side of the lesion, following unilateral damage which included dorsal prestriate cortex and posterior parietal cortex (IPL-PS lesions). Lesions which were restricted to the inferior parietal lobule (IPL lesions) did not produce significant OKN impairment. Visual tracking performance was not seriously disrupted following any unilateral lesion, but bilateral lesions (both IPL and IPL-PS) caused saccadic pursuit in both vertical directions in all four monkeys tested. Two of the four monkeys also had horizontal tracking impairments in both directions. These results indicate that in monkeys there are two distinct neural systems in the posterior association cortex which participate in the generation of slow eye movements.

KEYWORDS

Slow eye movements; visual tracking; slow pursuit; optokinetic nystagmus; association cortex; posterior parietal cortex; prestriate cortex; lesions.

INTRODUCTION

The neural systems which are involved in the control of eye movements are widely distributed across many areas of the nervous system and reside, in part, in several regions of the cerebral cortex as well as in some thalamic nuclei, the cerebellum, superior colliculus, pretectum, paramedian pontine reticular formation, and other midbrain and brainstem regions. The contributions of these areas vary greatly and include the direct motor control of the extraocular muscles, the generation and storage of internal programs of motor activity, and the processing

---

[1] Present address: Department of Anatomy, University of Mississippi Medical Center, Jackson, Mississippi 39216

[2] Present address: Department of Ophthalmology, Mayo Clinic and Foundation, Rochester, Minnesota 55905

of sensory information arising in the visual, vestibular, and somatosensory systems in order to provide the motor apparatus with the required parameters of the surrounding environment as well as to generate an internal neural replicate of this environment. Finally, the higher order neural process of selective attention plays a central role in eye movement control by separating out appropriate targets for eye movements from the potentially overwhelming amount of sensory information which continually impinges upon the nervous system (Robinson, 1975a; Raphan and Cohen, 1978; Daroff and Troost, 1978; Dell'Osso and Daroff, 1979; Young, 1977; Jung, 1977; Lynch, 1980a).

Within the cerebral cortex, the areas most directly involved in eye movement control are the frontal eye fields and the posterior association cortex, including the inferior parietal lobule and dorsal prestriate cortex. That posterior association cortex plays a role in eye movements has been suggested at least since 1876, when David Ferrier reported that electrical stimulation of parieto-occipital cortex in monkeys produced movements of the eyes toward the side opposite the hemisphere being stimulated. The experiments of Fleming and Crosby (1955) and Wagman (1964) have provided verification of this early observation.

Another line of evidence implicating posterior association cortex in the control of eye movements comes from behavioral-electrophysiological experiments in which the neural activity of single cells was recorded while animals performed learned oculomotor tasks. Neurons in area 7 have been observed which show no apparent sensory response to small visual stimuli, but which discharge vigorously before and during visually evoked saccadic and visual tracking eye movements while other neurons have been observed in which the sensory response to a visual stimulus is enhanced in conjunction with visually evoked eye movements (Mountcastle and colleagues, 1975; Lynch and colleagues, 1977a;Yin and Mountcastle, 1977; Sakata, Shibutani, and Kawano, 1978; Goldberg and Robinson, 1977; Robinson, Goldberg, and Stanton, 1978; see Lynch, 1980a, for review).

When parieto-occipital cortex is damaged in humans, the resulting symptoms often include disorders of voluntary and involuntary eye movement. Perhaps the most common is asymmetric optokinetic nystagmus following unilateral parieto-occipital lesion (Smith, 1963; Baloh, Yee, and Honrubia, 1980 a. In addition, oculomotor apraxia (an inability to look at a desired target without marked paralysis of eye movement) and disorders of slow pursuit including saccadic or "cogwheel" pursuit have been reported following posterior hemispheric damage in humans (Sharpe, Lo, and Rabonovitch, 1979; Baloh, Yee, and Honrubia, 1980 a,see Lynch, 1980a, for review).

A difficulty in the interpretation of clinical reports of behavioral deficits which follow brain damage in man is that disease and trauma rarely affect a single functional or anatomical entity in the brain, and consequently it is difficult to correlate a particular deficit with the loss of a particular neural structure or area. One attempt to overcome this difficulty has been to train subhuman primates to perform appropriate behavioral tasks and then observe the effect of precise, histologically confirmed brain lesions. The present experiments were designed to determine quantitatively the extent of disruption of slow eye movements in monkeys which is produced by experimental lesions of parieto-occipital association cortex. Slow eye movements were performed in a visual tracking task and during optokinetic stimulation. Oculomotor performance was studied before and after unilateral and bilateral cortical lesions. The results reported here have been discussed in a preliminary form at a symposium on vision (Lynch, 1980b) and in a theoretical paper (Lynch, 1980a).

METHODS

Eye position was recorded in 5 rhesus monkeys through Ag-AgCl pellet electrodes which were permanently implanted in the bony extra-orbital ridges. The electro-oculogram (EOG) signals from horizontal and vertical electrode pairs were amplified (bandwidth: dc-100 Hz), digitized at 10 msec intervals, and stored on magnetic disks. During recording sessions each monkey was seated in a plexiglas primate chair with its head rigidly fixed. Monkeys were returned to their home cages between recording sessions.

The monkeys were trained to fixate a small (0.1°) target light on a tangent 52° square rear-projection screen. When the target light was turned on under program control the monkey pulled an operant lever and held it back for 1-3 seconds while waiting for the target to dim. When the target dimmed slightly (after a randomly-selected delay), the monkey was required to push the lever forward within 500 msec in order to receive a liquid reward. The target was so small and the dimming so slight that the monkeys had to use central vision in order to detect the dim. After this task had been learned, the target could be positioned anywhere on the screen or moved in any direction, thus forcing the monkey to direct its gaze at any point in a 52° square or to execute saccadic eye movements of up to 24° or pursuit eye movements at velocities up to 40°/sec in either the horizontal or vertical plane. Parameters of the task were altered frequently in the course of the training to force the monkey to fixate accurately. The eye position signal was calibrated by measuring potential changes during saccadic eye movements between targets of a known distance.

Optokinetic nystagmus (OKN) was induced by placing the monkey at the center of a drum (122 cm diameter, 112 cm height) with alternating vertical black and white stripes (15° each) that could be rotated at angular velocities between 20°/sec and 160°/sec. The drum was lighted from above at a level of 4.7 foot-candles measured at the height of the monkey's eyes. All monkeys had strong, regular OKN in this stimulus situation. No drugs were used to enhance the monkeys' level of alertness. After eye movements had been measured during pursuit tasks and OKN stimulation for 10-20 days, cortical lesions were made under sterile conditions.

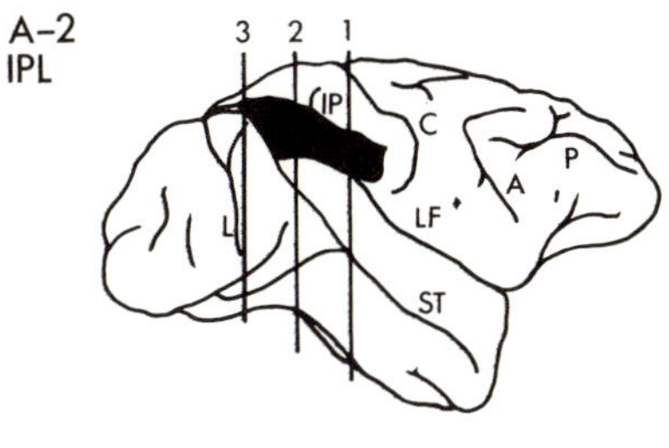

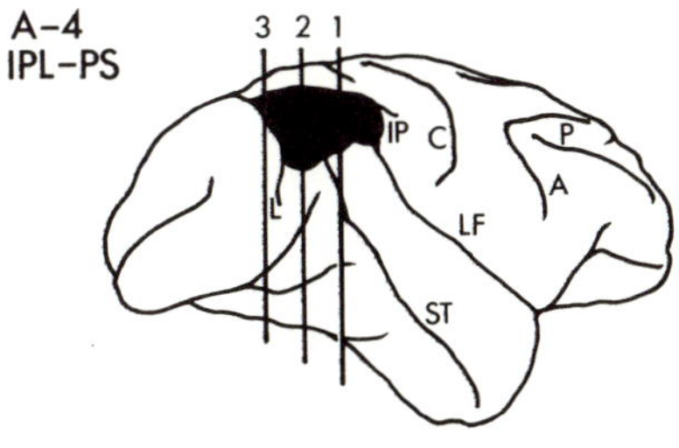

FIGURE 1. Representative cortical lesions. Two monkeys received lesions limited to the inferior parietal lobule (IPL), while 3 monkeys received lesions which included the inferior parietal lobule and adjacent dorsal prestriate cortex (IPL-PS). See McLaren and Lynch (in preparation) for complete reconstructions of the brains and the lateral geniculate nuclei. Sulci are indicated by letters: L, lunate; ST, superior temporal; LF, lateral fissure; IP, intraparietal; C, central; A, arcuate; P, principal.

Animals were anesthetized with sodium pentobarbital and cortex was removed by subpial aspiration. Three monkeys (A-3, A-4, and A-5) received unilateral lesions that included the inferior parietal lobule (area 7 of Brodmann) and the adjacent dorsal portion of pre-striate cortex (areas 18 and 19). These lesions were designated IPL-PS lesions. In two other monkeys (A-2 and A-6) the lesions included only the inferior parietal lobule (area &) and were designated IPL lesions. Representative lesions are illustrated in Figure 1.

Behavioral testing commenced the day following surgery and continued for 2-12 weeks. In four monkeys a second lesion, of approximately the same size as the first, was then made in a similar region of the opposite hemisphere and behavioral testing continued for another 2-4 weeks. At the end of the experiment monkeys were deeply anesthetized and sacrificed by intracardiac perfusion with normal saline followed by 10% buffered formalin. Brains were blocked in the stereotaxic plane, frozen, sectioned at 50 µm, and stained with cresylecht-violet. The sections were projected and traced and the extent of cortical damage and retrograde thalamic degeneration was reconstructed.

RESULTS

OKN was measured after unilateral lesions in 5 monkeys. The major deficit was a diminution of the mean velocity of the slow component of the OKN when the stimuli moved toward the side of the lesion, as illustrated in Figure 2. In this figure, eye position is plotted as a function of time during 80°/sec drum rotation. The top pair of traces depicts typical OKN in a normal monkey while the bottom pair of traces shows typical OKN following a left hemisphere IPL-PS lesion. The upper of each pair of traces shows OKN during right-to-left stimulus movement; the lower shows OKN during left-to-right movement.

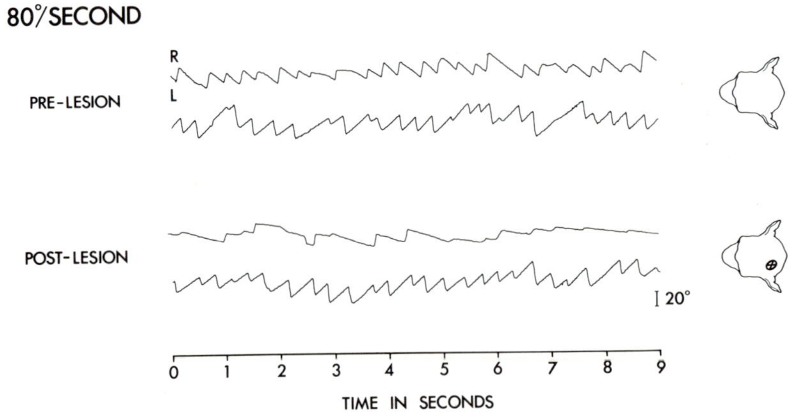

FIGURE 2. Eye position traces during OKN recorded before and after a left IPL-PS lesion (indicated by an X in the monkey head diagrams to the right of the traces). Stimulus velocity was 80°/sec. Monkey A-4.

Mean slow phase velocity over a 27-second OKN collection period was calculated by an interactive analysis program. Figure 3 shows mean slow phase eye velocity over days at 3 different drum velocities for a monkey before and after unilateral and bilateral IPL-PS lesions. After a unilateral IPL=PS lesion, mean slow-phase

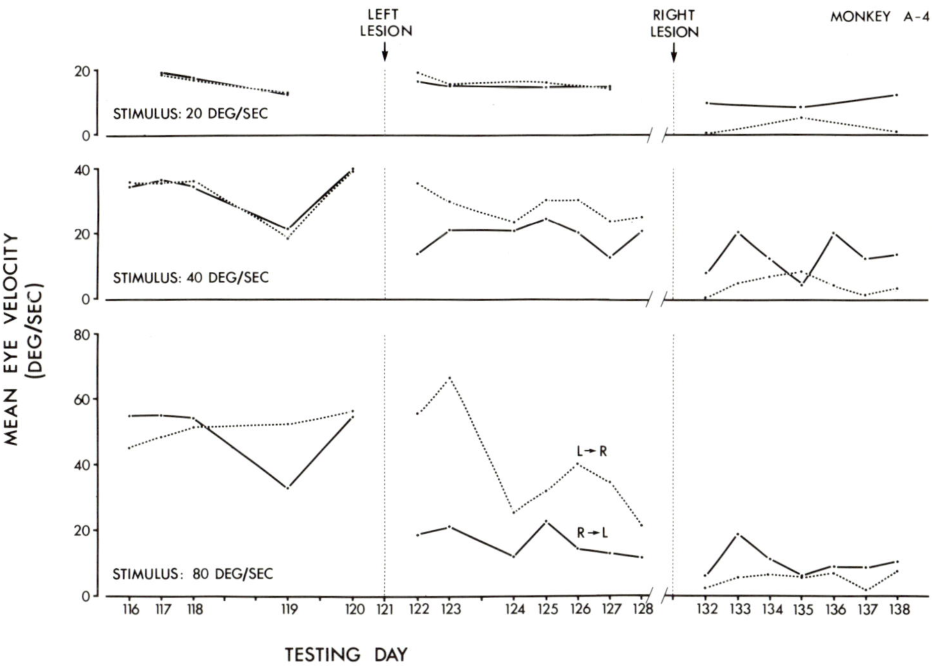

FIGURE 3. Mean slow phase velocity before and after unilateral ("LEFT LESION") and bilateral ("RIGHT LESION") IPL-PS lesions. Monkey A-4.

velocity was unchanged at 20°/sec, but at 40° and 80°/sec was more depressed when the stimuli moved from the monkey's right to left (toward the side of the lesion) than when the stimuli moved in the opposite direction. This reduction was statistically significant for the 3 monkeys which received IPL-PS lesions (t-test for paired samples), but not for 2 monkeys which received IPL lesions. Figure 3 also shows that following the second lesion, slow phase velocity was depressed in both directions even at the slowest stimulus velocity. This was characteristic of all 3 IPL-PS monkeys, while the 2 IPL monkeys had only mild and transient deficits following bilateral lesions. Monkey A-4 showed the least recovery following unilateral lesion of any IPL-PS monkey. A-3 and A-5 recovered to 75% of their mean pre-lesion slow phase velocity within 8 and 7 days, respectively, at 40°/sec stimulus velocity.

The monkeys were also trained in visual pursuit tasks. Horizontal and vertical eye position signals during a horizontal tracking task are illustrated in Figure 4. The pursuit target appeared under program control at one edge of the tangent screen and after a delay of 500 msec it either dimmed where it was or began to move across the screen at 10°, 20°, or 30°/sec. Each condition shows 10-15 superimposed EOG traces. One hundred fifty trials were given in random order and the eye position data were sorted and plotted at a later time. K indicates the time at which the operant lever was pulled; M indicates the point at which target movement began; and D indicates the time of dimming. After sufficient training, monkeys were able to accurately track the target with a high degree of reliability. Performance on the tracking task was not seriously impaired by unilateral IPL-PS or IPL lesions. The data illustrated in Figure 4 were collected 7 days after a unilateral IPL-PS lesion and are indistinguishable

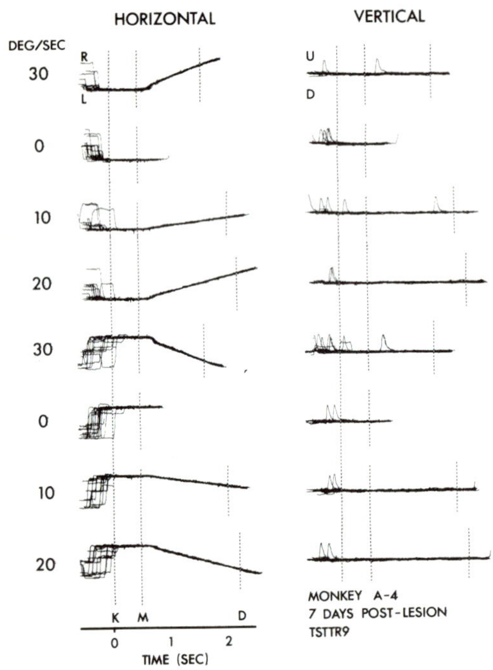

FIGURE 4. Superimposed EOG traces recorded during a horizontal visual pursuit task. K: lever pull; M: target movement; D: target dim. Monkey A-4, unilateral IPL-PS lesion.

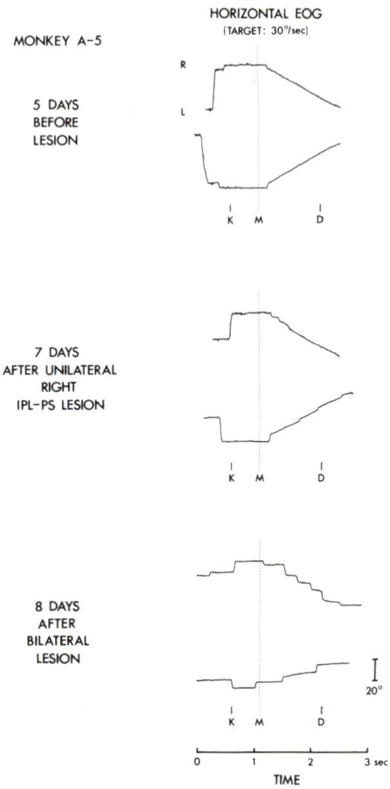

FIGURE 5. Typical EOG traces from a horizontal pursuit task. Monkey A-5, IPL-PS lesion. Reprinted by permission from Lynch, 1980a.

from pre-lesion data.

Visual tracking was markedly impaired, however, following bilateral lesions. Figure 5 shows representative eye position traces for monkey A-5 before lesion, after a unilateral IPL-PS lesion, and after bilateral lesion. Tracking accuracy was only slightly impaired after the first lesion, but after the second lesion the monkey was no longer able to generate smooth slow eye movements in response to a small moving target. All 4 monkeys which received bilateral lesions were similarly impaired in vertical pursuit. Two of these monkeys (A-5, IPL-PS lesion and A-2, IPL lesion) were impaired in horizontal pursuit. The monkey which received only a unilateral lesion had no tracking deficit, nor did 3 of the other 4 monkeys after their first lesions. A-5 had a brief tracking impairment when the target moved away from the side of the lesion (opposite in direction to the OKN deficits). This deficit persisted for about 5 days following a right IPL-PS lesion (see Figure 7 below).

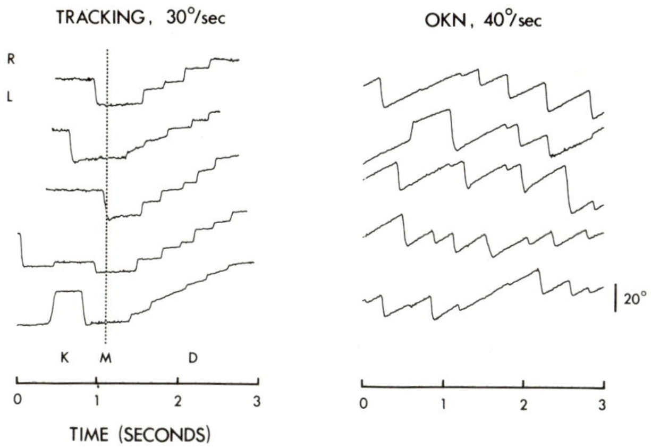

FIGURE 6. EOG traces during horizontal pursuit (left) and OKN (right) collected 17 days after bilateral IPL-PS lesion. Monkey A-5.

Figure 6 shows the oculomotor performance of monkey A-5 in a visual tracking task and during OKN after a bilateral IPL-PS lesion. At this time (17 days after the lesion), OKN performance had recovered to a considerable extent and the monkey was able to generate smooth slow phase eye movements which approximately matched the OKN stimulus velocity of 40°/sec. During the tracking task, however, the monkey was unable to match eye velocity to a target velocity of 30°/sec and could follow the target only with a series of small saccades.

The slow eye movements of visual pursuit and of optokinetic nystagmus are therefore seen to be affected differentially by cortical lesions and to recover at different rates. This dissociation between the effect of parieto-occipital lesions on the two types of eye movements is illustrated in another way in Figure 7. Monkey A-5 had a brief tracking deficit in only one direction following a unilateral IPL-PS lesion, as well as the usual OKN deficit. However, tracking was impaired when the target moved from right to left, while OKN slow phase velocity was depressed only in the opposite direction.

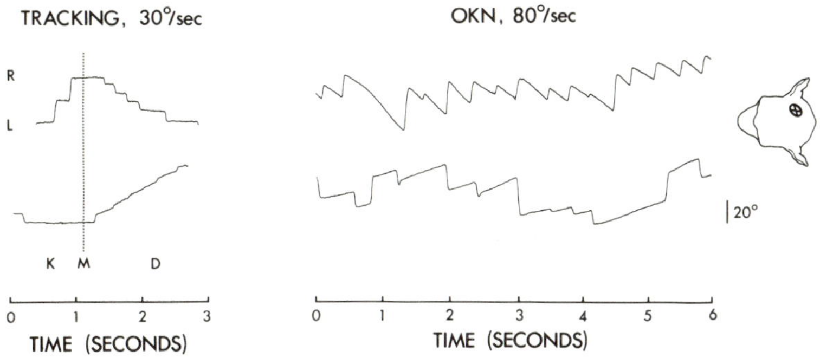

FIGURE 7. EOG traces recorded during tracking and OKN 4 days after right IPL-PS lesion. Monkey A-5.

DISCUSSION

Slow, smooth, conjugate eye movements are generated under a variety of conditions including the active tracking of a slowly moving visual target, optokinetic stimulation, angular acceleration of the head, caloric stimulation of the labyrinth, tracking of an unseen limb, tracking of a visual after-image, and the tracking of successively illuminated stationary points (Dell'Osso and Daroff, 1979; Young, 1977; Collewijn, 1972). The signal which is necessary to generate these slow eye movements is, in many cases, a retinal error ("slip") velocity which is reduced to zero when eye velocity matches target velocity (Robinson, 1975a. In some situations, however, afferent information from a non-visual modality or computed perceptual information is sufficient (Gauthier and Hofferer, 1976; Steinbach, 1976). Lesions of the central nervous system can impair the execution of some slow eye movements while leaving others intact. For example, the slow eye movements of vestibular nystagmus are usually normal following posterior hemispheric lesions in humans while the slow eye movements of optokinetic nystagmus are impaired toward the side of the lesion (Jung and Kornhuber, 1964).

The results reported here demonstrate that lesions limited to non-sensory, non-motor areas of the cerebral cortex of monkeys can disrupt the performance of at least two of these types of slow eye movements: visual pursuit and the slow phase of optokinetic nystagmus. The results tend to support Cords' hypothesis that the prestriate area is the site of the cortical mechanism of optokinetic nystagmus (Cords, 1926; Smith, 1963) and to argue against Cogan's proposal that posterior parietal cortex itself is essential for the generation of normal optokinetic nystagmus (Cogan, 1966). However, in the present series of experiments we have not yet made lesions restricted to only dorsal prestriate cortex and therefore a third possibility is also still open. It may be that the IPL-PS lesions were more effective in disrupting OKN than were the IPL lesions because the neural system concerned with optokinetic nystagmus is distributed across both posterior parietal and prestriate cortex. The IPL-PS lesions may thus have a greater effect on OKN simply because they destroy a larger proportion of this distributed system. While there is not at present any direct evidence in support of this last possibility, it cannot be dismissed until the experiment is actually performed because other functions, including visual spatial discriminations and some somatosensory discriminations, have been shown to be distributed across both of these cortical areas (Ungerleider and Mishkin, 1980; Moffett and colleagues, 1967; Ridley and Ettlinger, 1975; see Lynch, 1980a for review).

The OKN deficits which we have observed in monkeys have been considerably shorter in duration than those commonly observed in humans, where OKN may still be depressed months or even years after unilateral brain damage (Jung and Kornhuber, 1964). One possible explanation for this difference is that the directional properties of the cortical slow phase system may be more lateralized in humans than in monkeys, and that the OKN recovery in monkeys is mediated, at least in part, by a greater capacity for the remodelling of neural connections in the spared hemisphere. This hypothesis is supported by the observation in the present study that the OKN impairment following the second lesion in monkeys A-4 and A-5 was more profound and longer-lasting than that following the first lesion.

A second factor which may contribute to the rapid OKN recovery in monkeys is that while subcortical mechanisms undoubtedly contribute to the generation of OKN in both humans and monkeys this contribution appears to be greater in monkeys. Complete removal of striate cortex in monkeys is followed by initial abolition of OKN, but substantial recovery often occurs within a few months (ter Braak and van Vliet, 1963). In contrast, most (though not all) human patients who have been examined after complete destruction of the occipital lobe have failed to display optokinetic nystagmus (Brindley, Gautier-Smith, and Lewin, 1969; ter Braak,

Schenk, and van Vliet, 1971; see Baloh, Yee, and Honrubia, 1980a for review). The presence of recognizable, though somewhat abnormal, OKN following large bilateral cortical lesions in some animals in the present study also supports the possibility that subcortical structures play an important part in the generation of OKN, and that they may play a significant role in the relatively rapid recovery of OKN following unilateral cortical lesions in monkeys.

All four monkeys which received bilateral IPL or IPL-PS lesions in this study were impaired in their ability to generate smooth eye movements in tracking a vertically moving visual target. However, only two of these monkeys (A-5 and A-2) had deficits of horizontal tracking. One possible explanation of such an inconsistency would be that the lesions in A-5 and A-2 were larger than the others and encroached upon some adjacent or subjacent region concerned primarily with the control of horizontal tracking. This is certainly a reasonable possibility and must be carefully explored with further experiments. However, while A-5 did in fact have the largest IPL-PS lesion, A-2 had only a relatively small IPL lesion with no histological evidence of any subcortical damage.

A second possible explanation which must also be considered is that while parieto-occipital association cortex (POAC) is an important node in the distributed neural system subserving visual pursuit, other nodes in the system may play a relatively more important part in some individual monkeys than in others and consequently destruction of one of these nodes (e.g., POAC) may have a lesser effect in some individuals than in others. The distributed nature of some of the high-level processing mechanisms of oculomotor control has already been well established. For example, saccadic eye movements are relatively unimpaired by the destruction of either the frontal eye fields or the superior colliculus in monkeys, but when both of these structures are destroyed together saccadic eye movements are virtually abolished (Schiller, True, and Conway, 1979).

The observation that a given association cortex lesion may have a greater effect in some animals than in others has been frequently reported in private communications and in the published literature. Schwartz and Eidelberg (1968) have described a series of 11 monkeys in which unilateral parieto-occipital lesions were made. Most of these monkeys exhibited clear post-lesion extinction of the contralateral of two simultaneous somatosensory stimuli. This extinction persisted an average of more than 35 days. However, 1 of the 11 monkeys did not show any consistent pattern of extinction following the lesion. In a larger series, the same investigators (Eidelberg and Schwartz, 1971) reported that out of 30 monkeys which received similar lesions of areas PG and OA (equivalent to the IPL-PS lesions in the present study), 26 showed clear tactile extinction persisting for 5-90 days, but 4 did not show any such extinction. Similarly, Mishkin (personal communication) has recently completed a large series of monkeys in which the same area of infero-temporal association cortex was removed in each monkey. The monkeys were trained and tested on visual recognition tasks, and in spite of the histologically verified consistency of the amount and location of the tissue removed, the animals' post-operative performance deficits ranged from severe to nonexistent. While the actual basis for the inconsistency in the horizontal pursuit results in the present study is by no means certain, we propose that the distributed nature of higher neural processes is a well-established principle which must be routinely considered in contemporary investigations of the functional organization of association cortex and related neural systems.

Finally, the present results suggest that separate cortical mechanisms are involved in the generation of the slow eye movements of visual pursuit and optokinetic nystagmus. Unilateral cortical lesions which included prestriate cortex in addition to the inferior parietal lobule produced an OKN deficit when the stimuli moved toward the lesioned side but produced no consistent defect of active visual pursuit of a small target. Persistent horizontal tracking deficits were seen in two monkeys only after bilateral lesions. These results, together with the transient unidirectional tracking deficit in A-5, demonstrate that the slow eye movement system in monkeys is organized somewhat differently from that of humans, in which pursuit deficits are observed after unilateral hemispheric damage and in which the direction of the pursuit deficit is the same as that of the OKN slow phase deficit (Baloh, Yee, and Honrubia, 1980a; Sharpe, Lo, and Rabinovitch, 1979; Troost and colleagues, 1972).

ACKNOWLEDGEMENTS

The authors wish to thank Pamela Hammond, Jerome Allison, Lorri Lobeck, and Varie Lynch for assistance in the execution of these experiments and the preparation of the manuscript. This research was supported by NIH grants EY-2640, EY-5318, 5 SO1-RR-5530-14, and a grant from the Mayo Foundation.

PURSUIT DISORDERS

B. T. TROOST and L. A. ABEL

Ocular Motor Neurophysiology Laboratory, Veterans Administration Medical Center and Department of Neurology, Case Western Reserve University, Cleveland, Ohio, USA

ABSTRACT

We briefly review the normal physiology of human pursuit eye movement and emphasize cerebral disorders of visual tracking. Various methods for quantitation of pursuit eye movements are reviewed including the concept of pursuit gain.

The smooth pursuit system may be affected by diffuse cortical, basal ganglia, cerebellar and brainstem disease as well as focal cerebral lesions. Diffuse disease, inattention, aging changes and drugs may produce bilateral horizontal pursuit abnormality resulting in decreased gain.

Most asymmetric pursuit abnormalities caused by cerebral lesions produce a defect while tracking in a direction ipsilateral to the lesion. The responsible lesions in the studies reviewed, are in the parieto-occipital region. The finding of unidirectional pursuit abnormality would then suggest a posterior hemispheric lesion on the side toward which pursuit tracking was defective.

KEYWORDS

Pursuit eye movements; parieto-occipital cortex; "cogwheel" pursuit; asymmetric visual tracking; optokinetic nystagmus; ocular motor system.

INTRODUCTION

Human visual tracking of a moving target normally elicits eye movements which are clinically termed smooth pursuit. The majority of clinical and quantitative observations of human smooth pursuit eye movements have been made with the head fixed, even though normal tracking often uses a combination of head and eye movement. In most laboratory situations, actual visual tracking uses two types of eye movements: smooth pursuit and saccades. The smooth pursuit and saccadic subsystems differ functionally (Dodge, 1903; Westheimer, 1954; Rashbass, 1961; Dell'Osso and Daroff, 1974), anatomically (Astruc, 1971; Troost, Daroff, and Dell'Osso 1972 a & b; Baker and Berthoz, 1977), and physiologically (Robinson, 1964, 1965, and 1968 a & b; Dell 'Osso and Daroff, 1978). It was once believed that a visible, moving target was necessary to elicit a pursuit eye movement.

This lead to many reports of slow "pursuit" eye movements which paradoxically occurred in the absence of a visible stimulus (Deckert, 1964; Westheimer and Conover, 1954). Pursuit eye movements were also found to occur during tracking of an after-image (Steinbach, 1972; Kommerell and Klein, 1971; Kommerell and Taumer 1972; Heywood, 1972), imagined targets (Deckert, 1964; Lenox, Lange and Graham, 1970), with proprioceptive (Gauthier and Hofferer 1976; Lackner, 1975; Angel and colleagues 1971, 1972; Steinbach, 1969; Jordan, 1970), tactile and auditory input (Schmidt and Smith, 1971), and seemingly at will (Heywood, 1972; Steinman and colleagues, 1969). Additional understanding of these seeming paradoxes occurred when it was realized that tracking or pursuit eye movements might occur not just in response to a retinal velocity (or acceleration) error signal, but also in response to an internal idea or "percept" of target motion (Yasui and Young, 1975 a; Steinbach, 1976; Young, 1977). The role of target velocity or acceleration during tracking of unpredictable targets is still to be completely defined.

In reviewing recent clinical and normal studies of pursuit in humans, the primary emphasis will be upon cerebral pursuit disorders during tracking of visible targets. Various normal attributes of smooth pursuit have long been evaluated (Michael and Jones, 1966; St. Cyr and Fender, 1969; Young, 1971), but very few studies have attempted to measure abnormality in a quantitative fashion. Furthermore, the finding of some subtle abnormality in a widely disseminated disease such as multiple sclerosis without good clinical and/or clinico-pathologic correlation serves little purpose.

QUANTITATION OF PURSUIT

A subjective visual inspection of electro-oculographic records has been used for qualitative assessment of tracking attempts during standard electronystagmography (Benitz, 1970; von Noorden and colleagues, 1962, 1966; Covera and colleagues, 1963; Larmande and Deplace, 1973; Rodin, 1964; Bogacz and colleagues, 1977; Vedel-Jensen, 1966). Unfortunately, the nature and localization of central nervous system deficits was often imprecise and the ability to make a positive diagnosis of neurological abnormality was quite limited. Previous authors have also attempted to assess the effects of drugs using qualitative impressions of the efficacy of pursuit tracking (Rashbass, 1961; Norris, 1971; Frank and Kuhlo, 1970; Wilkinson, Kime and Purnell, 1974).

Further attempts have been made to quantitate pursuit function by a variety of methods such as counting the number or amplitude of saccades which occur during each sinusoidal target cycle (Yamazaki, 1970; Yamzaki and Ishikawa, 1973; Hartje and colleagues, 1978) or by determining the number of time pursuit velocity drops to zero (Holzman and colleagues, 1973; Shagrass and colleagues, 1976). The methodology of the last studies has been criticized because of the recording system employed and artifacts introduced (Troost and colleagues, 1974; Iacono and Lykken, 1981).

Most current analysis has applied a method for determining gain for the pursuit system, either by determining the ratio of the eye velocity to target velocity (Troost and colleagues, 1972 b; Schalen, 1980) or by determining how often the eye velocity approached or matched target velocity (Baloh and colleagues, 1976, 1977). Detection of phase lag (Thickbroom and Black, 1980) and spectral purity (Wolfe and colleagues, 1979) have also recently been employed. Other investigators have used aperiodic targets in humans (Bahill Bahill and colleagues, 1980). The use of such targets reduces predictability, but also introduces more saccades into the tracking record. Such unpredictable target waveforms have not been applied to the study of cerebral disease as yet.

Since a wide variety of targets have been used to study human pursuit, primarily sinusoids or ramps, no uniform definition of normal pursuit has emerged, but rather individual laboratories have identified their own standards for normalcy (Troost and colleagues, 1972 b; Baloh, 1976; Sharpe and Sylvester, 1978; Baloh and colleagues 1980 a). Most humans can track a sinusoidal target of 1 Hz with amplitude of 20° without intoducing saccades. During pursuit of constant velocity ramps, pursuit is interrupted by "catch-up" saccades at about 30° - 40°/second.

BIDIRECTIONAL PURSUIT DEFECTS

The smooth pursuit system is disrupted more than the saccadic system by alcohol, drugs, and fatigue (Rashbass, 1961; Wilkinson and colleagues, 1974; Flom and colleagues, 1976; Baloh and colleagues, 1976; Norris, 1971). A variety of central nervous system diseases may show smooth pursuit defects as an early ocular motor system abnormality (Zee and colleagues, 1976b; Troost and Daroff, 1977). Smooth pursuit is quite sensitive and is "broken-up", "fragmented" or "saccadic" in many patients with diffuse cerebral, cerebellar, and brainstem disease. In our previous study of progressive supranuclear palsy (Troost and Daroff, 1977) characteristic bilateral saccadic interruption of pursuit occurred in both horizontal directions. Gains determined for all target velocities in 6 such patients was from 0.2 to 0.5, gain being the ratio of eye velocity to target velocity.

The exact anatomy of cerebral pursuit control is still unknown. Previous schemes (Troost and Daroff, 1978) have depicted the smooth pursuit system as functioning primarily as an ipsilateral system, uncertain as to whether the actual anatomic connections had a double decussation or passed ipsilaterally from the parieto-occipital regions to the brainstem.

PURSUIT AND AGING

Before considering the effects of specific cerebral lesions on smooth pursuit, it is necessary to point out that physiological changes have been reported with aging. Sharpe and Sylvester (1978) studied 15 young volunteers (mean age 23) and 10 elderly volunteers (mean age 72). Horizontal smooth pursuit gain calculated as eye velocity/target velocity markedly changed with age. In the group of young subjects, gain exceed 0.96 at ramp velocities up to 30°/sec, but in the elderly group, the highest mean gain was 0.94 when tracking a 5°/sec target. Thereafter, the gain decreased more rapidly in the elderly where the gain was about 0.5, for a 30°/sec ramp compared to 0.96 for young normals who did not have a gain drop to 0.5 until a target velocity between 60° - 70°/sec. In the elderly smooth pursuit latencies were also significantly prolonged, and with increasing target speeds there were more saccades.

In another study of the effect of aging on smooth pursuit, Spooner and colleagues (1980), compared a control group of 25 people, aged 22 to 64 (mean age 42) with a group of patients who had symptoms of vertebrobasilar insufficiency (mean age 67). They also compared such patients against a control group of 14 elderly people (mean age 65). The smooth pursuit target moved in fixed-cycle constant velocity ramps. The authors compared the mode eye velocity (most frequently occurring velocity) in the three groups finding, (1) young normal subjects were consistently superior to both elderly groups and (2) while the group with vertebrobasilar system disease tended to be slightly worse than those of the elderly normal subjects, the differences were not significant. These two studies (Sharp and Sylvester, (1978); Spooner and colleagues, (1980) clearly suggest that age effects must be taken into consideration in any interpretation of a symmetrical impairment of smooth pursuit.

UNIDIRECTIONAL PURSUIT DEFECTS

Clinically important cerebral pursuit abnormalities should show marked asymmetry or be significantly different from age matched controls to provide useful information. No specific type of bilateral pursuit abnormality has been found to be characteristic of a specific cerebral disease process. Most of the asymmetrical pursuit abnormalities reported, occur in patients with unilateral cerebral disease, particularly in the posterior hemisphere. In our initial study of one patient with a left hemidecortication (Troost and colleagues, 1972 b), we found a marked drop in pursuit gain to 0.2 to 0.3 when ramp targets of 5° to 40°/sec moved to his left, but normal rightward pursuit.

Sharpe and colleagues (1979), studied ocular motor function after right or left hemidecortication performed at various ages in 5 patients. Every patient had subnormal pursuit velocities when tracking targets toward the side of the cerebral ablation. However, pursuit gain was greater than unity when tracking toward the blind field at ramp speeds up to 30°/sec. During fixation, the patients had jerk nystagmus beating toward the side of the cortical exterpation. Sharpe and Sylvester (1978) had previously indicated that individual pursuit velocities could exceed the speed of predictable targets in normal subjects, however, mean smooth eye movement velocities did not. The "pursuit defect" primary position horizontal jerk nystagmus would add a slow phase component to the tracking toward the normal hemisphere, but it is difficult to understand how this could produce a gain significantly greater than unity at rapid target velocities. The authors' reason that the smooth pursuit abnormality was not just an adaptation to the homonymous field defect is that asymmetric pursuit defects do not occur with homonymous defects caused by discrete optic tract, geniculocalcarine, or occipital cortical lesions (Kestenbaum, 1961; Daroff and Hoyt, 1971; Sharpe and Deck, 1978). Baloh (1977) reported briefly on 5 patients with fronto-parietal disease, indicating impairment of smooth pursuit with targets toward the side of the lesion in two, bilateral abnormality in one, and normal pursuit in another. All the patients, however, were on anticonvulsants and the extent of the lesions were not defined.

Paresis of ipsilateral pursuit after unilateral damage to the posterior hemisphere would suggest that horizontal pursuit is normally governed by the ipsilateral hemisphere (Troost and colleagues, 1972 b, Daroff and Troost, 1978), but as has been pointed out, approximately equal numbers of parietal neurons are active during ipsilateral, as well as, contralateral pursuit (Lynch, 1980a; Lynch and colleagues, 1977a).Sharpe and colleagues (1979), proposed that human control of ipsilateral pursuit by the extrastriate cortex of one hemisphere is dependent upon retinal information passing to either the ipsilateral or contralateral striate cortex. Therefore, asymmetric smooth pursuit in patients with hemianopia could be a manifestation of unilateral prestriate damage, or a type of disconnection syndrome, in which retinal velocity/acceleration information from the "seeing" hemisphere could not be passed to the "blind" or damaged hemisphere. This situation would be analogous to dyslexia without agraphia, a language disturbance from dominant hemispheric lesions which involve the occipital lobe and the splenium of the corpus callosum. In such a situation, there is a total right homonymous visual field loss but an intact left visual field. Unfortunately, the visual information passing to the intact right peristriate and striate cortex cannot be tranferred across the splenium of the corpus callosum to be interpreted by the "language centers" of dominant hemisphere. In theory, asymmetric pursuit could be present in the absence of a hemianopia, when one parietal "optomotor" region is disconnected from visual input from either homonymous visual field.

Along these lines, Larmande and colleagues (1980) discussed seven patients wiht unilateral occipto-parietal lesions. They found pursuit more severely impaired during tracking toward the lesion, but also some contralateral involvement agreeing that pursuit function is "fragile". They also found apparent gains of greater than unity in some instances of pursuit away from the lesion. The authors concluded that both hemispheres must be intact to produce unimpaired smooth pursuit, but that a single hemisphere could produce "some" pursuit movements in either direction. The bilateral parietal lobe activity during smooth pursuit figured prominantly in their explanation.

Foveal smooth pursuit and full field optokinetic nystagmus were quantitatively studied in two patients with cerebral lesions reported by Baloh and colleagues (1980). One patient was a 21-year-old man with a progressive parietal tumor, the other was an 80-year-old man with a left parieto-occipital infarction, which involved the splenium of the corpus callosum. The second patient had severe dysnomia and dyslexia but no receptive or expressive aphasia. Pursuit toward the damaged hemisphere was abnormal in both patients. Pursuit gain was calculated at the ratio of peak eye velocity to the peak velocity of sinusoidal targets. The pursuit abnormality consisted of reduced gain and "catch-up" saccades, similar to those reported in other human patients with posterior hemispheric disease (Troost and colleagues, 1972 b; Sharpe and colleagues, 1979). The pursuit gain toward the damaged hemisphere was approximately half that toward the normal hemisphere. The older patient had poorer pursuit than the young patient in a direction toward the normal hemisphere, but tracking was within normal range for his age (Sharpe and Sylvester, 1978; Spooner and colleagues, 1980). Both patients had optokinetic (OKN) abnormality and defects of the vestibulo-ocular reflex (VOR) gain modulation as discussed elsewhere in this symposium. The authors suggested that foveal smooth pursuit and full field OKN slow phases have, at least in part, different anatomic substrates.

What emerges from the relatively few quantitative studies of pursuit function in humans with posterior hemispheric disease is that the parietal cortex or subcortex must receive visual input to produce normal foveal pursuit, assuming an intact brainstem and cerebellum. In considering the multiplicity of conditions which can affect pursuit in both directions, only a significant directional asymmetry would be of clinical localizing value. Such asymmetry would strongly suggest parietal lobe dysfunction.

In view of the limited number of patients who have had quantitative eye movement studies, correlated with good clinical examination and pathological localization the time is ripe for additional study of cerebral pursuit defects. Such study should compare smooth pursuit function with predictable, as well as, unpredictable targets, and define possible coexistant abnormality of full field as well as foveal-parafoveal OKN and the ability to modulate the VOR gain.

EYE-HEAD COORDINATION IN PARKINSON'S DISEASE

C. KENNARD[1], W. H. ZANGEMEISTER[2], S. MELLORS, L. STARK and W. F. HOYT

Department of Physiological Optics and Engineering Science, University of California, Berkeley, California 94720 and Neuro-Ophthalmology Unit, Department of Neurology, Neurosurgery and Ophthlmology, University of California, San Francisco, California 94143, USA

ABSTRACT

Previous studies of eye movements in patients with Parkinson's disease have yielded contradictory results. Since eye movements are normally performed in association with head movements we have studied both eye movements and eye-head coordination in these patients. Eye movements were recorded by the infrared limbus reflection technique, and head movements by means of a light helmet attached to a low torque potentiometer. The stimuli were predictive and non-predictive step and ramp movements of a light spot. When moving their eyes and head naturally Parkinsonian patients rarely made head movements, and tended to follow the target with their eyes alone. When instructed to move their head to follow the target (forced condition) there was a prolonged delay of about 150 msec from the start of the saccade to the commencement of the head movements. These results are discussed in relation to the generalised motor disturbance found in extrapyramidal disease.

KEYWORDS

Parkinson's disease; eye-head coordination; saccades; smooth pursuit; bradykinesia; basal ganglia.

INTRODUCTION

Under normal circumstances head movements play an important role in alterations of gaze. This usually involves firstly an eye saccade to fixate the target on the fovea, followed by head rotation which, as a result of the vestibulo-ocular reflex, induces a counter rotation of the eye (Bizzi, Kalil and Tagliasco, 1971). Parkinson's disease is the commonest disorder of the extrapyramidal motor pathways and although several studies have investigated eye movements with the head fixed in these patients (Jones and Dejong 1971; Corin, Elizan and Bender, 1972; Shibasaki, Tsuji and Kuroiwa, 1979; Teravainen and Calne, 1980) none have concerned themselves with eye/head movements. The present study was, therefore, designed to investigate eye/head coordination in Parkinsonian patients similar to those already performed on normal subjects (Zangemeister, Jones and Stark, 1981a). In addition eye movements, in particular the saccadic trajectory, were studied with the head fixed.

---

[1] on leave from Dept. of Neurology, The London Hospital, London, England. Supported by an Alexander Pigott Wernher Fellowship and a Keeler Award.

[2] on leave from Dept. of Neurology, University of Hamburg, FRG. Supported by Deutsche Forschungs Gemeinschaft, Bonn, FRG

METHODS

Seven Parkinsonian patients (six males and one female, aged from 52 to 69 years, mean 61.7) were examined. They had had Parkinson's disease for between 2 and 11 years (mean 6) and were all taking antiParkinsonian drugs in the form of an l-Dopa preparation (Sinemet). Clinical examination showed them all to have Parkinson's disease of mild to moderate severity. Nine normal subjects were also examined, seven aged from 25 to 34 years, and two aged 58 to 62 years.

The techniques for eye and head movement measurements as used in our laboratory have recently been reported (Zangemeister, Jones and Stark, 1981). Briefly, the eye movement measurements are made with the infrared limbus reflection technique (Stark, Vossius and Young, 1962). The head movement measurement was made using mechanical linkages and a low torque potentiometer attached to a light plastic helmet that the subjects or patients wore while viewing the targets.

The target was a continuously illuminated bright dot of 20-arc min diameter, generated by a minicomputor, appearing on an oscilloscope screen, and was viewed by the subjects in a dimly lit room. Target displacements between 2 and 40° in predictable and unpredictable steps of different durations (0.1 to 2.0s) were used. Programmes giving unpredictable target steps in both amplitude and time, and ramps were used. The subjects were seated comfortably in front of the screen and were asked to follow the target with the head fixed (eye alone), then follow with 'natural' eye and head movements, and finally to force themselves to perform head movements as fast and as accurately as possible.

RESULTS

Eye alone

The mean latency of saccades to a predicted and unpredicted target shift was 238 $\pm$ 74 msec (n=60) and 240 $\pm$ 75 msec (n = 152), respectively, which was not significantly different to the normal controls 227 $\pm$ 59 msec (n = 79). In patients with predominantly unilateral Parkinsonism there was no difference in the latencies of saccades to the left and right.

TABLE 1 Analysis of Saccadic Trajectories: Frequency (%) of Over- and Under-shoots

	Dynamic Undershoot	Glissadic Undershoot	Static Undershoot	Dynamic Overshoot	Glissadic Overshoot	Static Overshoot	None
Parkinson's	0	9.3	52.4	7.3	21.8	11.3	6.7
Control	0	2.5	23.9	32.8	18.1	15.3	9.4

Analysis of saccadic trajectories (Table 1) showed that Parkinsonian patients had a much higher incidence of static undershoots, and a lower incidence of dynamic overshoots than the normal controls. The static undershoot usually resulted in one corrective saccade with a maximum of four. The intersaccadic latency of these corrective end saccades averaged 160 msec which would be adequate time for them to be the result of processing of feedback information. Hypometric saccades often appeared more frequently when the saccade was directed to the side of the maximal limb rigidity and bradykinesia.

Eye/Head Combined Movements

When the Parkinsonian patients were asked to follow predictable and unpredictable target shifts using natural head/eye movements they either made no head movement at all, or a very small amplitude movement (less than 25% of the full movement).

In the forced condition Parkinsonian patients made adequate head movements to similar target shifts. An analysis of the frequency of the different gaze types (see Zangemeister and Stark, this symposium) was made (Table 2).

TABLE 2 Frequency of Gaze Types

Type		Parkinsons (%)	Controls (%)
Type 1	(Synchronous eye/head EMG)	49	34
Type 2	(Head movement delayed)	33	4
Type 3	(Early head movement)	18	43
Type 4	(Late eye saccade)	0	19

49% of the gaze movements showed the normal coordinated eye/head movement (Type 1) with an eye saccade followed by a head rotation commencing immediately at the end of the saccade. Type 2 gaze movements were far commoner in Parkinsonian patients than in normal controls. In this gaze type the head movement is delayed, a pause occurring between the end of the saccade and the commencement of head movement. There was also a marked reduction of both Type 3 and 4 gaze movements in the Parkinsonian patients reflecting the unusual occurrence of a head movement before the commencement of the eye saccade. These results are further reinforced when the latency of both the eye and head movements were analysed. The responses to unpredictable targets resulted in an eye and head latency of 228 ± 84 msec and 377 ± 102 msec (n = 47) respectively. This is a significant (student t test $p < 0.01$) delay of the mean head latency by some 150 msec which is almost three times the normal delay (45 msec). With forced eye/head movements the head movement was often of slower than normal velocity and the velocity trace showed a "fragmented" maximum velocity curve (Fig 1A).

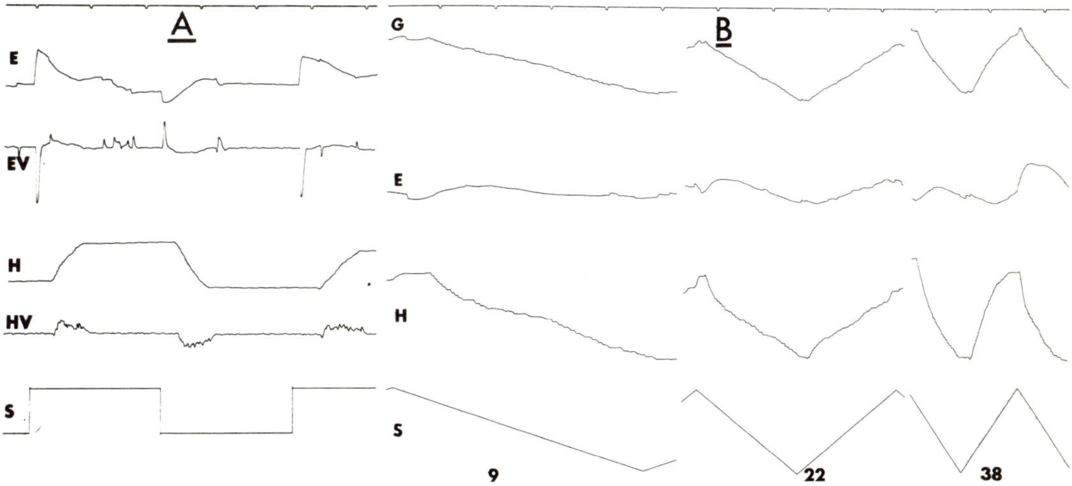

Fig. 1. Eye head movements in a Parkinson patient

A. Eye (E)/Head (H) movement recordings, with respective velocity (EV,HV) traces in response to 40°, stimulus (S) steps. This shows in particular the 'fragmented' head velocity curve.
B. Similar recording with eye/head tracking of smoothly moving target at velocities of 9, 22, 38°/sec. Note the fragmentation of the head movement. G = gaze; time marker 1 sec; upward movements are to the left.

Parkinsonian patients found considerable difficulty smoothly tracking a stimulus moving at a velocity of between 3 and 60°/sec with their head. The main abnormality was a fragmentation of the head movement as shown in Fig. 1B.

DISCUSSION

The clinical abnormalities found in Parkinson's disease, the major pathology of which is a loss of dopaminergic nigrostriatal neurones, are of both a positive type such as tremor, and a negative type such as the slowness of initiation and velocity of a movement (bradykinesia) (Martin, 1967). Studies of eye movements with the head fixed have shown prolonged saccadic latency (Corin, Elizan and Bender, 1972; Teräväinen and Calne, 1980; Shibasaki Tsuji and Kuroiwa, 1979) which was not found in the present study or that of Jones and Dejong (1971). This may relate to the severity of the disease which was mild to moderate in our patients, or the variation with time of a Parkinsonian patients' clinical disability. Saccadic velocities have usually been found to be normal in these patients (Teräväinen and Calne, 1980). The use of the infrared limbus reflection technique allowed a detailed analysis of the saccadic trajectory which showed a high incidence of hypometric saccades, well documented previously, with a corresponding diminution in the frequency of dynamic overshoots (Bahill, Clark and Stark, 1975 b). It would appear, therefore, that these two factors, prolonged saccadic latency and multiple step saccades, are the oculomotor equivalent of bradykinesia. It has been suggested that the reason for this is that the motor programme for saccades is defectively executed (Teräväinen and Calne 1980).

The lack of head rotation when the Parkinsonian patients were asked to 'naturally' follow the target, and the prolonged latency of head rotation under 'forced' conditions would both seem to be a further example of bradykinesia involving the neck musculature. Although accurate measurements of the peak velocities of head movement was not obtained, comparing the traces with normal controls some of the Parkinsonian patients appeared to have considerably slowed head movements. Of particular interest was the frequent fragmentation of the head movement occasionally seen in normals. This rapid oscillation at the midpoint of the trajectory may represent multiple switching of activity of the agonist and antagonist muscle, or just the agonist muscle alone. It is interesting in this context to compare rapid head movements with similar limb movements in Parkinson's disease. Hallett and Khoshbin (1980) showed that during rapid flexion of the elbow the Parkinsonian patient was unable to increase the amount of EMG activity in a burst, but instead increased the number of cycles of agonist/antagonist bursts. It is possible that the fragmented head movement may reflect a similar repetition of the agonist/antagonist muscle burst cycle.

The most widely advocated view of the role of the basal ganglia is that they "facilitate" movement by energising specific muscles for a particular movement. This includes selection of the muscle as well as inhibition of inappropriate muscles. It will, therefore, be most interesting to record the EMG from neck muscles in Parkinson patients to further understand the control signals which can only be inferred from analysis of head movement trajectories.

L.S. wishes to thank NASA-Ames Research Center for partial support (NCC 2-86).

DISCUSSION

K.Ciufreda. Dr.Sharpe showed in patients with unilateral parietal lobe lesions a smooth pursuit gain greater than unity in one direction of movement. How did you rule out summation of the jerk nystagmus with the pursuit, resulting in asymmetrical pursuit gain? Also, how did you rule out predictive effects associated with the predictive target input, especially at the turn-around points?

J.Sharpe. We could not distinguish between a linear descent of the pursuit and the nystagmus. It may simply be a semantic problem if pursuit can imbalance smooth eye movement control. It would give the appearance of nystagmus. Concerning the predictive effects, we never encountered persistently high gain in one direction among 35 control subjects, as we did in every one of our patients. Occasional smooth eye movements will exceed the velocity of predictable targets but if you run series of many ramps you don´t get mean gains that consistently exceed target velocity as we did in these patients. I don´t know whether this is an attempt to put the target on the seeing hemiretina. I don´t think that it is an adaptation to the hemianopia but it certainly helps to see if you have hemianopia.

L.Abel. We have reported a patient with a horizontal linear nystagmus due to a congenital tumour of the cerebellum and the brainstem, without hemianopia, and she also showed pursuit gain greater than unity in one direction. Since there was no visual problem at all, this would also argue against a hypothesis that high gain is an adapted behaviour.

T.Brandt. Dr.Sharpe, are you aware of the problem to incorporate depth perception concerning cerebral pursuit modulating VOR gain? The VOR gain is dependent upon the distance between the eye and the fixated target. In order for the VOR to maintain gaze in space constant, the gain must be greater for a target nearby as compared to distant targets. There is experimental evidence that convergence affects VOR gain.

J.Sharpe. Yes, gain goes up with vergence. There is another effect too, namely that vergence will dampen vestibular nystagmus. In our cases, we had our patients look at a screen at a fixed distance. In darkness, we monitored both eyes so that the patient was not converging. They were instructed to look roughly in the plane where the target had been for calibration. Whether they did this I don´t know, but at any rate we were looking for asymmetries and asymmetry would not be affected by imaginary depth of the target.

E.Keller. Dr.Goldberg, are the responses in frontal eye field cells (the pre-saccade type) similar to the response of collicular quasi visual cells? If so, would you say that the colliculus and the frontal eye fields are sending a similar command within the same time window to the burst generator in the pontine paramedian reticular formation?

M.Goldberg. Yes, I think that is right. The efferent connections of this part of the frontal eye fields go to the colliculus itself, and to at least three other areas that share collicular projections to the mesencephalic reticular formation. I would think then that the two organs in the normal work in concert to provide what we would consider to be a desired eye movement vector signal. I think that the colliculus has the same problem as the frontal eye field cells and that is to adjust the appropriateness of the eye movement direction according to recent eye movement since the retinal latency is much longer than this eye proprioceptive, probably corollary post-eye--movement-effect that we see.

L.Schalén. What is the optimal velocity range for smooth pursuit in the monkey? Dr.Lynch showed that the smooth pursuit had a normal gain for low velocities of the stimulus but was decreased for high velocities. We have found in patients that it is possible to discriminate between different locations of lesions according to how the gain varies. There is a decreased smooth pursuit velocity gain in patients with frontal lobe lesions when their pursuit is tested above the optimal velocity limits. For patients with posterior fossa lesions there is a decrease of gain already below the optimal limits for smooth pursuit.

J.Lynch. We tested the smooth pursuit over the range 6 to 40 degrees per second. We did not test at higher velocities.

D.Robinson. Our monkeys easily track peanuts at 120-125 degrees per second. I have seen some monkeys track at 230 degrees per second.

H.Bynke. Dr.Guiton, what was the time intervals between the operations and your examinations? Do these patients ever recover?

D.Guiton. There was no striking difference between examinations made four days and 14 days post surgery. Longterm patients improved considerably and were generally able to suppress their reflexive glance. Although they were able to make antisaccades they generally took considerably longer than a normal subject. One patient, who had been operated 22 years earlier, could suppress her reflexive glance but she took 100 milliseconds longer to generate an antisaccade compared to the normal population.

B.Cohen. From our studies of optokinetic nystagmus in the monkey it has been possible to simulate what was the contribution of the velocity storage mechanism and of the direct pathways. Velocity traces of optokinetic nystagmus and optokinetic afternystagmus in the monkey show an initial rapid rise from the stimulation apparently due predominantly to direct pathways, which then decrease their signals to about 20% of the response as the velocity storage mechanism charges up. This mechanism charges up with the time constant at the slow rise and reaches the level of the optokinetic afternystagmus. Up to the saturation level of the optokinetic afternystagmus about 80% is going to be produced by the vestibular nuclei of the brainstem. I would like to ask Dr.Lynch about the optokinetic saturation velocities in his monkeys and whether there was any change after parietal lobe lesions. At saturation velocity it takes longer to charge the storage mechanism and you now have a much larger contribution of the direct pathways. Therefore, at higher velocities one would certainly expect to see a larger component which might be affected by the critical lesion. Estimation of the cortex contribution to optokinetic nystagmus requires elimination or accounting for the activation of the vestibular nuclei. This can be done either by labyrinthectomy, or by looking at the initial rise in slow phase velocity.

J.Lynch. We had no opportunity to do parametric studies of afternystagmus. We did only one velocity (80 degrees per second) and at that stimulus velocity the afternystagmus was wiped out in monkeys with a slow phase deficit. This essentially mirrors their slow phase nystagmus deficit.

B.Cohen. It would be interesting to see the dynamic changes in the slow phase velocity because we know that the brainstem mechanisms can slowly charge up optokinetic nystagmus, and after 30-40 seconds you may have a significant amount of activation coming from this source.

J.Lynch. This type of registration requires a coil system instead of the EOG electrodes. Switching back and forth between light and darkness is sometimes a source of artefacts in the EOG recordings.

L.Stark. Dr.Abel´s remarks about the inadequacy of clinical studies of eye movements in schizophrenic patients need a comment. We have examined some of these patients, and they do have very abnormal smooth pursuit: they have both saccadic smooth pursuit and also a very high incidence of saccadic intrusions. While these are not pathognomic signs, they do explain with high precision recording what has been reported in the psychiatric and psychological literature.

L.Abel. Still, the investigations I cited seem to reflect mostly artefacts, e.g. intrusion by the EEG into the EOG. Many defects previously described can also be explained as attentional in origin. I do not disagree that the pursuit is poor: I just think that most of it is attentional.

L.Stark. We use changing numbers as the target to maintain the patients´ attention. They have to call out every time a number is switched.

L.Abel. It is still not clear that the attentional stage of schizophrenics is identical to normal counterparts. Also there is the matter of drugs...

J.Sharpe. I don´t think that the fact that it is an attentional defect undermines its value at all. We should also measure the spectrum of smooth pursuit velocities.

W.F.Hoyt. Can Dr.Goldberg make any suggestions about how we might test patients? Do you think that something like the antisaccade test could be put before some of our patients to test higher level decision making?

M.Goldberg. The antisaccade experiment is a wonderful experiment! As clinicians we are always faced with the fact that the patients with frontal lobe lesions can make perfectly good saccadic eye movements to visual targets. This may be due to the fact that they have an intact colliculus. What the frontal lobe patients classically is unable to do is to suppress inappropriate behaviour. The reason that frontal lobe patients are incontinent is that their frontal lobes don´t tell them to wait. Dr.Guiton has now shown us that the colliculus cannot wait. Instead of depending upon frontal signals, the brainstem has learned to be responsive to the collicular signal alone.

That system will make the saccade to an inappropriate target.

W.F.Hoyt. Smooth pursuit continues to be a depressing thing to work at clinically. Dr.Sharpe, how do you think we can use such recordings for interest or usefully?

J.Sharpe. I think that smooth pursuit is the most sensitive single indicator of brain function that the clinician has. If you have good pursuit then you are normal. Asymmetries in pursuit are very valuable in lateralization of brain disease, but of little or no value in localization along the anterior-posterior axis.

D.Guiton. I would like to emphasize that many patients can do the antisaccade task easily unless they are forced into a very tight timing situation. This is difficult to arrange at the bedside.

N.M.Henriksson. We have found that the vestibular gain was very much increased in patients with frontal cortical lesions on the left side. We found difficulties to initiate saccades to the right and to the left to about the same extent.

J.Sharpe. It is interesting that Dr.Guiton describe difficulty in making antisaccades in both directions from unilateral frontal lesion and yet one hemisphere exerts a predominant control of contralateral saccades. I wonder whether Dr.Guiton has an explanation for that.

D.Guiton. There is always the possibility of contralateral degeneration due to collaterals from the contralateral frontal eye field.

SECTION XI

Coordinator: G. Lennerstrand

FREE PAPERS: CENTRAL OCULAR MOTOR DISORDERS

LESION OF THE ABDUCENS NUCLEUS AS THE CAUSE OF A CONJUGATE GAZE PARALYSIS[1]

O. MEIENBERG*, J. A. BÜTTNER-ENNEVER** and
R. KRAUS-RUPPERT***

*Department of Neurology, University of Bern, Switzerland
**Brain Research Institute, University of Zürich, Switzerland
***Department of Pathology, University of Bern, Switzerland

ABSTRACT

Over a period of a few days a VIth and peripheral VIIth nerve paresis appeared in a 34-year-old woman on the right side, together with a gaze paretic nystagmus to the right. During the following six days a complete horizontal gaze paralysis to the right developed. A tumor destroying the abducens nucleus, and the immediately surrounding area was diagnosed as the cause of this disorder of conjugate horizontal gaze. This was confirmed by autopsy.

INTRODUCTION

Paralysis of conjugate lateral eye movements accompanying lesions of the pons is generally attributed to involvement of the paramedian pontine reticular formation (PPRF) known to be important in the generation of horizontal gaze (Bender and Shanzer, 1964; Büttner-Ennever and Henn, 1976; Cohen and others, 1968; Goebel and o 1971; Graybiel, 1977; Henn and others, 1978; Pierrot-Déseilligny and others, 1978, 1979). In the older literature, however, there were also some reports of cases with conjugate horizontal gaze paralysis in which only a minute lesion confined to the ipsilateral abducens nucleus was found on autopsy (Bennett and Savill, 1889; Blocq and Guinon, 1891; D'Espine and Démole, 1917; Garel, 1882). These observations have been confirmed experimentally in monkeys by Carpenter and others (1963). In the case we are reporting here, the combination of neurological signs, and especially the temporal sequence of their appearance, permitted the early diagnosis of a lesion which destroyed the VIth nerve nucleus, before it could be detected by other clinical means(CT-Scan etc.).

REPORT OF A CASE

A 34-year-old woman was admitted with a sixth and seventh nerve paresis on the right,which appeared some days previously.In primary gaze, the right eye was 15 degrees adducted.Abduction was possible to midposition only.Additionally, the adducting saccades of the opposite left eye were markedly slowed, but adduction was not restricted at that time. With the attempt to look to the right, a coarse

[1] A more detailed report of this case will be published in "Neuro-ophthalmology"

nystagmus appeared having smaller amplitudes on the right eye with the abduction paresis. DC-electro-oculography showed the characteristics of a gaze paretic nystagmus(of both eyes)with an exponential course of the slow phase slope. The VIIth nerve paresis was moderate and affected all three branches equally. Taste was preserved. Otherwise neurological findings were normal except for residual deficits in the lower extremities from an operated tumor of the conus terminalis. Within the six days following admission a left medial rectus paresis developed and the right facial nerve paresis became complete. Both eyes could no longer be moved to the right across the midline, neither voluntarily nor with oculocephalic manoeuvres.At rest both eyes showed a moderate conjugate deviation to the left, and the patient kept her head turned to the right for compensation.Convergence still was possible. Additionally a mild adduction deficit of the right eye was observed. Lid and vertical eye movements were normal as well as the pupillary reactions.Although during the following weeks a right palatal and pharyngeal paresis, a bilateral pterygoid paresis and a hypesthesia of the entire right side of the face appeared, and pyramidal signs in both lower extremities developed, several CT-Scans showed no abnormality. Finally a small tumor could be located in the pons by a vertebral arteriogram and a pneumoencephalogram. Radiotherapy was

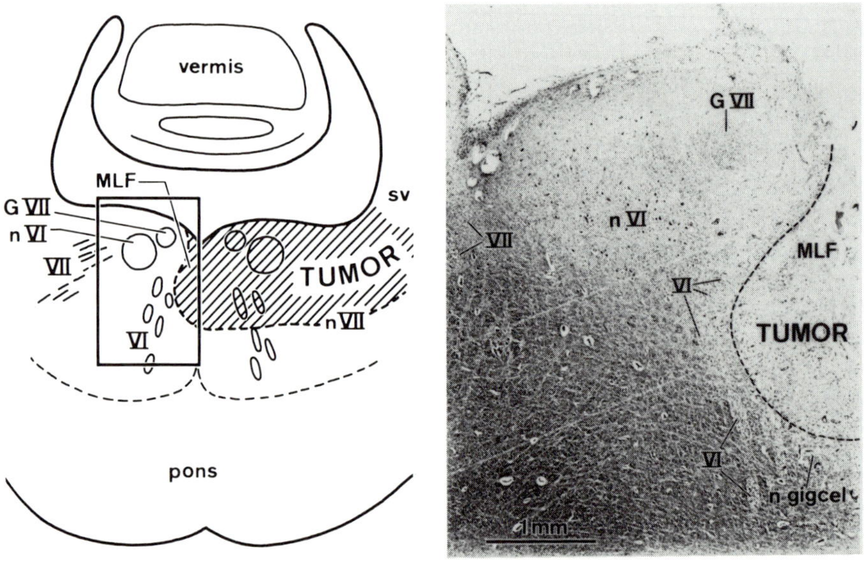

Fig. 1. Transverse section through the pons at the level of the abducens nuclei showing the intact VIth nucleus of the left side while the right nucleus is totally destroyed by a tumor as well as part of the right MLF. Some damage across the midline involves both MLF and the VIth nerve rootlets on the left to a minor degree. The inset is a low-power drawing to show the extent of the tumor. MLF = medial longitudinal fasciculus, n gigcel = nucleus gigantocellularis, n VI = abducens nucleus, VI = abducens nerve rootlets, G VII = genu of the facial nerve.

initiated. The patient died six months after the onset of symptoms. Autopsy revealed tumor masses in the pons, spinal cord, vertebrae and bones, a right axillary lymph node, liver, spleen and kidneys. Histologically the tumor was an undifferenciated lymphocytic lymphoma. The solitary tumor mass in the pons(Fig.1) completely destroyed the right upper medulla and lower pons. Right abducens nucleus, facial nucleus and nerve and facial knee and MLF were all totally destroyed. Caudal PPRF on the right side was damaged, but rostral PPRF was not.

DISCUSSION

Lesions strictly confined to the abducens nucleus lead to an ipsilateral paralysis of conjugate gaze, and not to a lateral rectus paralysis. The anatomical and physiological basis of this fact has been discussed already by Henn and Büttner, and by Baker and Spencer in this volume(see also there for references).

In our case the first signs were a simultaneously appearing right lateral rectus and peripheral facial paresis. This implies damage to the VIth nerve fascicle itself, since motoneurons and interneurons at least in the cat are intermingled throughout the abducens nucleus(Steiger and Büttner-Ennever, 1978).However, already at the initial stages there was a marked slowing of the adducting saccades of the left eye and a gaze paretic nystagmus to the right suggesting also some involvement of the abducens nucleus. Taking into consideration that the facial nerve knee bends closely around the abducens nucleus, that a complete conjugate gaze paresis developed within the following six days, that no other brain stem signs were present at this time, and finally that the tumor grew relatively slowly, one could assume that the tumor involved mainly the VIth nerve initially, but at an early stage the VI nerve nucleus as well.The late development of a mild right medial rectus paresis in this patient is to be expected on account of damage to the right MLF at the level shown in Fig. 1, where the axons of the internuclear neurons of the left abducens nucleus ascend to the oculomotor nucleus. Autopsy has shown in our patient that the right caudal PPRF also was destroyed by the tumor. From the clinical course, however, we can assume that the PPRF was affected at a later stage of the disease, and that the initial site of the tumor was associated mainly with the abducens nerve, probably near its exit from the VI nucleus close to the facial genu.An interesting question is whether it is possible to distinguish,by clinical examination, a horizontal gaze paresis due to a lesion of the VIth nucleus from a lesion of the PPRF. Some authors state that in pure PPRF-lesions, with no MLF-involvement, oculocephalic manoeuvres can still elicit eye movements toward the side of the gaze paresis(Cohen and others, 1968; Jaeger and others, 1981;Pierrot-Déseilligny and others, 1978, 1979) which is not found in the case of a lesion of the abducens nucleus.

The work was in part supported by Swiss National Science Foundation(J.A. B.-E.) Grant No: NF 3.58o.79 and 3.5o5.79.

COMPARISON OF OCULOMOTOR MOTONEURON AXON COLLATERALS IN MAMMALS

C. EVINGER*, R. SPENCER** and R. BAKER

*Department of Physiology & Biophysics, New York University Medical Center, New York, NY 10016, USA
**Department of Anatomy, Medical College of Virginia, Richmond, VA 23298, USA

One or more collaterals branch off the axon of most cat oculomotor motoneurons, arborize in the oculomotor nucleus and terminate in en passant and terminal boutons. Serial reconstruction of intracellularly stained (HRP) motoneurons at the electron microscope level demonstrates that these boutons are the site of synaptic contacts with oculomotor internuclear neurons (Fig. 1). The presence of oculomotor motoneuron axon collaterals is striking because no other cranial motoneurons possess them (Evinger, et al. in press).

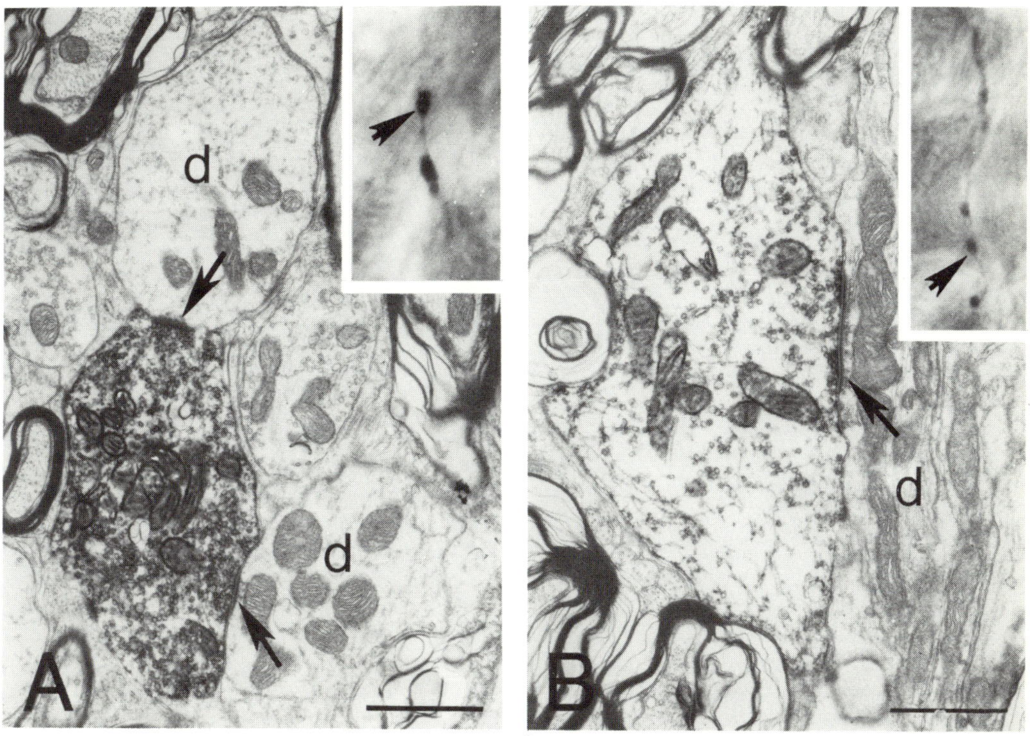

Fig. 1. Electron micrographs of terminal (A) and en passant (B) boutons of cat oculomotor axon collateral (arrows in light micrograph insets). d, dendritic profiles, calibrations 1 micron.

To determine whether oculomotor axon collaterals were unique to cats, antidromically identified rabbit, rat and guinea pig motoneurons were intracellularly stained with HRP (Fig. 2). Like cat motoneurons, the dendrites occupied about 1/3 of the nucleus and extended into the central gray and MLF (Figs. 2,3). Unlike cat motoneurons, however, collaterals were rare. None of the rabbit motoneurons (n=7, including a medial rectus motoneuron) exhibited collaterals. By contrast, all cat medial rectus motoneurons had collaterals (n=14). Only 30% of all guinea pig and rat motoneurons possessed collaterals (n=10) compared with 68% of all cat motoneurons (n=46). Besides their rarity, rodent collaterals differed in two other respects from cat collaterals. First, the terminal arborization was restricted. For example, a cat superior rectus motoneuron had two collaterals (Fig. 3; c) which divided into two or more secondary branches terminating in several boutons. Even though it is drawn at 4 times the magnification of the cat collateral (Fig. 3; c), the guinea pig collateral only extended 60 microns from the main axon. Second, rodent collaterals did not always occur in the oculomotor nucleus. In two of the three rodent motoneurons, the collaterals branched off the main axon near the exit of the third nerve from the brain and terminated in the ventral mesencephalic reticular formation. In cat motoneurons, the collaterals always occurred in or very near the oculomotor nucleus.

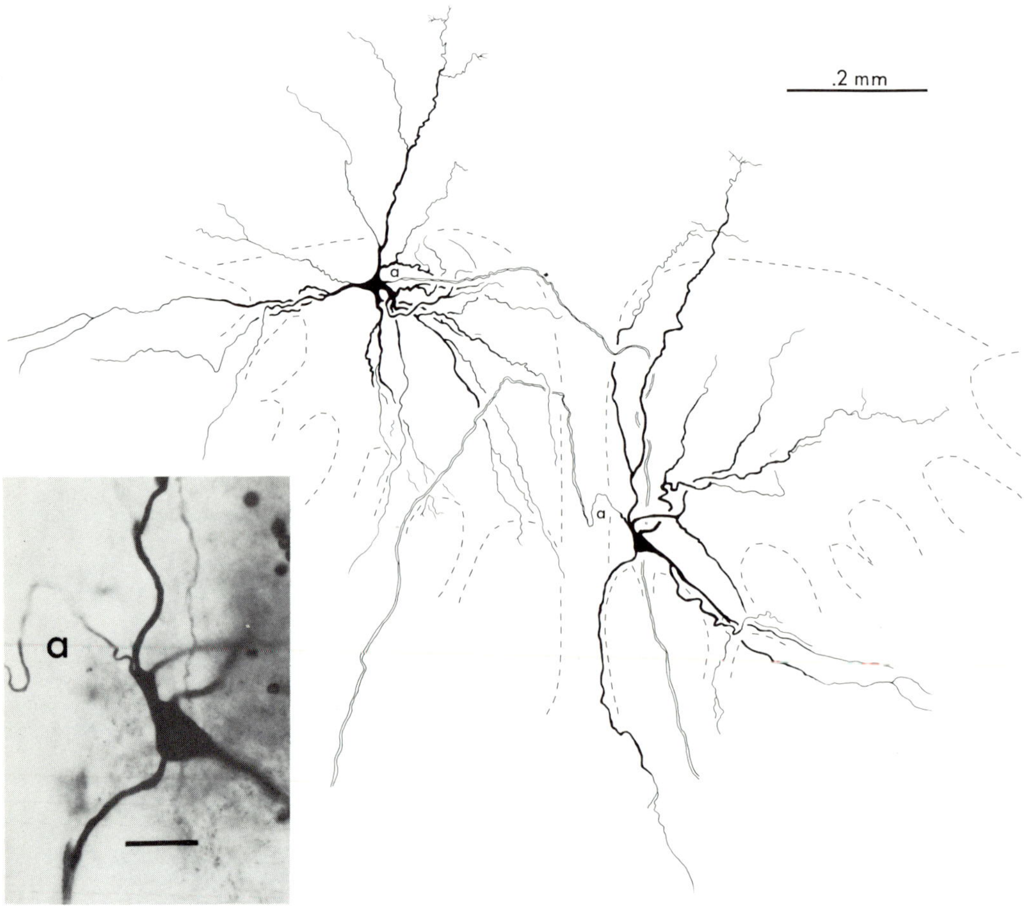

Fig. 2. Reconstruction of two rat superior rectus motoneurons and photomicrograph of one. a, axon, calibration is 30 microns.

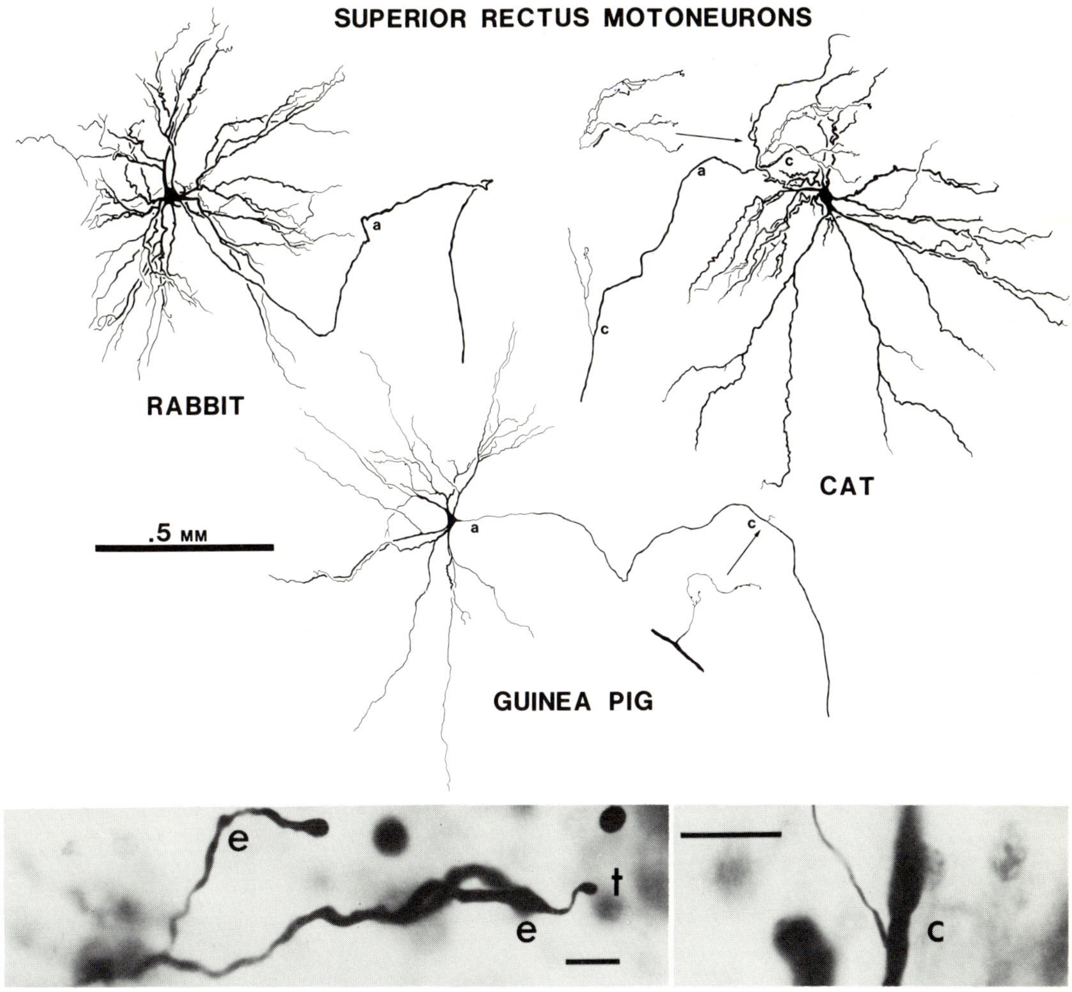

Fig. 3. Reconstruction of three superior rectus motoneurons. Photomicrographs of terminal (t) and en passant (e) boutons and collateral (c) of cat superior rectus. Calibration is 10 microns.

Since the difference in cat and rodent eye movements are inconsistent with convergent evolution, their collaterals are probably homologous. Perhaps collaterals originating in the ventral mesencephalic reticular formation are closer to the primitive condition than those in the nucleus. Since any neuron within the nucleus could generate motoneuron like activity by receiving the same inputs as motoneurons, the synapse of cat collaterals on oculomotor internuclear neurons seems superfluous. Neurons in the reticular formation could better use a direct motoneuron input to produce motoneuron like activity. During feline evolution these neurons may have migrated into the oculomotor nucleus. Perhaps the extensive collateralization in the cat underlies an ability not present in rodents and rabbits, e.g. smooth pursuit. On the other hand, the absence of collaterals in rabbit and their paucity in rodents relative to cats may reflect the shift from lateral to frontal eye positions.

Evinger, C., R. Baker, R.A. McCrea and R. Spencer. In W. Becker and A.F. Fuchs (Eds) Progress in Oculomotor Research, Elsevier, New York in press

DISTURBANCES OF THE OCULOMOTOR SYSTEM CAUSED BY HYDROCARBON SOLVENTS

L. M. ÖDKVIST, B. LARSBY, S. R. C. LIEDGREN and R. THAM

Department of Otolaryngology, University Hospital, Linköping, Sweden

Aliphatic and aromatic hydrocarbons can produce central nervous systems' symptoms e.g. headache, nausea, fatigue and vertigo. These symptoms are vague and an examination usually fails to unveil any signs. Vestibular and oculomotor tests have, however, shown positive findings caused by industrial solvents. In animal experiments rabbits rats have shown vestibular disturbances when exposed to solvents (Aschan and others, 1977; Larsby and others, 1976, 1978a, 1978b, 1981; Ödkvist and others, 1977, 1978, 1979, 1980a, 1980b; Tham and others, 1979, 1981). These disturbances have been registered as positional nystagmus or a diminished or exaggerated nystagmus response to a rotatory acceleration. A relatively high concentration of the solvent in blood is needed in the animal experiments to provoke the above mentioned symptoms. Already at a lower blood concentration styrene given to rabbits elicited an initial facilitation of the optokinetic response. The optokinetic fusion limit was studied and shown to return to the preintoxication value already half an hour after the exposure(Ödkvist and others, 1980a).

According to the chemical structure of carbon chain the industrial solvents can be divided into two main groups namely aliphatic and aromatic carbons. Two frequently used solvents, the aromatic styrene and the aliphatic trichloroethylene, were chosen for an investigation on humans. Healthy volunteers served as test subjects. Ten were given styrene and five trichloroethylene via a breathing valve and a mouth piece while performing exercise(50W) on an ergometer bicycle. The subjects were exposed to the solvents for about 1 hour. Electronystagmography was performed. The subjects were tested by sinusoidal oscillation in darkness, sinusoidal oscillation fixating a stable target, smooth pursuit movement test, optokinetic test, saccade test and visual suppression of rotatory nystagmus. Trichloroethylene did not give significant changes in the tests. The ten subjects exposed to styrene showed significant changes in the saccade and visual suppression tests due to solvent exposure. In the saccade test three parameters, the latency, maximum velocity and the accuracy of the saccade, were calculated. The latency was not altered by the exposure. The maximum velocity of the saccade was increased and there was a tendency for the test subjects to overshoot the target although the overshoot was not statistically significant. In the visual suppression test, where the subject is trying to fixate a target moving with him, the gain was significantly increased as the position of the eye divided by the position of the stimulus(chair).

People exposed to industrial solvents may suffer from a psychoorganic syndrome consisting of disturbances of the different psychophysiological function and develop neurastenia, personality changes and intellectual reduction(Axelsson and others, 1976). Eleven workers exposed to industrial solvents for many years and considered to suffer from a psychoorganic syndrome were tested with the same otoneurological test battery as the test persons. Six of the workers had a depression of the visual suppression ability as the main finding. Four out of eleven also had an increased saccade speed.

Results from animal experiments have revealed that intoxication with hydrocarbon solvents has an influence on the vestibulo-oculomotor reflex arc. The findings seem to indicate that the solvents block the inhibition of the vestibulo-oculomotor reflex presumably exerted by the cerebellum. The blood concentrations necessary to elicit oculomotor disturbances in animals were smaller than those who disturbed the vestibular function. Accordingly in human experiments styrene exposure did not elicit any positional nystagmus but caused an increased saccade speed and a diminished visual suppression of vestibular nystagmus. Some cerebellar clinical pathology in patients, suffering from a psychoorganic syndrome caused by solvents leads us to believe that this part of the brain might be the most vulnerable one. Some patients had a positional nystagmus but the most prominent pathology concerned the visual suppression test. It should be noted that the visual suppression of vestibular nystagmus is exerted by the cerebellum(Cohen, 1974; Precht, 1974; Fernandez and Fredrickson, 1964). Hence it may be deduced that the oculomotor disturbances exerted by hydrocarbon solvents may be mediated by cerebellar structures and that chronic brain damage due to solvents has one site of predilection in the cerebellum. Our findings compare well with the increased saccade speed and diminished visual suppression in patients with cerebellar lesions described by Wennmo and others(1981).

RAPID EYE MOVEMENTS IN PATIENTS WITH POSTERIOR FOSSA DISORDERS

C. WENNMO*, N. G. HENRIKSSON*, B. HINDFELT**, I. PYYKKÖ* and L. SCHALÉN*

Departments of Otolaryngology and Neurology**, University Hospital of Lund, Sweden*

ABSTRACT

To investigate the role of brainstem and cerebellum in control of rapid eye movements, 10 patients with pontine, 10 with medullary and 10 with cerebellar lesions were studied with electro-oculography. Characteristics of gaze in patients with pontine disorders were reduced velocities of all types of rapid eye movements whereas cases with medullary and cerebellar lesions showed preserved and even enhanced velocities in the quick components of postrotatory and optokinetic nystagmus. Our findings support the assumption that cerebellum is important for keeping the accurate velocity-amplitude relationship of rapid eye movements. If a cerebellar deficit occurs the velocity is too high for the amplitude whereas the velocity of rapid eye movements are reduced in pontine disorders.

KEYWORDS

Brainstem; medulla oblongata; cerebellum; rapid eye movements; amplitude-velocity relationship.

INTRODUCTION

Clinical evidence indicate that rapid eye movements are slowed in case of pontine disorder (Baloh et al., 1975; Bird & Leech, 1976; Wennmo & Hindfelt, 1980) and most investigators state that cerebellar disorders do not affect the velocity of these eye movements (Ellenberger et al., 1972: Baloh et al., 1975; Zee et al., 1976b;although this is a matter of persisting controversy (Daroff & Hoyt, 1971; Wadia & Swami, 1971). Patients with medullary lesions do probably exhibit a normal velocity of saccades though confirmation is sparse (Baloh et al., 1980; Corvera et al., 1980). Experimental results from single unit recordings in animals are generally agreed to show that the velocity of rapid eye movements is coded within neuronal units of the paramedian pontine reticular formation (PPRF) and that these units are active no matter whether the rapid eye movements are voluntarily or visually evoked (Cohen & Feldman, 1968; Cohen & Henn, 1972; Luschei & Fuchs, 1972; Keller, 1974; Henn & Cohen, 1976). With such an organization of neurons for velocity coding it would be expected that the two types of rapid eye movements would be disturbed to the same degree in case of a pontine lesion. Conversely, in patients with medullary or cerebellar lesions, the velocity of rapid eye movements would not be affected provided that the cerebellum or medulla do not participate in the velocity control. According to a few investigators, however, the velocity of quick components of vestibular nystagmus is coded not in the PPRF, but in the vestibular nuclei (Spiegel & Price, 1939), and recently units in the nucleus prepositus hypoglossi (Baker et al., 1975), another structure of the medulla, were found to be active during rapid eye movements. Recently also units active during rapid eye movements have been found in the cerebellum (Noda & Suzuki, 1979 a).

In humans, for easily obvious reasons, the location of structures which participate in eye velocity programming is not so well documented as in animals.

The present investigation was undertaken to evaluate the role of pons, medulla and cerebellum in ocular motor behaviour during performance of rapid eye movements in humans.

MATERIAL AND METHODS

Selection of cases

1. Ten patients (6 males, 4 females) with disorders located in pons, of whom 8 suffered from infarctions and 2 from tumours. Mean age 54.7 years (range 17-81).

2. Ten patients (7 males, 3 females) with lesions in medulla oblongata; 8 with lateral and 2 with medial medullary infarctions. Mean age 63.1 years (range 41-78).

3. Ten patients (5 males, 5 females) with cerebellar disease consisting of 5 patients with cerebellopathy, 2 tumours, 1 hematoma, 1 encephalitis and 1 with cerebellar manifestations of multiple sclerosis. Mean age 48.2 years (range 15-72).

4. Twenty healthy volunteers (10 males, 10 females) without previous neurological disease were used as controls. Mean age 48 years (range 23-72).

Test procedure

All tests were performed in ways previously described for this laboratory (Henriksson et al., 1980; Schalén, 1980).

Voluntary saccades were performed between light-emitting diode targets positioned 5, 10, 20, 40 and 60° apart.

Smooth pursuit were elicited by a target consisting of a moving light spot of 30 mm diameter projected on a horizontal screen and with a velocity of 5, 10, 20, 30, 40, 50 and 60° s^{-1}.

Vestibular nystagmus was induced by rotating patients in a revolving chair with an acceleration and deceleration of 120°s^{-2}. The velocity of the chair when fully accelerated was 120°s^{-1} and the test was performed in darkness.

Optokinetic nystagmus (OKN) was induced with the patient seated inside a drum of 180 cm diameter, the interior of which consisted of alternating black and white vertical stripes.

Recording of eye movements

The eye movements were recorded with an electro-oculographic technique using a d.c. coupled ink-jet writer (Siemens-Elema, Sweden). The electrodes were placed bitemporally at the outer canthi for recording of horizontal eye movements and monocularly above each eye for recording of vertical eye movements.

RESULTS

Velocities of voluntary saccades

Fig. 1 shows the mean values of the saccadic velocity for each group of patients. When the saccades for individual patients were analyzed separately, slowed saccades were found in 10 of 10 patients with pontine disorders but only in 6 of 10 patients with medullary disorders and in 2 of 10 patients with cerebellar disorders.

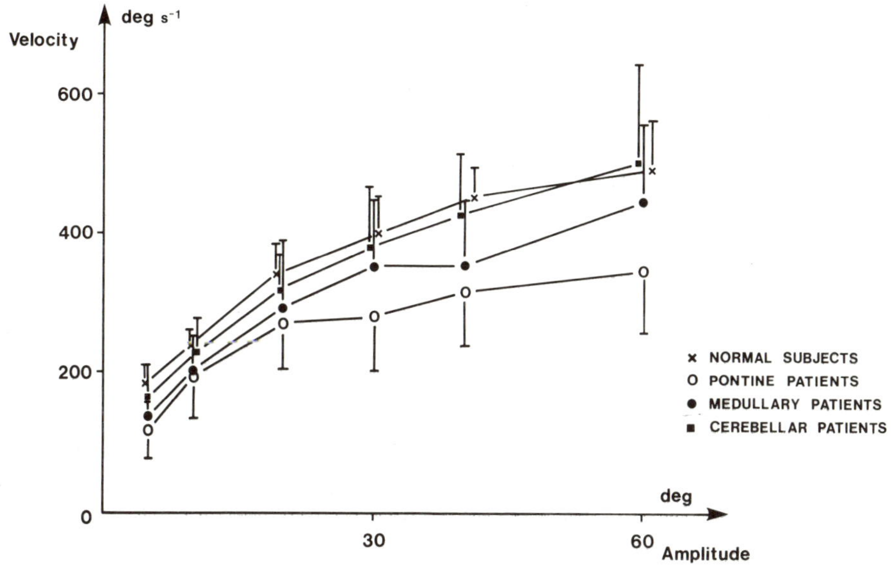

Fig. 1. Velocity-amplitude relationship of voluntary saccades. Controls and three different groups of patients (mean ± 1 SD).

Velocities of the quick components of nystagmus

Postrotatory responses. Patients with cerebellar or medullary disease exhibited a tendency towards enhanced velocities, although not significantly, when the groups as a whole were compared with the normal group. In contrast the mean peak velocities of the pontine group were reduced when compared to the normal group. When the quick components for individual patients were analyzed separately, 6 of 10 patients in the pontine lesion group exhibited reduced velocities while this was not seen in the medullary group and only in one patient in the cerebellar group. Increased velocities of the quick phase were found in one case of the medullary group and in 4 patients of the cerebellar group.

Optokinetic responses. The mean peak velocities of the quick component of optokinetic nystagmus in the different groups are depicted in Fig. 2. As for the rotatory responses an enhancement of the velocities in the cerebellar and medullary groups, but now significantly ($p < 0.05$, Student's t-test), compared with the normal group were found, while a reduction of the velocities were found in the group with pontine lesions. When the quick components for individual patients were analyzed separately, one of the 10 patients in the pontine lesion group had reduced velocity while this was not found in the medullary or cerebellar groups. Enhanced velocities were found in one patient in the medullary group and in 2 patients in the cerebellar group.

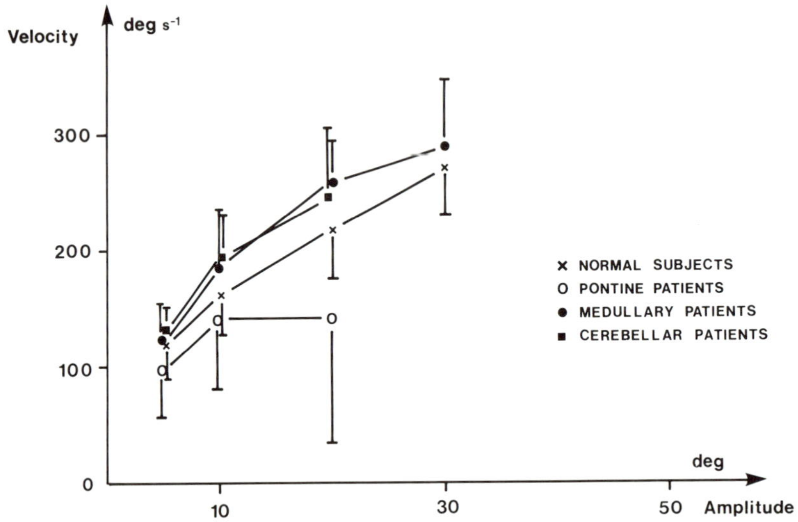

Fig. 2. Velocity-amplitude relationship of the quick components of optokinetic nystagmus. Groups and standard deviations as in Fig. 1.

DISCUSSION

The most likely explanation for the slowed saccades and slowed quick components of nystagmus found in our cases with pontine disorders, referring to the PPRF model, is a disturbance of neuronal units in the PPRF. The reduced velocities of voluntary saccades in patients with lesions in medulla oblongata may then be explained as follows: either the lesion encroaches upon pontine structures or, alternatively, some medullary areas are important for the velocity coding of rapid eye movements (Spiegel & Price, 1939; Baker et al., 1975). Considering the cerebellar group in which 2 of the patients exhibited reduced velocities, this may imply involvement of adjacent brainstem areas.

The enhanced velocities of the quick component of postrotatory and optokinetic nystagmus in case of cerebellar and medullary lesion indicate the importance of these regions for oculomotor function. Conventionally, neither cerebellum nor medulla oblongata influence the velocity coding of rapid eye movements. Our findings of enhanced velocities are therefore unexpected although there is some experimental support for them (Ron & Robinson, 1973). They could, by cerebellar stimulation in monkeys produce hypometric saccades with a velocity being the same as if the saccade was not hypometric and consequently much higher than in a normal saccade. We may then expect a patient with a cerebellar disorder to produce the same type of truncated eye movements with normal velocity but of too small an amplitude. Since the velocity is related to the amplitude this would simulate the increase in velocity which we actually found. The similar findings in cases with medullary lesions may be due to an impact on the pathways passing to or from the cerebellum. The enhancement we found in the rapid eye movements further illustrates the role of pontine, medullary and cerebellar structures in the control of eye movements.

MECHANISM OF OCULAR BOBBING

H. ISHIKAWA, S. SEKIMOTO, T. SUZUKI and M. INAGAKI

Department of Ophthalmology, Nihon University, School of Medicine, Itabashi-ku, Tokyo, Japan

ABSTRACT

A surviving case of a 40-year-old man with ocular bobbing caused by hypertensive pontine hemorrhage was reported. The mechanism of ocular bobbing was discussed with clinical course and electro-oculography.

KEYWORDS

Ocular bobbing; pons; pontine hemorrhage; vertical eye movement; eye movement disorder; medial longitudinal fasciculus; paramedian pontine reticular formation.

INTRODUCTION

Ocular bobbing is an abnormal vertical eye movement, characterized by abrupt downward jerks of the eyes followed by a slow return to the midposition. Generally, it has been well-known that this abnormal eye movement was caused by destructive lesions of the pons. However, its mechanism has not been clarified. In this presentation,we would like to introduce the surviving case of ocular bobbing and to discuss its mechanism.

CASE REPORT

A 40-year-old man was admitted to the Nihon University Hospital a few hours after onset of unconsciousness at January 9 in 1980. On admission, he was in semicoma with response to painful stimuli and his blood pressure was 190/70 mm Hg. The pupils were pinpoint and responded very sluggishly to light. The deep tendon reflexes were increased and bilateral Babinski responses were present. A computerized tomography was performed and high density area was observed in the bilateral tegmentum and basis of the pons.(Fig. 1) Therefore, it was diagnosed as the hypertensive pontine hemorrhage. On the third hospital day, typical ocular bobbing suddenly appeared. Spontaneous horizontal eye movement and oculo-cephalic reaction were absent. In the same day, a computerized tomography was performed again. Interestingly, it was defined that the high density area extended to the more dorsal portion of the pontine tegmentum.(Fig. 2)

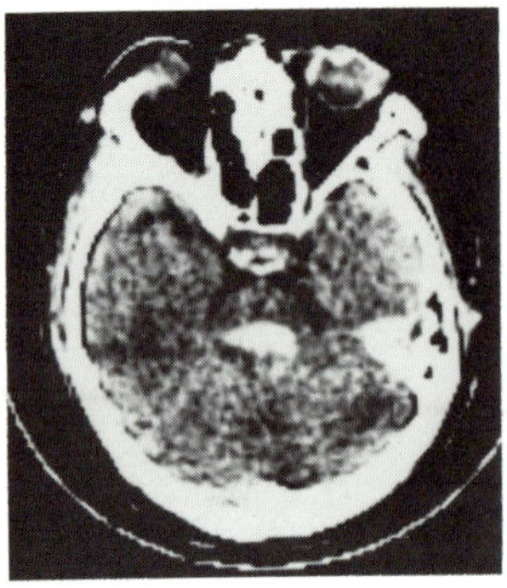

Fig. 1. CT scan on Jan. 9.

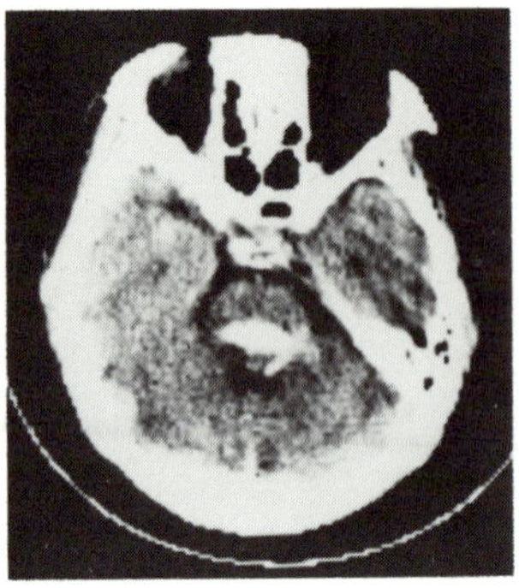

Fig. 2. CT scan on Jan. 11 when ocular bobbing appeared.

During the next four days, ocular bobbing persisted and after this disappearance, recovery of unconsciousness was present and left hemihypalgesia and facial weakness were observed.
50 days after onset, the abduction of the left eye improved, however, the adduction of both eyes and the abduction of the right eye had still been disturbed and it revealed so-called right "one and a half syndrome".(Fig. 3)
120 days after onset, these eye movement disorders almost improved except slight limitations of adduction and abduction of the right eye.

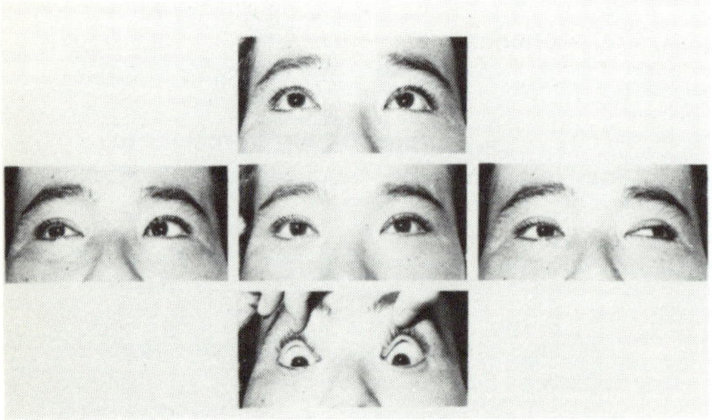

Fig. 3. Eye movements on 50 days after onset.

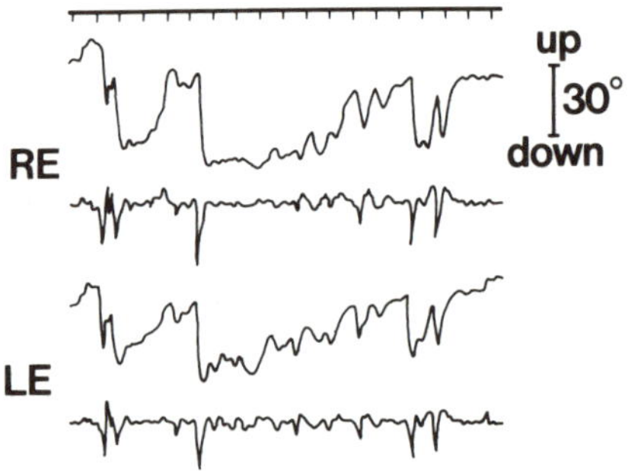

Fig. 4. DC-EOG of ocular bobbing.

DC-EOG Findings

Figure 4 shows DC-electro-oculogram of ocular bobbing. The upper two tracings represent position and velocity, respectively, from the right eye and the lower two tracings are from the left eye. As shown in this figure, both eyes were almost synchronous, but sometimes disjugate. The abnormal spontaneous vertical eye movement consisted of a quick downward component followed by a slow return to the midposition, sometimes lasting for 9 seconds. The synchronous record of ocular bobbing with DC-electro-oculography and cinematography was performed and the calibration of electro-oculography was measured. The results indicated that the downward velocity of ocular bobbing was about 300 degrees per second on the average and it was similar to that of normal downward saccade.

DISCUSSION

Ocular bobbing is a remarkable eye movement disorder in the pontine destruction first reported by Fisher (1964). Until now, many authors have reported. However, its mechanism has not been clarified, because the surviving case was very rare. (Hameroff and others, 1969; Susac and others, 1970; Newman and others, 1971; Boddie, 1972; Paty and others, 1972; Clarke and others, 1976) Fortunately, our case was surviving and we could observe the clinical course of this case in detail from the appearance of ocular bobbing to its improvement and investigate with DC-electro-oculography and cinematography. Therefore, we would like to discuss the mechanism of ocular bobbing.

In this case, ocular bobbing appeared just after onset of unconsciousness and horizontal eye movement was completely impaired. At the recovery stage, the disturbances of adductions of both eyes and abduction of the right eye had still remained. From these results, it was confirmed that bilateral destructions of the paramedian pontine reticular formation and medial longitudinal fasciculus played an important role in the generation of ocular bobbing. Additionally, from the electro-oculographical findings, the downward velocity of ocular bobbing was almost similar to that of normal downward saccade. Finally, it was detected with computerized tomography that ocular bobbing occurred when the lesion extended to the more dorsal portion of the pontine tegmentum. These results indicated that spontaneous downward saccadic eye movement was produced when horizontal eye movement was impaired completely and the inhibitory fibers of downward saccadic eye movement were destructed. These inhibitory fibers were considered to pass in the dorsal portion of the pontine reticular formation. And it was suggested that extreme downward deviation and slow return to the midposition were caused by destructions of the fibers of upward smooth pursuit eye movement passing through the bilateral medial longitudinal fasciculus as reported by Evinger and others. (1977) Furthermore, we could think that the fibers of vertical saccadic eye movement passed through the most dorsal portion of the pontine reticular formation. We presented our hypothesis about the mechanism of ocular bobbing. By studying such an abnormal eye movement accordingly, it is expected to confirm the pathway of vertical eye movement.

SACCADIC ABNORMALITIES IN DISEASES OF THE PERIPHERAL NERVOUS SYSTEM

S. E. FELDON*, L. STARK**, S. L. LEHMAN** and W. F. HOYT**

**Departments of Ophthalmology and Neurosurgery, University of Southern California, School of Medicine, Los Angeles, California, USA*
***Neuro-ophthalmic Unit, Departments of Neurology, Neurosurgery and Ophthamology, University of California, San Francisco, California, USA*

ABSTRACT

Typical oculographic patterns of saccadic eye movements are presented for two diseases of the peripheral nervous system -- myasthenia gravis and Guillain-Barre' syndrome. These eye movements are explained by intermittent conduction block, using computer simulations.

KEY WORDS

Peripheral nerve conduction, eye movements, myasthenia gravis, Guillain-Barre' syndrome, computer modeling, ophthalmoplegia, saccades.

INTRODUCTION

Two technological developments have facilitated a detailed study of eye movements in diseases of the peripheral nervous system -- control theory and high resolution oculography. Using control theory and experimental data, the pattern of neural activity for saccadic eye movements has been found to consist of a pulse-envelope of high frequency discharge to the agonist, followed by a step-envelope of higher tonic firing sufficient to hold the eye at the new position. The antagonist is completely inhibited during the pulse of agonist activity, after which it receives a lower step of tonic neural input. When saccadic movements become deficient, an increase in pulse width occurs to help bring the eyes to the intended target. With knowledge of both the theoretical input to the extraocular muscles and the exact behavioral output, as documented by infrared oculography, the mechanisms responsible for the degradation of saccadic responses in diseases of the peripheral nervous system can be investigated.

EYE MOVEMENT RECORDINGS

Horizontal eye movements in five patients with myasthenia gravis and three patients with Guillain-Barre' syndrome were studied. Four typical oculographic patterns were found which occurred independently in each eye. Three occurred during saccades (intra-saccadic) and one occurred after saccades (post-saccadic). The most unusual of these patterns was a series of small, rapid position changes separated by periods of little or no eye movement (Fig. 1a). This saccadic "stutter" produced a characteristic velocity recording with multiple peaks, each of which often reached higher peak velocities than would be predicted from normal isolated movements. A subtler intra-saccadic abnormality was a gradual slowing of saccadic velocity late in the eye movement, appearing oculographically as a gradual "decrescendo" of the velocity trace (Fig. 1b). Some saccades could only be characterized as "slow" (Fig. 1c). Immediately following saccades, a "backdrift" often occurred which was, in turn, followed by another saccade or drift toward the intended target position (Fig. 1d).

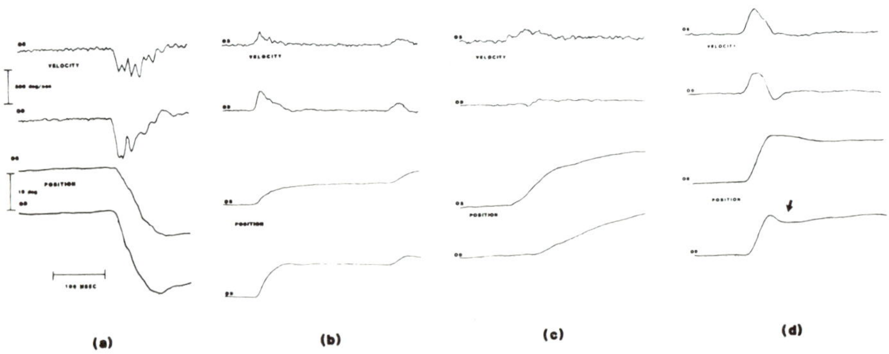

Fig. 1. Characteristic saccadic abnormalities in myasthenia gravis and Guillain-Barre′ syndrome are: a) "stutter", b) "decrescendo", c) "slow", and d) "backdrift" (arrow).

COMPUTER SIMULATIONS OF PERIPHERALLY DEGRADED SACCADES

Mechanisms of intra-saccadic oculomotor dysfunction. How can the four types of eye movements identified in both myasthenia gravis and Guillain-Barre′ syndrome be related mechanistically? "Stutter" has the most complex dynamics; therefore, any hypothesis explaining this oculomotor behavior may also account for the other observed patterns. "Stutter" or "multiple closely-spaced saccades" (Schmidt and co-workers, 1980) closely resemble overlapping saccades, previously reported to occur normally in fatigued individuals (Bahill and Stark, 1975). An altered central controller signal has been implicated in overlapping saccades, based upon the fit of each component to the "main sequence" (Bahill, Clark, and Stark, 1975a). Therefore, one interpretation of "stutter" could be that the extra effort needed to overcome the deficient excitation of the agonist muscle induces alterations in the central neural controller signal.

A second hypothesis to explain "stutter" would be necessary if the only response of the central neural controller to deficient eye movements were an increase in the pulse width of the controller signal. Because the pathophysiology of both myasthenia gravis and Guillain-Barre′ syndrome involves conduction block, the abnormal oculographic pattern in "stutter" could be explained by failure to faithfully conduct the central neural pulse envelope to the extraocular muscles. Favoring this latter, peripheral mechanism is the observation that "stutter" occurs independently in each eye, violating Herring's law of equal innervation. lso, the saccadic fragments have higher peak velocities and shorter durations than occur in centrally generated saccades. Finally, an hypothesis accounting for oculomotor behavior solely in terms of central controller signal would discount any primary effects of peripheral nervous system dysfunction on the eye movements.

To explore the possible role of peripheral conduction block in the eye movements of myasthenia gravis and Guillain-Barre′ syndrome, computer simulations of peripheral conduction block were obtained, using a modification of the model developed by Stark and co-workers (Cook and Stark, 1968; Clark and Stark, 1974). When the pulse width of the central neural signal to the extraocular muscles was prolonged, intermittent failure of the agonist muscle was sufficient to simulate the fractionation of saccades (Fig. 2a) seen clinically in "stutter". The number of subcomponents generated depended only upon the pulse width and the temporal spacing. We found that conduction failure had to be virtually complete in order to generate the separate saccadic subcomponents. Closer spacing or shorter intervals between conduction simulated "decresendo" (Fig. 2b). "Slow" movements could be simulated in many ways. In Figure 2c there was complete block early in the pulse of neural activity and there was no adaptive increase in pulse width.

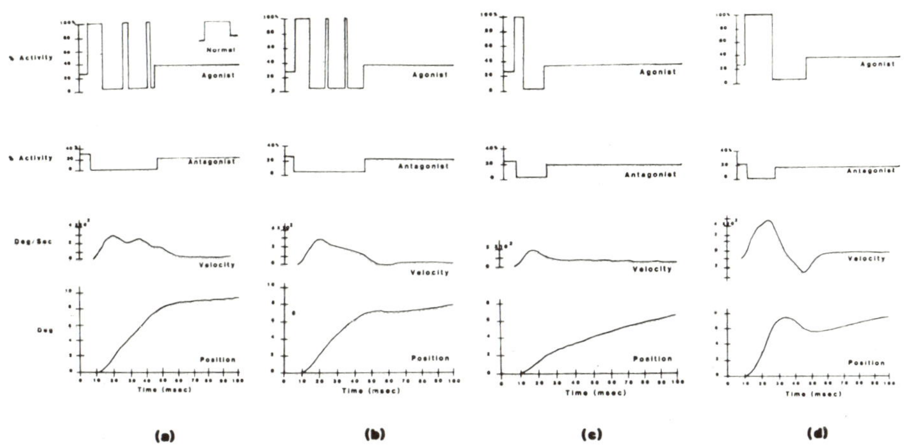

Fig. 2. Simulations of intermittent peripheral conduction block produce saccadic patterns similar to the oculographic abnormalities of: a) "stutter", b) "decrescendo", c) "slow", and d) "backdrift", seen in patients with myasthenia gravis and Guillain-Barre′ syndrome.

Mechanisms of post-saccadic oculomotor dysfunction. Having demonstrated that intra-saccadic oculomotor abnormalities in myasthenia gravis and Guillain-Barre′ syndrome can be explained by peripheral mechanisms, we now consider post-saccadic "backdrift". Post-saccadic backdrift is apparent clinically as "quiver" (Cogan, Yee, and Gittinger, 1976). Superficially, this eye movement resembles the normal, centrally programmed dynamic overshoot. However, attention to the oculographic recordings shows that there is no overshoot. Rather, these saccades are hypo- or normometric. If conduction fails just at the end of a centrally-programmed pulse of maximal innervation, the agonist may be incapable of holding the step-envelope of neural firing required for stable eye position. During the saccade, the antagonist is inhibited and, therefore, is capable of normal post-saccadic activation. Transiently, antagonist tone may exceed that in the agonist, causing the eye to drift backward (Fig. 2d). Refixation saccades or adjustments in agonist tone are necessary to bring the eye onto target. These corrective saccades, being centrally determined, are conjugate and, if multiple, may appear as nystagmus.

CONCLUSIONS

The saccadic patterns found in myasthenia gravis and Guillain-Barre′ syndrome can be simulated on the basis of intermittent peripheral conduction block to the extraocular muscles. The requirement that conduction block must be nearly complete may have implications for the pathophysiology of these diseases. Also, other neurologic disorders primarily affecting conduction to extraocular muscles may produce similar oculomotor abnormalities.

DISCUSSION

Dell′Osso commented that he thought that stutter and decrescendo (or closely-spaced saccades and saccades with discrete decelerations as Schmidt, Dell′Osso and Daroff called them) reflected central, adaptive innervation patterns rather than peripheral fatigue. He based this explanation on the seeming conjugacy of the phenomena and the response to tension -- the closely-spaced saccades still occurred only they now had larger amplitudes. He suggested that proprioceptive impulses triggered the closely-spaced saccades and indeed suggested that a role for extra ocular muscle proprioception was to trigger corrective saccades in the presence of neuromuscular junction blockade.

Feldon retorted that his myasthenic stutter and decrescendo were not conjugate. Stark commented that there are probably central causes of both binocular and monocular closely-related saccades and that they also may arise from peripheral disorders. All discussants were happy with this synthesis.

COMPOUND LIST OF REFERENCES

Abadi, R.V., D. Carden, and J. Simpson (1979). Controlling abnormal eye movements. Vision Res., 19, 961-963.

Abadi, R.V., D. Garden, and J, Simpson (1980). A new treatment for congenital nystagmus. Br. J. Ophthal., 64, 2-6.

Abadi, R.V., and M. Sandikcioglu (1974). Electrooculographic responses in a case of bilateral idiopathic nystagmus. Br. J. Physiol. Optics, 29, 73-85.

Abel, L.A., L.F. Dell´Osso, and R.B. Daroff (1978). Analog model for gaze-evoked nystagmus. IEEE Trans. Biomed. Engr. BME-25, 71-75.

Abel, L.A. , D. Schmidt, L.F. Dell´Osso. and R.B. Daroff (1978). Saccadic system plasticity in humans. Ann. Neurol., 4, 313-338.

Abel, L.A., L. Traccis, L.F. Dell´Osso, and C. Ansevin (In preparation). Downbeat nystagmus with three wave forms.

Abrahams, V.C. (1979). Proprioceptive influences from eye muscle receptors on cells of the superior colliculus. Prog. Brain Res., 50, 325-334.

Abramson, D.H. (1973). Latent nystagmus in identical twins. Arch. Ophthal., 89, 256-257.

Adamuk, E. (1870). Ueber die Innervation der Augenbewegungen. Zentr.Med. Wiss., 8, 65.

Adelstein, A.M., and J. Scully (1967). Epidemiological aspects of squint. Br. Med. J., 8, 334-338.

Adelstein, F. and C. Cüppers (1968). Probleme der operativen Schielbehandlung. Ber. dtsch. Ophthal. Ges., 69, 580-586.

Aichmair, H. and R. Mayr (1979). Elektronenmikroskopische Untersuchungen der Mitochondrien von Schielmuskeln.Albrecht v Graefes Arch.Ophthal.,186, 45-54.

Aihara, T., M. Miyata, and S. Ishkawa (1980). The lactate dehydrogenase isoenzyme pattern in the overacting inferior oblique muscle. J. Ped. Ophthal. and Strab., 15, 43-47.

Albano, J.E., and R.H. Wurtz (1981). The role of the primate superior colliculus, pretectum, and posterior-medial thalamus in visually-guided eye movements. In A. Fuchs and W. Becker (Eds.), Progress in Oculomotor Research, Elsevier Press, New York. pp 153-160.

Alpern, M. (1962). Accommodation: Evaluation of theories of presbyopia. In H. Davson (Ed.). The Eye Vol. 3, 1st Edition, Academic Press, New York.

Alpern, M., W.M. Kincaid, and M.J. Lubeck (1959). Vergence and accommodation. III. Proposed definitions of the AC/A ratios. Am. J. Ophthal., 48 (Pt.2), 141-148.

Alvarado, J.A., and C. van Horn (1975). Muscle cell types of the cat inferior oblique. In G. Lennerstrand and P. Bach-y-Rita (Eds.), Basic Mechanisms of Ocular Motility and Their Clinical Implications, Pergamon Press, Oxford. pp. 15-43.

Anderson, J.H., R.H.I. Blanks, and W. Precht (1978). Response characteristics of semicircular canal and otolith systems in cat. I. Dynamic responses of primary vesticular fibers. Exp. Brain. Res., 32, 491-507.
Anderson, J.H., and C. Pappas (1981). Changes in ocular torsion after lesions of the interstitial nucleus of Cajal (INC). Proc. New York Acad. Sci. In Press.
Anderson, J.H., W. Precht, and C. Pappas (1979). Changes in the vertical vestibulo-ocular reflex due to kainic acid lesions of the interstitial nucleus of Cajal. Neurosci. Letters, 14, 259-264.
Anderson, J.R. (1954). Latent nystagmus and alternating hyperphoria. Br. J. Ophthal. , 38, 217-231.
Angaut, P., and A. Brodal (1967). The projection of the "vestibulocerebellum" onto the vestibular nuclei in the cat. Arch. Ital. Biol., 105, 411-479.
Angel, R.W., and H. Garland (1972). Transfer of information from manual to oculomotor control system. J. Exp. Psychol., 96, 92-96.
Angel, R.W., H. Garland, and M. Fischler (1971). Tracking errors amended without visual feedback. J. Exp. Psychol., 89, 442-424.
Antony, J.H., R.A. Ouvrier, and G, Wise (1980). Spasmus nutans: A mistaken identity. Arch. Neurol., 37, 373-375.
Asanuma, H. (1975). Recent developments in the study of the columar arrangement of neurons within the motor cortex. Physiol. Rev., 55, 143-156.
Aschan, G., I. Bunnfors, D. Hydén, B. Larsby, L.M. Ödkvist, and R. Tham (1977). Xylene exposure. Electronystagmographic and gas chromatographic studies in rabbits. Acta oto-lar., 84, 370-376.
Aschoff, J.C., and B. Cohen (1971). Changes in saccadic eye movement produced by cerebellar cortical lesions. Expl. Neurol., 32, 123-133.
Aschoff, J.C., B. Conrad, and H.H. Kornhuber (1974). Acquired pendular nystagmus with oscillopsia in multiple sclerosis: A sign of cerebellar nuclei disease. J. Neurol. Neurosurg. Psychiat., 37, 570-577.
Aslin, R.N. (1977). Development of binocular fixation in human infants. J. Exp. Child. Psychol., 23, 47-56.
Asmussen, G., A. Kiessling, and F. Wohlrad (1971). Histochemische Charakterisierung der verschiedenen Muskelfasertypen in den äusseren Augenmuskeln von Säugetieren. Acta Anat.(Basel), 79, 526-545.
Astruc, J. (1971). Corticofugal connection of area 8 (frontal eye field) in Macaca mulatta. Brain Res., 33, 241-256.
Atkin, A., and M.B. Bender (1968). Ocular stabilisation during oscillatory head movements. Arch. Neurol., 19, 559-566.
Atkinson, J. (1979). Development of optokinetic nystagmus in the human infant and monkey infant: An analogue to development in kittens. In R.D. Freeman (Ed.), Developmental Neurobiology of Vision, Plenum Press, New York. pp. 277-287.
Atkinson, J., and O. Braddick (1976). Stereoscopic discrimination in infants. Perception, 5, 29-38.
Atkinson, J., O, Braddick, and J. French (1980). Infant astigmatism: Its disappearance with age. Vision Res., 20, 891-893.
Avanzini, G,. G. Floriano, P. Crenna, and S. Negri (1979). Alterations of ocular motility in cerebellar pathology, an electro-oculographic study. Arch. Neurol., 36, 274-280.
Axelson, O., M. Hane, and C. Hogstedt (1976). Neuropsychiatric illhealth in workers exposed to solvents - a case-control study. Läkartidningen, 73, 322-325.
Azzena, G.B., C. Desole, and G. Palmieri (1970). Cerebellar projections of the masticatory and extraocular muscle proprioception. Exp. Neurol., 27, 151-161.
Bach-y-Rita, P. (1972). Extraocular muscle inhibitory stretch reflex during active contraction. Arch. Ital. Biol., 110, 1-15.
Bach-y-Rita, P., C.C. Collins, and J.E. Hyde (1971). The Control of Eye Movements. Academic Press, New York and London.
Bach-y-Rita, P,. and F. Ito (1966a).Properties of stretch receptors in cat extra-ocular muscles. J. Physiol. (London). 186, 663-688.
Bach-Y-Rita, P., and F. Ito (1966b).In vivo studies on fast and slow muscle fibers in cat extraocular muscles. J. Gen. Physiol., 49, 1177-1198.

Bach-y-Rita, P., and G. Lennerstrand (1975). Absence of polyneuronal innervation in cat. J. Physiol., 244, 613-624.
Bach-y-Rita, P., G. Lennerstrand. J. Alvarado. K. Nichols, and C. McHolm (1977). Extraocular muscle fibers: Ultrastructural identification of iontoporetically labeled fibers contracting in response to succinylcholine. Invest. Ophthal. Vis. Sci., 161, 561-565.
Bach-y-Rita, P., and K. Murata (1964). Extraocular proprioceptive responses in the VI nerve of the cat. Quart. J. Exp. Physiol., 49, 407-416.
Bagolini. B. (1961). Diagnostic et possibilié de traitement de l'état sensorial du strabisme concomitant avec des instruments peu dissociants (test du verre strié et barre de filtres). Ann. Ocul., 194, 236-258.
Bagolini, B. (1967). Anomalous correspondence: Definition and diagnostic methods. Doc. Ophthal., 23, 346-398.
Bagolini, B., (1971). Anomalias sensoriales del estrabismo. Actas III Congreso del C.L.A.D.E., Mar del Plata, Argentina, pp. 359-377.
Bagolini, B., (1974). Sensory anomalies in strabismus. Br. J. Ophthal., 58, 313-318.
Bagolini, B. (1976a). Part I. Sensorial anomalies in strabismus (Suppression, anomalous correspondence, amblyopia). Doc. Ophthal., 41, 1-22.
Bagolini, B. (1976b). Part II. Sensorio-motorial anomalies in strabismus (anomalous movements). Doc. Ophthal., 41, 23-41.
Bagolini, B., and E.C. Campos (1977). Binocular campimetry in small-angle concomitant esotropia. Doc. Ophthal. Proc. Series, 14, 405-409.
Bagolini, B., and N.M. Capobianco (1965). Subjective space in comitant squint. Am. J. Ophthal., 59, 430-442.
Bahill, A.T., K.J. Ciuffreda, R.V. Kenyon, and L. Stark (1976). Dynamic and static violations of Hering's law of equal innervation. Am. J. Optom. Physiol. Optics, 53, 786-796.
Bahill, A.T., M.R. Clark, and L. Stark (1975a). The main sequence, a tool for studying human eye movements. Math. Biosci., 24, 191-204.
Bahill, A.T., M.R. Clark, and L. Stark (1975b). Dynamic overshoot in saccadic eye movements is caused by neurological control signal reversals. Exp. Neurol., 48, 107-122.
Bahill, A.T., M.J. Iandolo, and B.T. Troost (1980). Smooth pursuit eye movements in response to unpredictable target waveforms. Vision Res., 20, 923-931.
Bahill, A.T., and L. Stark (1975). Overlapping saccades and glissades are produced by fatique in the saccadic eye movement system. Exp. Neurol., 48, 95-106.
Baichenko, P.L., D.P. Matyushkin, and V.V. Suvorov (1967). Participation of fast and tonic oculomotor systems in stretch reflexes and labyrinthine reflexes of extraocular muscles. Fiziol. ZH. SSSR, 53, 82-90.
Baker, R., and A. Berthoz (1977). The Control of Gaze by Brainstem Neurons. Elsevier/North-Holland Biomedical Press, New York.
Baker, R., C. Evinger, and R.A. McCrea (1981). Some thoughts about the three neurons in the vestibular ocular reflex. In B. Cohen (Ed.), Recent Advances in Vestibular and Oculomotor Physiology. Ann. N.Y. Acad. Sci., In press.

Baker, R., M. Gresty, and A. Berthoz (1975). Neuronal activity in the prepositus hypoglossi nucleus correlated with vertical and horizontal eye movements in the cat. Brain Res., 101, 366-371.
Baker, R., and W. Precht (1972). Electrophysiological properties of trochlear motoneurons as revealed by IV nerve stimulation. Exp. Brain. Res., 14, 124-157.
Baker, R., W. Precht, and R. Llinas (1972). Mossy and climbing fiber projections of extraocular muscle afferents to the cerebellum. Brain Res., 38, 440-445.
Balaban, C.D., Y. Kawaguchi, and E. Watanabe (1981). Evidence of a collateralized climbing fiber projection from the inferior olive to the flocculus and vestibular nuclei in rabbits. Neurosci. Letters, 22, 23-29.
Baloh, R.W., and V. Honrubia (1979). Clinical Neurophysiology of the Vestibular System. F.A. Davis, Philadelphia.
Baloh, R.W., V. Honrubia, and H.R. Konrad (1976). Periodic alternating nystagmus. Brain, 99, 11-26.

Baloh, R.W., V. Honrubia, and A.W. Sills (1977). Eye-tracking and optokinetic nystagmus. Results of quantitative testing in patients with well-defined nervous system lesions. Ann. Otol. Rhino. Lar., 86, 108-114.

Baloh, R.W., H.R. Konrad, D. Dirks, and V. Honrubia (1976). Cerebellar-pontine angle tumors: Results of quantitative vestibulo-ocular testing. Arch. Neurol., 33, 507-512.

Baloh, R.W., H.R. Konrad, and V. Honrubia (1975). Vestibúlo-ocular function in patients with cerebellar atrophy. Neurol., 25, 160-168.

Baloh, R.W., H.R. Konrad, A.W. Sills, and V. Honrubia (1975). The saccade velocity test. Neurol.,25, 1071-1076.

Baloh, R.W., W.E. Kumley, A.W. Sills, V. Honrubia, and H.R. Konrad (1976). Quantitative analysis of smooth pursuit eye movements. Ann.Otol.Rhino. Lar., 85, 111-118.

Baloh, R.W., L. Langhofer. V. Honrubia, and R.D. Yee (1980). On-line analysis of eye movements using a digital computer. Aviat.Space Environ. Med., 51, 563-567.

Baloh, R.W., A. Sills, and V. Honrubia (1977). Eye tracking and optokinetic nystagmus. Results of quantitative testing in patients with well-defined nervous system lesions. Ann. Otol. Rhino. Lar., 86, 108-114.

Baloh, R.W., A.W. Sills, L. Solingen, and V. Honrubia (1977). Caloric testing. Ann. Otol. Rhino. Lar., 86, 1-30.

Baloh, R.W., J.W. Spooner, R.D. Yee, and V. Honrubia (1980). Visual-vestibular interaction in patients with infarction of the lateral medulla (Wallenberg´s syndrome). Presented at the Barany Society Meeting, New York 1980.

Baloh, R.W. , and J.W. Spooner (1981). Downbeat-nystagmus: A type of central vestibular nystagmus. Neurol., 31, 304-310.

Baloh, R.W., R.D. Yee, and E. Boder (1978). Eye movements in ataxia-telangiectasia. Neurol., 28, 1099-1104.

Baloh, R.W., R.D. Yee, and V. Honrubia (1978a). Internuclear ophthalmoplegia. I. Saccades and dissociated nystagmus. Arch. Neurol., 35, 484-489.

Baloh, R.W., R.D. Yee, and V. Honrubia (1978b). Internuclear ophthalmoplegia. II. Pursuit, optokinetic nystagmus and vestibulo-ocular reflex. Arch. Neurol., 35, 490-493.

Baloh, R.W., R.D. Yee, and V. Honrubia (1980a). Optokinetic nystagmus and parietal lobe lesions. Ann. Neurol., 7, 269-276.

Baloh, R.W., R.D. Yee, and V. Honrubia (1980b). Optokinetic asymmetry in patients with maldeveloped foveas. Brain Res., 186, 211-216.

Baloh, R.W., R.D. Yee, and V. Honrubia (1981). Eye movements in patients with Wallenberg´s syndrome. In press.

Baloh, R.W., R.D. Yee, J. Kimm, and V. Honrubia (1981). The vestibulo-ocular reflex in patients with lesions involving the vestibulo-cerebellum. Exp.Neurol.,72,141-152.

Balsam, M.H., and G.A. Gry (1959). Convergence-accommodation. Am. J. Optom. and Arch. Am. Acad. Optom., 36, 567-575.

Bárány, R. (1921). Zur Klinik und Theorie des Eisenbahn nystagmus. Acta Otolar., 3, 260 - 265.

Barmack, N.H. (1976). Measurements of stiffness of the extraocular muscles of the rabbit. J. Neurophysiol., 39, 1009-1019.

Barmack, N.H. (1977). Recruitment and suprathreshold frequency modulation of single extraocular muscle fibers in the rabbit. J. Neurophysiol., 40, 779-790.

Barmack, N.H., and D.T. Hess (1980a). Multiple-unit activity evoked in dorsal cap of inferior olive of the rabbit by visual stimulation. J. Neurophysiol.,43,151-164.

Barmack, N.H., and D.T. Hess (1980b). Eye movements evoked by microstimulation of dorsal cap of inferior olive in the rabbit. J. Neurophysiol., 43, 165-179.

Barmack, N,H, and V.E. Pettorossi (1978). Vestibular and optokinetic properties of neurons in the vestibular nuclei of rabbits. Soc. for Neurosci. Abstr. 4, 609.

Barmack, N.H., and J.I. Simpson (1980). Effects of microlesions of dorsal cap of inferior olive of rabbits on optokinetic and vestibulo-ocular reflexes. J. Neurophysiol., 43, 182-206.

Barnes. G.R. (1979). Vestibulo-ocular function during coordinated head and eye movements to acquire visual targets. J. Physiol., 287, 127-147

Barnes, G.R. (1980). Vestibular control of oculomotor and postural mechanisms Clin. Phys. Physiol. Meas., 1, 3?40.
Barnes, G.R. (1981). A procedure for the analysis of nystagmus and other eye movements. Naval Aerosp. Med. Res. Lab. Rept. In press.
Barnes, G.R., A.J. Benson, and A.R.J. Prior (1978). Visual-vestibular interaction in the control of eye movement. Aviat. Space Environ. Med., 49, 557-564.
Barnes, G.R., and R. Smith (1981). The effects on visual discrimination of image movement across the stationary retina. Aviat. Space Environ. Med.,52(8),466-472.
Barr, C.C. L.W. Schultheis and D.A. Robinson (1976). Voluntary, non-visual control of the human vestibulo-ocular reflex. Acta Oto-lar., 81, 365-375.
Barré, M.J.-A. (1927). Le nystagmus et le syndrome vestibulaire dans plusieurs cas personnels de syndrome de Babinski-Nagotte et de Wallenberg. Rev. Oto-Neuro-Ophthal., 5, 945-959.
Bartz, J. (1965). Eye and head movements in peripheral vision: Nature of compensatory eye movements. Science, 114, 1644-1645.
Bartz, A.E. (1966). Eye and head movement in peripheral vision. Science, New York, 152, 1644-1645.
Batini, C. (1979a). Properties of the receptors of extraocular muscles. Progr. Brain Res., 50, 301-314.
Batini, C. (1979b). Extraocular muscle input to the cerebellar cortex. Progr. Brain. Res., 50, 315-324.
Batini, C. and P. Buisseret (1974). Sensory peripheral pathway from extrinsic eye muscles. Arch. Ital. Biol., 112, 18-32.
Batini, C. and G. Horcholle-Bossavit (1979). Extraocular muscle afferents and visual input interactions in the superior colliculus of the cat. Progr. Brain Res., 50, 335-343.
Becker, W., O. Hoehne., K. Iwase, and H.H. Kornhuber (1972). Bereitschaftspotential pramatorische Positivierung und andere Hirnpotentials bei sakkadischen Augenbewegungen. Vision Res., 12, 421-436.
Behrens-Baumann, W., and U. Wölz (1978). Ergebnisse der "Fadenfixation" nach Cüppers bei Schielern mit schwankendem Winkel. Klin. Mbl. Augenheilk., 173, 814-824.
Behrens, F., and O.-J. Grüsser (1979). Smooth pursuit eye movements and optokinetic nystagmus elicited by intermittently illuminated stationary patterns. Exp. Brain Res., 37, 317-336.
Bender, M.B. (1946). Effects of barbiturates on ocular movements (nystagmus). Confinia Neurol., 7, 144-147.
Bender, M. B. (1960). Comments on the physiology and pathology of eye movements in the vertical plane. J. Nerv. Ment. Dis., 130, 456-466.
Bender, M.B. (1965). Oscillopsia. Arch. Neurol., 13, 204-213.
Bender, M.B. (1980). Brain control of conjugate horizontal and vertical eye movements. A survey of the structural and functional correlates. Brain, 103, 23-69.
Bender, M.B., and M. Feldman (1967). Visual illusions during head movements in lesions of the brainstem. Arch. Neurol., 17, 354-364.
Bender, M.B.., and S. Shanzer (1964). Oculomotor pathways defined by electrical stimulation and lesions in the brainstem of monkey. In M.B. Bender (Ed.), The Oculomotor System, Harper and Row, New York. pp 81-96.
Bender, M.B., and H.L. Teuber (1964). Nystagmoid movements and visual perception. Their inter-relation in monocular diplopia. Arch. Neurol. Psychiat., 55,511-529.
Benitz, J.T. (1970). Eye-tracking and optokinetic tests: Diagnostic significance in peripheral and central vestibular disorders. Laryngoscope (St Louis), 80, 834-848.
Bennett, H., and Th. Savill (1889). A case of permanent conjugate deviation of the eyes and head, the result of a lesion limited to the sixth nucleus; with remarks on associated lateral movements of the eyeballs, and rotation of the head and neck. Brain, 12, 102-116.
Benson, A.J. (1970). Interactions between semicircular canals and gravireceptors. In D.E. Busby (Ed.), Recent Advances in Aerospace Medicine. D. Reidel Publishing Co., Dordrecht-Holland. pp 249-261.
Benson, A.J. and G. Barnes (1978). Vision during angular oscillation: The dynamic interaction of visual and vestibular mechanisms. Aviat. Space Environ. Med., 49, 340-345.

Benson, A.J., and M.A. Bodin (1966). Interaction of linear and angular accelerations on vestibular receptors in man. Aerospace Med., 37, 144-154.

Benson, A.J., and M.A. Gresty (1980). In V.J. Wilson and G. Melville-Jones (Eds.), Mammalian Vestibular Physiology, Plenum Press, New York. p 288.

Bérard, V.P., N. Mouillac, R. Reydy, and A. Spielmann (1978). Surgical treatment of congenital nystagmus with horizontal torticollis. In R. Reinecke (Ed.), Strabismus, Grune & Stratton, New York. pp 169-175.

Bérard-Badier, M., .F. Pellissier, M. Toga, N. Mouillac, and P.V. Bérard (1978). Ultrastructural studies of extraocular muscles in ocular motility disorders. Albrecht v Graefes Arch. Ophthal., 208, 193-205.

Berman, N. (1977). Connections of the pretectum in the cat. J. Comp. Neurol., 174, 227-254.

Berthoz, A., K. Yoshida, and P.P. Vidal (1981). In B. Cohen (Ed.), Vestibular and Oculomotor Physiology. Ann. N.Y. Acad. Sci. In press.

Betz, W.J., J.H. Caldwell and R.R. Ribchester (1979). The size of motor units during post-natal development of rat lumbrical muscle. J. Physiol., 297, 463-478.

Bielschowski, A. (1938). Disturbances of the vertical motor muscles of the eye. Arch. Ophthal., 20, 175-200.

Bielschowsky, A. (1943). Lectures on Motor Anomalies. Dartmouth College Publications, Hanover, N.H. (reprinted 1956).

Bicas, H.E.A. (1978). Analysis of ocular mechanics. Arq.Bras.Oftal. 41(3), 116-124.

Bird, A.C., and J. Leech (1976). Inernuclear Ophthalmoplegia. An electrooculographic study of peak angular saccadic velocities. Br. J. Ophthal., 60, 645-651.

Birukow, G. (1937). Untersuchungen über den optischen Drehnystagmus und über die Sehschärfe des Grasfrosches (Rana temporaria). Z. vergl. Physiol., 25, 92-142.

Bizzi, E. (1968). Discharge of frontal eye field neurons during saccadic and following eye movements in unanesthetized monkeys. Exp. Brain Res., 6, 69-80.

Bizzi, E. (1975). Central control of eye and head movements in monkeys. In G. Lennerstrand and P. Bach-y-Rita (Eds.), Basic Mechanisms of Ocular Motility and Their Clinical Implications, Pergamon Press, Oxford. pp 469-471.

Bizzi, E., R. Kalil, and V. Tagliasco (1971). Eye head coordination in monkeys. Science, 173, 452-454.

Bizzi, E. and P.H. Schiller (1970). Single unit activity in the frontal eye fields of unanesthetized monkeys during eye and head movement. Exp. Brain Res., 10, 151-158.

Bjerver, K. and B.P. Silfverskiöld (1968). Lateropulsion and imbalance in Wallenberg´s syndrome. Acta Neurol. Scand.,44, 91-100.

Björk, A., and E. Kugelberg (1953). The electrical activity of the muscles of the eye and eyelids in various postitions and during movement. Electroen. Neurophysiol., 5, 595-602

Blair, S., and M. Gavin (1979). Modification of the macaques vestibulo-ocular reflex after ablation of the cerebellar vermis. Acta Oto-lar., 88, 235-243.

Blakemore, C., and M. Donaghy (1980). Coordination of head and eyes in the gaze changing behaviour of cats. J. Physiol., 300, 317-335.

Blakemore, C. and R.C. van Sluyters (1974). Reversal of the physiological effects of monocular deprivation in kittens: Further evidence for a sensitive period. J. Physiol., 237, 195-216.

Blanks, R.H.I., and W. Precht (1981). Mossy fiber responses of Purkinje cells in the cerebellar flocculus of the alert, pigmented rat during optokinetic and vestibular stimulation. Soc. Neuroscience. In press.

Blanks, R.H.T., R. Volkind, W. Precht, and R. Baker (1977). Responses of cat prepositus hypoglossi neurons to horizontal angular acceleration. Neuroscience, 2, 391-403.

Bleuler, P.E. (1885). Zur Casuistik der Herderkrankungen der Brücke mit besonderer Berücksichtigung der Störungen der combinierten seitlichen Augenbewegungen. Dissertation Universität Bern. Leipzig: Hirschfeld.

Blocq, P., and G. Guinon (1891). Sur un cas de paralysie conjugée de la sixième paire. Arch. Med. Exp. Anat. Path. (Paris), 3, 74-89.

Boddie, H.G. (1972). Ocular bobbing and opsoclonus.Two abnormal spontaneous eye movements occuring in the same patient: cas report. J. Neurol. Neurosurg. Psychiat., 35, 739-742.

Bogacz, J., C. Mendilaharsu, and S.A. de Mendilalaharsu (1977). Electro-oculographic study of saccadic pursuit eye movements in patients with brain lesions. Electroen. Neurophysiol., 42, 23-30.

Bond, H.W., and P. Ho (1970). Solid miniature silver-silver chloride electrodes for chronic implantation. Electroen. Neurophysiol., 28, 206-208.

Bormiolo, S.P., S. Sartores, M. Vitadello, and S. Schiaffano (1980). "Slow" myosins in vertebrate skeletal muscle. J. Cell Biol., 85, 672-682.

Bormiolo, S.P., P. Torresan, S. Sartores. G. Moschini, and S. Schiaffano (1979). Immunohistochemical identification of slow tonic fibers in human extrinsic eye muscles. Invest. Ophthal., 18, 303-306.

Bortolami, R., E. Manno. M.L. Lucchi, E. Callegari, V. De Pasquale, and G. Lalatta Costerbosa (1979). Labelled trigeminal ganglion cells after injection of horse-radish peroxidase in the extraocular muscles and IIIrd nerve of the lamb. Boll. Soc. Ital. Biol. Sper., 55, 1206-1209.

Bouis, D., P. Baude, and G. Vossius (1975). Ein neues Gerät zur Messung der Augenbewegung. Biomedizinische Technik, 20, Ergänzungsband, 305-306.

Brain, W.R. (1926). On the rotated or "cerebellar" posture of the head. Brain, 49, 61-76.

Braitenberg, Van , and R.P. Atwood (1958). Observations on the cerebellar cortex. J. Comp. Neurol., 109, 1-33.

Brandt, D., and C. Leeson (1966). Structural differences of fast and slow fibers in human extraocular muscle. Am. J. Ophthal., 62, 478.

Brandth, S.E., and A.J. Karten (1977). Direct accessory optic projections to the vestibulo-cerebellum: A possible channel for oculomotor control systems. Exp. Brain Res., 28, 73-84.

Brandt, Th., and W. Büchele (1979). Ocular myasthenia: Visual disturbance of posture and gait. Agressologie, 20, 195-196.

Brandt, Th., J. Dichgans, and E. Koenig (1973). Differential effects of central versus peripheral vision on egocentric and exocentric motion perception. Exp. Brain Res., 16, 476-491.

Brandt, Th., J. Dichgans, and W. Buechele (1974). Motion habituation: Inverted self motion perception and optokinetic after-nystagmus. Exp. Brain Res., 21, 337-352.

Brecha, N., and H.J. Karten (1979). Accessory optic projections upon oculomotor nuclei and vestibulocerebellum. Science , 203, 913-916.

Breinin, G.M.(1971). The structure and function of extraocular muscle appraisal of the duality concept. Am. J. Ophthal., 72, 1.

Brindley, G.S., P.C. Gautier-Smith, and W. Lewin (1969). Cortical blindness and the functions of the non-geniculate fibres of the optic tracts. J. Neurol. Neurosurg. Psychiat., 32, 259-264.

Brindley, G., and P. Merton (1960). The absence of position sense in human eye. J. Physiol., 153, 127-130.

Brogden, R.N. , T.M. Speight, and G.S. Avery (1974). Baclofen: a preliminary report of its pharmacological properties and therapeutic efficacy in spaticity. Drugs, 8, 1-14.

Brooke, M.H., and K.K. Kaiser (1970). Muscle fiber types: How many and what kind? Arch. Neurol. Psychiat. (Chic.), 23, 369-379.

Brown, M.D., M.A. Cotter, O. Hudlická, and G. Vrbová (1976). The effects of different patterns of muscle activity on capillary density, mechanical properties and structure of slow and fast rabbit muscles. Pflügers Arch, 361, 241-50.

Browne, J.S. (1975). The responses of muscle spindles in sheep extraocular muscles. J. Physiol. 251, 483-496.

Brunner, H. (1921). Über Inversion des experimentellen optokinetischen Nystagmus. Monatsschr. Ohrenheilkd., 55, 574-582.

Brunner, H. (1933). Zur Klinischen der Inversion des optokinetischen Nystagmus. Albrecht v Graefes Arch. Ophthal., 129, 30-56.

Buller, A.J., J.C. Eccles and R.M. Eccles (1960). Differentiation of fast and slow muscles in the cat hindlimb., J. Physiol., 150, 399-416.

Buller, A.J., and D.M. Lewis (1965). Further observations on the differentiation of skeletal muscles in kitten hindlimb. J. Physiol., 176, 355-370.

Buchtel, H.A. (1970). Visual-learning deficits following cerebellar damage in rats. J. Comp. Physiol. Pshchol., 72, 296-305.

Buettner, U.W., U. Büttner, and V. Henn (1978). Transfer characteristics of neurons in the vestibular nuclei of the alert monkey. J. Neurophysiol., 41, 1614-1628.

Buettner, U.W., and U. Büttner (1979). Vestibular nuclei activity in the alert monkey during suppression of vestibular and optokinetic nystagmus. Exp. Brain Res., 37, 581-593.

Buffon, G.L. de (1746). Dissertation sur les causes du strabisme, ou des yeux louches. Memoires de l´Academic Royale des Sciences, Paris.

Buisseret, P. (1979). Does extraocular proprioception influence the development of visual processes and the oculomotor system? Progr. Brain Res., 50, 345-352.

Buisseret, P., and L. Maffei (1977). Extraocular proprioceptive projections to the visual cortex. Exp. Brain Res., 28, 421-425.

Burian, H.M. (1941). Fusional movements in permanent strabismus. Arch. Ophthal., 26, 626-650.

Burian, H.M., and G.K. von Noorden (1974). Binocular Vision and Ocular Motility, The C. V. Mosby Co., St Louis, 420-423.

Burke, R.E., D.N. Levine, P. Tsairis, and F.E. Zajac (1973). Physiological types and histochemical profiles in motor units of the cat gastrocnemius. J. Physiol., 234, 723-748.

Burns, S., and J. Wallman (1981). Relation of single unit properties to the oculomotor function of the nucleus of the basal optic root (Accessory optic system) in chickens. Exp. Brain Res., 42, 171-180.

Bushnell, M.C., M.E. Goldberg, and D.L. Robinson (1981). Behavioural enhancement of visual responses in monkey cerebral cortex: I. Modulation in posterior parietal cortex related to selective visual attention. J. Neurophysiol., In press.

Bushnell, M.C., and M.E. Goldberg (1979). The monkey frontal eye fields have a neuronal signal that precedes visually guided saccades. Soc. Neuroscience Abstr., 5, 779.

Büchele, W., D. Degner, and Th. Brandt (1980). Thresholds for object-motion perception raised by concurrent head-movements. Pflügers Arch. Suppl., 384, R 33, 131.

Büttner-Ennever, J.A. (1977). Pathways from the pontine reticular formation to structures controlling horizontal and vertical eye movements in the monkey. In Baker and Berthoz (Eds.), Control of Gaze by Brain Stem Neurons. Developments in Neuroscience, 1, Amsterdam: Elsevier/North Holland. pp 89-98.

Büttner-Ennever, J.A. (1979). Organization of reticular projections onto oculomotor neurones. In R. Granit and O. Pompeiano (Eds.), Reflex Control of Posture and Movement, Prog.Brain Res., 50, 619-630. Amsterdam: Elsevier.

Büttner-Ennever, J.A., and K. Akert (1981). Medial rectus subgroups of the oculomotor nucleus and their abducens internuclear input in the monkey. J. Comp. Neurol., 197, 17 -27.

Büttner-Ennever, J.A., and U. Büttner (1978). A cell group associated with accessory oculomotor nuclei in the rostral mesencephalic reticular formation of the monkey. Brain Res., 151, 31-47.

Büttner-Ennever, J.A., U. Büttner, B. Cohen, and G. Baumgartner (1981). Vertical gaze paralysis and the rostral interstitial nucleus of the medial longitudinal fasciculus (rostral iMLF). Brain, In press.

Büttner-Ennever, J.A., and V. Henn (1976). An autoradiographic study of the pathways from the pontine reticular formation involved in horizontal eye movements. Brain Res., 108, 155-164.

Büttner, U., J.A. Büttner-Ennever, and V. Henn (1977). Vertical eye movement related unit activity in the rostral mesencephalic reticular formation of the alert monkey. Brain Res., 130, 239-252.

Büttner, U., and W. Waespe (1981). Vestibular nerve activity in the alert monkey durin vestibular and optokinetic nystagmus. Exp. Brain Res., 41, 310-315.

Campos, E.G., and B. Bagolini (1978). Der senso-motorische Aspekt des anomalen Binokularsehens: die anomale Fusionsbewegungen. In G. Kommerell (Ed.), Symposium Deutsche Ophthalmologische Gesellschaft über Neurophysiologie und Klinik der Augenbewegung Störungen, Springer, Berlin. pp 335-340.

Campos, E.C., and T. Catellani (1978). Further evidence for the fusional nature of the compensation (or "eating up") of prisms in concomitant strabismus. Int. Ophthal., 1, 57-62.

Campos, E.C., and M.R. Zanasi (1978). Die anomale Fusionsbewegungen: der senso-motorische Aspekt des anomalen Binokularsehens. Albrecht v Grafes Arch. Ophthal., 205, 101-111.

Carmichael, E.A., M.R.Dix, C.S. Hallpike, and J.D. Hood (1961. Some further observations upon the effect of unilateral cerebral lesions on caloric and rotational nystagmus. Brain, 84, 571-584.

Carpenter, M.B. (1971). Central oculomotor pathways. In P. Bach-y-Rita, C.C. Collins and J.E. Hyde (Eds.), The Control of Eye Movements, Academic Press, New York and London. pp 67-103.

Carpenter, M.B. (1976). Human Neuroanatomy. Seventh ed. Williams and Wilkins, Baltimore, p 416.

Carpenter, M.B., J.W. Harbison, and P. Peter (1970). Accessory oculomotor nuclei in the monkey: Projections and effects of discrete lesions. J. Comp.Neurol.,140,131-154.

Carpenter, M.B., R.E. Mc Masters, and G.R. Hanna (1963). Disturbances of conjugate horizontal eye movments in the monkey. I.Physiological effects and anatomical degeneration resulting from lesions of the abducens nucleus and nerve. Arch. Neurol., 8, 231-247.

Carpenter, M.G., B.M. Stein, and P. Peter (1972). Primary vestibulocerebellar fibers in the monkey: distribution of fibers arising from distinctive cell groups in the vestibular ganglia. Am. J. Anat., 135, 221-250.

Carpenter, R.H.S. (1977). Movement of the Eyes. Pion Ltd., London.

Carter, D.B. (1965). Fixation disparity and heterophoria following prolonged wearing of prisms. Am. J. Optom. and An. Acad. Optom., 42, 141-152.

Caussé, R. (1936). Diagnostic différentiel entre le nystagmus congénital et le nystagmus vestibulaire. Ann. d'Oto-Laryngol.,55, 661-676.

Cazin, L., W. Precht, and J. Lannou (1980a). Optokinetic responses of vestibular nucleus neurons in the rat. Pflügers Arch., 384, 31-38.

Cazin, L., W Precht, and L. Lannou (1980b). Optokinetic responses of vestibular nucleus neurons in the rat. Pflügers Arch., 384, 19-29.

Cazin, L., W. Precht, and J. Lannou (1980c). Firing characteristics of neurons mediating optokinetic responses to rat's vestibular neurons. Pflügers Arch., 386, 221-230.

Chan, C., L. Kearny, and G. Mellvill Jones (1979). Tibialis anterior response to sudden ankle displacements in normal and parkinsonian subjects. Brain Res., 173, 303-314.

Charman, W.N. (1979). Speckle movement in laser refraction. I. Theory. Am. J. Optom. and Physiol. Opt., 56, 219-227.

Charman, W.N., and H. Whitefoot (1979). Speckle motion in laser refraction. II. Experimental. Am. J. Optom. and Physiol. Opt., 56, 295-304.

Cheng, M., and J.S. Outerbridge (1975). Optokinetic nystagmus during selective retinal stimulation. Exp. Brain Res., 23, 129-139.

Chiarandini, D.J., and J. Davidowitz (1979). Structure and function of extraocular muscle fibers. In J.A. Zadunaisky and H. Davson (Eds.)., Current Topics in Eye Research, Vol. 1, Academic Press, New York. pp 91-142.

Christoff, N. (1974). A clinicopathologic study of vertical eye movements. Arch. Neurol., 31, 1-8.

Chubb, M.C., and A.F. Fuchs (1981). The role of the dentate nucleus and Y-group in the generation of vertical smooth eye movements. In B. Cohen (Ed.), Recent Advances in Oculomotor and Vestibular Physiology, Ann.N.Y. Acad.Sci., In press.

Chubb, M.C., and A.F. Fuchs (1981). Monkey dentate nucleus and Y-group neurons with activity related to vertical vestibular stimuli and smooth eye movements. Ann. N.Y. Acad. Sci., In press.

Chun, K.S., and D.A. Robinson (1978). A model of quick phase generation in the vestibulo-ocular reflex. Biol. Cybernetics, 28, 209-221.

Ciancia, A.O. (1962). La esotropia con limitación bilateral de la abducción el lactante. Arch. Oftal. B. Air., 37, 207.

Ciuffreda, K.J., A.T. Bahill, R.V. Kenyon, and L. Stark (1976). Eye movements during reading: case reports. Am. J. Optom. Physiol. Opt., 389-395.

Ciuffreda, K.J., S. Goldrich, and C. Neary (1980). Auditory biofeedback as a potentially important new tool in the treatment of nystagmus. J. Am. Optom. Assn., 51, 615-617.

Ciuffreda, K.J., S. Goldrich, and C. Neary (1981). Eye movement auditory biofeedback treatment of nystagmus. Proc. Ninth Annual Northeast Biomed. Engn. Conf. (Rutgers), 198-200.

Ciuffreda, K.J., S. Goldrich, and C. Neary (In press). Use of eye movement auditory biofeedback in the control of nystagmus. Am. J. Optom. Physiol. Optics.

Ciuffreda, K.J., R.N. Kenyon, and L. Stark (1978a). Increased saccadic latencies in amblyopic eyes. Invest. Ophthal., 17, 697-702.

Ciuffreda, K.J., R.V. Kenyon, and L. Stark (1978b). Processing delays in amblyopic eyes; evidence from saccadic latencies. Am. J. Optom. Physiol. Opt., 55, 187-196.

Ciuffreda, K.J., R.V. Kenyon, and L. Stark (1979a). Different rates of functional recovery of eye movement during orthoptics treatment in adult amblyope. Invest. Ophthal., 18, 213-219.

Ciuffreda, K.J., R.V. Kenyon, and L. Stark (1979b). Abnormal saccadic substitution during small-amplitude pursuit tracking in amblyopic eyes. Invest. Ophthal., 18, 506-516.

Ciuffreda, K.J., R.V. Kenyon, and L. Stark (1979c). Suppression of fixational saccades in strabismic and anisometropic amblyopia. Ophthalmic Res., 11, 33-39.

Ciuffreda, K.J., R.V. Kenyon, and L. Stark (1979d). Saccadic intrusions in strabismus. Arch. Ophthal., 97, 1673-1679.

Ciuffreda, K.J., R.V. Kenyon, and L. Stark (1979e). Fixational eye movements in amblyopia and strabismus. J. Am. Optom. Assn., 50, 1251-1258.

Ciuffreda, K.J., R.V. Kenyon, and L. Stark (1980). Increased drift in amblyopic eyes. Br. J. Ophthal., 64, 7-14.

Ciuffreda, K.J., and L. Stark (1975). Descartes´ law of reciprocal innervation. Am. J. Optom. Physiol. Opt., 52, 663-673.

Clark, M.R., and L. Stark (1974). Control of human eye movements. II. A model for the extraocular plant mechanism. Math. Biosci., 6, 108-116.

Clarke, C., and R. Stern (1976). Ocular bobbing with survival. J. Neurol. Neurosurg. Psychiat., 39, 58-60.

Cochran, S.L., and W. Precht (1980). Electrophysiological characterization of the basal optic region in the anuran. Proc. Internat. Union of Physiolog. Sci., 14, 1100.

Cochran, S.L., W. Precht, and N. Dieringer (1980). Direction-selective neurons in the frog´s visual system. Soc. Neurosci. Abstr., 6, 121.

Cochran, S.L., W. Precht, and N. Dieringer (1981). Responses of sensory relay neurons and extraocular motoneurons to optokinetic stimulation in the frog. Soc. Neurosci. Abstr., In press.

Cogan, A.I. (1976a). Role of compensation in the development and performance of the binocular sensory-motor system. In V.D. Glezer (Ed.), Mechanisms of identification of visual images. Problems in Physiol. Opt., 14, Nauka, Leningrad, pp. 61-78.

Cogan, A.I. (1976b). Visual efficiency and the binocular system of man. Doctoral dissertation. (Unpublished).

Cogan, D.G. (1948). Neurology of the Ocular Muscles. C.C. Thomas, Springfield.

Cogan, D.G. (1954). Ocular dysmetria: flutterlike oscillations of the eyes and opsoclonus. Arch. Ophthal., 51, 318-335.

Cogan, D.G. (1956). Neurology of the Ocular Muscles. C.C. Thomas, Springfield.

Cogan, D.G. (1966). Neurology of the Visual System. C.C. Thomas, Springfield.
Cogan, D.G. (1966). Congenital ocular motor apraxia. Can. J. Ophthal., 1, 253-260.
Cogan, D.G. (1968). Down-beat-nystagmus. Arch. Ophthal., 80, 757-768.
Cogan, D.G. (1974). Paralysis of downgaze. Arch. Ophthal., 91, 192-199.
Cogan, D.G., and R.D. Adams (1953). A type of paralysis of conjugate gaze (ocular motor apraxia). Arch. Ophthal., 50, 434-442.
Cogan, D.G., R.D. Yee, and J. Gittinger (1976). Rapid eye movements in myasthenia gravis. I. Clinical observations. Arch. Ophthal., 94, 1083-1085.
Cohen, B. (1974). The vestibulo-ocular reflex arc. Handbook of sens. Physiol. VI/I, Springer. pp 477-540.
Cohen, B. and M. Feldman (1968). Relationship of electrical activity in pontine reticular formation and lateral geniculate body to rapid eye movements. J. Neurophysiol., 31, 806-817.
Cohen, B., and V. Henn (1972). The origin of the quick phases of nystagmus in the horizontal plane. Bibl. Ophthal., 82, 36-55.
Cohen, B., and V. Henn (1972). Unit activity in the pontine reticular formation associated with eye movements. Brain Res. 46, 403-410.
Cohen, B., V. Henn, T. Raphan, and D. Dennett (1981). Role of velocity storage in visual-vestibular interactions in humans. In B. Cohen (Ed.). Recent Advances in Oculomotor and Vestibular Physiology, Ann. N.Y. Acad. Sci. In press.
Cohen, B., A. Komatsuzaki, and M.B. Bender (1968). Electro-oculographic syndrome in monkeys after pontine reticular formation lesions. Arch. Neurol., 18, 78-92.
Cohen, B., V. Matsuo, and T. Raphan (1977). Quantitative analysis of the velocity characteristics of optokinetic nystagmus and optokinetic after-nystagmus. J. Physiol., 279, 321-344.
Cohen, B., T. Uemera, and S. Takemori (1973). Effects of labyrinthectomy on optokinetic nystagmus and optokinetic after-nystagmus. Equilibrium Res., 3, 88-93.
Collewijn, H. (1969). Optokinetic eye movements in the rabbit: Input-output relations. Vis. Res., 9, 117-132.
Collewijn, H. (1972). An analog model of the rabbit´s optokinetic system. Brain Res., 36, 71-88.
Collewijn, H. (1975a). Oculomotor areas in the rabbit´s midbrain and pretectum. J. Neurobiol., 6, 3-22.
Collewijn, H. (1975b). Direction-selective units in the rabbit´s nucleus of the optic tract. Brain Res., 100, 489-508.
Collewijn, H. (1977). Eye- and head-movements in freely moving rabbits. J. Physiol., 266, 471-498.
Collewijn, H., and A.F. Grootendorst (1978). Adaptation of the rabbit´s vestibulo-ocular reflex to modified visual input: Importance of stimulus conditions. Arch. Ital. Biol., 116, 273-280.
Collewijn, H., and A.F. Grootendorst (1979). Adaptation of optokinetic and vestibulo-ocular reflexes to modified visual input in the rabbit. In R. Granit and O. Pompeiano (Eds.), Reflex Control of Posture and Movement. Prog. Brain Res., Vol. 50, Elsevier, Amsterdam. pp 772-781.
Collewijn, H., and H.J. Kleinschmidt (1975). Vestibulo-ocular and optokinetic reactions in the rabbit: Changes during 24 hours of normal and abnormal interaction. In G. Lennerstrand and P. Bach-y-Rita (Eds.), Basic Mechanisms of Ocular Motility and Their Clinical Implications. Pergamon Press, Oxford. pp 477-483.
Collewijn, H., A.J. Martins, and R.M. Steinman (1981a). Natural retinal image motion: Origin and change. In B. Cohen (Ed.), Recent Advances in Oculomotor and Vestibular Physiology. Ann. N.Y. Sci. In press.
Collewijn, H., A.J. Martins, and R.M. Steinman (1981b). The time course of adaptation of human compensatory eye movements. Documenta Ophthal. In press.
Collewijn, H., F. Van der Mark, and T.C. Jansen (1975). Precise recording of human eye movements. Vision Res., 15, 447-450.
Collewijn, H., A.M. Verhagen, and A.F. Grootendorst (1980). Adaptation of the vestibulo-ocular reflex in albino rabbits by selective exposure of the anterior sector of the visual field. Brain Res., 192, 305-312.

Collewijn, H., B.J. Winterson, and M.F.W. Dubois (1978). Optokinetic eye movements in albino rabbits: Inversion in anterior visual field. Science, 199, 1351-1353.

Collins, C.C. (1971). Orbital mechanics. In P. Bach-y-Rita and C.C. Collins (Eds.), The Control of Eye Movements, Academic Press, N.Y. pp 283-325.

Collins, C.C. (1975). The human oculomotor control system. In G. Lennerstrand and P. Bach-y-Rita (Eds.), Basic Mechanisms of Ocular Motility and Their Clinical Implications. Pergamon Press, Oxford. pp 145-180.

Collins, C.C. (1976). Human oculomotor control. Proc. 1975 Winter Computer Simulation Conference, Sacramento, California. pp 69-76.

Collins, C.C. (1978). Length-force recording strabismus forceps.In C.Souza-Dias (Ed.), Smith-Kettlewell Symposium on Basic Sciences in Strabismus: Mechanical and Tonic Factors on Strabismus Diagnosis and Sugery, Annex to the V Congress of the Conselho Latino-Americano de Estrabismo (C.L.A.D.E.), October 16-17, 1976, Guaruja-Brasil. Ificinas das Edicoes Loyola, Sao Paolo. pp 7-19.

Collins, C.C., M.R. Carlson, A.B. Scott, and A, Jampolsky (1981). Extraocular muscle force in normal human subjects. Invest. Ophthal. Vis. Sci., 20(5), 652-664.

Collins, W.E., D.J. Schroeder, N. Rice, R.A. Mertens, and G. Kranz (1970). Some characteristics of optokinetic eyemovement patterns: A comparative study. Aerospace Med., 41, 1251-1262.

Conley, M., and K.V. Fite (1980). Optokinetic nystagmus in the domestic pigeon. Brain Behv. Evol., 17, 89-102.

Conrad, H.G., and H. Treumer (1981). Zum Wirkungsprofil der Fadenoperation. Klin. Mbl. Augenheilk., 178, 174.

Cook,G., and L. Stark (1968). The human eye-movement mechanism; Experiments, modeling and model testing. Arch. Ophthal., 97, 428-436.

Cooper, S., P.M. Daniel, and D. Whitteridge (1953). Nerve impulses in the brain stem of the goat. Responses with long latencies obtained by stretching the extrinsic eye muscles. J. Physiol., 120, 491-513.

Cooper, S., P.M. Daniel, and D. Whitteridge (1955). Muscle spindles and other sensory endings in the extrinsic eye muscles; The physiology and anatomy of these receptors and of their connections with the brain stem. Brain, 78, 564.

Corbin, K.A., and R.K. Oliver (1942). The origin of fibres to the grapelike endings in the insertion third of the extraocular muscles. J. Comp. Neurol., 77, 171-186.

Cords, R. (1926). Optisch-motorische Feld und optisch-motorische Bahn. Albrecht v Graefes Arch. Ophthal., 117, 58-113.

Correia, M.J., and K.E. Money (1970). The effect of blockage of all six semicircular canal ducts on nystagmus produced by linear acceleration in the cat. Acta Oto-lar., 69, 7-16.

Costenbader, F.D. (1961). Infantile esotropia. Trans. Am. Ophthal. Soc., 59, 397.

Corvera, J., L.D. Benitez, G. Lopez-Rios, and M. T. Rabiela (1980). Vestibular and oculomotor abnormalities in vertebrobasilar insufficiency. Ann. Otol., 89,370-376.

Covera, J., G. Torres-Courtney, and G. Lopez-Rios (1973). The neurological significance of alterations of pursuit eye movements in the pendular eye tracking test. Ann. Otol. Rhinol. Lar., 82, 1-13.

Cowan, W.M., L. Adamson, and T.P.S. Powell (1961). An experimental study of the avian visual system. J. Anat., 95, 545-563.

Coyle, J.T., M.E. Molliver, and M.J. Kuhar (1978). In situ injection of kainic acid: A new method for selectively lesioning neuronal cell bodies while sparing axons of passage. J. Comp. Neurol., 180, 301-324.

Crane, H.D. (1978). Binocular motor adjustments for far and near vision. Opt. Soc. Am. Annual Meeting Oct-Nov., 1359.

Crawford, W.A. (1960). Visual acuity and moving objects: The coordination of eye and head movements. Flying Personnel Research Committee Memo 159c. R.A.F. Inst. of Aviation Medicine, Farnborough, Hants, England

Crone, R.A. (1973). The control of eye movement. Diplopia, American Elsevier Publ. Co., Inc., N.Y.

Crone, R.A., and S. Hardowijoto (1979). What is normal binocular vision? Documenta Ophthal, 47(1), 163-199.

Crone, R.A., and C.M.J. Velzboer (1956). Statistics on strabismus in the Amsterdam youth. Arch. Ophthal., 55, 455-470.

Crosby, E.C. (1953). Relations of brain centers to normal and abnormal eye movements in the horizontal plane. J. Comp. Neurol., 99, 437-479.

Cüppers, C. (1974). The so-called Fadenoperation. II. Congr. I.S.A. Marseillc 1974, Diff. Gen. Libr. Paris-Marseille. p. 395.

Currier, R.D. (1969). Syndromes of the medulla oblongata. In P.J. Vinken and G.W. Bruyn (Eds.), Handbook of Clinical Neurology, Vol. 2, North-Holland Publ. Co., Amsterdam. pp 217-237.

Curtis, D.R., C.J. Game, G.A. Johnston, and R.M. McCulloch (1974). Central effects of b-(p-chorophenyl)-gamma-aminobutyric acid. Brain Res., 70, 493-499.

Dale, R.T., A.W. Kirby, and R.S. Jampel (1978). Square wave jerks in Friedeich´s ataxia. Am. J. Ophthal., 85, 400-406.

Darlot, C., J. Lopez-Barneo, and D. Tracey (1981). Asymmetrics of vertical vestibular nystagmus in the cat. Exp. Brain Res., 41, 420-426.

Daroff, R.B. (1970). Ocular motor manifestations of brainstem and cerebellar dysfunction. In J.L. Smith (Ed.), Neuro-Ophthalmology, Vol. V., Huffman Publ. Co., Hallandale, Florida. pp 104-118.

Daroff, R.B., and L.F. Dell´Osso (1974). Periodic alternating nystagmus and the shifting null. Can. J. Oto-lar., 3, 367-371.

Daroff, R.B., and L.F. Dell´Osso (1979). Nystagmus, a contemporary approach. In H.S. Thompson, R.B. Daroff. J.S. Glaser, L. Frisén and M.D. Sanders (Eds.), Topics in Neuro-Ophthalmology, 4.4, Williams and Wilkins Comp., Baltimore, Maryland. pp 286-297.

Daroff, R.B., and W.F. Hoyt (1971). Supranuclear disorders of ocular control systems in man: Clinical, anatomical and physiological correlations, In P. Bach-y-Rita, C.C. Collins and J.E. Hyde (Eds.), The Control of Eye Movements. Academic Press, N.Y. pp. 175-235.

Daroff, R.B., W.F. Hoyt, M.D. Sanders, and L.R. Nelson (1968). Gaze-evoked eyelid and ocular nystagmus inhibited by the near reflex: Unusual ocular motor phenomena in a lateral medullary syndrome. J. Neurol. Neurosurg. Psychiat., 31, 362-367.

Daroff, R.D., and B.T. Troost (1978). Supranuclear disorders of eye movements. In T.D. Duane (Ed.), Clinical Ophthalmology, Vol. 2. Harper and Row,Hagarstown, Maryland, Chapt. 10. pp 1-4.

Daroff, R.B., B.T. Troost, and L.F. Dell´Osso (1978). Nystagmus and related ocular oscillations. In J.S. Glaser (Ed.). Neuro-Ophthalmology, Harper and Row, Hagarstown, Maryland. pp 219-243.

David, N.J., E.A. Mackey, and J.L. Smith (1968). Further observations in progressive supranuclear palsy. Neurology, 18, 349-356.

Davidoff, R.A., and E.S. Sears (1974). The effects of Lioresal on synaptic activity in the isolated spinal cord. Neurology, 24, 957-967.

Davidowitz, J., D.J. Chiarandini. G.H. Philips, and G.M. Breinin (1981). Structural variations along the length of multiply innervated muscle fibers in rat inferior rectus - A serial analysis. Proc. 39th Electron Microscopy Soc. of Am. Meeting. Atlanta, Georgia, 500-501.

Davidowitz, J., G.H. Philips, and G.M. Breinin (1977). Organization of the orbital surface layer in rabbit superior rectus. Invest. Ophthal., 16, 711-729.

Davidowitz, J., G.H. Philips, and G.M. Breinin (1980). Variation of mitochondrial volume along multiply innervated fibers in rabbit extraocular muscle. Tissue & Cell, 12, 449-457.

de Decker, W., and H. Henning (1979). Fixationsverbessernde Fadenoperation als Früheingriff in Klinik und Tierversuch. Klin. Mbl. Augenheilk., 174, 200-206.

Deckert, G.H. (1964). Pursuit eye movements in the absence of a moving visual stimulus. Science, 143, 1192-1193.

Deecke, L., B. Grozinger, and H.H. Kornhuber (1976). Voluntary finger movement in man: Cerebral potentials and theory. Biol. Cybernetics, 23, 99-119.

Degner, D., and Th. Brandt (1981). Interaction between self and object motion perception. Pflügers Arch. Suppl. 389, R 30, 118.

DeJong, J.D., and G. Melville Jones (1971). Akinesia, hypokinesia, and bradykinesia om the oculomotor system of patients with Parkinson´s disease. Exp. Neurol., 32, 58-68.

DeJong, J.D., B. Vianney, B. Cohen, V. Matsuo, and T. Uemura (1980). Midsagittal pontomedullary brain stem section: Effects on ocular adduction and nystagmus. Exp. Neurol., 68, 420-442.

Dell´Osso, L.F. (1973a). Fixation characteristics in hereditary congenital nystagmus. Am. J. Optom. and Arch. Am. Acad. Optom., 50, 85-90.

Dell´Osso, L.F. (1973b). Improving visual acuity in congenital nystagmus. In J.L. Smith and J.S. Glaser (Eds.), Neuro-Ophthalmology Symposium of the University of Miami and Bascom Palmer Eye Institute, Vol. 7, 9, C.V. Mosby Company, St Louis, Missouri. pp 98-106.

Dell´Osso, L.F. (1976). Functional definitions and classification of congenital nystagmus waveforms. Invited paper, Ophthal. Digest, 38, 19-27.

Dell´Osso, L.F. (1980). Nystagmus and other ocular motor oscillations. In S. Lessell and J.T.W. van Dalen (Eds.), Neuro-Ophthalmology, Vol. 1, 11, Excerpta Medica, Amsterdam, The Netherlands. pp 146-177.

Dell´Osso, L.F., L.A. Abel, and R.B. Daroff (1977). "Inverse latent" macro square-wave jerks and macro saccadic oscillations. Ann. Neurol., 2, 57-60.

Dell´Osso, L.F., L.A. Abel, R.B. Daroff, and B. T. Troost (1981). Absence of VOR suppression in the presence of intact pursuit. Invest. Ophthal. Vis. Sci. Supplement, 20, 57.

Dell´Osso, L.F., and R.B. Daroff (1974). Functional organization of the ocular motor system. Aerospace Med., 45, 873-875.

Dell´Osso, L.F., and R.B. Draoff (1975). Congenital nystagmus waveforms and foveation strategy. Doc. Ophthal., 39, 155-182.

Dell´Osso, L.F., and R.B. Daroff (1976). Braking saccade: A new fast eye movement. Aviat. Space Environ. Med., 47, 435-437.

Dell´Osso, L.F., and R.B. Daroff (1978). Eye movement characteristics and recording techniques. I. J.S. Glaser (Ed.), Neuro-Ophthalmology. pp. 185-200.

Dell´Osso, L.F., and R.B. Daroff (1979). Eye movement characteristics and recording techniques. In T.A. Duane (Ed.), Clinical Ophthalmology, Volume 2, Neuro-ophthalmology, Harper and Row, Hagerstown, Maryland, Chapter 9.

Dell´Osso, L.F., and R.B. Daroff (1981). Clinical disorders of ocular movement. In B.L. Zuber (Ed.). Models of Oculomotor Behaviour and Control. C.R.C. Press, West Palm Beach, Florida. In press.

Dell´Osso, L.F., and J.T. Flynn (1979). Congenital nystagmus surgery: A quantitative evaluation of the effects. Arch. Cphthal., 97, 462-469.

Dell´Osso, L.F., J.T. Flynn, and R.B. Daroff (1974). Hereditary congenital nystagmus. Arch. Ophthal., 92, 366-374.

Dell´Osso, L.R., G. Gauthier, G. Liberman, and L. Stark (1972). Eye movement recordings as a diagnostic tool in a case of congenital nystagmus. Am. J. Optom. and Arch. Am. Acad. Optom., 49, 3-13.

Dell´Osso, L.F., D. Schmidt, and R.B. Daroff (1979). Latent, manifest latent, and congenital nystagmus. Arch. Ophthalmol., 97, 1877-1885.

Dell´Osso, L.F., B.T. Troost, and R.B. Daroff (1975). Macro square wave jerks. Neurol., 25, 975-979.

Demer, J.L. (1981). The variable gain element of the vestibulo-ocular reflex is common to the optokinetic system of the cat. Brain. Res. In press.

Demer, J.L., and D.A. Robinson (1981). Effect of reversible lesions of the inferior olive(IO)on gain of the vestibulo-ocular reflex(VOR). Supplement to: Invest. Ophthal. Visual Sci., 20, 57.

D´Espine, A., and V. Démole (1917). Tubercules de la protubérance. Arch. Med. Enf. (Paris), 20, 355-359.

Dichgans, J. (1969). Congenitaler und früherworbener Nystagmus: Nystagmographische, statistische und genetische Untersuchungen. Habilitationsschrift. Freiburg i. Br.

Dichgans, J. (1977). Optokinetic nystagmus as dependent on the retinal periphery via the vestibular nucleus. In R.Baker and A.Berthoz (Eds.), Control of Gaze by Brain Stem Neurons. Developments in Neuroscience. Elsevier/North Holland. pp 261-267.

Dichgans, J. (1979). Visual-vestibular interaction in the control of eye movement. In R. Schmidt and D. Zambarbieri (Eds.), Eye Movement Analysis in Neurological Diagnosis. Italian National Research Council. pp 123-155.

Dichgans, J., E. Bizzi, P. Morasso, and V. Tagliasco (1973). Mechanisms underlying recovery of eye-head coordination following bilateral labyrinthectomy in monkeys. Exp. Brain Res., 18, 548-562.

Dichgans, J., E. Bizzi, P. Morasso, and V. Tagliasco (1974). Mechanisms underlying recovery of eye-head coordination following bilateral labyrinthectomy in monkeys. Brain Res., 71, 225-232.

Dichgans, J., and T. Brandt (1979). Visual-vestibular interaction: Effects of self-motion preception and postural control. In R. Held. H.W. Leibowitz and H.L. Teuber (Eds.), Handbook of Sensory Physiology, Vol. VII, Springer Verlag, Berlin. pp 755-804.

Dichgans, J., and R. Jung (1975). Oculomotor abnormalities due to cerebellar lesions. In G. Lennerstrand and P. Bach-y-Rita (Eds.), Basic Mechanisms of Ocular Motility and Their Clinical Implications, Pergamon Press, Oxford. pp 281-298.

Dichgans, J., and H.H. Kornhuber (1964). Eineseltene Art des hereditären Nystagmus mit autosomal-dominantem Erbgang und besonderem Erscheinungsbild. Acta genet., Basel, 14, 240-250.

Dichgans, J., B. Nauck, and W. Wolpert (1973). The influence of attention, vigilance and stimulus area on optokinetic and vestibular nystagmus and voluntary saccades. In V. Zikmund (Ed.), The Oculomotor System and Brain Functions, Butterworths, London.

Dichgans, J. C.L. Schmidt, and W. Graf (1973). Visual input improves speedometer function of vestibular nuclei in goldfish. Exp. Brain Res., 18, 319-322.

Dichgans, J., G.M. v. Reutern, and U. Römmelt (1978). Impaired suppression of vestibulo nystagmus by fixation in cerebellar and non-cerebellar patients. Arch. Psychiat. Nervenkr., 226, 183-199.

Dieringer, N., A.R. Blight, and W. Precht (1980). Optokinetic nystagmus of head and eye in the frog. Proc. Internat. Union of Physiol. Sci., 14, 1221.

Dietert, S.E. (1965). The demonstration of different fiber types of muscle fibers in human extraocular muscle by electron microscopy and cholinesterase staining. Invest. Ophthal, 1, 51-54.

Dobson, V., D.L. Mayer, and C.P. Lee (1980). Visual acuity screening of preterm infants. Invest. Ophthal. & Vis. Sci., 19/12, 1498-1505.

Docen, W. (1961). Latenter Nystagmus bei Strabismus concomitans alternans.In Ber. 63. Zusammenkunft Dtsch. Ophthalmol. Ges., Bergmann, München. pp 486-490.

Donaldson, I.M.L. (1979). Responses in cat suprasilvian cortex (Clare-Bishop area) to stretch of extraocular muscles. J. Physiol., 296, 60-61.

Donaldson, I.M.L., and R.A. Dixon (1980). Excitation of units in the lateral geniculate and contiguous nuclei of the cat by stretch of extrinsic ocular muscles. Exp. Brain Res., 38, 245-255.

Donaldson, I.M.L., and A.C. Long (1980). Interactions between extraocular proprioceptive and visual signals in the superior colliculus of the cat. J. Physiol., 298, 85-110.

Doslag, M.J., L.F. Dell´Osso, and R.B. Daroff (1981). Intermittent occurrence of overshoot dysmetria, flutter, flutter dysmetria, and macro saccadic oscillations. In preparation.

Dow, R.S., and E. Manni (1964). The relationship of the cerebellum to extraocular movements. In M.B. Bender (Ed.), The Oculomotor System, Harper and Row, N.Y., pp. 280-302.

Dubois, M.F.W., and H. Collewijn (1979). Optokinetic reactions in man elicited by localized retinal stimuli. Vision Res., 19, 1105-1115.

Duensing, F., and K.P. Schaefer (1958). Die Aktivitär einzelner Neurons im Bereich der Vestibulariskerne bei Horizontalbeschleunigungen unter besonderer Berücksichtigung des vestibulären Nystagmus. Arch.Psychiat.Nervenkr., 198, 225-252.

Dufossé, M., M. Ito, P.J. Jastreboff, and Y. Miyashita (1978). A neuronal correlate in rabbit´s cerebellum to adaptive modification of the vestibulo-ocular reflex. Brain Res., 150, 611-616.

Dufossé, M., M. Ito, and Y. Miyashita (1978). Diminution and reversal of eye movements induced by local stimulation of rabbit cerebellar flocculus after partial destruction of the inferior olive. Exp. Brain Res., 33, 139-141.

Duke-Elder, S. (1971). System of Ophthalmology, XII, 760, Henry Kimpton, London.

Duke-Elder, W.S., and K. Wyber (1973). System of Ophthalmology. Vol. 6. Ocular motility and strabismus. The C.V. Mosby Co., St. Louis.

Duncan, G.W., S.W. Parker, and C.M. Fisher (1975). Acute cerebellar infarction in the PICA territory. Arch. Neurol., 32, 364-368.

Durston. J.H. (1974). Histochemistry of primate extraocular muscles and the changes of denervation. Br. J. Ophthal., 58, 193-216.

Easter, S.S. (1972). Pursuit eye movements in goldfish (Carassius auratus). Vision Res., 12, 673-688.

Easton, R.A. (1971). Inhibition from cat eye muscle stretch. Brain Res., 25, 633-637.

Eckmiller, R., and M. Mackeben (1980). Pre-motor single unit activity in the monkey brain stem correlated with eye velocity during pursuit. Brain Res., 184, 210-214.

Eidelberg, E., and A.S. Schwartz (1971). Experimental analysis of the extinction phenomenon in monkeys. Brain, 94, 91-108.

Ellenberger, C., J.L. Keltner, and M.H. Stroud (1972). Ocular dyskinesia in cerebellar disease. Brain, 95, 685-692.

Enoch, J.M., and C.E. Windson (1968). Remission of nystagmus following fitting contact lenses to an infant with aniridia. Am. J. Ophthal., 66, 333-335.

Erlandson, R.F., and D.G. Fleming (1974). Uncertainty sets associated with saccadic eye movements: Basis of satisfaction control. Vision Res., 14, 481-486.

Estanol, B., R. Romero, and J. Covera (1979). Effects of cerebellectomy on eye movements in man. Arch. Neurol., 36, 281-284.

Evarts, E.V. (1968). Relation of pyramidal tract activity to force exerted during voluntary movement. J. Neurophysiol., 31, 14-27.

Evarts, E.V., and R. Granit (1976). Relations of reflexes and intended movements. Progr. in Brain Res., 44, 1-14.

Evinger, C., R. Baker, R.A. McCrea, and R. Spencer (1981). In W. Becker and A.F. Fuchs (Eds.), Progress in Oculomotor Research, Elsevier, N.Y. In press.

Evinger, C., and A.R. Fuchs (1979). Saccadic, smooth pursuit, and optokinetic eye movements of the trained cat. J. Physiol., 285, 209-229.

Evinger, L.C., A.F. Fuchs, and R. Baker (1977). Bilateral lesions of the medial longitudinal fasciculus in monkeys: Effects on the horizontal and vertical components of voluntary and vestibular induced eye movements. Exp.Brain Res., 28, 1-20.

Feldbaum, A. (1965). Optimal control systems. Academic Press, N.Y.

Feldman, R.G., M. Kelly-Hayes, J.P, Conomy, and J.M. Foley (1978). Baclofen for sparticity in multiple sclerosis. Neurol., 28, 1094-1098.

Feldon, S.E., and J.W. Langston (1977). Square-wave jerks: A disorder of microsaccades? Neurol., 27, 278-281.

Fernandez, C., and J.M. Fredrickson (1964). Experimental cerebellar lesions and their effect on vestibular function. Acta oto-lar. Suppl.,192, 52-62.

Fernandez, C., and J.M. Goldberg (1971). Physiology of peripheral neurons innervating semicircular canals of the squirrel monkey. II. Response to sinusoidal stimulation and dynamics of peripheral vestibular system. J. Neurophysiol., 34, 661-675.

Ferrier, D. (1875). Experiments on the brains of monkeys. Phil. Trans., London, (Croonian Lecture), 165, 433-488.

Ferrier, D. (1876). The function of the brain. Emith-Elder and Co., London.

Fillenz, M. (1955). Responses in the brain stem of the cat to stretch of extrinsic ocular muscles. J. Physiol., 128, 182-199.

Fincham, E.F., and J. Walton (1957). The reciprocal actions of accommodation and convergence. J. Physiol., 137, 488-508.

Fiorentini, A., C. Ghez, and L. Maffei (1972). Physiological correlates of adaptation to a rotated visual field. J. Physiol., 227, 313-322.

Fisher, C.M. (1964). Ocular bobbing. Arch. Neurol., 11, 543-546.

Fisher, C.M. (1967). Some neuro-ophthalmological observations. J. Neruol. Neurosurg. Psychiat., 30, 383-392.

Fisher, C.M., W.E. Karnes, and C.S. Kubik (1961). Lateral medullary infarction: The pattern of vascular occlusion. J. Neuropath. exp. Neurol., 20, 323-379.

Fisher, C.M., E.H. Picard, A. Pollak, P. Dalal, and R.G. Ojemann (1965). Acute hypertensive cerebellar hemmorhage: Diagnosis and surgical treatment. J. Nerv. Ment. Dis., 140, 38-57.

Fisher, T. (1902). Congenital nystagmus in father and child. Br. Med. J., 2, 694.

Fleming, D.G., Vossius, G.W., G. Bowman, and E.L. Johnson (1969). Adaptive properties of the eye tracking system as revealed by moving head and open loop studies. Ann. N.Y. Acad. Sci., 156, 825-850.

Fleming, J.F.R., and E.C. Crosby (1955). The parietal lobe as an additional motor area. J. Comp. Neurol., 103, 486.

Flom, M.C. (1960a). On the relationship between accommodation and accommodative convergence: I. Linearity. Am. J. Optom. and Arch. Am. Acad. Optom., 37, 474-482.

Flom, M.C. (1960b). On the relationship between accommodation and accommodative convergence. III. Effects of orthoptics. Am. J. Optom. and Arch. Am. Acad. Optom., 37, 619-632.

Flom, M.C., B. Brown, J.Adams, and T.R. Jones (1976). Alcohol and marijuana effects on ocular tracking. Am. J. Optom. Physiol. Optics, 53, 764-773.

Flynn, J.T., and L.F. Dell´Osso (1979). Congenital nystagmus surgery. Invited paper. Ophthal. AAO, 86, 1414-1425.

Foley, J.M., and W. Richards (1972). Effects of voluntary eye movements and convergence on the binocular appreciation of depth. Percept and Psychophys.,11 (6),423-425.

Forssman, B. (1971). Hereditary studies of congenital nystagmus in a Swedish population. Ann. Human. Genet., 35, 119-138.

Forssman, B., and B. Ringnér (1971). Prevalence and inheritance of congenital nystagmus in a Swedish population. Ann. Human. Genet., 35, 139-147.

Forsythe, W.J. (1955). Congenital hereditary vertical nystagmus. J. Neurol. Neurosurg. Psychiat., 18, 196-198.

Francois, J., G. Verriest, and A. de Rouck (1955). L´achromatopsie congénitale. Docum. Ophthal., 9, 338-424.

Frank, M.C., and W. Kuhlo (1979). Die Wirkung des Alkohols auf die raschen Blickzielbewegungen (Saccaden) beim Menschen. Arch. Psychiat. Nervenkr., 213, 238-245.

Freeman. W. (1922). Paralysis of associated lateral movements of the eyes. Arch. Neurol. Psychiat., 7, 454-487.

Freeman, W. (1925). The relationship of the radix mesencephalica trigemini to the extraocular muscles. Arch. Neurol. Psychiat., 14, 111-113.

Freeman, W., H.H. Ammerman, and M. Stanley (1943). Syndromes of the pontile tegmentun. Arch Neurol. Psychiat., 50, 462-471.

Fricker, S.J. (1971). Dynamic measurements of horizontal eye motion. Invest. Ophthal., 10, 724-732.

Frisén, L. (1978). Lateropulsion of the eyes. A localizing brainstem sign. J. Neurol., 218, 171-177.

Fry, G.A. (1941). An analysis of the relationship between phoria, blur, break and recovery findings at the near point. Am. J. Optom.Arch.Am.Acad.Optom., 18, 393-402.

Fuchs, A.F. (1971). The saccadic system. In P. Bach-y-Rita. C.C. Collins and J.E. Hyde (Eds.), The Control of Eye Movements. Academic Press, N.Y. pp 343-362.

Fuchs, A.F., and H.H. Kornhuber (1969). Extraocular afferents to the cerebellum of the cat. J. Physiol., 200, 713-722.

Fuchs, A.F., and E.S. Luschei (1970). Firing patterns of abducens neurons of alert monkeys in relationship to horizontal eye movement. J. Neurophysiol., 33, 382-392.

Fukai, S., J. Tsutsui, and Y. Nakamura (1976). Abnormal pursuit movements of the fellow eye in amblyopia with strabismus. In S. Moore, J. Mein and L. Stockbridge (Eds.), Orthopics: Past, Present and Future. Stratton Intern. Med. Book Corp.,N.Y.

Fukuda, H., Y. Kudo, and H. Ono (1977). Effects of beta- (p-chlorophenyl)-GABA (baclofen) on spinal synaptic activity. Europ. J. Pharm., 44, 17-24.

Fukuda, J., S.M. Highstein, and M. Ito (1972). Cerebellar inhibitory control of the vestibulo-ocular reflex investigated in rabbit IIIrd nucleus. Exp. Brain Res., 14, 511-526.

Fukuda, T. (1959). The unidirectionality of the labyrinthine reflex in relation to the unidirectionality of the optokinetic reflex. Acta Oto-lar., 50, 507-516.

Fukushima, K., N.G. Pitts, and B.W. Peterson (1978). Direct excitation of neck motoneurons by interstitiospinal fibers. Exp. Brain Res., 33, 565-581.

Gacek, R.R. (1969). The course and central termination of first order neurons supplying vestibular end organs in the cat. Acta oto-lar., Suppl. 254, 1-66.

Gacek. R.R. (1971). Anatomical demonstration of the vestibulo-ocular projections in the cat. Acta oto-lar., Suppl. 293.

Gardner, E.P., and A.F. Fuchs (1975). Single unit responses to natural vestibular stimuli and eye movements in deep cerebellar nuclei of the alert rhesus monkey. J. Neurophysiol., 38, 627-649.

Garel, J. (1882). Nouveau fait de paralysie de la sixième paire avec déviation conjugée dans un cas d'hémiplégie alterne. Revue Med. (Paris), 2, 593-599.

Gauthier, G.M. (1970). Bio-engineering studies of cerebellar influences on oculomotor control. Ph.D. Thesis, Univ. of Illinois. Chicago.

Gauthier, G.M., and J.-M. Hofferer (1976). Eye tracking of self-moved targets in the absence of vision. Exp. Brain Res., 26, 121-139.

Gauthier, G.M., J. Hoefferer, W.F. Hoyt, and L. Stark (1979). Visual-motor adaptation: Quantitative demonstration in patients with posterior fossa involvment. Arch. Neurol., 36, 155-160.

Gauthier, G.M., and D.A. Robinson (1975). Adaptation of the human vestibulo-ocular reflex to magnifying lenses. Brain Res., 92, 331-335.

Gauthier, G.M., and L. Stark (1979). Cerebellar stimulation and eye movement in cats. Math. Biosci., 46, 37-58.

Gay, A.J., N. Newman, and M.H. Stroud (1969). Vestibular studies on a case of congenital nystagmus. Lancet, 2, 694-695.

Ghelarducci, B., S.M. Highstein, and M. Ito (1977). Origin of the preoculomotor projections through the brachium conjunctivum and their functional roles in the vestibulo-ocular reflex. In R. Baker and A. Berthoz (Eds.), Control of Gaze by Brain Stem Neurons, Elsevier/North-Holland, Amsterdam. pp. 167-176.

Ghelarducci, B., M. Ito, and N. Yagi (1975). Impulse discharges from flocculus Purkinje cells of alert rabbits during visual stimulation combined with horizontal head rotation. Brain Res., 87, 66-72.

Giolli, R.A. (1961). An experimental study of the accessory optic tracts (transpeduncular tracts and anterior accessory optic tracts) in the rabbit. J. Comp. Neurol., 117, 77-95.

Giolli, R.A. (1963). An experimental study of the accessory optic system in the Synomolgus monkey. J. Comp. Neurol., 121, 89-108.

Giolli, R.A., R.H.I. Blanks, and Sang Pham (1981). Projections of medial terminal nucleus of accessory optic system to pretectum in pigmented rat. Soc.Neurosci.Abstr.

Goddé-Jolly, D., and A. Larmande (1973). Les nystagmus. Masson U. Cie (Ed.), Paris.

Goebel, H.H., A. Komatsuzaki, M.B. Bender, and B. Cohen (1971). Lesions of the pontine tegmentum and conjugate gaze paralysis. Arch. Neurol., 24, 431-440.

Goldberg, J.M., and C. Fernandez (1981). Physiological mechanisms of the nystagmus produced by rotations about an earth horizontal axis. Ann. N.Y. Acad.Sci. In press.

Goldberg, M.E., and M.C. Bushnell (1980). Role of the frontal eye fields in visually guided saccades. In A. Fuchs and W. Becker (Eds.), Progress in Oculomotor Research. Elsevier, N.Y., pp 185-192.

Goldberg, M.E., and M.C. Bushnell (1981a). Enhancement of visual responses in monkey cerebral cortex: II. Modulation in frontal eye fields specifically related to saccades. J. Neurophysiol. In press.

Goldberg, M.E., and M.C. Bushnell (1981b). The role of the frontal eye fields in visually guided saccades. In A. Fuchs and W. Becker (Eds.), Progress in Oculomotor Research. Elsevier, N.Y. In press.

Goldberg, M.E., and D.L. Robinson (1977). Visual responses of neurons in monkey inferior parietal lobule: The physiological substrate of attention and neglect. Neurology, 27, 350.

Goldberg, M.E., and R.H. Wurtz (1972a). Activity of superior colliculus in behaving monkey. I. Visual receptive fields of single neurons. J. Neurophysiol, 35, 542-559.

Goldberg, M.E., and R.H. Wurtz (1972b). Activity of superior colliculus in behaving monkey. II. Effect of attention on neuronal responses. J. Neurophysiol.,35, 560-574.

Goldberg, S.J., C.D. Hull, and N.A. Buchwald (1974). Afferent projections in the abducens nerve. An intracellular study. Brain Res., 68, 205-214.

Goldberg, S.J.,G. Lennerstrand, and C.D. Hull (1976). Motor unit responses in the lateral rectus muscle of the cat: Intracellular current injection of abducens nucleus neurons. Acta Physiol. Scand., 96, 58-63.

Goldrich, S.G. (1981). Emergent textural contours: A new technique for visual monitoring in nystagmus, oculomotor dysfunction, and accommodative disorders. Am. J. Optom. Physiol. Optics. In press.

Goldstein, J.H., and F. Greenstein (1971). Eye-hand coordination in strabismus. In P. Fells (Ed.), The First Congress of the International Strabismological Association, C.V. Mosby Co., St. Louis.

Gonshor, A., and G. Melville Jones (1971). Plasticity in the adult human vestibulo-ocular reflex arc. Proc. Can. Fed. Biol. Soc., 14, 11.

Gonshor, A., and G. Melville Jones (1976a). Short-term adaptive changes in the human vestibulo-ocular reflex arc. J. Physiol., 256, 361-379.

Gonshor, A., and G. Melville Jones (1976b). Extreme vestibulo-ocular adaptation induced by prolonged optical reversal of vision. J. Physiol., 256, 381-414.

Graefe, A. von (1854). Über Doppelsehen nach Schieloperationen und Incongruenz der Netzhäute. Albrecht v Graefes Arch. Ophthal.,1, 82-120.

Granit, R. (1977). The Purposive Brain. The MIT Press, Cambridge, Mass.

Granit, R., and O. Pompeiano (Eds.), (1979). Reflex Control of Posture and Movement. Progr. in Brain Res., 50.

Grant, G. (1966). Infarction localization in a case of Wallenberg's syndrome. A neuroanatomical investigation with comments on structures responsible for nystagmus, impairment of taste and deglutition. J. Hirnforsch., 8, 419-429.

Grasse, K.L., and M.S. Cynader (1980). Directional selectivity in the medial terminal nucleus of the cat. Soc. Neurosci. Abstr., 6, 122.

Graybiel, A.M. (1977). Direct and indirect preoculomotor pathways of the brainstem: An autoradiographic study of the pontine reticular formation in the cat. J. comp. Neurol., 175, 37-78.

Graybiel, A.M. (1977). Organization of oculomotor pathways in the cat and rhesus monkey. In R. Baker and A. Berthoz (Eds.), Control of Gaze by Brain Stem Neurons, Elsevier, Amsterdam, 1.

Graybiel, A.M., and E.A. Hartwieg (1974). Some afferent connections of the oculomotor complex in the cat: An experimental study with tracer techniques. Brain Res., 81, 543-551.

Green, A.E., and J. Wallman (1978). Rapid change in gain of vestibulo-ocular reflex in chickens. Neurosci. Abstr., 4, 163.

Gresty, M.A. (1974). Coordination of head and eye movements to fixate continuous and intermittent targets. Vision Res., 14, 395-403.

Gresty, M.A. (1977). Eccentric head positions reveal dissorders of conjugate eye movements. J. Neurol. Neurosurg. Psychiat., 40, 992-1002.

Gresty, M.A., J.J. Ell, and L.J. Findley (1981). Acquired pendular nystagmus. Brain. In press.

Gresty, M.A., L.J. Findley, and P. Wade (1980). Mechanism of rotary eye movements in opsoclonus. Br. J. Ophthal., 64, 923-925.

Gresty, M.A.and G.M. Halmagyi (1979). Abnormal head movements. J. Neurol.Neurosurg. Psychiat., 42, 705-714.

Gresty, M.A., and G.M. Halmagyi (1980). Head shaking in congenital nystagmus. In B. Cohen (Ed.), Vestibular and Oculomotor Physiology. Ann. N.Y. Acad. Sci. In press.

Gresty, M.A., G.M. Halmagyi, and J. Leech (1978). The relationship between head and eye movement in congenital nystagmus with head shaking: Objective recordings of a single case. Br. J. Ophthal., 62, 533-535.

Gresty, M.A., K. Hess, and J. Leech (1977). Disorders of the vestibulo-ocular reflex producing oscillopsia and mechanisms compensating for loss of labyrinthine function. Brain, 100, 693-716.

Gresty, M.A., and J. Leech (1977). Coordination of head and eye movements in pursuit of predictable and random target motion. Aviat. Space and Environm. Med., 48, 741-744.

Grüsser, O.-J., M. Pause, and U. Schreiter (1979). Three methods to elicit sigma-optokinetic nystagmus in Java monkeys. Exp. Brain Res., 35, 519-526.

Guedry, F.E. (1965). Orientation of the rotation axis relative to gravity: Its influence on nystagmus and the sense of rotation. Acta Oto-lar., 60, 30-48.

Guedry, F.E., M.J. Lentz, and R.M. Jell (1979). Visual-vestibular interactions. I Influence of peripheral vision on suppression of the vestibulo-ocular reflex and visual acuity. Aviat. Space Environm. Med., 50, 205-211.

Guibor, G.P. (1950). The use of atropine in the treatment of motor defects. In J.H. Allen (Ed.), Strabismus Ophthalmic Symposium. The C.V. Mosby Co. St. Louis. pp.316-322.

Guillain, G., R. Thurel, and I. Bertrand (1933). Examen anatomo-pathologique du cas de myoclonies vélo-pharyngo-oculo-diaphragmatiques associées à des myoclonies squelettiques synchrones. Rev. Neurologique, 2, 801.

Guillery, R.W., V.A. Casagrande, and M.D. Oberdorfer (1974). Congenitally abnormal vision in Siamese cats. Nature, 252, 195-199.

Guitton, D., and T. Kirkham (1978). Vertical oculomotor deficits following MLF lesions in man and monkey are similar. Neurosci. Abstr., 4, 163.

Haase. W., C. Malchartzeck, and J. Rickers (1978). Ergebnisse der Fadenoperation nach Cüppers. Klin. Mbl. Augenheilk., 192, 313.

Haddad, G.M., J.L. Demer, and D.A. Robinson (1980). The effect of lesions of the dorsal cap of the inferior olive on the vestibulo-ocular and optokinetic systems of the cat. Brain Res., 185, 265-275.

Haddad, G., A. Friendlich, and D.A. Robinson (1977). Compensation of nystagmus after VIII nerve lesions in vestibulocerebellectomized cats. Brain Res., 135, 192-196.

Hagström, L., G. Hörnsten, and B.P. Silfverskiöld (1969). Oculostatic syndrome. Acta Neurol. Scand., 45, 568-582.

Halldén, U. (1952). Fusional phenomena in anomalous correspondence. Acta Ophthal., Kbh. Suppl., 37, 1-93.

Hallett, P.E. (1978). Primary and secondary saccades to goals defined by instructions. Vision Res., 18, 1279-1296.

Hallett, P.E., and B.D. Adams (1980). The predictability of saccadic latency in a novel voluntary oculomotor task. Vision Res., 20, 329-339.

Hallett, M., and S. Khoshbin (1980). A physiological mechanism of bradykinesia. Brain, 103, 301-314.

Halmagyi, G.M., W.A. Evans, and J.M. Hallinan (1978). Failure of downward gaze. The site and nature of the lesion. Arch. Neurol., 35, 22-26.

Halmagyi, G.M., and M.A. Gresty (1979). Clinical signs of visual-vestibular interaction. J. Neurol. Neurosurg. Psychiat., 42, 931-939.

Halmagyi, G.M., M.A. Gresty, and W.P.R. Gibson (1979). Ocular tilt reaction with peripheral vestibular lesion. Ann. Neurol., 6, 80-83.

Halmagyi, G.M., M.A. Gresty, and J. Leech (1980). Reversed optokinetic nystagmus (OKN): Mechanism and clinical significance. Ann. Neurol., 7, 429-435.

Halmagyi, G.M., P. Rudge, M.A. Gresty, R.J. Leigh, and D.S. Zee (1980). Treatment of periodic alternating nystagmus. Ann. Neurol., 8, 609-611.

Halsey, J.H., R. Ceballos, and E.C. Crosby (1967). The supranuclear control of voluntary lateral gaze. Neurology, 17, 928-933.

Hamann, K.-U. (1979). Systematische Abweichung sakkadischer Augenbewegungen beim Wallenberg-Syndrom. Ophthalmologica Basel, 178, 373-380.

Hameroff, S.B., R. Garcia-Mullin, and J. Eckholdt (1969). Ocular bobbing. Arch. Ophthal., 82, 774-780.

Hammarberg, C., (1974). The histochemical appearance of developing muscle fibres in the gastrocnemius, soleus and anterior tibial muscles of the kitten, as viewed in serial sections stained for lipids and succinic dehydrogenase. Acta Neurol. Scand., 50, 285-301.

Hammarberg, C., and J.-O. Kellerth (1975a). The postnatal development of some twitch and fatigue properties of the ankel flexor and extensor muscles of the cat. Acta Physiol. Scand., 95, 166-178.

Hammarberg, C., and J.-O. Kellerth (1975b). Studies of some twitch and fatigue pro-properties of different motor unit types in the ankle muscles of the adult cat. Acta Physiol. Scand., 95, 231-242.
Hanson, J., and G. Lennerstrand (1977). Contractile and histochemical properties of the inferior oblique muscle in the rat and in the cat. Acta Ophthal., 55, 88-102.
Hanson, J., G. Lennerstrand, and K. Nichols (1980). The postnatal development of the inferior oblique muscle of the cat. III. Fiber sizes and histochemical properties. Acta Physiol. Scand., 108, 61-71.
Harcourt, B. (1970). Hereditary nystagmus in early childhood. J. Med. Genet.,7, 253-256.
Harris, C.S. (1965). Perceptual adaptation to inverted, reversed, and displaced vision. Psychol. Rev., 72, 419-444.
Harrison, R., D. Hoefnagel, and J.N. Hayward (1960). Congenital total color blindness. Arch. Ophthal., 64, 65-72.
Harrison. M.D., and C. Ozahinoglu (1975). Positional vertigo. Arch. Otol.,101, 675-678.
Hartje, W., D. Steinhauser, and M. Kerschensteiner (1978). Diagnostic value of saccadic pursuit eye movement in screening for organic cerebral dysfunction. J. Neurol., 217, 253-260.
Hausser, C.O., F. Robert, and N.Giard (1980). Balint´s syndrome. Canad. J. Neurol. Sci., 7, 157-161.
Hayhow, W.R. (1959). An experimental study of the accessory optic fiber system in the cat. J. Comp. Neurol., 113, 281-313.
Hayhow, W.R., C. Webb, and A. Jervie (1960). The accessory optic fiber system in the rat. J. Comp. Neurol., 115, 187-215.
Heilman, K.M., and E. Valenstein (1972). Frontal lobe neglect in man. Neurology, 22, 660-664.
Hellström-Hoddevik, G., A. Brodal, and F. Walberg (1975). The reticulovestibular projection in the cat. An experimental study with silver impregnation methods. Brain Res., 94, 383-399.
Helmholtz, H. (1911). Handbuch der physiologischen Optik. Vol. 111, 47.
Helveston, E.M. (1978). Reoperations in strabismus.Presentation at Strabismus Symposium, American Academy of Ophthalmology and Otolaryngology Meeting, October 25, 1978. Abstr. in Ophthal., 85, 66-67.
Hemmes, G.D. (1924). Over hereditarien Nystagmus. Wageningen: H. Veenman und Zonen.
Henn, V., U. Büttner, and J. Büttner-Ennever (1978). Supranukleäre Störungen der Okulomotorik - physiologische und anatomische Grundlagen. In G. Kommerell (Ed.) Disorders of Ocular Motility, Neurophysiological and Clinical Aspects. J.F. Bergmann, München. pp. 129-141.
Henn, V., and B. Cohen (1973). Quantitative analysis of activity in eye muscle motoneurons during saccadic eye movements and positions of fixation. J. Neurophysiol., 36, 115-124.
Henn, V., and B. Cohen (1976). Coding of information about rapid eye movements in the pontine reticular formation of alert monkeys. Brain Res., 108, 307-325.
Henn, V., B. Cohen, and L.R. Young (1980). Visual-vestibular interaction in motion perception and the generation of nystagmus. Neurosci. Res. Progr. Bull., 18,459-651.
Hennerici, M., and C. Fromm (1981). Isolated complete gaze palsy: An unusual ocular movement deficit probably due to a bilateral parapontine reticular formation (PPRF) lesion. Neuro-Ophthal., 1, 165-173.
Hennessy, R.T., and H.W. Leibowitz (1970). Subjective measurement of accommodation with laser light. J. Opt. Soc. Am., 60, 1700-1701.
Hennessy, R.T., and H.W. Leibowitz (1972). Laser optometer incorporating Badal principle. Behav. Res. Methods and Instru., 4, 237-239.
Henoch, E.H. (1864). Tuberculose de corpora quadrigemina. Berliner Klinische Wochenschrift, No 13, March 21, 125-127.
Henriksson. N.G., I. Pyykkö, L. Schalén, and C. Wennmo (1980). Velocity patterns of rapid eye movements. Acta Oto-lar., 89, 504-512.
Henson, D.B. (1978). Corrective saccades: Effects of altering visual feedback. Vision Res., 18, 63-67.
Henson, D.B., and R.E. North (1980). Adaptation to prism-induced heterophoria. Am. J. Optom. Physiol.Optics, 57, 129-137.

Hepp, K., and V. Henn (1981). On the generation of rapid eye movements in the brainstem and cerebellum. In J. Szentagothai, M. Palkovits and J. Hamori (Eds.), Regulatory Functions of the CNS. Motion and Organization Principles. Adv. Physiol. Sci., 1, Budapest. pp 235-243.

Hepp. K., V. Henn. and J. Jaeger (1981). Eye movement related neurons in the cerebellar nuclei of the alert monkey. Exp. Brain Res., In press.

Hering, E. (1868). Die Lehre vom binokularen Sehen. Engelmann, Leipzig.

Hering, E. (1977). Theory of Binocular Vision, 1868, translated by B. Bridgeman and L. Stark, Plenum Press, New York.

Herishany, Y., and J.A. Sharpe (1981). Normal square wave jerks. Invest. Ophthal. Vis. Sci., 20, 268-272.

Heywood, S. (1971). Voluntary control of smooth eye movements and their velocity. Nature, 238, 408-410.

Heywood, S. (1973). Pursuing stationary dots: Smooth eye movements and apparent movement, Perception, 2, 181-195.

Hikosaka, O., and Y. Igusa (1980). Axonal projection of prepositus hypoglossi and reticular neurons in the brainstem of the cat. Exp. Brain Res., 39, 441-451.

Hikosaka, O., Y. Igusa, and H. Imai (1980). Inhibitory connections of nystagmus-related reticular burst neurons with neurons in the abducens, prepositus hypoglossi and vestibular nuclei in the cat. Exp. Brain Res., 39, 301-311.

Hikosaka, O., M. Maeda, S. Nakao, H. Shimazu, and Y. Shinoda (1977). Presynaptic impulses in the abducens nucleus and their relation to postsynaptic potentials in motoneurons during vestibular nystagmus. Exp. Brain Res., 27, 355-376.

Hirsch, M.J., M. Alpern, and H. Schultz (1948). The variation of phoria with age. Am. J. Optom. Arch. Am. Acad. Optom., 25 (11), 535-541.

Hitzig, E. (1874). Physiologische und klinische Untersuchungen über das Gehirn. A. Hirschwald, Berlin.

Hixon. W.C. (1974). Frequency response of the oculo-vestibular system during yaw oscillation. Report NAMRL 1212, U.S. Naval Aerosp. Med. Res. Lab., Pensacola,Fla.

Hoddevik, G.H. (1978). The projection from nucleus reticularis tegmenti pontis onto the cerebellum in the cat. A study using the methods of anterograde degeneration and retrograde axonal transport of horseradish peroxidase. Anat. Embryol.,153,227-242.

Hoffman, F.B., and A. Bielschowsky (1900). Über die der Villkuf Entzogenen Fusions-Bewegungen der Augen. Arch. Ges. Physiol., 80, 1-40.

Hoffmann, K.-P. (1979). Optokinetic nystagmus and single cell responses in the nucleus tractus opticus after early monocular deprivation in the cat. In R.D. Freeman (Ed.), Developmental Neurobiology of Vision, Plenum Publ. Corp., N.Y. pp 63-72.

Hoffmann. K.-P. (1981). Neuronal responses in the cat´s nucleus of the optic tract related to optokinetic nystagmus. In A. Fuchs and W. Becker (Eds.), The Neuronal Control of Eye Movements, In press.

Hoffmann, K.-P., K. Behrend, and A. Schoppmann (1976). A direct afferent visual pathway from the nucleus of the optic tract to the inferior olive in the cat. Brain Res., 115, 150-153.

Hoffmann, K.-P., and A. Schoppmann (1975). Retinal input to direction selective cells in the nucleus tractus opticus of the cat. Brain Res., 99, 359-366.

Hoffmann, K.-P., and A. Schoppmann (1981). A quantitative analysis of the direction-specific response of neurons in the cat´s nucleus of the optic tract. Exp. Brain Res., 42, 1-12.

Hofstetter, H.W. (1945). The zone of clear single binocular vision. Am. J. Optom. Arch. Am. Acad. Optom., 22 (7), 301-333.

Hoggelen, J.F., and H. Collewijn (1971). Effect of cerebro/cortical and collicular ablations upon the optokinetic reactions in the rabbit. Documenta ophth.,30,227-239.

Holmes, G. (1921). Palsies of the conjugate ocular movements. Br. J. Ophthal.,5,241-250.

Holmes, G. (1922). Clinical symptoms of cerebellar disease. Lancet, July 8, 59-65.

Holmes, G. (1931). Ocular palsies. Br. Med. J., 2, 1165-1167.

Holmes, G. (1938). The cerebral integration of ocular movements. Br.Med.J.,2, 107-112.

Holzman, R.S., L.R. Proctor, and D.W. Hughes (1973). Eye tracking patterns in schizophrenia. Science, 181, 179-181.

Honrubia, V. (1979). Optokinetic nystagmus. In R. Schmid and D. Zambarieri (Eds.), Eye Movement Analysis in Neurological Diagnosis. Ital. Nat. Res. Council. pp 71-96.

Honrubia, V., R.W. Baloh, and C.G.Y. Lau (1977). The patterns of eye movements during physiological vestibular nystagmus in man. Trans. Am. Acad. Ophthal. Oto-lar., 84, 339-347.

Honrubia, V., W.L. Downey, D.P. Mitchell, and P.H. Ward (1968). Experimental studies on optokinetic nystagmus. II. Normal humans. Acta Oto-lar., 65, 441-448.

Honrubia, V., B.J. Scott, and P.H. Ward (1967). Experimental studies on optokinetic nystagmus. I. Normal cats. Acta Oto-lar., 64, 388-402.

Hood. J.D. (1967). Observations upon the neurological mechanism of optokinetic nystagmus with especial reference to the contribution of peripheral vision. Acta Oto-lar., 63, 208-215.

Hood, J.D. (In press). Further observations on the phenomenon of rebound nystagmus. In B. Cohen (Ed.), Recent Advances in Oculomotor and Vestibular Physiology, Ann. N.Y. Acad. Sci.,New York.

Hoogenraad, T.V., F.G. Jennekens, and K.E. Tan (1977). Histochemistry of inferior oblique muscle in a case of congenital third nerve palsy. Doc. Ophth.,44, 187-192.

Hooten, K., E. Myers, R. Worrall, and L. Stark (1979). Cyclovergence: The motor response to cyclodisparity. Graefes Arch. Ophthal., 210, 65-68.

Hörnsten, G. (1974a).Wallenberg´s syndrome. Part I. General symptomatology, with special reference to visual disturbances and imbalance. Acta Neurol.Scand., 50,434-446.

Hörnsten, G. (1974b).Wallenberg´s syndrome. Part II. Oculomotor and oculostatic disturbances. Acta Neurol. Scand., 50, 447-468.

Horsley, V. (1909). The Cavendish Lecture. West London Med. J., 14.

Hotson, J.R. (1979). A basis for pathologic fixation instability in normal subjects. Neurosci. Abstr., 1249.

Hotson, J.R. (1981). Cerebellar control of fixation eye movements. Neurology. In press.

Hoyt, W.F., and R.B. Daroff (1971). Supranuclear disorders of ocular control systems in man; clinical, anatomical and physiological correlations. In P. Bach-y-Rita, C.C. Collins and J.E. Hyde (Eds.), The Control of Eye Movements, Academic Press, New York/London. pp 175-235.

Hoyt, W.F., and L. Frisén (1975). Supranuclear ocular motor control. Some clinical considerations. In G. Lennerstrand and P. Bach-y-Rita (Eds.), Basic Mechanisms of Ocular Motility and Their Clinical Implications, Pergamon Press, Oxford.pp 379-392.

Hoyt, W.F., and J.R. Keane (1970). Superior oblique myokymia: Report and discussion on five cases of benign intermittent uniocular microtremor. Arch. Ophthal.,84,461-467.

Hoyt, C., D.K. Mousel, and A.A. Weber (1980). Transient supranuclear disturbances of gaze in healthy neonates. Am. J. Ophthal., 89, 708-713.

Hsu, F.K., V.V. Krishnan, and L.Stark (1976). Simulation of ocular dysmetria using a sampled-data model of the human saccadic system. Anns.Biomed. Eng., 4, 321-329.

Hubel, D.H., and T.N. Wiesel (1965). Binocular interaction in striate cortex of kittens reared with artificial squint. J. Neurophysiol., 28, 1041-1059.

Hubel, D.H., and T.N. Wiesel (1970). The period of susceptibility of the physiological effects of unilateral eye closure in kittens. J. Physiol., 206, 419-436.

Hubel, D.H., and T.N. Wiesel (1971). Aberrant visual projections in the Siamese cat. J. Physiol., 218, 33-62.

Hung, G., K.J. Ciuffreda, and J. Semmlow (1981). Response components of the human near response. Submitted for publication.

Hung, G., and J.L. Semmlow (1980). Static behaviour of accommodation and vergence: Computer simulation of an interactive dual feedback system. IEEE Trans. Biomed. Eng., BME-27, 439-447.

Hung, G., J.L. Semmlow, and K.J. Ciuffreda (1981). The cominance of control components in the oculomotor near triad. Submitted for publication.

Hyvärinen, J., and J. Poranen (1974). Function of the parietal associative area 7 as revealed from cellular discharges in alert monkeys. Brain, 97, 673-692.

Iacono, W.G., and D.T. Lykken (1981). Two-year retest stability of eye tracking performance and a comparison of electro-oculographic and infrared recording techniques: Evidence of EEG in the electro-oculogram. Psycholphysiol., 18, 49-55.

Igarashi, M., H. Miyata, Y. Kato, W.K. Wright, and J.K. Levy (1975). Optokinetic nystagmus after cerebellar uvulonodulectomy in squirrel monkeys. Acta Oto-lar., 80, 180-184.

Irvine, S.R. (1936). Histology of the extraocular muscles. Arch. Ophthal., 62, 847.

Isch, F. (1957). Formes de début et séquelles du syndrome rétroolivaire de Dejerine. Rev. Neurol., 97, 350-365.

Ishikawa, S. (1978). Latent nystagmus and its etiology. In R. Reinecke (Ed.), Strabismus. Grune & Stratton, N.Y., pp 203-214.

Ito. M. (1972a). Neural design of the cerebellar motor control system. Brain Res., 40, 81-84.

Ito. M. (1972b). Cerebellar control of the vestibular neurons: Physiology and pharmacology. In A. Brodal and O. Pompeiano (Eds.), Basic Aspects of Central Vestibular Mechanisms, Elsevier Publ. Co., Amsterdam. pp 377-390.

Ito, M. (1977). Neuronal events in the cerebellar flocculus associated with an adaptive modification of the vestibulo-ocular reflex of the rabbit. In R. Baker and A. Berthoz (Eds.), Control of Gaze by Brain Stem Neurons. Elsevier, Amsterdam. pp 391-398.

Ito, M., (1978). Recent advances in cerebellar physiology and pathology. Adv. Neurol., 21, 59-84.

Ito, M., P.J. Jastreboff, and Y. Miyashita (1979). Adaptive modification of the rabbit´s horizontal vestibulo-ocular reflex during sustained vestibular and optokinetic stimulation. Exp. Brain Res., 37, 17-30.

Ito, M., and Y. Miyashita (1975). The effects of chronic destruction of the inferior olive upon visual modification of the horizontal vestibulo-ocular reflex of rabbits. Proc. Jpn. Acad., 50, 716-720.

Ito, M., N. Nisimaru, and M. Yanamoto (1973). Specific neural connections for the cerebellar control of vestibulo-ocular reflexes. Brain Res., 60, 238-243.

Ito, M., N. Nisimaru, and M. Yamamoto (1976). Pathways for the vestibulo-ocular reflex excitation arising from semicircular canals of rabbits. Exp. Brain Res., 24, 257-271.

Ito, M., N. Nisimaru, and Y. Yamamoto (1977). Specific patterns of neuronal connections involved in the control of the rabbit´s vestibulo-ocular reflexes by cerebellar flocculus. J. Physiol., 265, 833-854.

Ito, M., N. Nisimaru, and K. Shibuki (1979). Destruction of inferior olive induces rapid depression in synaptic action of cerebellar Purkinje cells. Nature, 277, 568-569.

Ito, M., I. Orlov, and I. Shimoyama (1978). Reduction of the cerebellar stimulus effect of rat Deiter´s neurons after chemical destruction of the inferior olive. Exp. Brain Res., 33, 143-145.

Ito, M., T. Shiida, N. Yagi, and M. Yamamoto (1974a). The cerebellar modification of rabbit´s horizontal vestibulo-ocular reflex induced by sustained head rotation combined with visual stimulation. Proc. Jpn. Acad., 50, 85-89.

Ito. M., T. Shiida, N. Yagi, and M. Yamamoto (1974b). Visual influence on rabbit horizontal vestibulo-ocular reflex presumably effected via the cerebellar flocculus. Brain Res., 65, 170-174.

Itoh, K. (1977). Efferent projections of the pretectum in the cat. Exp. Brain Res., 30, 89-105.

Jacobs, L., P.J. Anderson, and M.B. Bender (1973). The lesions producing paralysis of downward but not upward gaze. Arch. Neurol., 28, 319-323.

Jaeger, J., V. Henn. W. Lang. T.S. Miles. and W. Waespe (1981). Vestibular unit activity in monkeys with horizontal gaze palsy. In A.L. Fuchs and W. Becker (Eds.), Progress in Oculomotor Research. Elsevier, Amsterdam. In press.

Jampal, R.J. (1959). Representation of the near response on the cerebral cortex of the macaque. Am. J. Ophthal., 48, 573-581.

Jampel, R.S. (1981). Ocular torsion and the primary retinal meridians. Am. J. Ophthal., 91, 14-24.

Jampolsky, A.J. (1956). Esotropia and convergent fixation disparity. Am.J. Ophthal., 41, 825-833.

Jampolsky, A.J. (1970). Ocular divergence mechanisms. Trans. Am. Ophthal.Soc., 68, 730.

Jampolsky, A.J. (1971). Systems of strabismus surgery. Actas III Congreso del Consejo Latino Americano de Estrabismo, Mar del Plata, Argentina. pp 433-443.

Jampolsky A.J. (1971). A simplified approach to strabismus diagnosis. In Symposium on Strabismus: Trans. New Orleans Acad. Ophthal., C.V. Mosby Co., St. Louis. pp 34-92.

Jampolsky, A.J. (1977).When should one operate for congenital strabismus? In R.J. Brockhurst (Ed.), Controversy in Ophthalmology, W.B. Saunders Co, Philadelphia. p. 416.

Jampolsky A.J., and H.E.A. Bicas (1975). Balance of tonic and mechanical forces in strabismus surgery. Presented at Pan Am. Congr. of Ophthal., Puerto Rico.

Javal, E. (1896). Manuel theorique et pratique du strabisme. Masson & Cie, Paris.

Jenkyn, L.R., G. Margolis, and A.G. Reeves (1978). Reflex vertical gaze and the medial longitudinal fasciculus. J. Neurol. Neurosurg. Psychiat., 41, 1084-1091.

Jones, E.G., and T.P.S. Powell (1970). An anatomical study of converging sensory pathways within the cerebral cortex of the monkey. Brain, 93, 793-820.

Jones, G.M., and J.D. DeJong (1971). Dynamic characteristics of saccadic eye movements in Parkinson´s disease. Exp. Neurol., 31, 17-31.

Jones, R. (1977). Anomalies of disparity detection in the human visual system. J. Physiol., 264, 621-640.

Jones, R., and K.E. Kerr (1971). Motor responses to conflicting asymmetrical vergence stimulus information.Am. J. Optom. Arch. Am. Acad. Optom., 48 (12), 989-1000.

Jordan, S. (1970). Ocular pursuit movement as a function of visual and proprioceptive stimulation. Vision Res., 10, 775-780.

Judge, S.J., and F.A. Miles (1981). Gain changes in accommodative vergence induced by alteration of the effective interocular separation. In A.F. Fuchs and W. Becker (Eds.), Progress in Oculomotor Research, Elsevier, New York. In press.

Judge, S.J., B.J. Richmond, and F.C. Chu (1980). Implantation of magnetic search coils for measurement of eye position: An improved method. Vision Res.,20,535-538.

Jung, R. (1977). Perception, consciousness and visual attention. In P.A. Buser and A. Rougel-Buser (Eds.), Cerebral Correlates of Conscious Experience Inserum Symposium No 6, North-Holland Publ. Co. pp 15-36.

Jung, R., and H.H. Kornhuber (1964). Results of electronystagmography in man: The value of optokinetic, vestibular, and spontaneous nystagmus for neurologic diagnosis and research. In M.B. Bender (Ed.), The Oculomotor System, Harper & Row, New York. pp 428-482.

Jung, R., and H.H. Kornhuber (1976). Eye tracking of self-moved targets in the absence of vision. Exp. Brain Res., 26, 121-139.

Jürgens, R., W. Becker, and H.H. Kornhuber (1981). Natural and drug-induced variations of velocity and duration of human saccadic eye movements: Evidence for a control of the neural pulse generator by local feedback. Biol. Cyber., 39, 81-96.

Kamei, T., and H.H. Kornhuber (1974). Spontaneuous and head shaking nystagmus in normals and in patients with central lesions. Canad. J. Oto-lar., 3, 372-380.

Kasai, T., and D. Zee (1978). Eye-head coordination in labyrinthine defective humans. Brain Res., 144, 123-141.

Kase, M., D.C. Miller, and H. Noda (1980). Discharges of Purkinje cells and mossy fibers in the cerebellar vermis of the monkey during saccadic eye movements and fixation. J. Physiol., 300, 539-555.

Kase, M., H. Noda, D.A. Suzuki, and D.C. Miller (1979). Target velocity signals of visual tracking in vermal Purkinje cells of the monkey, Science, 205, 717-720.

Käser, O. (1942). Nystagmus als rezessiv geschlechtsgeb. Merkmal in 4 Generationen. Schweiz. Med. Wschr., 72, 846-850.

Kawano, K., and M. Sasaki (1981). Neurons in the posterior parietal association cortex of the monkey activated during optokinetic stimulation. Neurosci. Letters, 22, 239-244.

Kawano, K., M. Sasaki, and M. Yamashita (1980). Vestibular input to visual tracking neurons in the posterior parietal association cortex of the monkey. Neurosci. Letters, 17, 55-60.

Keane, J.R. (1975). Ocular skew deviation. Arch. Neurol., 185, 185-190.

Keiner, E.C.J.F. (1978). Spontaneous recovery in microstrabismus. Ophthalmologica, 177, 280-283.

Keiner, C.B.J., and C.O. Roelofs (1955). Optomotor reflexes and nystagmus. In M. Niihoff (Ed.), La Haye, Vol. I. p. 224. Cited after D. GoddéJolly and A. Larmande (1973). Les Nystagmus, Vol. I. Ch. VIII, Masson u. Cie., Paris. p 632.

Keller, E.L. (1974). Participation of medial pontine reticular formation in eye movement generation in monkey. J. Neurophysiol., 37, 316-332.

Keller, E.L. (1981). Brain stem mechanisms in saccadic control. In A.F. Fuchs and W. Becker (Eds.), Progress in Oculomotor Research, Elsevier, New York. In press.

Keller, E.L., and W.F. Crandall (1981). Neural activity in the nucleus reticularis tegmenti pontis in the monkey related to eye movements and visual stimulation. Anns. N.Y. Acad. Sci., In press.

Keller. E.L., and P.D. Daniels (1975). Oculomotor related interaction of vestibular and visual stimulation in vestibular nucleus cells in alert monkeys. Exp. Neurol., 46, 187-198.

Keller, E.L., and B.Y. Kamath (1975). Characteristics of head rotation and eye movement-related neurons in alert monkey vestibular nucleus. Brain Res., 100, 182-187.

Keller, E.L., and W. Precht (1979a).Visual-vestibular responses in vestibular nuclear neurons in intact and cerebellectomized, alert cat. Neuroscience, 4, 1599-1613.

Keller, E.L., and W. Precht (1979b).Adaptive modification of central vestibular neurons in response to visual stimulation through reversing prisms. J. Neurophysiol., 42, 896-911.

Keller, E.L., and D.A. Robinson (1971). Absence of a stretch reflex in extraocular muscles of the monkey. J. Neurophysiol., 34, 908-919.

Kennard, M.A., and L. Ectors (1938). Forced circling movements in monkeys following lesions of the frontal lobes. J. Neurophysiol., 1, 45-54.

Kent, P.R. (1958). Convergence-accommodation. Am. J. Optom. Arch.Am. Acad. Optom., 35, 393-406.

Kenyon, R.V., K.J. Ciuffreda, W. Hoyt, and F. Hsu (1977). Voluntary nystagmus is saccadic: Motor mechanisms. Am. Acad. Optom. , Birmingham, Alabama.

Kenyon, R.V., K.J. Ciuffreda, and L. Stark (1976). Binocular eye movements during accommodative vergence. Ass. Res. Vision Ophthal., Sarasota, Florida.

Kenyon, R.V., K.J. Ciuffreda, and L. Stark (1978). Binocular eye movements during accommodative vergence. Vision Res., 18, 546-555.

Kenyon, R.V., K.J. Ciuffreda, and L. Stark (1980a). Dynamic vergence eye movements in strabismus and amblyopia: Symmetric vergence. Invest. Ophthal.Vis.Sci.,19,60-74.

Kenyon, R.V., K.J. Ciuffreda, and L.Stark (1980b). An unexpected role for normal accommodative vergence in strabismus and amblyopia. Am.J. Optom. Physiol. Opt., 57, 566-577.

Kenyon, R.V., K.J. Ciuffreda, and L. Stark (1980c). Unequal saccades during vergence. Am. J. Optom. Physiol. Opt., 57, 586-594.

Kenyon, R.V., K.J. Ciuffreda, and L. Stark (1981). Dynamic vergence eye movements in strabismus and amblyopia: Asymmetric vergence. Br. J. Ophthal., 65, 167-176.

Kenyon, R.V., and L. Stark (1981). Unequal saccades with equal innervation when saccades are summated onto ongoing vergence or smooth pursuit eye movements. Math. Biosci. Accepted for publication.

Kestenbaum, A. (1961). Clinical Methods of Neuro-ophthalmologic Examination, Grune and Stratton, New York. pp. 366.

King, W.M., and A.F. Fuchs (1979). Reticular control of vertical saccadic eye movements by mesencephalic burst neurons. J. Neurophysiol., 42, 861-876.

King, W.M., A.F. Fuchs, and M. Magnin (1981). Vertical eye movement-related responses of neurons in midbrain near interstitial nucleus of Cajal. J. Neurophysiol., 46, 549-562.

King, W.M., S. G. Lindberger, and A.F. Fuchs (1976). Responses of fibers in medial lontitudinal fasciculus (MLF) of alert monkeys during horizontal and vertical eye movements evoked by vestibular or visual stimuli. J. Neurophysiol., 39, 1135-1149.

King, W.M., W. Precht, and N. Dieringer (1980a). Afferent and efferent connections of cat omnipause neurons. Exp. Brain Res., 38, 395-403.

King, W.M., W. Precht, and N. Dieringer (1980b).Synaptic organization of frontal eye field and vestibular afferents to interstitial nucleus of Cajal in the cat. J. Neurophyisol., 43, 912-928.

King-Smith, P.E., and L.A. Riggs (1978). Visual sensitivity to controlled motion of a line or edge. Vision Res., 18, 1509-1520.

Kirchmair, H. (1958). Über den erblichen Nystagmus und über eine besondere benigne Form des angeb. Nystagmus. Med. Klinik, 53, I, 928-930.

Knoll, H.A. (1966). Measuring ametropia with a gas laser; a preliminary report. Am. J. Optom. and Arch. Am. Acad. Optom., 43, 415-418.

Kohler, J. (1951). Über Aufbau und Wandlungen der Wahrnehmungswelt. Sitzber. Öster. Wiss., 227, 118.

Kohler, I. (1956). Die Methode des Brillenversuches in der Wahrnehmungs-Psychologie mit Bemerkungen zur Lehre der Adaptation. Z. exp. angew. Psychol., 3, 381-417.

Komatsuzaki, A. J. Alpert, H.H. Harris, and B. Cohen (1972). Effects of mesencephalic reticular formation lesions on optokinetic nystagmus. Exp. Neurol., 34, 522-534.

Kommerell, G. (1974). Nystagmusoperation zur Korrektur verschiedener Kopfzwangshaltungen. Klin. Mbl. Augenheilk., 164, 172-191.

Kommerell, G. (1978). Beziehungen zwischen Strabismus und Nystagmus. In G. Kommerell (Ed.), Disorders of Ocular Motility; Neurophysiological and Clinical Aspects, Bergmann, München. pp 367-373.

Kommerell, G., and W.F. Hoyt (1973). Lateropulsion of saccadic eye movements. Electro-oculographic studies in a patient with Wallenberg´s syndrome. Arch Neurol., 28, 313-318.

Kommerell, G., and U. Klein (1971). Über die Visuelle Regelung der Okulomotorik: Die Optomotorische Wirkung Exzenterischer Nachbilder. Vision Res., 11, 905-920.

Kommerell, G., D. Olivier, and H. Theopold (1976). Adaptative programming of phasic and tonic components in saccadic eye movements. Investigations in patients with abducens palsy. Invest. Ophthal., 15, 657-660.

Kommerell, G., and R. Taumer (1972). Investigations of the eye tracking system through stabilized retinal images. Bibl. Ophthal., 82, 288-297.

Kompf, D., T. Pasik, P. Pasik, and M.B. Bender (1979). Downward gaze in monkeys. Stimulation and lesion studies. Brain, 102, 527-558.

Kornhuber, H.H. (1960). Über Begleitschielen und latenten Nystagmus aus neurol. Sicht. Sitzber. Rhein.-Westf. Augenärzte, 102, 45-48.

Kornhuber, H.H. (1971). Motor function of the cerebellum and basal ganglia: The cerebellocortical saccadic (ballastic) clock, the cerebellonuclear hold regulator and the basal ganglia ramp (voluntary speed smooth movement) generator. Kybernetic, 8, 157-162.

Kosaka, K.Z. (1912). Zur Frage der physiologischen Natur der zerebralen Trigeminuswurzel. Folia Neurobiol., 6, 1-16.

Kretzer-Stein, J. (1971). Nystagmogr. u. statist. Unters. über den latenten Nystagmus. Inauguarl-Dissertation, Freiburg.

Kretzschmar, S. (1955). La fausse correspondance rétinienne. Doc. Ophthal., 9, 46-208.

Krill, A. (1977). Hereditary Retinal and Chorioidal Disease. Vol. I, II, Harper and Row, Hagerstown, Maryland.

Krishnan, V.V., and L. Stark (1977). A heuristic model for the human vergence eye movement system. IEEE Trans. BME, 250, 347-366.

Kugelberg, E. (1976). Adaptive transformation of rat soleus motor units during growth. Histochemistry and contraction speed. J. Neurol. Sci., 27, 269-289.

Kunzle, H., and K. Akert (1977). Efferent connections of cortical area 8 (frontal eye field) in Macaca fascicularis. A reinvestigation using the autoradiographic technique. J. Comp. Neurol., 173, 147-164.

Kurtzberg, D., and H.G. Vaughan, Jr. (1977). Electrophysiological observations on the visuomotor system and visual neurosensorium. In J.E. Desmedt (Ed.), Visual Evoked Potentials in Man: New Developments, Clarendon Press, Oxford. pp 314-331.

Kuypers, H.G.J.M., and D.G. Lawrence (1976). Cortical projections to the red nucleus and the brain stem in rhesus monkey. Brain Res., 4, 151-188.

Kyrieleis (1931). Kurses, Hb. d. Ophthal., 6, 701, Berlin.

Lackner, J.R. (1975). Pursuit eye movement elicited by muscle afferent information. Neurosci. Letters, 1, 25-28.

Lamontagne, C. (1973). A new experimental paradigm for the investigation of the secondary system of human visual motion perception. Perception, 2, 167-180.

Lang, J. (1967). Der kongenitale oder frühkindliche Strabismus. Ophthalmologica, Basel, 154, 201.

Lang, J. (1978). Nystagmusprobleme in der Praxis. Klin. Mbl.Augenheilk., 172, 410-413.
Lanman, J., E. Bizzi, and J. Allum (1978). The coordination of head and eye movement during smooth pursuit. Brain Res., 153, 39-53.
Lannou, J., L. Cazin, W. Precht, and M. Toupet (1981). Optokinetic, vestibular, and optokinetic-vestibular responses in albino and pigmented rats. Pflügers Arch. In press.
Larmande, A.M., and M.P. Deplace (1973). L´epreuve de poursuite pendulair. Principe et technique. Arch. Ophthal., 33, 269-278.
Larmande, P., and Autret, A. (1980). Influence du cervelet sur les mouvements ovulaires voluntaires. Rev. Neurol. Paris, 136, 259-269.
Larmande, P., S. Prier, M. Masson, and J. Cambier (1980). Perturbations de la poursuite oculaire et lesions parieto-occipitales unilaterales. Rev.Neurol.Paris, 136, 345-353.
Larsby, B., L.M. Ödkvist, D. Hydén, and S.R.C. Liedgren (1976). Disturbances of the vestibular system by toxic agents. Acta Physiol. Scand. Suppl., 440, 108.
Larsby, B., L.M. Ödkvist, D. Hydén, B. Eriksson, R. Tham, and S.R.C. Liedgren (1981). Optokinetic disturbances caused by styrene. An experimental study in rabbits. Proc. Neuroequilibriometric Soc.
Larsby, B., R. Tham, L.M. Ödkvist, D. Hydén, I. Bunnfors, and G. Aschan (1978a). Exposure of rabbits to styrene. Electronystagmographic findings correlated to the styrene level in blood and cerebrospinal fluid. Scand. J. Work Environ. Health, 4, 60-65.
Larsby, B., R. Tham, L.M. Ödkvist, B. Norlander, D. Hydén, G. Aschan, and A. Rubin (1978b). Exposure of rabbits to methylchloroform: Vestibular disturbances correlated to blood and cerebrospinal fluid levels. Int. Arch. Occup. Environ. Health., 41, 7-15.
Latto, R., and A. Cowey (1971). Fixation changes after frontal eye-field lesions in monkeys. Brain Res., 30, 25-36.
Lau, C.G.Y., V. Honrubia, and R.W. Baloh (1978). The patterns of eye movement trajectories during physiological nystagmus in humans. In J.D. Hood (Ed.), Vestibular Mechanisms in Health and Disease, VI. Extraordinary Meeting of the Barany Soc., Academic Press, London. pp 37-44.
Lau, C.G.Y., V. Honrubia, and R.W. Baloh (1981). A model for visual vestibular interaction. In T. Gualtierotti (Ed.), Vestibular Function and Morphology, Springer Verlag, New York.
Lau, C.G.Y., V. Honrubia, H.A. Jenkins, R.W. Baloh, and R.D. Yee (1978). Linear model for visual-vestibular interaction. Aviat. Space Environ., 49 (7), 880-885.
Lawwill, T. (1968). Local adaptation in functional amblyopia. Am. J. Ophthal., 65(6), 903-906.
Leech, J., M. Gresty. K. Hess, and P. Rudge (1977). Gaze failure, drifting eye movements, and centripetal nystagmus in cerebellar disease. Br. J. Ophthal., 61, 774-781.
Lehman, S. and L. Stark (1981). Simulation of linear and non-linear eye movement models. Cybernetics. In press.
Leichnetz, G.R. (1980). An anterogradely-labeled cortico-oculomotor pathway in the monkey demonstrated with HRP gel and TMB neurohistochemistry. Brain Res., 198, 440-44
Leichnetz, G.R. (1981). The prefrontal cortico-oculomotor trajectories in the monkey: A possible explanation for the effects of stimulation/lesion experiments on eye movement. J. Neurol. Sci. In press.
Leigh, R.J., S.A. Newman, S.E. Folstein, and A.G. Lasker (1981). Disturbed ocular motor control in Huntington´s disease. Neurosci. Abstr., 7. In press.
Leigh, R.J., and D.S. Zee (1980). Eye movements of the blind. Invest. Ophthal. Vis. Sci., 19, 328-331.
Leigh, R.J., and D.S. Zee (1982). The Neurology of Eye Movements. F.A. Davis, Philadelphia.
Le Liever, W.C., and H.O. Barber (1981). Observations on optokinetic nystagmus in patients with congenital nystagmus. Oto-lar. Head Neck Surg., 89, 110-116.
Lennerstrand, G. (1974). Electrical activity and isometric tension in motor units of the cat´s inferior oblique muscle. Acta Physiol. Scand., 91, 458-474.

Lennerstrand, G. (1975). Motor units in eye muscles. In G. Lennerstrand and P. Bach-y-Rita (Eds.), Basic Mechanisms of Ocular Motility and Their Clinical Implications, Pergamon Press, Oxford. pp. 119-143.

Lennerstrand. G (1979). Contractile properties of extraocular muscle in Siamese cat. Acta Ophthal., 57, 1030-1038.

Lennerstrand, G. (1980). Histochemical studies on the inferior oblique muscle of Siamese cats and domestic cats with unilateral lid suture. Exp.Eye Res.,30,619-629.

Lennerstrand, G., and P. Bach-y-Rita (1974). Spindle responses in pig eye muscles. Acta Physiol. Scand., 90, 795-797.

Lennerstrand, G., and P. Bach-y-Rita (1975). Basic Mechanisms of Ocular Motility and Their Clinical Implications, Pergamon Press, Oxford.

Lennerstrand, G., and J. Hanson (1978a). The postnatal development of the inferior oblique muscle of the cat. I. Isometric twitch and tetanic properties. Acta Physiol. Scand., 103, 132-143.

Lennerstrand, G., and J. Hanson (1978b). The postnatal development of the inferior oblique muscle of the cat. II. Effects of repetitive stimulation on isometric tension responses. Acta Physiol. Scand., 103, 144-153.

Lennerstrand, G., and J. Hanson (1979). Contractile properties of extraocular msucles in cats reared with monocular lid closure and artificial squint. Acta Ophthal., 57, 591-599.

Lennerstrand, G., and K. Nichols (1977). Morphology of motor units in cat extraocular muscle. Acta Ophthal., 55, 913-918.

Lenox, J.R., A.F. Lange, and K.R. Graham (1970). Eye movement amplitudes in imagined pursuit of a pendulum with eyes closed. Psychophysiol., 6, 773-777.

Lettvin, J.Y., H.R. Maturana, W.S. McCulloch, and W.H. Pitts (1959). What the frog´s eye tells the frog´s brain. Proc. I.R.E., 47, 1940-1951.

Lewis, P.M. (1940). Ocular complications of meningococcal meningitis, observation in 350 cases. Am. J. Ophthal., 23, 617-632.

Lisberger, S.G., C. Evinger, G.W. Johanson, and A.F. Fuchs (1981). Relationship between eye acceleration and retinal image velocity during foveal smooth pursuit in man and monkey. J. Neurophysiol. In press.

Lisberger, S.G., and A.F. Fuchs (1977). Role of the primate flocculus in smooth pursuit eye movments and rapid behavioural modification of the vestibulo-ocular reflex. In R. Baker and A. Berthoz (Eds.), Control of Gaze by Brain Stem Neurons, Biomed. Press, Elsevier/North-Holland, Amsterdam. pp 381-389.

Lisberger, S.G., and A.F. Fuchs (1978). Role of primate flocculus during rapid behavioural modification of vestibulo-ocular reflex. I. Purkinje cell activity during visually guided horizontal smooth-pursuit eye movements and passive head rotation. J. Neurophysiol., 41, 733-763.

Lisberger, S.G., and F.A. Miles (1980). Role of primate medial vestibular nucleus in long-term adaptive plasticity of vestibulo-ocular reflex. J. Neurophysiol., 43, 172-145.

Lisberger, S.G., F.A. Miles, L.M. Optican, and B.B. Eighmy (1981). Optokinetic response in monkey: Underlying mechanisms and their sensitivity to long-term adaptive changes in vestibulo-ocular reflex. J. Neurophysiol, 45, 869-890.

Llinas, R., K. Walton, D.E. Hillman, and C. Sotelo (1975). Inferior olive: Its role in motor learning. Science, 190, 1230-1231.

Llinas, R., and J.W. Wolfe (1977). Functional linkage between the electrical activity in the vermal cerebellar cortex and saccadic eye movements. Exp. Brain Res., 29, 1-14.

Loewer-Sieger, D.H. (1962). Amblyopie. Een studie over de kenmerken en de behandeling. J. Ruysendaal, Amsterdam.

Lømo, T., R.H. Westgaard, and H. Dahl (1974). Contractile properties of muscle: Control by pattern of muscle activity in the rat. Proc. Soc. Lond. B.,187, 99-103.

Lopez-Barneo, J., C. Darlot, and A. Berthoz (1979). Functional role of the prepositus hypoglossi nucleus in the control of gaze. Prog. Brain Res., 50, 667-679.

Lorente de No, R. (1933). Vestibulo-ocular reflex. Arch. Neurol. Psychiat.,30,245-291.

Ludvigh, E., P. McKinnon, and L. Zartzeff (1964). Temporal course of the relaxation of binocular duction (fusion) movements. Arch. Ophthal., 71, 389-399.

Luschei, E.S., and A.F. Fuchs (1972). Activity of brain stem neurons during eye movements of alert monkey. J. Neurophysiol., 35, 445-461.

Lynch, J.C.(1980a). The functional organization of posterior parietal association cortex. Behav. Brain Sci., 3, 485-534.

Lynch. J.C.(1980b). The role of parieto-occipital association cortex in oculomotor control. Exp. Brain Res., 41, A32.

Lynch, J.C., V.B. Mountcastle, W.H. Talbot, and T.C.T. Yin (1977a).Parietal lobe mechanisms for directed visual attention. J. Neurophysiol., 40, 362-389.

Lynch, J.C., V.B. Mountcastle, W.H. Talbot, and T.C.T. Yin (1977b).Parietal lobe mechanisms for directed visual attention. J. Neurophysiol., 60, 362-389.

Mabuchi, M., and T. Kusama (1970). Mesodiencephalic projections to the inferior olive and the vestibular and hypoglossal nuclei. Brain Res., 17, 133-136.

Maciewicz, R.J., E. Eagen, C.R.S. Kaneko, and S.M. Higstein (1977). Vestibular and medullary brain stem afferents to the abducens nucleus in the cat. Brain Res., 123, 229-240.

Mackensen, G. (1958). Reaktionszeitmessungen bei amblyopie. Albrecht von Graefes. Arch. Ophthal., 159, 636-642.

Maddox, E.C. (1886). Investigations on the relationship between convergence and accommodation of the eyes. J. Anat., 20, 475-505, 565-584.

Maddox, E.C (1893). The Clinical Use of Prism, 2nd Ed., Wright, Bristol. pp. 83.

McCrea, R.A., R. Baker, and J. Delgado-Garcia (1979). Afferent and efferent organisation of the prepositus hypoglossi nucleus. Prog. Brain Res., 50, 653-665.

McCrea, R., K. Yoshida, A. Berthoz, and R. Baker (1980). Eye movement related activity and morphology of second order vestibular neurons terminating in the cat abducens nucleus. Exp. Brain Res., 40, 468-473.

McCrea, R.A., K. Yoshida, C. Evinger, and A. Berthoz (1981). In A. Fuchs and W. Becker (Eds.). Progress in Oculomotor Research, Biomed. Press, Elsevier/North-Holland, Amsterdam. In press.

McElligott, J.G., (1979). Purkinje cell activity in the vermal cerebellum of the cat during trained saccadic eye movements and fixations. Soc. Neurosci. Abstr., 5, 104.

McLean, S., and J.P. Caffey (1928). Endemic meningococcus meningitis; Clinical manifestations in infancy and in early childhood. Am. J. Dis. Child., 35, 357-387.

Maekawa, K., and M. Kimura (1980). Mossy fiber projections to the cerebellar flocculus from the extraocular afferents. Brain Res., 191, 313-325.

Maekawa, K., and M. Kimura (1981). Electrophysiological study of the nucleus of the optic tract that transfers optic signals to the nucleus reticularis tegmenti pontis - the visual mossy fiber pathway to the cerebellar flocculus. Brain Res., 211, 456-462.

Maekawa, K., and J.I. Simpson (1973). Climbing fiber responses evoked in vestibulocerebellum of rabbit from visual system. J. Neurophysiol., 36, 649-666.

Maekawa, K., and T. Takeda (1975). Mossy fiber responses evoked in the cerebellar flocculus of rabbits by stimulation of the optic pathway. Brain.Res., 98, 590-595.

Maekawa, K., and T. Takeda (1978). Origin of the mossy fiber projection to the cerebellar flocculus from the optic nerves in rabbits. Integrative Control Functions of the Brain, Kodansha Scientific. Tokyo; Elsevier, Amsterdam, 1, 93-95.

Maekawa, K., T. Takeda, and M. Kimura (1981). Neural activity of nucleus reticularis tegmenti pontis - The origin of visual mossy fiber afferents to the cerebellar flocculus of rabbits. Brain Res., 210, 17-30.

Maffei, L., and A. Fiorentini (1977). Oculomotor proprioception in the cat. In R. Baker and A. Berthoz (Eds.), Control of Gaze by Brain Stem Neurons,Biomed.Press, Elsevier North-Holland, Amsterdam. pp 477-481.

Magnus, R. (1924). Körperstellung, Springer, Berlin.

Manas, L. (1958). The effect of visual training upon the ACA ratio. Am. J. Optom. and Arch. Am. Acad. Optom., 35, 428-437.

Manas. L., and P. Shulman (1954). The variation in the accommodative-convergence accommodation (ACA) ratio upon periodic testing. Am. J. Optom. and Arch. Acad. Optom., 31, 385-395.

Manni, E., R. Bortolami, and C. Desole (1966). Eye muscle proprioception and the semilunar ganglion. Exp. Neurol., 16, 226-236.

Manni, E., R. Bortolami, and C. Desole (1968). Peripheral pathway of the eye muscle proprioception. Exp. Neurol., 22, 1-12.

Manni, E., R. Bortolami, and P.L. Deriu (1970a). Presence of cell bodies of the afferents from the eye muscles in the semilunar ganglion. Arch. Ital. Biol., 108, 106-120.

Manni, E., R. Bortolami, and P.L. Deriu (1970b). Superior oblique muscle proprioception and the trochlear nerve. Exp. Neurol., 26, 543-550.

Manni, E., R. Bortolami, V.E. Pettorossi, M.L. Lucchi, and E. Callegari (1981). A direct trigemino-oculomotor pathway. In A.F. Fuchs and W. Becker (Eds.), Progress in Oculomotor Research, Elsevier, Amsterdam. In press.

Manni, E., C. Desole, and G. Palmieri(1970). On whether eye muscle spindles are innervated by ganglion cells located along the oculomotor nerve. Exp. Neurol., 28, 333-343.

Manni, E., G. Palmieri, and R. Marini (1971a). Peripheral pathway of the proprioceptive afferents from the lateral rectus muscle of the eye. Exp.Neurol.,30, 46-53.

Manni, E.,G. Palmieri, and R. Marini (1971b). Extraocular muscle proprioception and the descending trigeminal nucleus. Exp. Neurol., 33, 195-204.

Manni, E., G. Palmieri, and R. Marini (1972a). Pontine trigeminal terminations of the proprioceptive afferents from the eye muscles. Exp. Neurol., 36, 310-318.

Manni, E., G. Palmieri, and R. Marini (1972b). Mesodiencephalic representation of the eye muscle proprioception. Exp. Neurol., 37, 412-421.

Manni, E., G. Palmieri, and R. Marini (1974). Central pathway of the extraocular muscle proprioception. Exp. Neurol., 42, 181-190.

Manni, E., G. Palmieri, R. Marini, and V.E. Petterossi (1975a). Trigeminal influences on extensor muscles of the neck. Exp. Neurol., 47, 330-342.

Manni, E., G. Palmieri, R. Marini, and V.E. Pettorossi (1975b). New observations on the representation of the eye muscle proprioception in the descedning trigeminal nucleus. Experientia, 31, 944-945.

Manni, E., and V.E. Pettorossi (1976). Somatotopic organization of the eye muscle afferents in the semilunar ganglion. Arch. Ital. Biol., 114, 178-187.

Maraini, G., and L. Pasino (1964). Variations in the fusional movements in cases of small-angle convergent strabismus with harmonious anomalous retinal correspondence. Br. J. Ophthal., 48, 439-443.

Marg , E. (1964). The accessory optic system. Ann. N.Y. Acad. Sci., 117, 35-52.

Marini, R., and R. Bortolami (1979). Somatotopic organization of second order neurons of the eye muscle proprioception. Arch. Ital. Biol., 117, 45-57.

Marini, R., and R. Bortolami (1980). Somatotopic representation of eye muscle proprioception within the superior colliculus of the lamb. Exp. Neurol., 69, 226-238.

Markham, C.H., W. Precht, and H. Shimazu (1966). Effect of stimulation of interstitial nucleus of Cajal on vestibular unit activity in the cat. J. Neurophysiol., 29, 493-507.

Marlow, F.W. (1924). The relative position of rest of the eyes and the prolonged occlusion test. F.A. Davis, Philadelphia.

Martin, J.P. (1967). The Basal Ganglia and Posture. Pitman Med. Publ., London.

Martinez, A.J., A.W. Biglan, and D.A. Hiles (1980). Structural features of extraocular muscles of children with strabismus. Arch. Ophth., 98, 533-539.

Martinex, A.J., S. Hay, and K.W. McNeer (1976). Extraocular muscles, light microscopy and ultrastructural features. Acta Neuropath., Berlin, 34, 237.

Masterton, R.B.,K. K. Glendenning, and K.A. Hutson (1979). Preservation of trapezoid body fibers after biochemical ablation of superior olives with kainic acid. Brain. Res., 173, 156-159.

Matsuo, V. (1981). Velocity storage in vertical optokinetic and vestibular nystagmus and visual-vsetibular interaction. Ph.D. Thesis, City University of New York.

Matsuo, F., and E.T. Ajax (1979). Palatal myoclonus and denervation suprasensitivity in the central nervous system. Ann. Neurol., 5, 72-78.

Matsuo, V., and B. Cohen (1981). Effect of static head position on the duration of vertical optokinetics after-nystagmus (OKAN) in monkeys. Soc. for Neurosci. Abstr., 7, 39.

Matsuo, V., B. Cohen, T. Raphan, V. Dejong, and V. Henn (1979). Asymmetric velocity storage for upward and downward nystagmus. Brain Res., 176, 159-164.

Mayr, R. (1971). Structure and distribution of fibre types in the external eye muscles of the rat. Tissue & Cell, 3, 433.462.

Mays, L.E., and J.G. McElligott (1976). Neuron-11: A computer system for relating neuronal spike trains to physiological and behavioural data. Behav. Res. Methods Instru., 8, 325-328.

Mays, L.E., and D.L. Sparks (1980). Saccades are spatially, not retinocentrically, coded. Science, 208, 1163-1165.

Mehdorn, E., G. Kommerell, and O. Meienberg (1979). Primary position vertical nystagmus: 'directional preponderance' of the pursuit system. Graefes Arch. Klin. Ophth., 209, 209-217.

Meienberg, O., W.H. Zangemeister, M. Rosenberg, W.F. Hoyt and L. Stark (1981). Saccadic eye movement strategies in patients with homonymous hemianopia. Ann. Neurol., 9, 537-544.

Melamed, E., and B. Larsen (1979). Cortical activation periods during saccadic eye movements in humans: Localization by focal cerebral blood flow increases. Ann. Neurol., 5, 79-88.

Melvill Jones, G. (1977). Plasticity in the adult vestibulo-ocular reflex arc. Phil. Trans. R. Soc. Lond., 278, 319-334.

Melvill Jones. G., and P. Davies (1976). Adaptation of cat vestibulo-ocular reflex to 200 days of optically reversed vision. Brain Res., 103, 551-554.

Merillees, N.C.R., S. Sutherland, and W. Hayhow (1950). Neuromuscular spindles in man. Anat. Rec., 108, 23.

Merwarth, H.R., and E. Feiring (1939). Modifications of induced nystagmus by acute cerebral lesions. Preliminary report. Brooklyn Hosp. J., 1, 99-106.

Michael, J.A., and G. Melvill Jones (1966). Dependence of visual tracking capability upon stimulus predictability. Vision Res., 6, 707-716.

Michalski, A., M. Kossut, and B. Zernicki (1977). The ocular following reflex elicitied from the retinal periphery in the cat. Vision Res., 17, 713-736.

Mikami, A., H. Noda, and N. Suzumura (1981). Discharges of parafloccular units during eye movements. Suppl. to: Invest. Ophthal. Vis. Sci., 20, 57.

Miles, F.A., and D.J. Braitman (1980). Long-term adaptive changes in primate vestibulo-ocular reflex. II Electrophysiological observations on semicircular canal primary afferents. J. Neurophysiol., 43, 1426-1436.

Miles, F.A., D.J. Braitman, and B.M. Dow (1980). Long-term adaptive changes in primate vestibulo-ocular reflex. IV. Electrophysiological observations in flocculus of adapted monkeys. J. Neurophysiol., 43, 1477-1493.

Miles, F.A., and B.B. Eighmy (1980). Long-term adaptive changes in primate vestibulo-ocular reflex. I. Behavioural observations. J. Neurophysiol., 43, 1406-1425.

Miles, F.A., and J.H. Fuller (1974). Adaptive plasticity in the vestibulo-ocular responses of the rhesus monkey. Brain Res., 80, 512-516.

Miles, F.A., J.H. Fuller, D.J. Braitman, and B.M. Dow (1980). Long-term adaptive changes in primate vestibulo-ocular reflex. III. Electrophysiological observations in flocculus of normal monkeys. J. Neurophysiol., 43, 1437-1476.

Miles, F.A., and S.G. Lisberger (1981a). Plasticity in the vestibulo-ocular reflex: A new hypothesis. Ann. Rev. , 4, 273-299.

Miles, F.A., and S.G. Lisberger (1981b). The "error" signals subserving adaptive gain control in the primate vestibulo-ocular reflex. Ann. N.Y. Acad. In press.

Milla, P.J., and A.D. Jackson (1977). A controlled trial of Baclofen in children with cerebral palsy. J. Int. Med. Res., 5, 398-404.

Miller, J.E. (1971). Recent histologic and electron microscopic findings in extraocular muscle.Trans. Am. Acad. Ophth. and Otol., 75, 1175.

Miller, J.E. (1975). Aging changes in extraocular muscle. In G. Lennerstrand and P. Bach-y-Rita (Eds.), Basic Mechanisms of Ocular Motility and Their Clinical Implication, Pergamon Press, Oxford.pp 47-61.

Mills, R.P., and P.D. Swanson (1978). Vertical oculomotor apraxia and memory loss. Ann. Neurol., 4, 149-153.

Mishra. R.K., and S.P. Gupta (1962). Ocular complications of Tuberculous Meningitis. J. Ind. Med. Ass., 38, 513-518.

Mitchell, D.E. (1980). The influence of early visual experience on visual perception. In: C.S. Harris (Ed.), Visual Coding and Adaptability, Lawrence Erlbaum Assoc., Hillsdale, N.J. pp 1-50.

Mitchell, D.E., M. Cynader, and J.A. Movshon (1977). Recovery from the effects of monocular deprivation in kittens. J. Comp. Neurol., 176, 53-63.

Miyashita, Y. (1981). Differential roles of the climbing and mossy fiber visual pathways in vision-guided modification of the vestibulo-ocular reflex. In H. Flohr and W. Precht (Eds.), Lesion-Induced Neuronal Plasticity in Sensimotor Systems, Springer Verlag, pp 305-313.

Miyashita, Y., M. Ito, P.J. Jastreboff, K. Maekawa, and S. Nagao (1980). Effect upon eye movements of rabbits induced by severance of mossy fiber visual pathway to the cerebellar flocculus. Brain Res., 198, 210-215.

Moberg, A., L. Preber, B.P. Silfverskiöld, and S. Vallbo (1962). Imbalance, nystagmus and diplopia in Wallenberg´s syndrome. Acta Oto-lar., 55, 269-282.

Moffett,A., G. Ettlinger, H.B. Morton, and M.F. Piercy (1967). Tactile discrimination performance in the monkey: The effect of ablation of various subdivisions of posterior parietal cortex. Cortex, 3, 59-96.

Mohindra, I., R. Held, J. Gwiazda, and S. Brill (1978). Astigmatism in infants. Science, 202, 329-331.

Mohler, C.W., M.E. Goldberg, and R.H. Wurtz (1973). Visual receptive fields of frontal eye field neurons. Brain Res., 61, 385-389.

Mohler, C.W., and R.H. Wurtz (1977). Role of striate cortex and superior colliculus in visual guidance of saccadic eye movements in monkeys. J. Neurophysiol,40,74-94.

Money, K.E., and J.W. Scott (1962). Functions of separate sensory receptors of non-auditory labyrinth of cat. Am. J. Physiol., 202, 1211-1220.

Montarolo, P.G., W. Precht, and P. Strata (1981). Functional organization of the mechanisms subserving the optokinetic nystagmus in the cat. Neurosci., 6, 231-246.

Montarolo, P.G., F. Baschi, and P. Strata (1981). Are the climbing fibres essential for the Purkinje cell inhibitory action? Exp. Brain Res., 42, 215-218.

Montgomery, N., K. Fite, and L. Bentson (1979). The anuran accessory optic system: Neuroanatomical analysis. Soc. Neurosci. Abstr., 5, 798.

Moorey, A.J. (1956). Some ocular sequelae of tuberculous meningitis. A preliminary survey. Am. J. Ophthal., 41, 753-768.

Morales-Garcia, C., J.L. Cardenas, C. Arriagada and J. Otte (1978). Clinical significance of rebound nystagmus in neuro-otological diagnosis. Ann. Otol.Rhinol.Lar. 87, 238-242.

Morasso, P., E. Bizzi, and J. Dichgans (1973). Adjustment of saccade characteristics during head movements. Exp. Brain Res., 16, 492-500.

Morgan, B., and B.J. Frost (1981). Visual response characteristics of neurons in nucleus of basal optic root of pigeons. Exp. Brain Res., 42, 181-188.

Morgan Jr, M.W. (1941). Analysis of clinical data. Am. J. Optom. Arch.Am. Acad. Optom., 21(12), 477-491.

Morgan, M.W. (1944). Accommodation and its relationship to convergence. Am. J. Optom. and Arch. Am. Acad. Optom., 21, 183-195.

Morgan, M.W. (1954). The ciliary muscular force required for accommodation.. J. Physiol., 128, 219-229.

Mountcastle, V.B. (1976). The world around us: Neural commant functions for selective attention (The F.O. Schmit Lecture in Neuroscience, 1975). Neurosci.Res. Prog. Bull.14, Suppl., pp 1-47.

Mountcastle, V.B., J.C. Lynch,A. Georgopoulos, H. Sakata, and C. Acuna (1975). The posterior parietal association cortex of the monkey: Command functions for operations within extrapersonal space. J. Neurophysiol., 38, 871-908.

Mowrer, O.H. (1932). Concerning the normal functions of the vestibular apparatus. Ann. Otol. Rhinol. Lar., 41, 412-421.

Mühlendyck, H. (1979). The Faden operation in the treatment of congenital nystagmus. In R. Reinecke (Ed.), Strabismus, Grune & Stratton, New York. pp 235-248.

Mühlendyck, H., and S.A. Ali (1978). Histological and structural studies on the ring-bands in human extraocular muscles.Albrecht v Graefes Arch. Ophthal.,208, 177-191.

Mühlendyck, H., and H.J. Linnen (1975). Die operative Behandlung nystagmusbedingter schwankender Schielwinkel mit der Fadenoperation nach Cüppers. Klin. Mbl. Augenheilk., 167, 273-290.

Mukuno, K. (1966). The fine structure of human extraocular muscles. J. Electron. Micro., 15, 227-236.

Mukuno, K. (1968). The fine structure of human extraocular muscles report 2. The classification of muscle fibers. Acta Soc. Ophthal. Jap., 71, 909-918.

Mukuno, K. (1969). Electron microscopic studies of the extraocular muscles under pathologic conditions. Acta Soc. Ophthal. Jap., 72, 1678-1690.

Mukuno, K., S. Ishikama T. Toga, and M. Humiko (1976). Histopathological study on the overacting inferior oblique muscles with special reference to "central core" within the muscle fibers. Jap. J. Ophthal., 20, 166.

Mulch, G., and W. Lewitzki (1977). Spontaneous and positional nystagmus in healthy persons demonstrated only by electronystagmography: Physiological spontaneous nystagmus or "funtional scar"? Arch. Otol. Rhinol. Lar., 215, 135-145.

Muratore, R., and D.S. Zee (1979). Pursuit after-nystagmus. Vision Res.,19,1057-1059.

Murphy, B.J. (1978). Pattern thresholds for moving and stationary gratings during smooth eye movements. Vision Res., 18, 521-530.

Naegele, J.R., and R. Held (1980). Monocular optokinetic nystagmus shows directional asymmetry in human infants. Invest. Ophth. Vis. Sci. Suppl., p. 210.

Nagel, W.A. (1902). Einige Beobachtungen an einem Fall von totaler Farbenblindheit. Arch. Augenheilk., 44, 153-163.

Nashner, L.M. (1976). Adapting reflexes controlling the human posture. Exp. Brain. Res., 26, 59-72. .

Nettleship, E. (1909). On some hereditary diseases of the eye. Transact. Ophth. Soc. Unit. Kingd., 29, 57-198.

Neville, B.G.R., B.D. Lake, R. Stephens, and M.D.Sanders (1973). A neurovisceral storage disease with vertical supranuclear ophthalmoplegia and its relationship to Neimann-Pick disease. Brain, 96, 97-120.

Newman, N.M., H. Day, and M.J. Aguilar (1978). Paralytic pontine exotropia: A case report with clinicopathologic confirmation. In G. Kommerell (Ed.), Disorders of Ocular Motility, Neurophysiological and Clinical Aspects.Bergmann,München.pp 183-188.

Newman, N., A. Gay, M.H. Stroud, and J. Brooks (1970). Defective rapid eye movements in progressive supranuclear palsy. Brain, 93, 775-784.

Newman, N., A.J. Gay, and M.P. Heilbrun (1971). Disjugate ocular bobbing: Its relation to midbrain, pontine, and medullary function in a surviving patient. Neurology, 21, 633-637.

Nicholson, H. (1924). On the presence of ganglion cells in the III, IV and VI nerves of man. J. Comp. Neurol., 37, 31-36.

Nicolai, H. (1959). Differenzen zwischen optokinetischem Rechts- und Linksnystagmus bei einseitiger Schiel-Amblopie. Klin. Mbl. Augenheilk., 134, 245-250.

Noda, H., and D.A. Suzuki (1978). Purkinje cell activity in the monkey flocculus during smooth pursuit eye movement. Neurosci. Abstr., 4, 167.

Noda, H., and D.A. Suzuki (1979a). The role of the flocculus of the monkey in saccadic eye movements. J. Physiol., 294, 317-334.

Noda, H., and D.A. Suzuki (1979b). Processing of eye movement signals in the flocculus of the monkey. J. Physiol., 294, 349-364.

Norris, H. (1971). The action of sedatives on brainstem oculomotor systems in man. Neuropharmacol., 10, 181-191.

Norton,E.W., and D.G. Cogan (1954). Spasmus nutans. Arch. Ophthal., 52, 442-446.

Nyström, B. (1968a). Histochemistry of developing cat muscles. Acta Neurol. Scand., 44, 405-439.

Nyström, B (1968b). Mechanical and electrical responses to single shocks in developing cat leg muscles following tetanization. Acta Physiol. Scand., 74, 207-225.

Ochs, A.L., L. Stark, W.F. Hoyt, and D. D'Amico (1979). Opposed adducting saccades in convergence-retraction nystagmus. Brain, 102, 497-508.

Ödkvist, L.M., B. Larsby, and S.R.C. Liedgren (1977). Influence of industrial solvents on the vestibular system. XI World Congress in Otorhinolaryngology, Buenos Aires, Argentina.

Ödkvist, L.M., B. Larsby, R. Tham. S.R.C. Liedgren, and G. Aschan (1978). Positional nystagmus by industrial solvents. In J.D. Hood (Ed.), Vestibular Mechanisms in Health and Disease, Academic Press, London. pp 188-194.

Ödkvist, L.M., B. Larsby, R. Tham, and G. Aschan (1979). On the mechanism of vestibular disturbances caused by industrial solvents.Adv.Otol.Rhinol.Lar.,25,167-172.

Ödkvist, L.M., B. Larsby, J.M. Fredrickson, S.R.C. Liedgren, and R. Tham (1980a). Vestibular and oculomotor disturbances caused by industrial solvents. J. Oto-lar., 9, 1, 53-59.

Ogle, K.N., T.G. Martens, and J.A. Dyer (1967). Oculomotor Imbalance in Binocular Vision and Fixation Disparity, Henry Kimpton, London.

Ohm, J. (1929). Zur Tätigkeit des Augenmuskelsenders. 2. Bd. Nichtberufliches Augenzittern, Selbstverlag, Bottrop.

Ohm, J. (1930). Das Augenzittern der Albinos. Arch. Augenheilk., 103, 216-234.

Ohm, J. (1936). Zur Augenzitternk.: über die Bed. der Aufmerksamkeit beim lat. Nystagmus. Albrecht v Graefes Arch. Ophthal., 136, 229-255.

Ohm, J. (1938). Heilung des Augenzitterns bei 2 Geschwistern mit Farbblindheit. Arch. Augenheilk., 95, 200-205.

Ohm, J. (1958). Nystagmus und Schielen bei Sehschwachen und Blinden. Enke, Stutgart.

O'Neill, J.F. (1967). Strabismus in congenital Rubella. Arch. Ophth., 77, 450-454.

Ono, H., S. Nakamizo, and M. Steinback (1978). Nonadditivity of vergence and saccadic eye movements. Vision Res., 18, 545-565.

Optican, L.M. (1978). Cerebellar-dependent adaptive control of the saccadic eye movement system . (Doctoral dissertation), Johns Hopkins University, Baltimore, Maryland.

Optican, L.M., and F.A. Miles (1979). Visually induced adaptive changes in oculomotor control signals. Soc. Neurosci. Abstr., 5, 380.

Optican, L.M., and D.A. Robinson (1980). Cerebellar-dependent adaptive control of primate saccadic system. J. Neurophysiol., 44, 1058-1076.

Optican, L.M., D.S. Zee. F.A. Miles, and S.G. Lisberger (1980). Oculomotor deficits in monkeys with floccular lesions. Soc. Neurosci. Abstr., 6, 474.

Orrison, W.W., and W.G. Robertson (1979). Congenital ocular motor apraxia. Arch. Neurol., 36, 29-31.

Osorio, I., and R.B. Daroff (1980). Absence of REM and altered NREM sleep in patients with spinocerebellar degeneration and slow saccades. Ann. Neurol., 7, 277-280.

Oyster, C.W., J.I. Simpson, E.S. Takahashi, and R.E. Sookak (1980). Retinal ganglion cells projecting to the rabbit accessory optic system. J. Comp.Neurol.,190,49-61.

Oyster, C.W., E. Takahashi, and H. Collewijn (1972). Direction-selective retinal ganglion cells and control of optokinetic nystagmus in the rabbit. Vision Res., 12, 183-193.

Ozawa, T., K. Cheng-Minoda, J. Davidowitz, and G.M. Breinin (1969). Correlation of potential and fiber types in extraocular muscle. Documenta Ophth., 26, 192-210.

Packwood, J., and B. Gordon (1975), Stereopsis in normal domestic cat, Siamese cat, and cat raised with alternate monocular occlusion. J. Neurophysiol., 38,1485-1499.

Panum, P.L. (1858). Physiologische Untersuchungen über das Sehen mit zwei Augen, Schwerssche Buch Handlung, Kiel.

Parinaud, H. (1883). Paralysie des mouvements associen des yeux. Arch. Neurologie (Paris), 5, 145-172.

Parks, M.M. (1977). Operate early for congenital strabismus. In R. J. Broackhurst (Ed.), Controversy in Ophthalmology, W.B. Saunders Co., Philadelphia. p.423.

Pasik, P., T. Pasik, and M.B. Bender (1960). Oculomotor function following cerebral hemidecortication in the monkey. A study with special refernce to optokinetic and vestibular nystagmus. Arch. Neurol., 3, 298-305.

Pasik, P,. and T. Pasik (1964a). Oculomotor functions in monkeys with lesions of the cerebrum and the superior colliculi. In M. Bender (Ed.), The Ocular Motor System. Harper and Row, New York. pp. 40-80.

Pasik, P., and T. Pasik (1964b). Optokinetic nystagmus. An unlearned response altered by section of chiasma and corpus callosum in monkeys. Nature, 203, 609-611.

Pasik, P., T. Pasik, and M.B. Bender (1969). The pretectal syndrome in monkeys. I. Disturbances of gaze and body posture. Brain, 92, 521-534.

Paty, D.W., and H. Sherr (1972). Ocular bobbing in bromism. A case report. Neurology, 22, 526-527.

Pedersen, P., and C.L. Schmidt (1978). Ein Analysator zur halbautomatischen, quantitativen Nystagmusauswertung. Arch. Otol. Rhinol. Lar., 219, 425.

Pedersen, R.A., B.T. Troost, L.A. Abel, and D. Zorub (1980). Intermittent downbeat nystagmus and oscillopsia reversed by suboccipital craniectomy. Neurology, 30, 1239-1242.

Pellionisz, A., and R. Llinas (1980). Tensorial approach to the geometry of brain function. Neurosci., 5, 1125-1136.

Penfield, W., and H. Jasper (1954).Epilepsy and the functional anatomy of the human brain. Little, Brown and Co., Boston. pp 269-270, 370-371.

Perenin, M.T., and M. Jeannerod (1978). Visual function within the hemianopic field following early cerebral hemidecortication in man. I. Spatial localization. Neuropsychologica, 16, 1-13.

Perryman, J.H., and G.M. Breinin (1971). Coordination of the recti muscles in the cat. Invest. Ophthal., 10, 78-86.

Peterman, A.F., and R.G. Siekert (1960). The alteral medullary (Wallenberg) syndrome: Clinical features and prognosis. Med. Clin. N. Am., 44, 887-896.

Peterson, G.M., and R.Y. Moore (1980). Selective effects of kainic acid on diencephalic neurons. Brain Res., 202, 165-182.

Pettorossi, V.E., and G.M. Filippi (1981). Muscle spindle autogenetic inhibition in the extraocular muscles of the lamb. Arch. Ital. Biol. In press.

Pierrot-Deseilligny, C., S. Prier, M. Masson, and J. Cambier (1978). Enregistrement des mouvements oculaires chez l´homme lors de lésions unilatérales de la formation réticulaire pontine paramédiane. Contribution à la physiologie du regard latéral à partir de deux observations. Rev. Neurol. (Paris)., 134, 355-366.

Pierrot-Deseilligny,C., F. Chain, F. Gray, R. Escourolle, and P. Castaigne (1979). Paralysies supranucléaires de la latéralité d'origine protubérantielle. Rev. Neurol. (Paris), 135, 741-762.

Pinhas, I., A. Pinhas, Y. Goldhammer, and J. Braham (1978). Progressive supranuclear palsy: Electromyographic examinations of eye muscles. Acta Neurol. Scand., 58, 304-308.

Pola, J., and D.A. Robinson (1978). Oculomotor signals in the medial longitudinal fasciculus of the monkey. J. Neurophysiol., 41, 245-259.

Pola, J., and H.J. Wyatt (1980). Target position and velocity: The stimuli for smooth pursuit eye movements. Vision Res., 20, 523-534.

Pompeiano, O., T. Mergner, and N. Corvaja (1978). Commissural, perihypoglossal and reticular afferent projections to the vestibular nuclei in the cat. An experimental anatomical study with the method of the retrograde transport of horseradish peroxidase. Arch. Ital. Biol., 116, 130-172.

Pompeiano, O., and F. Walberg (1958). Descending connections to the vestibular nuclei, an experimental study in the cat. J.Comp. Neurol., 108, 465-503.

Poppel, E., R. Held, and D. Forst (1973). Residual visual function after brain wounds involving the central visual pathways in man. Nature, 243, 295-596.

Potashner, S.J. (1979). Baclofen: Effects on amino acid release and metabolism in slices of guinea pig cerebral cortex. J. Neurochem., 32, 103-109.

Pratt-Johnson, J.A. (1976). Sensory basis for prismotherapy in esotropia. In P.Fells (Ed.), Proc. Second Congress of the I.S.A., Diffusion générale du Librairie, Marseille. pp 274-280.

Precht, W. (1974). The physiology of the vestibular nuclei. Handbook of Sensory Physiology VI/I, Springer. pp 353-416.
Precht, W. (1981). Visual-vestibular interaction in vestibular neurons: Functional pathway organization. In B. Cohen (Ed.), Recent Advances in Oculomotor and Vestibular Physiology. Ann. N.Y. Acad. Sci., In press.
Precht, W., and L. Cazin (1979). Functional deficits in the optokinetic system of albino rats. Exp. Brain Res., 37, 183-186.
Precht, W., P.G. Montarolo, and P. Strata (1980). The role of the crossed and uncrossed retinal fibers in mediating the horizontal optokinetic nystagmus in the cat. Neurosci. Letters, 17, 39-42.
Precht, W., J.I. Simpson, and R. Llinas (1976). Responses of Purkinje cells in rabbit nodulus and uvula to natural vestibular and visual stimuli. Pflügers Arch., 367, 1-6.
Precht, W., and P. Strata (1980). On the pathway mediating optokinetic responses in vestibular nuclear neurons. Neurosci., 5, 777-787.
Quéré, M.A., G. Chargeau, and A. Pecherau (1978). L´association chirurgie du fil-chirurgie classic dans le cure operatoire des esotropies. Bull. Soc. Ophth. de France, 78, 373.
Rahn, A.C., and B.L. Zuber (1971). Cerebellar evoked potentials resulting from extra-ocular muscle stretch.Evidence against a cerebellar origin.Exp.Neurol., 31,230-238.
Raphan, T., and B. Cohen (1978). Brainstem mechanisms for rapid and slow eye movements. Ann. Rev. Physiol., 40, 527-552.
Raphan, T., and B. Cohen (1980). Integration and its relation to ocular compensatory movements. Mt. Sinai J. Med., 47, 410-417.
Raphan, T., B. Cohen, and V. Henn (1981). Effects of gravity on rotatory nystagmus in monkey. In B. Cohen (Ed.), Recent Advances in Oculomotor and Vestibular Physiology. Ann. N.Y. Acad. Sci., In press.
Raphan, T., B. Cohen, and V. Matsuo (1977). A velocity-storage mechanism responsible for optokinetic nystagmus (OKN), optokinetic after-nystagmus (OKAN) and vestibular nystagmus. In R. Baker and A. Berthoz (Eds.), Control of Gaze by Brain Stem Neurons, Biomed. Press, Elsevier, Amsterdam. pp 37-47.
Raphan, T., V. Matsuo, and B. Cohen (1979). Velocity storage in the vestibulo-ocular reflex arc VOR. Exp. Brain Res.,35, 229-248.
Raphan, T., W. Waespe, and B. Cohen (1981). Vestibular nerve activity induced by off-vertical axis rotation. Neurosci. Abstr., In press.
Rashbass, C. (1961). The relationship between saccadic and smooth tracking eye movements. J. Physiol., 159, 326-338.
Rashbass, C., and G. Westheimer (1961). Disjunctive eye movements. J. Physiol., 159 (2), 339-360.
Reason, J.T., and J.J. Brand (1975). Motion Sickness, Academic Press, London.
Reese, W.S., and J.C. Yaskin (1941). Preservation of convergence with paralysis of all lateral movements in a case of intramedullary tumor of the pons. Am. J. Ophthal,24, 544-549. .
Reinecke, R.D., and K. Simons (1975). Phoria and EOM afference: Preliminary support for a new theory. In G. Lennerstrand and P. Bach-y-Rita (Eds.), Basic Mechanisms of Ocular Motility and Their Clinical Implications. Pergamon Press,Oxford,pp.113-117.
Richards, W. (1970). Stereopsis and Stereoblindness. Exp. Brain Res., 10 (4), 380-388.
Richards , W. (1977). Stereopsis with and without monocular contours. Vision Res., 17, 967-969.
Ridley, R.M., and E. Ettlinger (1975). Tactile and visuo-spatial discrimination performance in the monkey: The effects of total and partial posterior parietal removals. Neuropsychologia,13, 191-206.
Ringel, S.P., W.B. Wilson, M.T. Barden, and K.K. Kaiser (1978). Histochemistry of human extraocular muscle. Arch. Ophth. , 96, 1067.
Ritchie, L. (1976). Effects of cerebellar lesions on saccadic eye movements. J. Neurophysiol., 39, 1246-1256.
Roberts, T.D.M. (1967). Neurophysiology of postural mechanisms. Butterworths,London.
Robinson, D.A. (1963). A method of measuring eye movement using a scleral search coil in a magnetic field. IEEE Trans. Biomed. Electron. BME, 10, 37-145.
Robinson, D.A. (1964). The mechanics of human saccadic eye movement. J. Physiol., 174, 245-264.

Robinson, D.A. (1964). The mechanics of human saccadic eye movement. J. Physiol., 174, 245-264.

Robinson, D.A. (1965). The mechanics of human smooth pursuit eye movement. J. Physiol., 180, 569-591.

Robinson, D.A. (1968a). Eye movement control in primates, Science, 161, 1219-1224.

Robinson, D.A. (1968b). The oculomotor control system: A review. Proc. IEEE, 56, 1032-1049.

Robinson, D.A. (1970). Oculomotor unit behaviour in the monkey. J. Neurophysiol. 33, 393-404.

Robinson, D.A. (1972). Eye movements evoked by collicular stimulation in the alert monkey. Vision Res., 12, 1795-1808.

Robinson, D.A. (1973). Models of the saccadic eye movement control system. Kybernetik, 14, 71-83.

Robinson, D.A. (1975a). Oculomotor control signals. In G. Lennerstrand and P. Bach-y-Rita (Eds.), Basic Mechanisms of Ocular Motility and Their Clinical Implications, Pergamon Press, Oxford. pp.337-374.

Robinson, D.A. (1975b). How the ocular motor system repairs itself. Invest. Ophth., 14, 413-415.

Robinson, D.A. (1976). Adaptive gain control of vestibulo-ocular reflex by the cerebellum. J. Neurophysiol., 39, 954-969.

Robinson, D.A. (1977). Linear addition of optokinetic and vestibular signals in the vestibular nucleus. Exp. Brain Res., 30, 447-450.

Robinson, D.A., and A.F. Fuchs (1969), Eye movements evoked by stimulation of frontal eye fields. J. Neurophysiol., 32, 637-648.

Robinson, D.L., M.E. Goldberg, and G.B. Stanton (1978). Parietal association cortex in the primate: Sensory mechanisms and behavioural modulations. J. Neurophysiol., 41, 910-932.

Robinson, D.A.,D. O'Meara, A.B. Scott, and C.C. Collins (1969). The mechanical components of human eye movements. J. Appl. Physiol., 26, 548-553.

Rodieck, R.W. (1979). Visual pathways. Ann. Rev. Neurosci., 2, 193-225.

Rodin, E.A. (1964). Impaired ocular pursuit movements. Arch. Neurol., 10, 327-330.

Roelofs, C.O. (1928). Nystagmus latens. Arch. Augenheilk., 98, 401-447.

Ron, S., and D.A. Robinson (1973). Eye movements evoked by cerebellar stimulation in the alert monkey. J. Neurophysiol., 36, 1004-1022.

Ron, S., D.A. Robinson, and A.A. Skavenski (1972). Saccades and the quick phase of nystagmus. Vision Res., 12, 2015-2022.

Rosenberg, M.A., J.A. Sharpe, and W.F. Hoyt (1975). Absent vestibulo-ocular reflexes and acute supratentorial lesions. J. Neurol. Neurosurg. Psychiat., 38, 6-10.

Ryan, S.J., F.M. Blanton. and G.K. von Noorden (1965). Surgery of congenital cataract. Am. J. Ophthal., 60, 583-587.

Sachais, B.A., J.N. Logue, and M.S. Carey (1977). Baclofen, a new antispasmotic drug, a controlled, multicenter trial in patients with multiple sclerosis. Arch. Neurol., 34, 422-428

Sakata, H., H. Shibutani, and K. Kawano (1978). Parietal neurons with dual sensitivity to real and induced movements of visual target. Neursci. Letters, 9, 165-169.

Sakimoto, T. (1968). Electron microscopic studies on human extraocular muscles. J. Electron. Micro., 4, 227.

Sasaki, K. (1963). Electrophysiological studies on oculomotor neurons of the cat. Jap. J. Physiol., 13, 287-302.

Saye, A. and J.P. Frisby (1975). The role of monocular conspicuous features in facilitating stereopsis from random dot stereograms. Perception, 4, 159-171.

Schairer, J.O., and M.V.L. Bennett (1977). Adaptive gain control in vestibulo-ocular reflex of goldfish. Neurosci. Abstr., 3, 157.

Schairer, J.O., and M.V.L. Bennett (1978). VOR gain changes produced by target rotation without head movement in goldfish. Neurosci. Abstr., 4, 167.

Schairer, J.O., and M.V.L. Bennett (1980). Cerebellectomy in goldfish prevents adaptive gain control of the VOR affecting the optokinetic system. In T. Gualtierotte (Ed.), Neuroscience Satellite Symposium on Vestibular Function and Morphology. Springer-Verlag, New York. In press.

Schalen, L. (1980). Quantification of tracking eye movements in normal subjects. Acta Oto-lar., 90, 404-413.

Schiller, P.H., and F. Koerner (1971). Discharge characteristics of single units in superior colliculus of the alert rhesus monkey. J. Neurophysiol., 34, 920-936.

Schiller. P.H., S.D. True, and J.L. Conway (1979). Effects of frontal eye field and superior colliculus ablations on eye movements. Science, 206, 590-592.

Schiller, P., S.D. True, and J.L. Conway (1980). Deficits in eye movements following frontal eye-field and superior colliculus ablations. J. Neurophysiol.,44,1175-1189.

Schlag, J., M. Schlag-Rey, C.K. Peck, and J.P. Joseph (1980). Visual responses of thalamus neurons depending on the direction of gaze and the position of targets in space. Exp. Brain Res., 40, 170-184.

Schlag-Rey, M., and J. Schlag (1980). Saccade-related neurons in primate thalamus. Soc. Neurosci. Abstr., 6, 317.

Schmid, R., D. Zambarbieri, and G. Magenes (1981). Modifications of vestibular nystagmus produced by fixation of visual and non-visual targets. In B. Cohen (Ed.), Recent Advances in Oculomotor and Vestibular Physiology.Proc.N.Y.Acad.Sci.In press.

Schmidt, D., L.A. Dell'Osso, and L.A. Abel (1980). Normal saccadic structure of voluntary nystagmus. Arch. Ophthal., 95, 1399-1404.

Schmidt, J.G., and K.U. Smith (1971). Feedback analysis of eye tracking of auditory and tactual stimuli. Am. J. Optom., 48, 204-209.

Schor, C.M. (1975). A directional impairment of eye movement control in strabismus amblyopia. Invest. Ophthal., 14, 692.

Schor, C.M. (1979a). The influence of rapid prism adaptation upon fixation disparity. Vision Res., 17, 757-765.

Schor, C.M. (1979b). The relationship between fusional vergence eye movements and fixation disparity. Vision Res., 19, 1359-1367.

Schor, C.M. (1980). Fixation disparity: A steady state error. Am. J. Physiol. Opt. Optom., 57, 618-631.

Schor, C.M. (1981). Directional anisotropies of pursuit tracking and optokinetic nystagmus in abnormal binocular vision. In D. Fender and B. Cooper (Eds.), Ocular Motor Symposium, Cal-Tech Press, Pasadena, California. pp 83-104.

Schor, C., and D.L. Levi (1979). Abnormal optokinetic nystagmus of amblyopic eyes. Suppl. Invest. Ophthal. Vis. Sci., 18, 201.

Schor,C., and D.L. Levi (1980). Disturbances of small field horizontal and vertical optokinetic nystagmus in amblyopia. Invest. Ophthal. Vis. Sci., 19, 668-684.

Schor, C., and V. Narayan (1981). The influence of field size upon the spatial frequency response of optokinetic nystagmus. Vision Res. , In press.

Schor, C.M., and V. Narayan (1982). Graphical analysis of prism adaptation, convergence accommodation and accommodative convergence. Am.J.Optom. Physiol. Opt., 59, In press.

Schor, C.M., and C.W. Tyler (1981). Spatio-temporal properties of Panum´s fusional area. Vision Res., 21, 683-692.

Schwartz, A.S., and E. Eidelberg (1968). "Extinction" to bilateral simultaneous stimulation in the monkey. Neurology, 18, 61-68.

Schwindt, P.C., W. Precht, and A. Richter (1974). Monosynaptic excitatory and inhibitory pathways from medial midbrain nuclei to trochlear mononeurons. Exp. Brain Res., 20, 223-238.

Scott, A.B. (1980). Botulinum toxin injection into extraocular muscles as an alternative to strabismus surgery. Ophthalmology, 87, 1044-1049.

Scott, A.B., and C. Collins (1973). Division of labor in human extraocular muscle. Arch. Ophthal., 90, 319-322.

Scott, A.B., A.L. Rosenbaum, and C.Collins (1973). Pharmacologic weakening of extraocular muscles. Invest. Ophthal., 12, 232-233.

Scott, W.E. (1977). Office use of prisms. In Symposium on Strabismus. Trans. of the New Orleans Acad. of Ophthal., C.V. Mosby, St. Louis.

Scott, W.E, and D.E. Braverman (1977). Surgical treatment of dissociated vertical deviations. J. Ped. Ophthal., 14, 337-342.

Segarra, J.M. (1970). Cerebrovascular disease and beaviour. I. The syndrome of the mesencephalic artery. Arch. Neurol., 22, 408-418.

Selhorst, J.B., L. Stark, A.L. Ochs, and W.F. Hoyt (1976a). Disorders in cerebellar ocular motor control. I. Saccadic overshoot dysmetria an oculographic, control system and clinico-anatomical analysis. Brain, 99, 497-508.

Selhorst, J.B., L. Stark, A.L. Ochs, and W.F. Hoyt (1976b). Disorders in cerebellar ocular motor control. II. Macrosaccadic oscillation an oculographic, control system and clinico-anatomical analysis. Brain, 99, 509-522.

Semmlow, J.L., and D. Heerema (1979). The synkinetic interaction of convergence accommodation and accommodative convergence. Vision Res., 19, 1237-1242.

Semmlow, J.L., and G. Hung (1979). Accommodative and fusional components of fixation disparity. Invest. Ophthal. Vis. Sci., 18, 1082-1086.

Semmlow, J.L., and G. Hung (1981). Experimental evidence for separate mechanisms mediating accommodative convergence and convergence accommodation. Documenta Ophthal. In press.

Semmlow, J.L., and R. Jaeger (1972). Modelling the visual motor triad: An example of a multiple intput-output biocontrol system. Proc. 24th ACEMB, Bal Harbor,Florida.

Semmlow, J.L., and N. Venkiteswaran (1976). Dynamic accommodative vergence in binocular vision. Vision Res., 16, 403-411.

Semmlow, J.L., and P. Wetzel (1979). Dynamic contributions of binocular vergence components. J. Optom. Soc. Am., 69, 639-645.

Shagrass, C., R.A. Roemer, and A. Amadeo (1976). Eye-tracking performance and engagement of attention. Arch. Gen. Psychiat., 33, 121-125.

Sharpe, J.A., and H. Deck (1978). Destruction of the internal sagittal stratum and normal smooth pursuit. Ann. Neurol., 4, 473-476.

Sharpe, J.A., M.E. Goldberg, A.W. Lo, and Y.O. Herishanu (1981). Visual-vestibular interaction in multiple sclerosis. Neurology, 31, 427-433.

Sharpe, J.A., Y.O. Herishanu, and O.B. White (1982). Cerebral square wave jerks. Neurology, In press.

Sharpe, J.A., and A.W. Lo (1981). Voluntary and visual control of the vestibulo-ocular reflex after cerebral hemidecortication. Ann. Neurol., 10, 164-172.

Sharpe, J.A., A.W. Lo, and H.E. Rabinovitch (1979). Control of the saccadic and smooth pursuit systems after cerebral hemidecortication. Brain, 102, 387-403.

Sharpe, J.A., M.A. Rosenberg, W.F. Hoyt, and R.B. Daroff (1974). Paralytic pontine exotropia - a sign of acute unilateral pontine gaze palsy and internuclear ophthalmoplegia. Neurology, 24, 1076-1081.

Sharpe, J.A., and T.O. Sylvester (1978). Effect of aging on horizontal smooth pursuit. Invest. Ophthal. Vis. Sci., 17, 465.468.

Shea, S.L., R. Fox, R.N. Aslin, and S.T. Dumais (1980). Assessment of stereopsis in human infants. Invest. Ophthal. Vis. Sci, 19, 1400-1404.

Sheard, C (1930). Zones of ocular comfort. Am. J. Optom, 7, 9-25.

Sherman, S.M. (1972). Development of interocular alignment in cats. Brain Res.,37, 187-203.

Sherrington, C.S. (1918). Observations on the sensual role of the proprioveptive nerve supply of the extrinsic eye muscles. Brain, 41, 332-343.

Shibasaki. H., S. Tsuji, and Y. Kuroiwa (1978). Oculomotor abnormalities in Parkinson´s disease. Arch. Neurol., 36, 360-364.

Shimazu, H.S., and W. Precht (1965). Tonic and kinetic responses of cat´s vestibular neurons to horizontal angular acceleration. J. Neurophysiol., 28, 991-1013.

Shimizu, N., M. Mizuni, M. Naito, and M. Yoshida (1981). The interaction between accuracy of gaze with and without head movements in patients with cerebellar ataxia. In B. Cohen (Ed.), Recent Advances in Oculomotor and Vestibular Physiology. Ann. N.Y. Acad. Sci., In press.

Shy, G.M., W.K. Engel, J.E. Somers, and T. Wanko (1963). Nemalin myopathy. Brain, 89, 793.

Sills, A.W., V. Honrubia, H.R. Konrad, and R.W. Baloh (1975). A rapid optokinetic nystagmus test: Comparison with standard testing. ORL., 82, 223-231.

Simpson, J.I., and K.E. Alley (1974). Visual climbing fiber input to rabbit vestibulo-cerebellum: A source of direction-specific information. Brain Res.,82,302-308.

Simpson, J.I., R.E. Soodak, and R. Hess (1979). The accessory optic system and its relation to the vestibulo-cerebellum. In R. Granit and O. Pompeiano (Eds.), Reflex Control of Posture and Movement. Prog. Brain Res., 50, 715-724. Elsevier-North Holland, Amsterdam.

Skavenski, A.A. (1972). Inflow as a source of extraretinal eye position information. Vision Res., 12, 221-229.

Skavenski, A.A., S.M. Blair, and G. Westheimer (1981). The effect of habituating vestibular and optokinetic nystagmus on each other. J. Neurosci., 1, 351-357.

Skavenski, A.A., R. Hansen, R.M. Steinman, and B.J. Winterson (1979). Quality of retinal image stabilization during small natural and artificial body rotations in man. Vision Res., 19, 675-683.

Skavenski, A.A., and D.A. Robinson (1973). Role of abducens neurons in vestibulo-ocular reflex. J. Neurophysiol., 36, 724-738.

Skavenski, A.A., and R.M. Steinman (1970). Control of eye position in the dark. Vision Res., 10, 193-203.

Smith, J.L. (1963). Optokinetic nystagmus. C.C. Thomas, Springfield. Illinois.

Smith, P. (1876). Bilateral deviations of the eyes. Ophthal. Hosp. Rep.,9-10,428-433.

Smith, R.S., and W.K. Ovalle (1973). Varieties of fast and slow extrafusal muscle fibers in amphibian hind limb muscles. J. Anat., 116, 1-24.

Smithburn. K.C., G.F. Kempf, L.G. Zerfasrand, and L.H. Gilman (1930). Meningococcic meningitis: Clinical study of 144 epidemic cases. J. Am. Med.Ass., 95, 776-780.

Sogg, R.L., and W. Hoyt (1962). Intermittent vertical nystagmus in a father and son. Arch. Ophthal., 68, 515-517.

Sommerkamp, H. (1928). Das Substrat der Daververkurzung am Froschmuskel. Arch. Exp. Path. Pharmac., 128, 99.

Spencer, R.F., C. Evinger, and R. Baker (1981). Soc. Neusosci. Abstr., In press.

Spencer, R.F., and K.W. McNeer (1978). Structural alterations in overacting inferior oblique muscles. Arch. Ophthal., 98, 128-133.

Spencer, R.F., and J.D. Porter (1981). The innervation and structure of extraocular muscles in the monkey in comparison to the cat. J. Comp. Neurol, 198, 649-665.

Spiegel, E.A., and J.B. Price (.1939). Origin of the quick component of labyrinthine nystagmus. Arch. Oto-lar., 30, 576-588.

Spielmann, A., and J. Laulan (1978). Action of recessions and resections when associated with Cüppers Fadenoperation in esotropia. Statistical results. In R. Reinecke (Ed.), Strabismus, Grune & Stratton, N.Y., p 355.

Spiller, W.G. (1905). The importance in clinical diagnosis of paralysis of associated movements of the eyeballs (Blicklaehmung), especially of upward and downward associated movements. J. Nerv. Ment. Dis., 32, 417-488, 497-530.

Sprague, J.B., S. Moore, H.Eggers, and P.H. Knapp (1980). Dissociated vertical deviation. Treatment with the Fadenoperation of Cüppers. Arch. Ophthal.,98, 465.

St. Cyr, G.J., and D.H. Fender (1965).Nonlinearities of the human oculomotor system: Gain. Vision Res., 9, 1235-1246.

Stanton, G.B. (1980). Afferents to oculomotor nuclei from area "Y" in Macaca mulatta: An anterograde degeneration study. J. Comp. Neurol., 192, 377-385.

Stark, L. (1967). Three nonexclusive hypotheses on the physiology of the cerebellum with six appended remarks on varied topics in neurophysiology. Presented at Salisan Conference on the Cerebellum, Neurosciences Program, Salisan, Oregon.

Stark. L, (1968). Neurological control systems. Plenum Press, N.Y.

Stark. L., A.T. Bahill, K.J. Ciuffreda, R.V. Kenyon, and S. Phillips (1977). Neuro-optometry: An evolving specialty clinic. Am. J. Optom. Physiol. Opt., 54, 85-96.

Stark. L, R.V. Kenyon, V.V. Krishnan, and K.J. Ciuffreda (1980). Disparity vergence: A proposed name for a dominant component of binocular vergence eye movements. Am. J. Optom. Physiol. Opt., 57, 606-609.

Stark, L., G. Vossius, and L.R. Young (1962). Predictive control of eye tracking movements. IEEE Trans. Hum. Fact. Electr., HFE-3, 52-57.

Steele, J.C., J.C. Richardson, and J. Olszewski (1964). Progressive supranuclear palsy. Arch. Neurol., 10, 333-359.

Steer, R.W. (1967). The influence of angular and linear acceleration and thermal stimulation on the human semicircular canals. Sc.D. Thesis. M.I.T. Press, Cambridge, Massachusetts, MVT-67-3.

Steiger, H.-J., and A.J. Büttner-Ennever (1978). Relationship between motoneurons and internuclear neurons in the abducens nucleus: A double retrograde tracer study in the cat. Brain Res., 148, 181-188.

Steiger, H.-J., and J.A. Büttner-Ennever (1979). Oculomotor nucleus afferents in the monkey demonstrated with horeradish peroxidase. Brain Res., 160, 1-15.

Stein, B.M., and M.B. Carpenter (1967). Central projections of portions of the vestibular ganglia innervating specific parts of the labyrinth in the rhesus monkey. Am. J. Anat., 120, 281-318.

Steinbach, M.J. (1969). Eye tracking of self-moved targets: The role of efference. J. Exp. Psychol., 82, 366-376.

Steinbach, M.J. (1976). Pursuing the perceptual rather than the retinal stimulus. Vision Res., 16, 1371-1376.

Steinbach, M.J., and R. Held (1968). Eye tracking of observer-generated target movements. Science, 161, 187-188.

Steinbach, M.J., and D.G. Pierce (1972). Release of pursuit eye movements using after-images. Vision Res., 12, 1307-1311.

Steinman, R.M., and H. Collewijn (1980). Binocular retinal image motion during active head rotation. Vision Res., 20, 415-429.

Steinman, R.M., A.A. Skavenski, and R.V. Sandbury (1969). Voluntary control of smooth pursuit velocity. Vision Res., 9, 1167-1171.

Stibbe, E.P. (1929). Sensory component of the motor nerves of the eye. J. Anat., 64, 112-113.

Stoper, A.E. (1967). Vision during pursuit movement: The role of oculomotor information. Ph. D. Thesis, Brandis University.

Stoper, A.E. (1973). Apparent motion of stimuli presented stroboscopically during pursuit movement of the eye. Percept. Psychophysiol., 13, 201-211.

Stratton, G.M. (1897). Vision without inversion of the retinal image. Psychol. Rev., 4, 341-360, 463-481.

Sugie, N., and M. Wakakuwa (1970). Visual target tracking with active head rotation. IEEE Trans. Systems Sci. Cybernetics, 6, 103-109.

Susac, J.O., W.F. Hoyt, R.B. Daroff, and W. Lawrence (1970). Clinical spectrum of ocular bobbing. J. Neurol. Neurosurg. Psychiat., 33, 771-775.

Swan, K.C. (1947). A squint syndrome. Arch. Ophthal., 37, 149-154.

Szentagothai, J. (1943). Die zentrale Innervation der Augenbewegungen. Arch. Psych. Nervenkr., 116, 721-760.

Tait, E.F. (1951). Accommodative convergence. Am.J. Ophthal., 34, 1093-1108.

Takahashi, M., M. Igarashi, and J.L. Homick (1977). Effect of otolith end organ ablation on horizontal optokinetic nystagmus, and optokinetic after-nystagmus in the squirrel monkey. ORL, 39, 74-81.

Takahashi, M., T. Uemura, and T. Fujishiro (1980). Studies on vestibulo-ocular reflex by means of active head movements. Acta Oto-lar., 90, 115-124.

Takahashi, M., T. Uemura, and T. Fujishiro (1981). Optokinetic reactions during free head rotations. Acta Oto-rhino-lar., 43, 39-49.

Takemori, S., and B. Cohen (1974). Loss of visual suppression of vestibular nystagmus after flocculus lesions. Brain Res., 72, 213-224.

Takemori, S., and L. Suzuki (1977). Cerebellar contribution to oculomotor function. ORL, 39, 209-217.

Tauber, E.S., and A. Atkin (1968). Optomotor responses to monocular stimulation: Relation to visual system organization. Science, N.Y., 160, 1365-1367.

Teller, D.Y. (1979). The forced-choice preferential looking procedure: A psychophysical technique for use with human infants. Infant. Behav. Devel., 2, 135.

Terasawa, K., K. Otani, and J. Yamada (1979). Descending pathways of the nucleus of the optic tract in the rat. Brain Res., 173, 405-417.

Teräväinen, H (1968). Electron microscopic and histochemical observations on different types of nerve endings in the extraocular muscles of the rat. Z. Zellforsch., 90, 372-388.

Teräväinen, H., and D.B. Calne (1980). Studies of Parkinsonian movement: 1. Programming and execution of eye movements. Acta Neurol. Scand., 62, 137-148.

Ter Braak, J.W.G. (1936). Untersuchungen über optokinetischen Nystagmus. Arch. Neerl. Physiol., 21, 309-376.

Ter Braak, J.W.G., V.W.D. Schenk, and A.G.M. VanVliet (1971). Visual reactions in a case of long-lasting cortical blindness. J. Neurol. Neurosurg. Psychiat., 34, 140-147.

Ter Braak, J.W.G., and A.G.M. VanVliet (1963). Subcortical optokinetic nystagmus in the monkey. Psychiat. Neurol. Neurochir., 66, 277-283.

Tham, R., B. Larsby, L.M. Ödkvist, B. Norlander, D. Hydén, G. Aschan, and Å. Bertler (1979). The influence of trichloroethylene and related drugs on the vestibular system. Acta Pharmac. Tox., 44, 336-342.

Tham, R., B. Larsby, B. Eriksson. I. Bunnfors, L.M. Ödkvist, and S.R.C. Liedgren (1981). Electronystagmographic findings in rats exposed to styrene or toluene. Acta Oto-lar., In press.

Thickbroom, G.W., and J.L. Black (1980). Eye motion kinetics in moving target pursuit: A system for detection of oculomotor abnormalities in neurological disorders. Int. J. Biomed. Comput., 11, 427-439.

Thomas, A., H. Schaefer, and F. Bertrand (1933). Paralysie de l´abaissement du regard, paralysie des infergyres. hypertonie des superogyres et des releveurs du regards. Rev. Neurol., 40, 535-542.

Thompson, R.H. (1929). Occlusion of the posterior inferior cerebellar artery. A clinical study of four cases. Arch.Neurol. Psychol., 22, 530-546.

Tigges, J., J. Bos, and M. Tigges (1977). An autoradiographic investigation of the subcortical visual system in chimpanzees. J. Comp. Neurol., 172, 367-380.

Tigges, J., and M. Tigges (1969). The accessory optic system in Erinacues (insectivora) and Galago (primates). J. Comp. Neurol., 137, 59-70.

Toates, F.M. (1974). Vergence eye movements. Documenta ophth., 37, 153-214.

Tomlinson, R.D., and D.A.Robinson (1981). Is the vestibulo-ocular reflex cancelled by pursuit? In W. Becker and A.F. Fuchs (Eds.), Progress in Oculomotor Research, Elsevier, New York, In press.

Tozer, F.M. (1912). On the presence of ganglion cells in the roots of III, IV and VI cranial nerves. J. Physiol., 45, 15-16.

Traub, M., J. Rothwell, and C. Marsden (1980). Anticipatory postural reflexes in Parkinson´s disease and other akinetic-rigid syndromes and in cerebellar ataxia. Brain, 103, 393-412.

Travers, T.B. (1936). The comparison between the results obtained by various methods employed for the treatment of concomitant strabismus. G. Pulman & Sons, London.

Trojanowski, J.Q., and S.H. Wray (1980). Vertical gaze ophthalmoplegia: Selective paralysis of downgaze. Neurology, 30, 605-610.

Troost, B.T., and R.B. Daroff (1977). The ocular motor defects in progressive supranuclear palsy (PSP). Ann. Neurol., 2, 397-403.

Troost, B.T., R.B. Daroff, and L.F. Dell´Osso (1972a). Hemispheric control of eye movements. I. Quantitative analysis of refixation saccades in a hemispherectomy patient. Arch. Neurol., 27, 441-448.

Troost, B.T., R.B. Daroff, and L.F. Dell´Osso (1972b). Hemispheric control of eye movements. II. Quantitative analysis of smooth pursuit in a hemispherectomy patient. Arch. Neurol., 27, 449-452.

Troost, B.T., R.B. Daroff, and L.F. Dell´Osso (1974). Eye tracking patterns in schizophrenia. Science, 184, 1202-1203.

Troost, B.T., R.B. Daroff, and L.F. Dell´Osso (1976). Quantitative analysis of the ocular motor deficit in progressive supranuclear palsy (PSP). Trans. Am. Neurol. Ass., 101, 60-64.

True, S., P. Schiller, and J. Conway (1979). Eye movement control: The effects of joint superior colliculus and frontal eye field stimulation. Abstr. Soc. Neurosci., 5, 389.

Uemara, T., Y. Arai, and C. Shimazaki (1980). Eye-head coordination during lateral gaze in normal subjects. Acta Oto-lar., 90, 191-198.

Uemara, T., and B. Cohen (1973). Effects of vestibular nuclei lesions on vestibulo-ocular reflexes and posture in monkeys. Acta Oto-lar., Suppl., 315, 1-71.

Ungerleider, L.G., and M. Mishkin (1980). Two cortical visual systems. In D.J. Ingle, R.J.W. Mansfield, and M.A. Goodale (Eds.), Advances in the Analysis of Visual Bevaiour, MIT Press, Cambridge, Massachusetts.

Updyke, B.V. (1977). Topographic organization of the projections from the cortical areas 17, 18 and 19 onto the thalamus, pretectum and superior colliculus in the cat. J. Comp. Neurol., 173, 81-122.

Van Bogaert, L., and I. Bertrand (1928). Sur les myoclinies associées synchrones rhythmiques par lesions en foyer du bronc cérébral. Revue Neurol., 1,203.

Van Die, G., and H. Collewijn (1981). Optokinetic nystagmus in man: Role of central and peripheral retina and occurence of asymmetries. Human Neurobiol., In press.

Van Gisbergen, J.A.M., D.A.Robinson, and S. Gielen (1981). A quantitative analysis of saccadic eye movements by burst neurons. J. Neurophysiol., 45, 417-442.

Van Hof-Van Duin, J. (1976). Early and permanent effects of monocular deprivation on pattern discrimination and visuomotor behaviour in cats. Brain Res.,111,261-276.

Van Hof-Van Duin, J. (1978a). Asymmetry of optokinetic nystagmus observed in normal kittens and light deprived cats. In G. Kommerell (Ed.), Disorders of Ocular Motility,Neurophysiological and Clinical Aspects, Bergmann Verlag, München, pp. 363-366.

Van Hof-Van Duin, J. (1978b). Direction preference of optokinetic responses in monocularly tested normal kittens and light-deprived cats. Arch. Ital. Biol., 116, 471-477.

Van Sluyters, R.C., and D.L. Stewart (1974a). Binocular neurons of the rabbit´s visual cortex: Receptive field characteristics. Exp.Brain Res., 19, 166-195.

Van Sluyters, R.C., and D.L. Stewart (1974b). Binocular neurons of the rabbit´s visual cortex: Effects of monocular sensory deprivation. Exp.Brain Res.,19,196-204.

Van Vliet, A.G.M. (1973). On the central mechanism of latent nystagmus. Acta Ophthal., 51, 772-781.

Van Vliet, A.G.M. (1978). Optokinetic nystagmus in a case of cortical blindness. Documenta Ophth. Proc. Ser., 17, 435-438.

Vedel-Jensen, N. (1966). Pathologic ocular fixation instability. Acta Ophthal., 44, 481-492.

Vennmo, C. , and B. Hindfelt (1980). Eye movements in brainstem lesions. Acta Oto-lar., 90, 230-236.

Verhage, J.W.C. (1942). Eine klinische Studie über den latenten Nystagmus. Ophthalmologica, 103, 209-224.

Verhoeff,F.H. (1941). Occlusion hypertropia. Arch.Ophthal., 25, 780-795.

Vetterli, A., and V. Henn (1981). Congenital horizontal gaze palsy in two brothers. In A. Huber and D. Klein (Eds.), 6th Intern. Congress Neurogenetics Neuro-Ophthal., Elsevier, Amsterdam, In press.

Vilis, T., and J. Hore (1980). Changes in saccade duration during cerebellar dysmetria. Soc. Neurosci. Abstr., 6, 468.

Vilis, T., and J. Hore (1981). Characteristics of saccadic dysmetria in monkeys during reversible lesions of the medial cerebellar nuclei. J. Neurophysiol., In press.

Von Noorden, G. (1961). Reaction time in normal and amblyopic eyes. Arch Ophthal., 66, 694-703.

Von Noorden, G.K., (1973). Experimental amblyopia in monkeys. Further behavioural observation and clinical correlations. Invest. Ophthal., 12, 721-726.

Von Noorden, G.K., and G. Mackensen (1962). Pursuit movements of normal and amblyopic eyes. Am. J. Ophthal., 53, 325-336.

Von Noorden, G.K., and T.J. Preziosi (1966). Eye movement recordings in neurological disorders. Arch. Ophthal., 76, 162-171.

Von Reutern, G.M., and J. Dichgans (1977). Augenbewegungsstörungen als cerebellare Symptome bei Kleinhirnbruckenwinkeltumoren. Arch. Psychiat. Nervenkr.,223, 117-130.

Waardenburg, P.J. (1970). Remarkable facts in human albinism and leukism. van Gorcum, Assen, Holland.

Wadia, N.H., and R.K. Swami (1971). A new form of heredo-familial spino-cerebellar degeneration with slow eye movements. Brain, 94, 359-374.

Waespe, W., U. Büttner, and V. Henn (1981). Visual-vestibular interaction in the flocculus of the alert monkey. I. Input activity. Exp. Brain Res., 43, 337-348.

Waespe, W., and V. Henn(1977a). Neuronal activity in the vestibular nuclei of the alert monkey during vestibular and optokinetic stimulation. Exp. Brain Res., 27, 523-538.

Waespe, W., and V. Henn (1977b). Vestibular nuclei activity during optokinetic after-nystagmus (OKAN) in the alert monkey. Exp. Brain Res., 30, 323-330.

Waespe, W., and V. Henn (1978). Conflicting visual-vestibular stimulation and vestibular nucleus activity in alert monkeys. Exp. Brain Res., 23, 203-211.

Waespe, W., and V. Henn (1981). Visual-vestibular interaction in the flocculus of the alert monkey. II. Purkinje cell activity. Exp. Brain Res., 43, 349-360.

Wagman, I.H. (1964). Eye movements induced by electric stimulation of cerebrum in monkeys and their relationship to bodily movement. In M.B. Bender (Ed.), The Oculomotor System, Harper and Row, New York, pp. 18-39.

Walberg, F. (1974). Descending connections from the mesencephalon to the inferior olive: An experimental study in the cat. Exp. Brain Res., 21, 145-156.

Walberg, F., T. Nordby, K.-P. Hoffmann, and H. Holländer (1981). Olivary afferents from the pretectal nuclei in the cat. Anat. Embryol., 161, 291-304.

Wall, C., D.P. O´Leary, and F.O. Black (1978). Systems analysis of vestibulo-ocular system response using white noise rotational stimuli. In J.D. Hood (Ed.), Vestibular Mechanisms in Health and Disease, Academic Press, London, pp.157-164.

Walley, R.E. (1967). Receptive fields in the accessory optic system of the rabbit. Exp. Neurol., 17, 27-43.

Waltz, A.G. (1961). Dyspraxias of gaze. Arch. Neurol., 5, 638-647.

Warwik, R. (1964). Oculomotor organization. In M.B. Bender (Ed.), The Oculomotor System, Harper and Row, New York, pp. 173-202.

Waterhouse, B.D., and J.G. McElligott (1980). Simple spike activity of Purkinje cells in the posterior vermis of awake cats during spontaneous saccadic eye movements. Brain Res. Bull., 5, 159-168.

Weiskrantz, L., E.K. Warrington, M.D. Sanders, and J. Marshall (1974). Visual capacity in the hemianopic field following a restricted occipital ablation. Brain, 97, 709-728.

Welch, K., and P. Stuteville (1958). Experimental production of neglect in monkeys. Brain, 81, 341-347.

Wernicke, C. (1877). Ein Fall von Ponserkrankung. Arch. Psychiat., 7, 513-538.

Westheimer, G. (1954). Eye movement responses to a horizontally moving visual stimulus. Arch. Ophthal., 52, 932-941.

Westheimer, G. (1955a). The relationship between accommodation and accommodative convergence. Am. J. Optom. and Arch. Am. Acad. Optom., 32, 206-212.

Westheimer, G. (1955b). The inconstancy of the ACA ration. Am. J. Optom. and Arch. Am. Acad. Optom., 32, 435-436.

Westheimer, G., and S. Blair (1973). Oculomotor defects in cerebellectomized monkeys. Invest. Ophthal., 12, 618-621.

Westheimer, G., and S.M. Blair (1974). Functional organization of primate oculomotor system revealed by cerebellectomy. Exp. Brain Res., 21, 463-472.

Westheimer, G., and D.W. Conover (1954). Smooth eye movements in the absence of a moving visual stimulus. J. Exp. Psychol., 47, 283-284.

Westheimer, G., and S.P. McKee (1975). Visual acuity in the presence of retinal image motion. J. Optom. Soc. Am., 65, 847-850.

Westheimer, G., and D. Mitchell (1969). The sensory stimulus for disjunctive eye movements. Vision Res., 9, 749-755.

White, J.C. (1969). Familial periodic nystagmus, vertigo and ataxia. Arch. Neurol., 20, 276-280.

Wiesel, T.N., and D.H. Hubel (1963a). Effects of visual deprivation on morphology and physiology of cells in the cat´s lateral geniculate body. J. Neurophysiol., 26, 978-992.

Wiesel, T.N., and D.H. Hubel (1963b). Singlecell responses in striate cortex of kittens deprived of vision in one eye. J. Neurophysiol., 26, 1003-1017.

Wiesel, T.N., and D.H. Hubel (1965a). Comparison of the effects of unilateral and bilateral eye closure on cortical unit responses in kittens. J. Neurophysiol., 28, 1029-1040.

Wiesel, T.N., and D.H. Hubel (1965b).Extent of recovery from the effects of visual deprivation in kittens. J. Neurophysiol., 28, 1060-1072.

Wilkinson, I.M.S., R. Kime, and M. Purnell (1974). Alcohol and human eye movement. Brain, 97, 785-792.

Wilson, V.J., and G. Mellvill Jones (1979). Mammalian Vestibular Physiology., Plenum Press, New York.

Winckler, G. (1956). L'innervation proprioceptive des muscles extrinséques du globe oculaire chez l'homme. C.R. Ass. Anat., 43, 848-857.

Wist, E.R., Th. Brandt, and S. Krafczyk (1981). Oscillopsia and retinal slip: Evidence supporting a clinical test. Brain, In press.

Witkop, C.J., J.D. Wiswander, D.R. Bergsma. P.L. Workman, and J.G. White (1972). Tyrosinase-pos. oculo-cutaneous albinism among the zuni and the brandy-wine triracial isolate. Am. J. Physiol. Anthrop., 36, 397-406.

Wolfe, J., E.J. Engleken, J.W. Olson, and J.P. Allen (1978). Crosspower spectal density analysis of pursuit tracking. Ann. Otol. Rhinol. Lar., 87, 837-884.

Wood, C.C., P.D. Spear, and J.J. Braun (1973). Direction-specific deficits in horizontal optokinetic nystagmus following removal of visual cortex in the cat. Brain Res., 80, 231-237.

Woollard, H.H. (1931). The innervation of the ocular muscles. J. Anat., 65, 215.

Worth, C. (1903). Squint: Its causes, pathology and treatment. J. Bale, Sons and Danielson, London.

Wright, K.A. (1981). A new binocular fixation test for amblyopia. Arch.Opthal,In press.

Wuerthele, S.M., K.L. Lovell, M.F. Jones, and K.E. Moore (1978). A histological study of kainic acid-induced lesions in the rat brain. Brain Res., 149, 489-497.

Wurtz, R.H., and J.E. Albano (1980). Visual-motor function of the primate superior colliculus. Ann. Rev. Neurosci., 3, 189-226.

Wurtz, R.H., and M.E. Goldberg (1971). Superior colliculus cell responses related to eye movements in awake monkeys. Science, 171, 82-84.

Wurtz, R.H., and M.E. Goldberg (1972a). Activity of superior colliculus in behaving monkey. III. Cells discharging before eye movements. J. Neurophysiol.,35, 575-586.

Wurtz, R.H., and M.E. Goldberg (1972b). Activity of superior colliculus in behaving monkey. IV. Effects of lesions on eye movements. J. Neurophysiol., 35, 587-596.

Wurtz, R.H., and C.W. Mohler (1976a). Organization of monkey superior colliculus: Enhanced visual response of superficial layer cells. J. Neurophysiol.,39,745-762.

Wurtz, R.H., and C.W. Mohler (1976b). Enhancement of visual responses in monkey striate cortex and frontal eye fields. J. Neurophysiol., 39, 766-772.

Wybar, K. (1969). Diagnostic and therapeutic problems in nystagmus. Br. J. Ophthal., 53, 224-229.

Yagi, T., M. Shimizu, S. Sekine, T. Kamio, and J.I Suzuki (1981). A new neuro-otological test for detecting cerebellar dysfunction. In B. Cohen (Ed.), Recent Advances in Oculomotor and Vestibular Physiology, Ann. N.Y. Acad. Sci., New York. In press.

Yamamoto, M., I. Shimoyama, and S.M. Highstein (1978). Vestibular nucleus neurons relaying excitation from the anterior canal to the oculomotor nucleus. Brain Res., 148, 31-42.

Yamazaki, A (1979). Abnormalities of smooth pursuit and vestibular eye movements in congenital jerk nystagmus. In K. Shimizu (Ed.), Ophthalmology, Vol. 2, Excerpta Med., Amsterdam, Oxford. pp. 1162-1165.

Yamazaki, A. (1970). Electrophysiological study on saccades during fixation and small pursuit movement in neurological disorders. Acta Soc. Ophthal. Jap., 74, 244-252.

Yamazaki, A., and S. Ishikawa (1973). Horizontal and vertical smooth pursuit eye movements. Jap. J. Ophthal., 103, 244-252.

Yamazaki, A., and D.S. Zee (1979). Rebound nystagmus: EOG analysis of a case with a floccular tumor. Br. J. Ophthal., 63, 782-786.

Yarbus, A.L. (1967). Eye Movements and Vision, Plenum Press, New York.

Yasui, S., and L.R. Young (1975a). Perceived visual motion as effective stimulus to pursuit movement system. Science, 190, 906-908.

Yasui, S., and L.R. Young (1975b). Eye movements during after-image tracking under sinusoidal and random vestibular stimulation. In. G. Lennerstrand and P. Bach-Y-Rita (Eds.), Basic Mechanisms of Ocular Motility and Their Clinical Implications, Pergamon Press, Oxford. pp. 509-513.

Yee, R.D., R.W. Baloh, and V. Honrubia (1980). Study of congenital nystagmus; Optokinetic nystagmus. Br. J. Ophthal., 64, 926-932.

Yee, R.D., R.W. Baloh, V. Honrubia, C.G.Y. Lau, and H.A. Jenkins (1979). Slow build-up of optokinetic nystagmus associated with downbeat nystagmus. Invest. Ophthal. Vis. Sci., 18, 622-629.

Yee, R.D., R.W. Baloh, V. Honrubia, and H.A. Jenkins (1981). Pathophysiology of optokinetic nystagmus. In V. Honrubia and M.A.B. Brazier (Eds.), Nystagmus and Vertigo: Clinical Approaches to the Patient with Dizziness. UCLA Forum in Medical Sciences, Vol. 24, Academic Press, New York. In press.

Yee, R.D., R.W. Baloh, V. Honrubia, and Y.S. Kim (1981). A study of congenital nystagmus;Vestibular nystagmus. J. Otol-lar., 10, 89-98.

Yee, R.D., E.K. Wong,R.W. Baloh, and V. Honrubia (1976). A study of congenital nystagmus waveforms. Neurology, 26, 326-333.

Yin, T. C.-T., and V.B. Mountcastle (1977). Visual input to the visuomotor mechanisms of the monkey's parietal lobe. Science, 197, 1381-1383.

Yinon, U. (1976). Age dependence of the effect of squint on cells in kittens'visual cortex. Exp. Brain Res., 27, 151-157.

Yoshida, K., A. Berthoz, P. Vidal, and R.A. McCrea (1981). In A. Fuchs and W. Becker (Eds.), The Neuronal Control of Eye Movements. Biomed. Press. Elsevier/North Holland, Amsterdam. In press.

Yoshida, K., R. McCrea,A. Berthoz, and P.P. Vidal (1979). Soc. Neurosci.Abstr.,5,391.

Yoshida, K., R. McCrea, A. Berthoz, and P.P. Vidal (1982). J. Neurol. In press.

Young, L.R. (1971). Pursuit eye tracking movements. In P. Bach-y-Rita, C.C. Collins and J.E. Hyde (Eds.), The Control of Eye Movements, Academic Press, New York, pp 429-443.

Young, L.R. (1977). Pursuit eye movement - what is being pursued? In R.Baker and A. Berthoz (Eds.), The Control of Gaze by Brain Stem Neurons, Biomed. Press, Elsevier/North Holland, New York, pp 29-36.

Young, L.R. and V. Henn (1975). Nystagmus induced by pitch and yaw rotation of monkeys. Fortschritte der Zoologie, 23, 235-246.

Young, L.R., and L. Stark (1963). Variable feedback experiments testing a sampled data model for eye tracking movements. IEEE Transactions of the Professional Technical Group on Human Factors in Electronics, HFE-4.

Zangemeister, W.H., A. Jones, and L. Stark (1981a). Dynamics of head movement trajectories: Main sequence relationship. Exp. Neurol., 71, 76-91.

Zangemeister,W.H., L. Stark, O. Meienberg, and T. Waite (1981b). Neural control of head rotation: Electromyographic evidence. J. Neurol. Sci., In press.

Zangemeister, W.H., S. Lehman, and L. Stark (1981c). Simulation of head movement trajectories: Model and fit to main sequence. Biol. Cybern., 41, 19-32.

Zangemeister, W.H., S. Lehman, and L. Stark (1981d). Sensitivity analysis and optimization for a head movement model. Biol. Cybern., 41, 33-45.

Zangemeister, W.H., O. Meienberg, L.Stark, and W.F. Hoyt (1981e). Eye head coordination in homonymous hemianopia. J. Neurol., In press.

Zangemeister, W.H., A. Muller-Jansen, and S. Zschocke (1979). Benign encephalitis: Electro-oculographic analysis of opsoclonus. J. Neurol., 222, 95-108.

Zangemeister, W.H., and L. Stark (1981). Dynamics of active head movements and eye-head coordination. In B. Cohen (Ed.), Recent Advances in Oculomotor and Vestibular Physiology. Ann. N.Y. Acad. Sci., New York. In press.

Zaret, C.R., M.M. Behrens, and H.M. Eggers (1980). Congenital ocular motor apraxia and brain stem tumor.Arch. Ophthal., 98, 328-330.

Zee, D.S. (1981). Ocular motor control: The cerebellum. In S. Lessell and J.T.W. van Dalen (Eds.), Neuro-Ophthalmology, Vol. 2, Excerpta Med., Amsterdam. In press.

Zee, D.S., A.R. Friendlich, and D.A. Robinson (1974). The mechanisms of downbeat nystagmus. Arch. Neurol., 30, 227-237.

Zee, D.S., R.J. Leigh, and F. Mathieu-Millaire (1980). Cerebellar control of ocular gaze stability. Ann. Neurol., 7, 37-40.

Zee, D.S., L.M. Optican. J.D. Cook, D.A. Robinson, and W.K. Engel (1976a). Slow saccades in spinocerebellar degeneration. Arch. Neùrol., 53, 243-251.

Zee, D.S., R.D. Yee, D.G. Cogan, D.A. Robinson, and W.K. Engel (1976b). Ocular motor abnormalities in hereditary cerebellar ataxia. Brain, 99, 207-234..

Zee, D.S., R.D. Yee, and D. Robinson (1976c). Optokinetic responses in labyrinthine-defective human beings. Brain Res., 113, 423-428.

Zee, D.S., and D.A. Robinson (1979). A hypothetical explanation of saccadic oscillations. Ann. Neurol., 5, 405-414.

Zee, D.S., A. Yamazaki, and G. Gücer (1978). Ocular motor abnormalities in trained monkeys with floccular lesions. Neurosci. Abstr., 4, 168.

Zee, D.S., A. Yamazaki, P. Butler, and G. Gücer (1981). Effect of ablation of flocculus and paraflocculus on eye movement in primate. J. Neurophysiol., In press.

Zee. D.S., R.D. Yee, and H.S. Singer (1977). Congenital oculomotor apraxia. Brain, 100, 581-600.

Zeevi, Y.Y., E. Peli, and L. Stark (1979). Study of eccentric fixation with secondary visual feedback. J. Opt. Soc. Am., 69, 669-675.

Zikmund, V. (1966). Oculomotor activity during visual imagery of a moving stimulus pattern. Stud. Psychol., 8, 254-272.

ABBREVIATIONS

ABV	anomalous binocular vision
ACA	accommodative convergence-accommodation (ratio)
ACEM	anticipatory compensatory eye movement
AMF	anomalous fusional movements
AOS	accessory optic system
ARC	anomalous retinal correspondance
AR	accommodation response
AS	acceleration saturation
BC	brachium conjunctivum
BHF	blind hemifield
nBOR	nucleus of the basal optic root
CAC	convergence accommodation - convergence (ratio)
CEM	compensatory eye movement
CF	climbing fibers
CN	congenital nystagmus
CNS	central nervous system
CR	convergence response
CRT	cathod ray tube
CSF	cerebrospinal fluid
CT	computer assisted tomography
CV	circularvection
DC	direct current
D	diopter
DTN	dorsal terminal nucleus (of AOS)
DV	dorsal vermis
DVD	dissociated vertical deviation
E/H	eye displacement/head velocity
EMG	electromyogram
EOG	electro-oculogram
EOM	extraocular muscle
ENG	electronystagmogram
EPSP	excitatory postsynaptic potential
ERG	electroretinogram
ET	esotropia
Fd	"Faden" operation
FEF	frontal eye field
FM	frequency modulation
FP	fixation point
HRP	horse-radish peroxidase
INC	interstitial nucleus of Cajal
IPL	inferior parietal lobe
IPL-PS	inferior parietal lobe pre-striate cortex
IPSP	inhibitory postsynaptic potential
LED	light emitting diod
LGN	lateral geniculate nucleus
LH	left hypertropia
LMR	left medial rectus
LN	latent nystagmus
LP	lumbar puncture
LTN	lateral terminal nucleus (of AOS)
MF	mossy fibers
MIF	multiply innervated fibers
MLF	medial longitudinal fasciculus
iMLF	interstitial nucleus of the medial longitudinal fasciculus
riMLF	rostral interstitial nucleus of the medial longitudinal fasciculus
MLN	manifest latent nystagmus
MP	motor potential
MRF	mesencephalic reticular formation
MSWS	macro square wave jerks
MTN	medial terminal nucleus (of AOS)

N	nystagmus
NBV	normal binocular vision
NFM	normal fusional movements
NOT	nucleus of the optic tract
NRC	normal retinal correspondance
NRTP	nucleus reticularis tegmenti pontis
OK	optokinetic
OKAN	optokinetic after nystagmus
OKN	optokinetic nystagmus
OKR	optokinetic response optokinetic reflex
OSL	orbital surface layer
OVAR	off-vertical axis rotation
POAC	parietooccipital association cortex
P-cell	Purkinje cell
PMP	premotion positive waves
PPRF	paramedian pontine reticular formation
Pt	pretectal
PVS	pursuit velocity saturation
SCC	semicircular canals
SEM	slow eye movements
SHF	seeing hemifield
SIF	singly innervated fibers
SPV	slow phase velocity
SR	sarcoplasmic reticulum
SVN	superior vestibular nucleus
SWS	square wave jerks
TVP	tonic-vestibular-pause (cells)
VC	vestibulo cerebellum
VD	vertical deviation
VER	visual evoked response
Vn	vestibular neurons
VN	vestibular nucleus
VOR	vestibulo-ocular reflex vestibular-ocular response
VVOR	vertical vestibulo-ocular reflex
XT	exotropia

SUBJECT INDEX